# CONTEMPORARY EXTENSILE EXPOSURES IN ORTHOPAEDIC SURGERY

# CONTEMPORARY EXTENSILE EXPOSURES IN ORTHOPAEDIC SURGERY


***Ronald P. Williams, PhD, MD, FACS***

Assistant Professor
Department of Orthopaedics
University of Texas Health Science Center
San Antonio, Texas

***James D. Heckman, MD***

Chairman
Department of Orthopaedics
University of Texas Health Science Center
San Antonio, Texas



Williams & Wilkins
A WAVERLY COMPANY

BALTIMORE • PHILADELPHIA • LONDON • PARIS • BANGKOK
BUENOS AIRES • HONG KONG • MUNICH • SYDNEY • TOKYO • WROCLAW

ISBN 0-683-09190-5
90000>
9 780683 091908

*Editor:* Darlene Barela Cooke
*Managing Editor:* Frances M. Klass
*Production Coordinator:* Cindy Park
*Copy Editor:* Jennifer D. Weir
*Designer:* Susan Blaker
*Composition:* Mario Fernández, Donna Smith
*Manufacturing:* Edwards Brothers



351 West Camden Street
Baltimore, Maryland 21201-2436 USA

Rose Tree Corporate Center
1400 North Providence Road
Building II, Suite 5025
Media, Pennsylvania 19063-2043 USA



Accurate indications, adverse reactions, and dosage schedules for drugs are provided in this book, but it is possible that they may change. The reader is urged to review the package information data of the manufacturers of the medications mentioned.

*Printed in the United States of America*

First Edition,

**Library of Congress Cataloging-in-Publication Data**

Williams, Ronald P.
Contemporary extensile exposures in orthopaedic surgery / Ronald P. Williams, James D. Heckman; illustrator, Rusty Jones.
p. cm.
Includes index.
ISBN 0-683-09190-5
1. Orthopedic surgery—Atlases. 2. Cutdown (Surgery)—Atlases.
I. Heckman, James D. II. Title.
[DNLM: 1. Extremities—surgery. 2. Orthopedics—methods. 3. Surgery, Operative—methods.
WE 190 W726c 1996]
RD733.2.W55 1996
617.4'71'00222—dc20
DNLM/DLC
for Library of Congress 96-22442
CIP



Call our customer service department at **(800) 638-0672** for catalog information or fax orders to **(800) 447-8438**. For other book services, including chapter reprints and large quantity sales, ask for the Special Sales department.

To purchase additional copies of this book or for information concerning American College of Sports Medicine certification and suggested preparatory materials, call **(800) 486-5643.**

Canadian customers should call **(800) 268-4178**, or fax **(905) 470-6780**. For all other calls originating outside of the United States, please call **(410) 528-4223** or fax us at **(410) 528-8550**.

***Visit Williams & Wilkins on the Internet:*** **http://www.wwilkins.com** or contact our customer service department at **custserv@wwilkins.com**. Williams & Wilkins customer service representatives are available from 8:30 am to 6:00 pm, EST, Monday through Friday, for telephone access.

97 98 99 00 01
1 2 3 4 5 6 7 8 9 10

# Dedication

This work is dedicated to the students, residents, fellows, and surgeons who spend the time and energy to observe and study anatomy for the benefit of their patients.

# PREFACE

In 1950, Arnold K. Henry published his text, *Extensile Exposure Applied to Limb Surgery*, which has provided the basic description of surgical exposure of the bones of the appendages. His underlying principle was to place the incisions so the major nerves and vessels were avoided. Therefore, the surgeon was taught to "cut down to the bone and stay there." The use of surgical resection, chemotherapy, and radiation for the treatment of limb tumors and the improvement in techniques of managing limb trauma led to the recognition of the critical role of preserving the circulation to the bone and soft tissue envelope during limb salvage. Manchot and Taylor and coworkers provided a detailed description of the blood supply to the soft tissues. Clinical experience has shown that preservation of this blood supply can improve the outcome of elaborate surgical dissections by minimizing complications caused by soft tissue ischemia.

This text describes approaches that are modifications of the "internervous plane" dissections of Henry. These approaches are designed to minimize the damage to the blood supply to the soft tissues. In addition, the text elaborates on the principles of compartment resection that allow the preservation of a functional limb with minimal complications. The approaches are designed to be combined as necessary to provide true "extensile" exposure. Exposure of the spine is also included and the text describes a safe and functional approach to the entire axial and appendicular skeleton.

# ACKNOWLEDGMENT

The authors thank Theresa Hill for her organization, dedication, and patience, which allowed the creation of this book.

# CONTRIBUTORS

James D. Heckman, MD
Chairman
Department of Orthopadeics
University of Texas Health Science Center
San Antonio, Texas

Jay D. Mabrey, MD
Assistant Professor of Orthopaedic Surgery
University of Texas Health Science Center
Chief, Orthopaedic Service
Audie L. Murphy Memorial VA Hospital
Director, Adult Reconstruction Service, University Hospital
San Antonio, Texas

Robert C. Schenck, Jr., MD
Associate Professor
Department of Orthopaedics
University of Texas Health Science Center
San Antonio, Texas

Lorence W. Trick, MD
Clinical Professor
Department of Orthopadeics
University of Texas Health Science Center
San Antonio, Texas

Ronald P. Williams, PhD, MD, FACS
Assistant Professor
Department of Orthopadeics
University of Texas Health Science Center
San Antonio, Texas

# CONTENTS

## VIII
## SURGICAL APPROACHES TO THE WRIST AND HAND 159



## IX
## SURGICAL APPROACHES TO THE PELVIS 187



## X
## SURGICAL APPROACHES TO THE HIP 237

*Jay D. Mabrey and Lorence W. Trick*



## XI
## SURGICAL APPROACHES TO THE THIGH AND FEMUR 273

# XII
## SURGICAL APPROACHES TO THE KNEE 291

*Robert C. Schenck, Jr.*



# XIII
## SURGICAL APPROACHES TO THE LEG 317



# XIV
## SURGICAL APPROACHES TO THE FOOT AND ANKLE 335



## INDEX 373

# INTRODUCTION

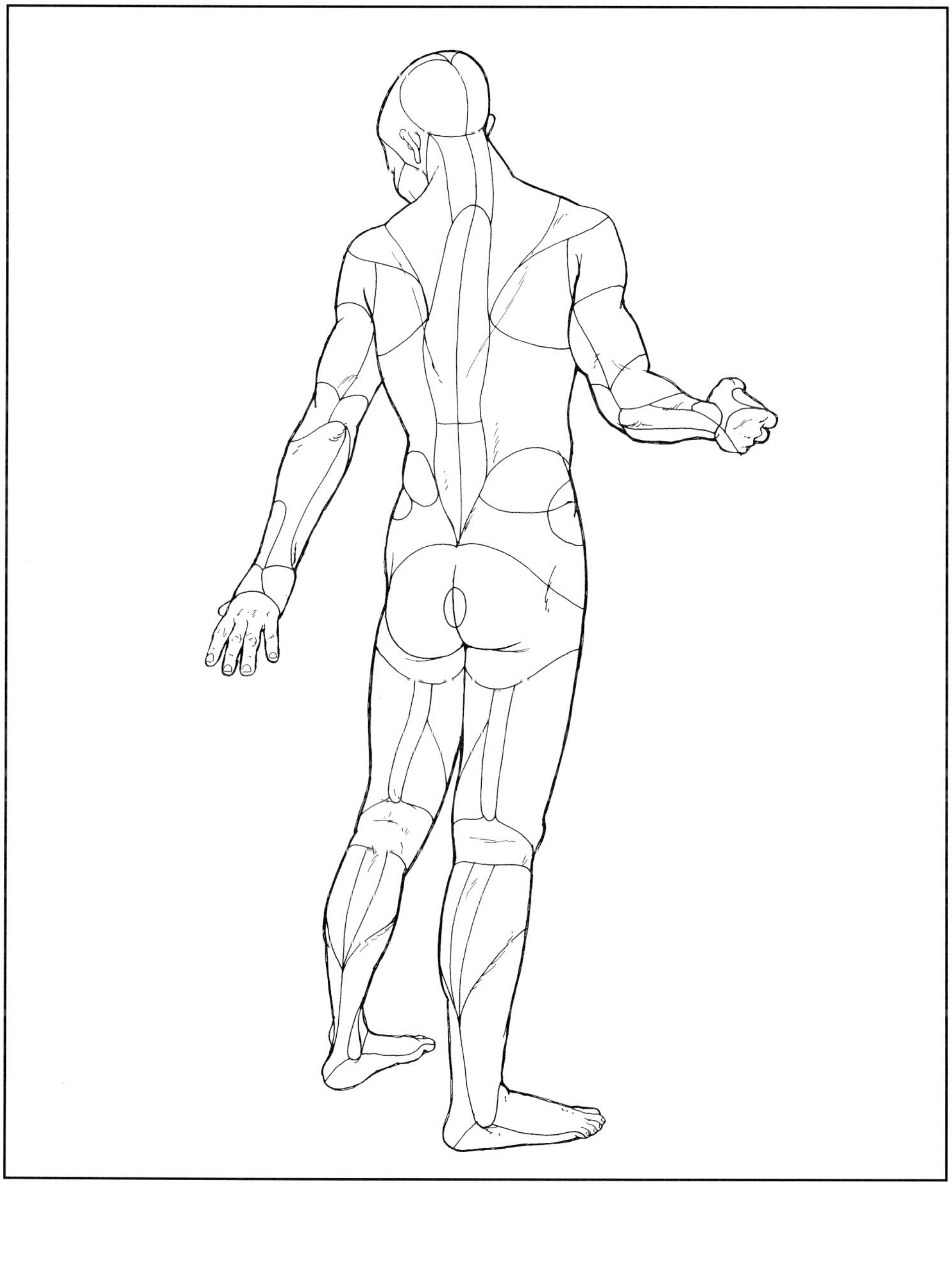

As our skills in orthopaedic surgery have evolved, our interest in surgical reconstruction of more complex problems has increased. Just as this has led to exciting success, it has also led to catastrophic failure.

One factor that commonly determines success or failure of orthopaedic procedures is the survival of the soft tissue envelope. In limb salvage for malignancies, the use of radiation and chemotherapy seriously compromises the survival of the soft tissue flaps, making the placement of the extensile incisions a critical factor in determining the outcome. Similarly, in trauma surgery, the mechanical destruction of the soft tissues, including muscle, fascia, and skin as well as vascular and nerve trunks, has limited the use of early bony reconstruction because of the fear of wound breakdown and infection.

Improved understanding of the blood supply to the soft tissues has now made it possible to design surgical dissections along intervascular planes. This concept, popularized by Henry (1), can now be used to design more extensive surgical dissections that maintain soft tissue viability. The work of Taylor and Palmer (2), Manchot (3), and others has refined our understanding of the vascular supply to the trunk and limbs so that improved techniques of incision placement and dissection result in decreased risk of wound complications.

These authors have demonstrated that the concept of *angiosomes* is a valid way to map the blood supply to the soft tissues. An angiosome is a defined region of soft tissue supplied with blood by a parallel artery and vein. The cutaneous vessels supplying an angiosome follow a constant route and distribution to the skin, fascia, and each angiosome is relatively autonomous and dependent on its vascular pedicle.

The cutaneous vessels arise from the nearest vascular trunk, and thus, their distribution can be envisioned as parallel to the named arterial branches. They are classed as "direct" or "indirect" by their pattern of dispersal from the trunk of origin (Int-1). The most common type in the extremities is the indirect musculocuta-

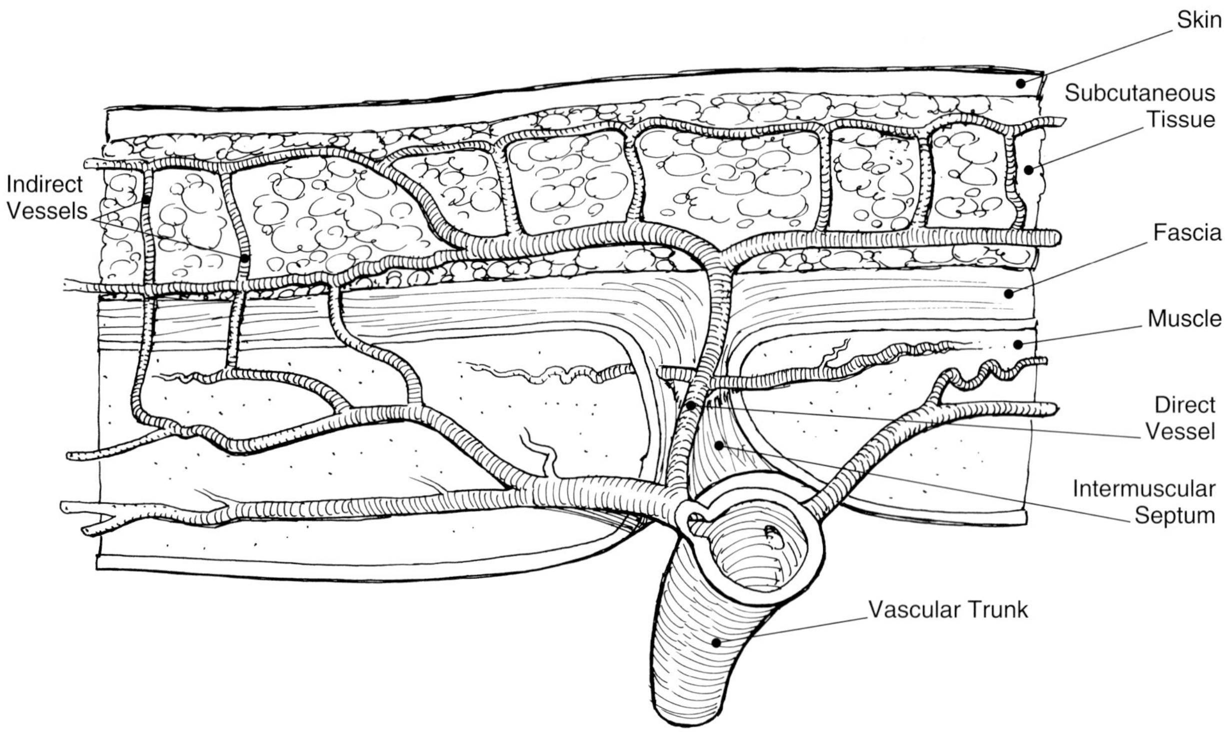


**FIGURE INT–1**

neous vessels that perforate the muscle and continue through the fascia to disperse in the subcutaneous tissue. Indirect vessels also follow the intermuscular septa to distribute to the overlying skin. In addition, *relay arteries* (Int-2) run parallel to the cutaneous nerves and are proportional in size to the size of the nerve. For example, the greater saphenous nerve has a large cutaneous artery and vein in intimate contact throughout its distribution.

The loose skin overlying the subcutaneous extremity joints (knees, elbows) receives a direct blood supply from all of the collateral trunks anastomosing about the joint (Int-3). These vessels also supply the joint capsule and periosteum. The body surface can, therefore, be divided into vascular territories analogous to the dermatomes.

Because the cutaneous vessels run in the deep adipose layer after perforating the investing fascia, the subcutaneous fat must be respected as a vessel transporter to the skin. Large, extensile dissections should begin with placement of the incision from the skin *through* the fascia without dissection of the subcutaneous space. Soft tissue flaps created for extensile exposure should be mobilized deep to the investing fascia. The skin incisions should be placed along the perimeter of the angiosomes to maximize collateral circulation to the wound.

# Back

The vascular supply to the skin of the back is divided into numerous small territories. Beginning at the midline are superior and inferior territories supplied by dorsispinal branches of the intercostal and lumbar arteries, respectively. Laterally,

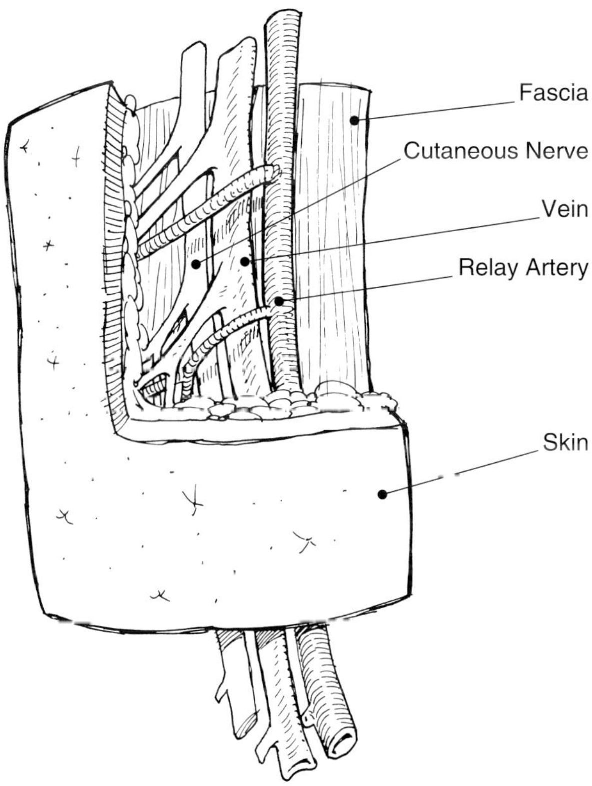


**FIGURE INT–2**

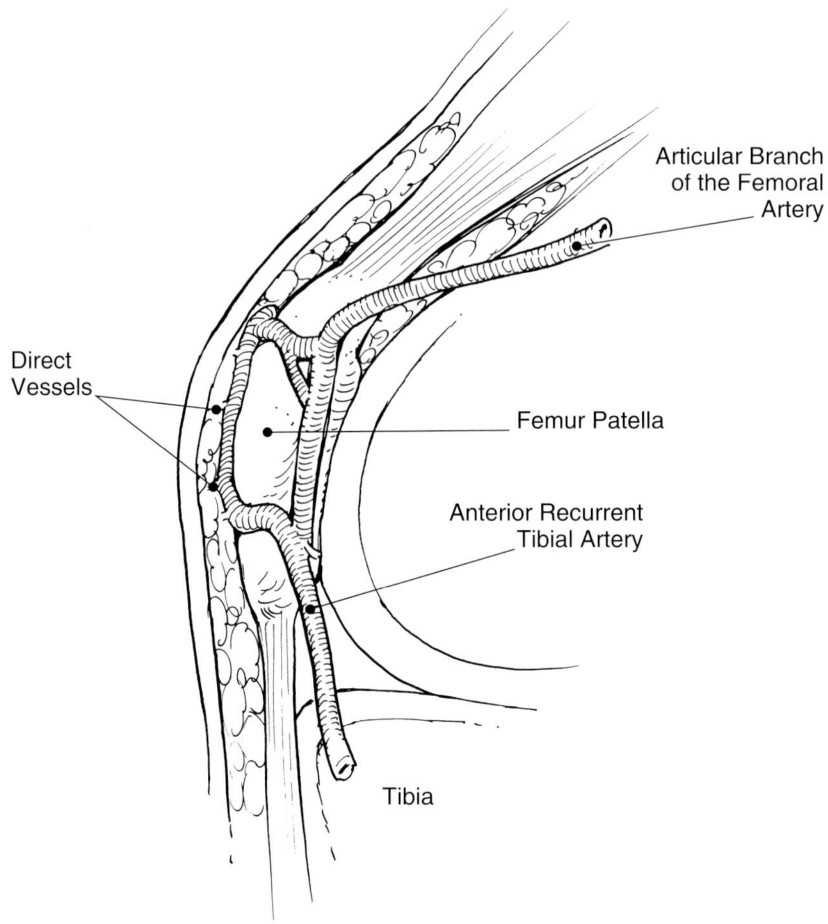


**FIGURE INT–3**

overlying the trapezius and the superior scapula are the zones of the transverse cervical artery and suprascapular artery. The subscapular artery supplies the upper portion of the lateral chest wall and the intercostal arteries supply the lateral abdominal wall (Int-4).

## Upper Extremity

The transverse cervical and suprascapular arteries supply the acromial region. A large territory in the anterior and lateral deltoid region is supplied by the axillary system through the thoracoacromial trunk and posterior humeral circumflex arteries (Int-4 and Int-5).

The anterior arm is divided into medial, middle, and lateral territories supplied by the brachial artery muscular branches to the biceps brachii, and profunda brachii, respectively. The dorsal arm is supplied laterally by direct and muscular branches of the profunda brachii. A small medial territory is supplied by medial collateral branches of the brachial artery. There is a plexus of collateral vessels about the elbow, each sending cutaneous branches to a number of small, poorly defined territories.

The volar forearm is supplied by the radial and ulnar arteries. The dorsal forearm is supplied medially by the continuation of the ulnar territory and centrally

1. Ophthalmic
2. Superficial Temporal
3. Occipital
4. Sternomastoid
5. Deep Cervical
6. Transverse Cervical
7. Suprascapular
8. Post. Humeral
9. Subscapular
10. Dorsopspinal
11. Profunda Brachii
12. Brachial
13. Radial Recurrent Ulnar
14. Post. Recurrent Ulnar
15. Post. Interosseous
16. Ulnar
17. Ant. Interosseous
18. Dorsal Carpal
19. Ulnar
20. Post. Interosseous
21. Lumbar
22. Lumbar
23. Superficial Circumflex Iliac
24. Superior Gluteal
25. Inf. Gluteal
26. Int. Pudendal
27. Perforating Profunda Femoris
28. Perforating Profunda Femoris
29. Adductors
30. Perforating Profunda Femoris
31. Popliteal
32. Gastrocnemius
33. Saphenous
34. Gastrocnemius
35. Dorsal Pedis
36. Medial Plantar

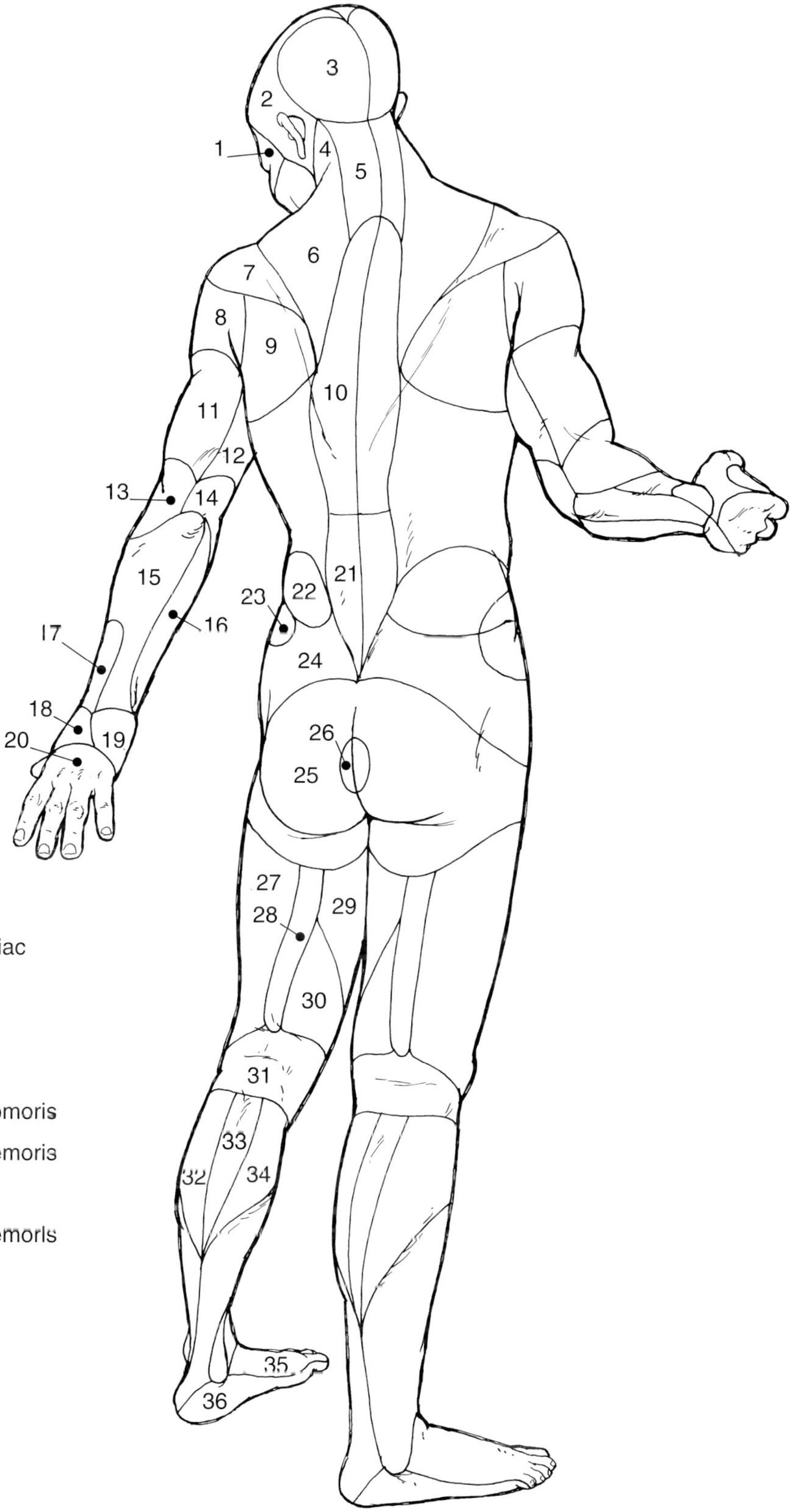


**FIGURE INT–4**

1. Ophthalmic
2. Superficial Temporal
3. Occipital
4. Sternomastoid
5. Facial
6. Thyroid
7. Transverse Cervical and Suprascapular
8. Deltoid
9. Circumflex Humeral
10. Thoracic Branches
11. Brachial
12. Profunda Brachii
13. Brachial
14. Epicondylar
15. Epitrochlear
16. Radial
17. Ulnar
18. Deep Palmar
19. Superficial Palmar
20. Internal Mammary
21. External Mammary
22. Intercostal
23. Superior Epigastric
24. Lumbar
25. Superior Epigastric
26. Deep Epigastric
27. Ext. Sup. Pudendal
28. Ext. Inf. Pudendal
29. Superficial Circumflex Iliac
30. Femoral
31. Vastus Lateralis
32. Superficial Femoral
33. Adductor
34. Lateral Articular
35. Medial Articular
36. Genus Descendens
37. Ant. Tibial
38. Post. Tibial
39. Peroneal
40. Dorsal Pedis
41. Medial Plantar

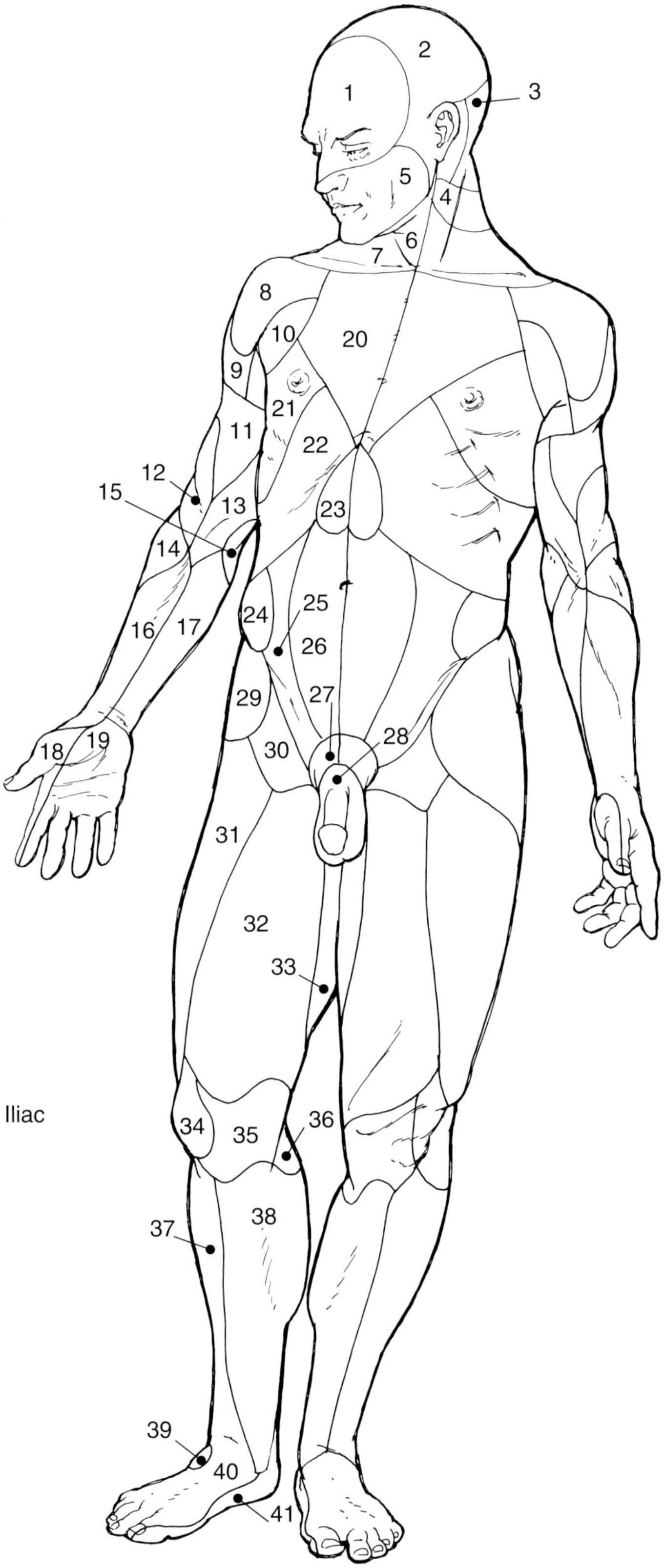


**FIGURE INT-5**

and laterally by the posterior interosseous artery. The distal, lateral third is supplied by the anterior interosseous artery.

In the palmar surface of the hand, the radial artery supplies the skin of the thenar eminence, thumb, and lateral index finger. The ulnar artery supplies the remaining skin through the superficial arch and digital vessels. The dorsal hand has two territories, the medial supplied by the dorsal branch of the ulnar artery and the lateral by the dorsal carpal and posterior interosseous branches of the radial artery. The dorsal skin of the fingers is supplied by the digital vessels from the ulnar system.

## Lower Extremity

In the gluteal region, the lumbar arteries extend over the iliac crest distally for 4 to 5 cm. The superolateral gluteal region is supplied by the superficial iliac circumflex artery. The superior gluteal artery supplies the middle third of the buttock and the inferior gluteal artery provides the blood supply to the distal and lateral buttock, extending laterally to the posterior edge of the trochanter.

The inguinal region has a large lateral territory supplied by the superficial iliac circumflex artery and two small territories supplied by the femoral and pudendal arteries.

There are three large, vertically oriented territories on the anterior thigh. The middle territory is supplied by the superficial femoral artery. The medial territory is supplied by the adductor muscle branches from the profunda femoris. Muscular branches from the profunda femoris supply the lateral territory (Int-4 and Int-5).

The dorsal surface of the thigh is divided into four longitudinal territories. The two lateral territories are supplied by the perforating branches of the profunda femoris. The middle territory is supplied by the longitudinal artery of the inferior gluteal nerve. The medial territory is supplied by the muscular branches of the profunda femoris. Thus, the profunda system supplies the major blood supply to the skin of the thigh.

The knee is analogous to the elbow with multiple small, poorly defined angiosomes. The lateral skin is supplied by the lateral genicular vessels, the posterior territory by the medial genicular vessels, and the anterior and medial skin by the descending genicular branch of the femoral artery. The anterolateral leg is supplied by the anterior tibial artery, from the subcutaneous border of the tibia to the fibula. The posterior tibial artery supplies the medial leg from the tendon Achilles to the tibial crest. The posterior calf is supplied proximally by muscular branches from the gastrocnemius and distally by the lesser saphenous vessels. The dorsum of the foot is provided by the dorsalis pedis artery. The lateral border is supplied by the peroneal artery. The plantar surface is supplied by the medial and lateral plantar vessels.

# References

1. Henry AK. Exposure of the humerus and femoral shaft. Br J Surg 12:84–91, 1925.
2. Taylor G, Palmer J. The vascular territories (angiosomes) of the body: experimental study and clinical applications. Br J Plast Surg 40:113–141, 1987.
3. Manchot C; Ristic J, Morain W, trans. The Cutaneous Arteries of the Human Body. New York: Springer-Verlag, 1983.

# I

# SURGICAL APPROACHES TO THE CERVICAL SPINE

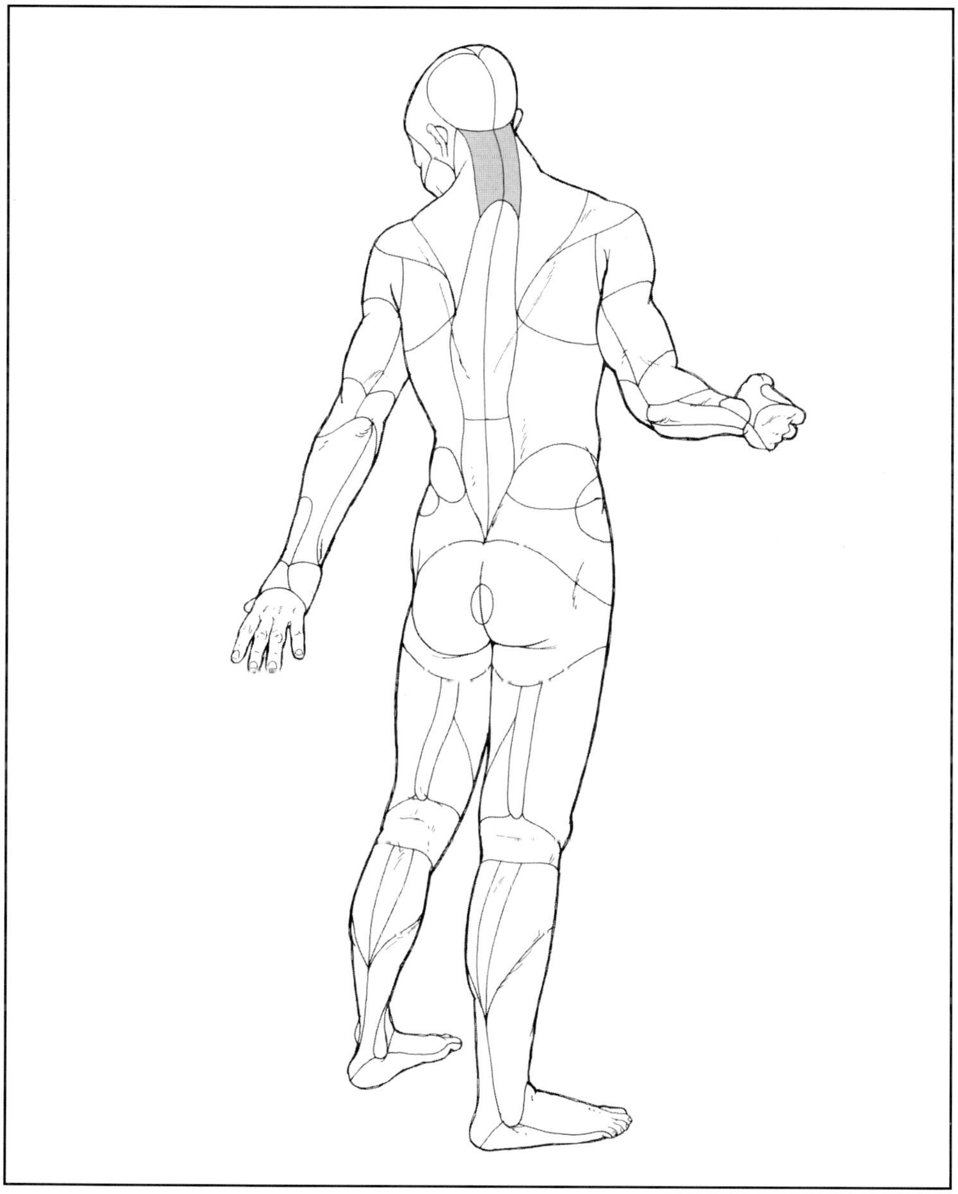

# General Principles and Complications

The cervical spine can be approached through either an anterior or posterior route. The specific approach should be dictated by the location of the pathologic process. The anterior approaches provide direct access to the vertebral bodies, vertebral arteries, and transverse processes. The posterior approach provides access to the spinous processes, laminae, and facet joints. In planning the approach, the surgeon must always assess the stability of the spine and anticipate the need to use hardware to stabilize it. A standard anterior approach, through a transverse incision, provides adequate access to the third through seventh cervical vertebrae. Exposure of the upper cervical vertebrae and base of the skull requires more extensive dissection with significantly more morbidity. The anterior surgical approaches require that the surgeon be intimately familiar with the anatomy of the neck, especially the fascial planes, blood vessels, and nerves. The major concerns with the anterior approach are avoidance of injury to the cranial nerve branches, especially nerves IX through XII; the esophagus; cervical sympathetic trunk; internal carotid artery and vein; and branches of the external carotid artery (I-1) (1).

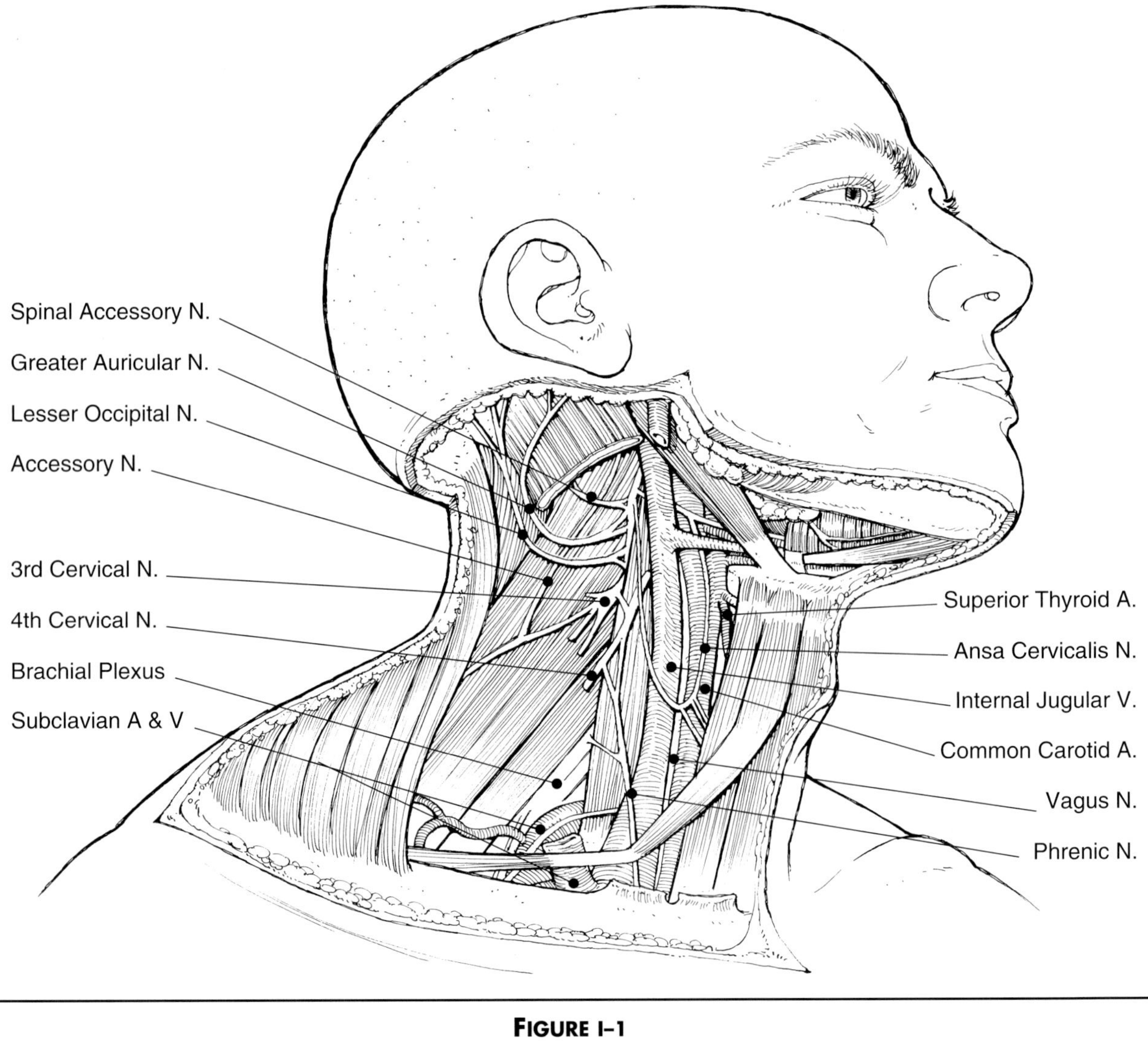


**FIGURE I–1**

The face and neck have a copious blood supply, and therefore, viability of skin flaps is of minimal concern as long as the extensile dissection is carried out deep to the platysma muscles. Oblique incisions are preferred because they are parallel to the skin tension lines and produce minimal scarring. The posterior approach allows wider exposure of the spinal canal with less loss of stability. It also provides access to the laminae and facets for placement of instrumentation and fusion.

The most serious complications of the anterior approach are injury to the upper cervical cord, inadvertent disruption of the vertebral artery, esophageal laceration, and laryngeal or pharyngeal edema causing airway obstruction. The more frequent complications include Horner's syndrome and vocal cord weakness. Other potential complications include hemorrhage from the carotid artery branches or internal jugular system and air embolism. The major risk of the posterior approach is injury to a vertebral artery. Each vertebral artery is encased in the transverse foramina as it ascends through the neck. These arteries lie at the lateral limits of the posterior approach (I-2). Inadvertent injury to the vessel can produce uncontrollable bleeding, and acute ligation of the vertebral artery may precipitate brainstem ischemia, causing either a stroke or death.

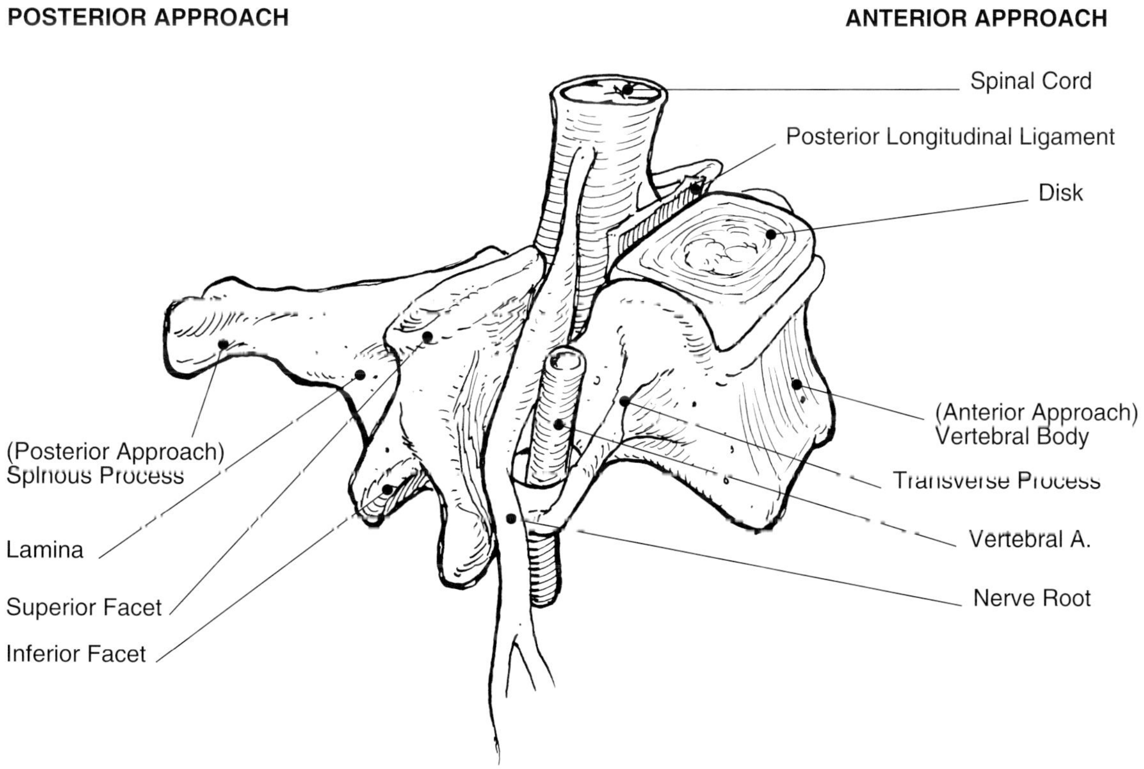


**FIGURE I-2**

## Surgical Anatomy

The neck is divided into the anterior and posterior triangles by the large (I-3), obliquely oriented sternocleidomastoid muscle. Palpable surface landmarks help to localize the cervical spine levels. The transverse process of the atlas (first cervical vertebra) is palpable caudal and anterior to the mastoid process of the skull. The third cervical vertebra underlies the hyoid bone, the fourth is deep to the upper margin of the thyroid cartilage, and the sixth cervical vertebra is deep to the cricoid cartilage. The most cephalad posterior bony prominence below the skull is the spinous process of the second cervical vertebra.

The investing fascial layers of the neck divide it into discrete compartments. Recognizing and preserving these compartments can protect the vital structures and minimize complications. There are three fascial layers: superficial (investing),

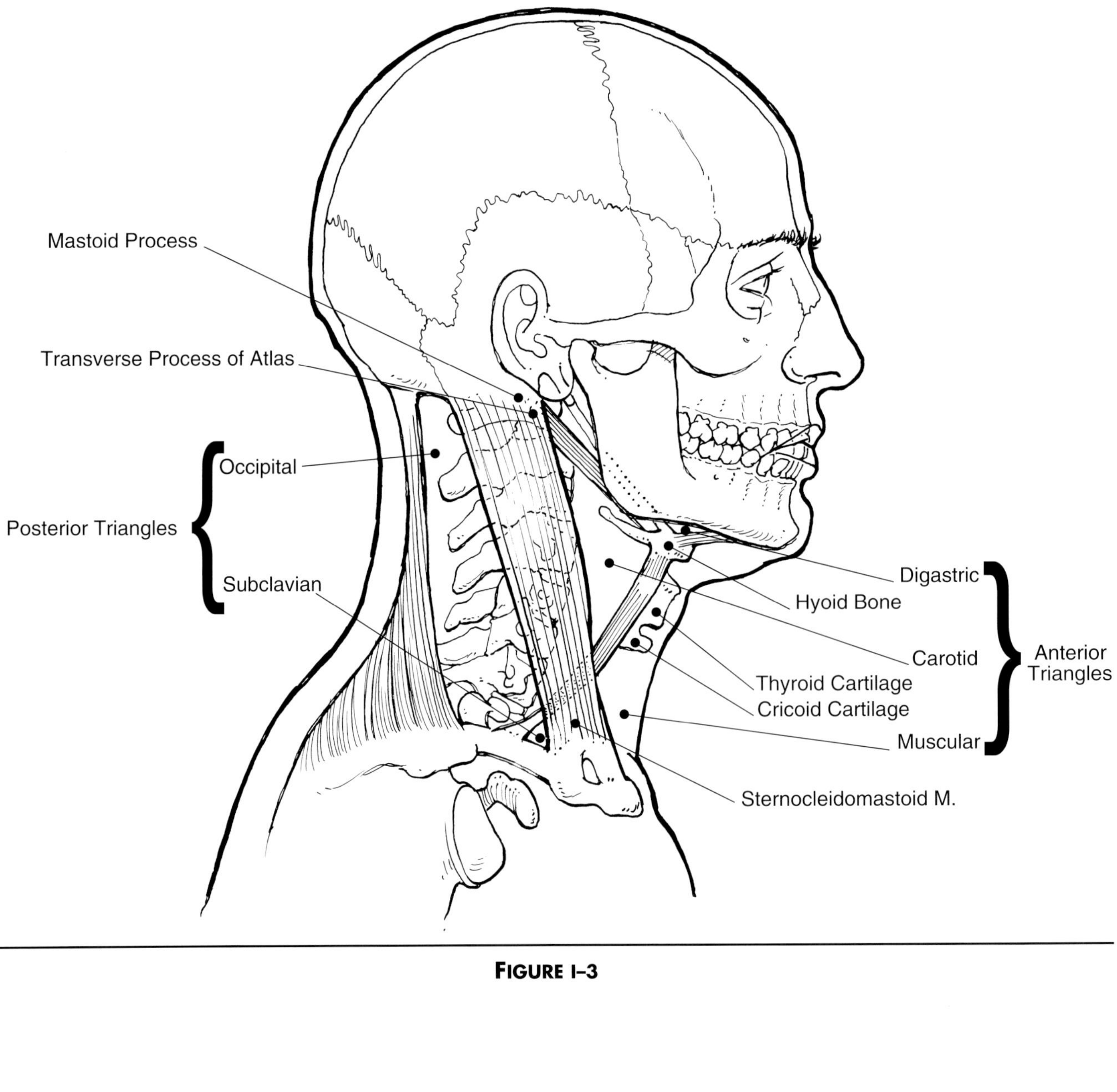


**FIGURE I–3**

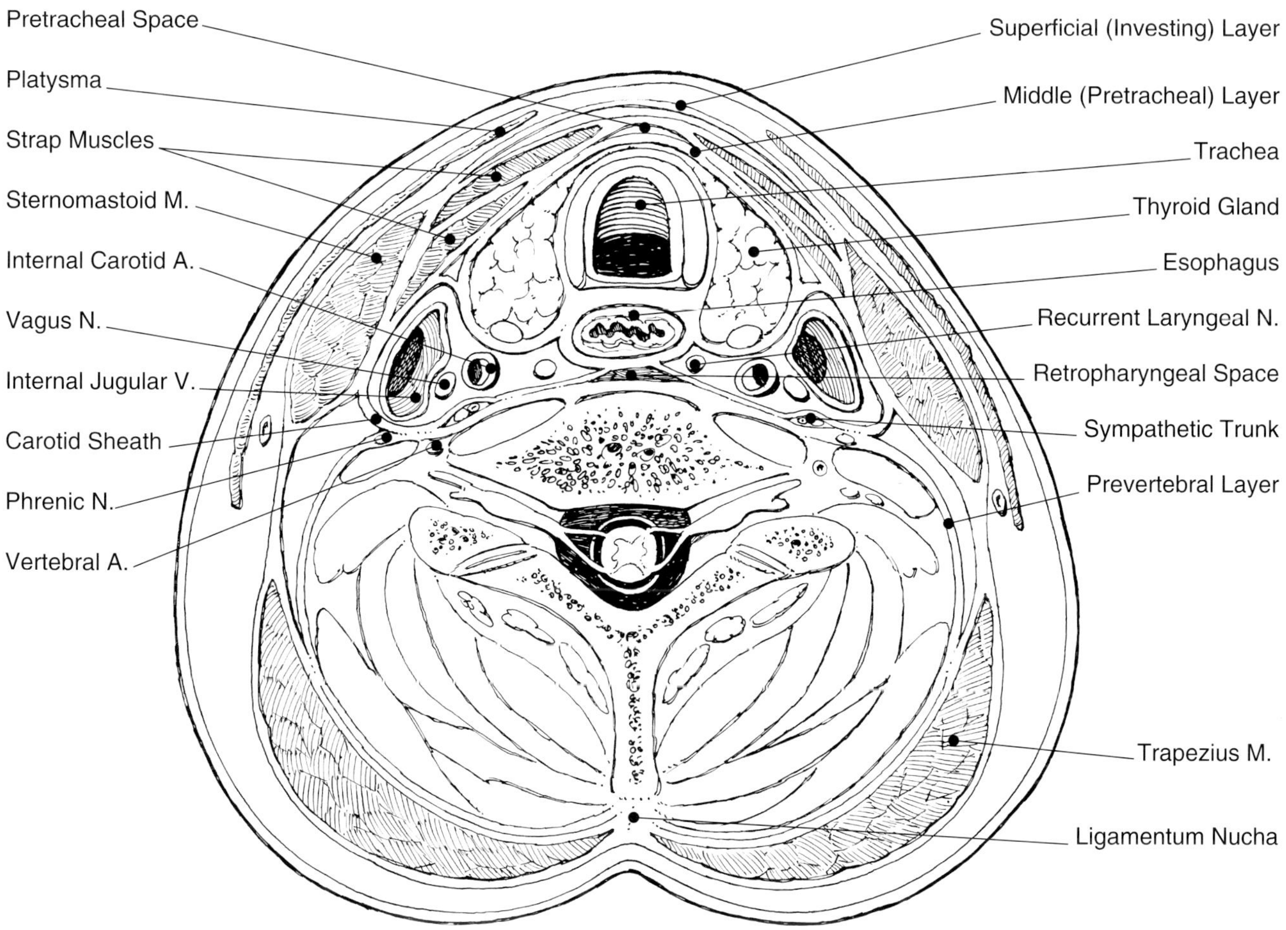


**FIGURE I-4**

middle (pretracheal), and prevertebral (I-4). The superficial layer adheres to the tips of the spinous processes posteriorly and engulfs the trapezius, sternocleidomastoid, and platysma muscles. At its caudal extent, it adheres to the clavicle and cephalad to the hyoid and the inferior edge of the mandible. The superficial veins of the neck lie external to this superficial layer of fascia.

The middle (pretracheal) fascial layer is a thin, delicate membrane in the anterior cervical triangle. It encompasses the infrahyoid "strap" muscles and blends with the carotid sheath (I-5). It bounds the "visceral compartment" which contains the trachea, esophagus, recurrent laryngeal nerve, and thyroid gland. The prevertebral fascia adheres to the tips of the spinous processes and engulfs the intrinsic muscles of the neck, thus making up the floor of the posterior cervical triangle. It covers the scalenus muscles and the muscles directly anterior to the vertebral bodies. It also encapsulates the trunks of the brachial plexus and the phrenic nerve, which lie on the anterior surface of the anterior scalene. The cervical sympathetic trunk lies on the external surface of the pretracheal fascia, just anterior to the longus colli muscle. The space between the esophagus and prevertebral fascia extends from the base of the skull into the posterior mediastinum and is known as the retropharyngeal space. The potential space anterior to the trachea and deep to the infrahyoid "strap" muscles extends from the thyroid cartilage into the anterior mediastinum and is called the pretracheal space (I-6).

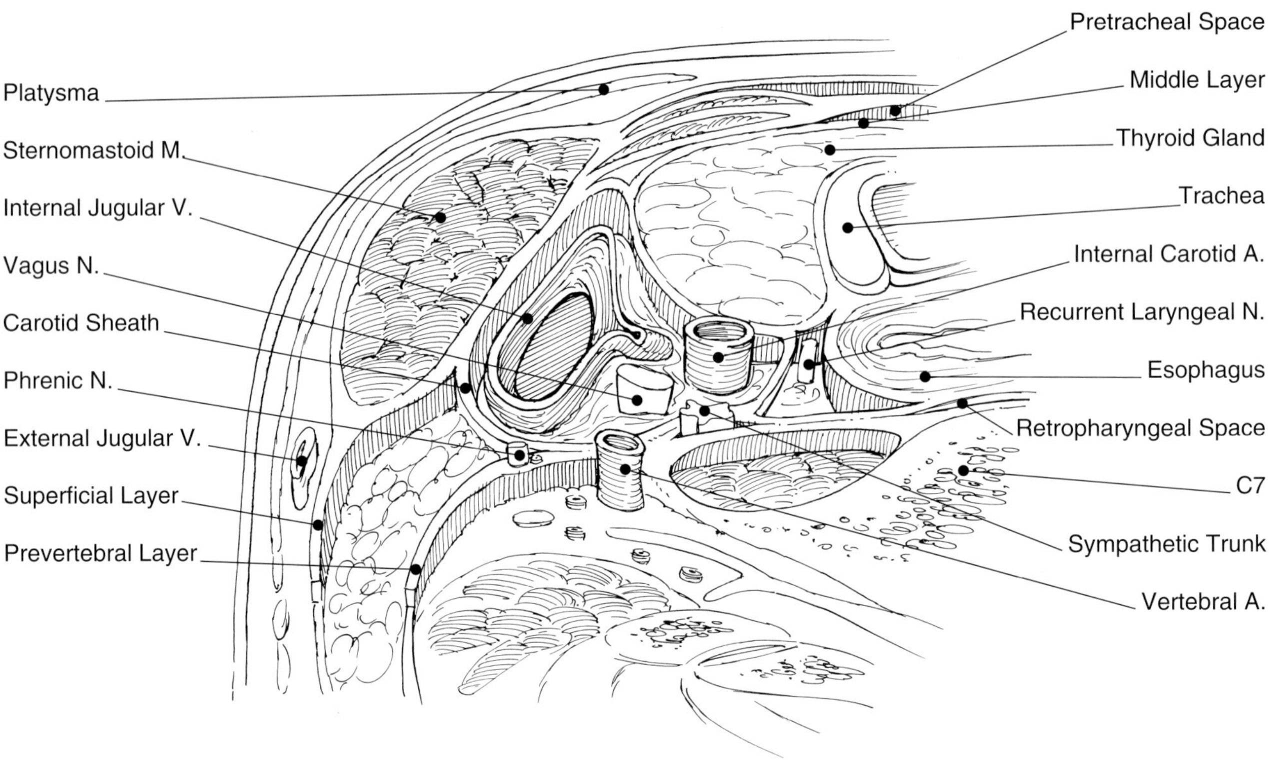


**FIGURE I–5**

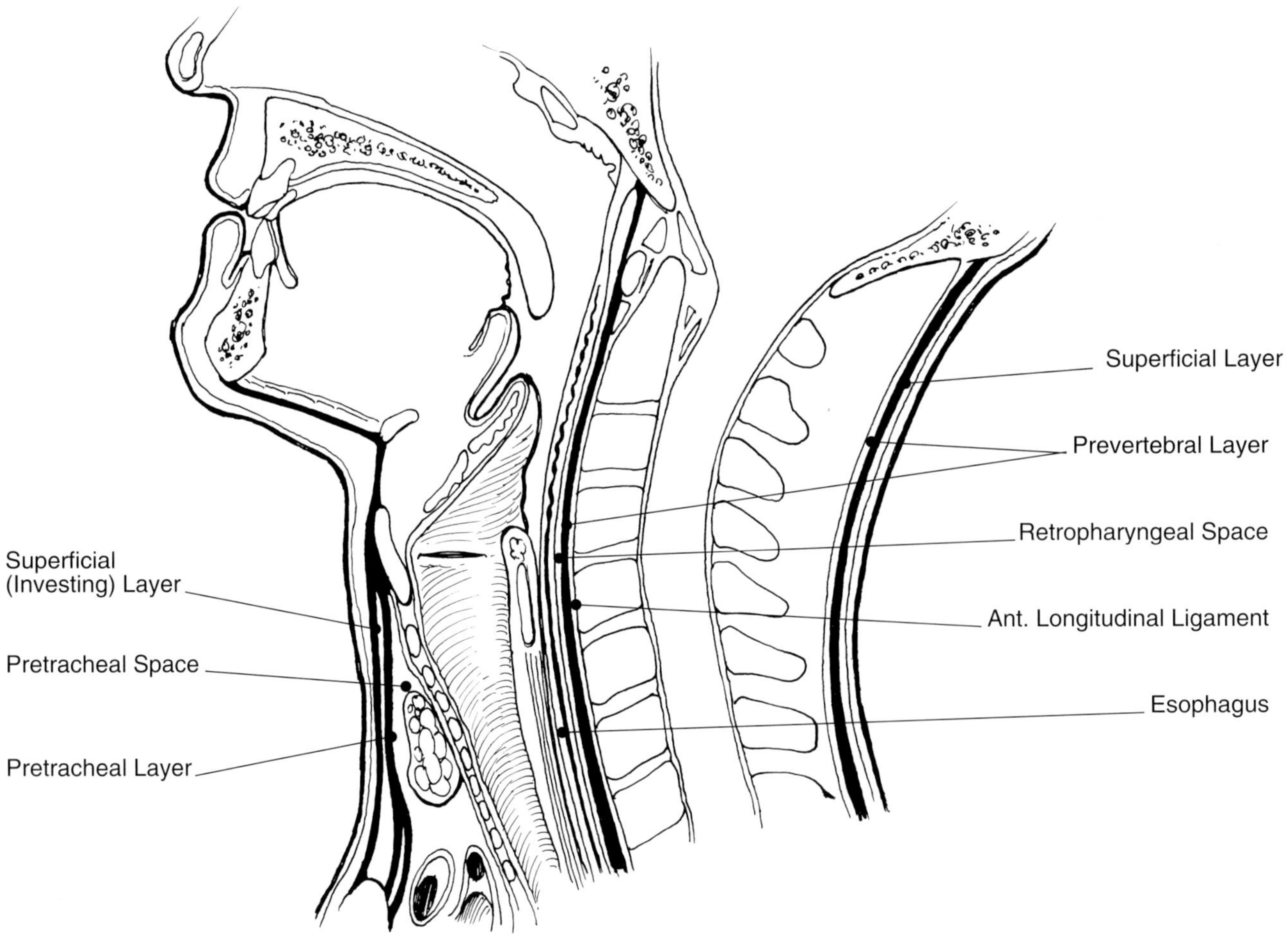


**FIGURE I–6**

In the posterior neck, the tips of the spinous processes are covered by the ligamentum nuchae. Extending laterally is the trapezius muscle, which spans from the base of the skull into the thorax. Just lateral to the cephalad border of the trapezius at the level of the second cervical vertebra are the greater occipital nerve and artery. At the caudal end of the neck, the rhomboideus minor and serratus posterior superior muscles originate from the spinous processes. Just deep to these is the splenius capitis muscle that extends from the spinous processes to the base of the skull. In the same plane is the splenius cervicis muscle that extends from the upper thoracic vertebra to the first three cervical vertebrae (I-7A and I-7B).

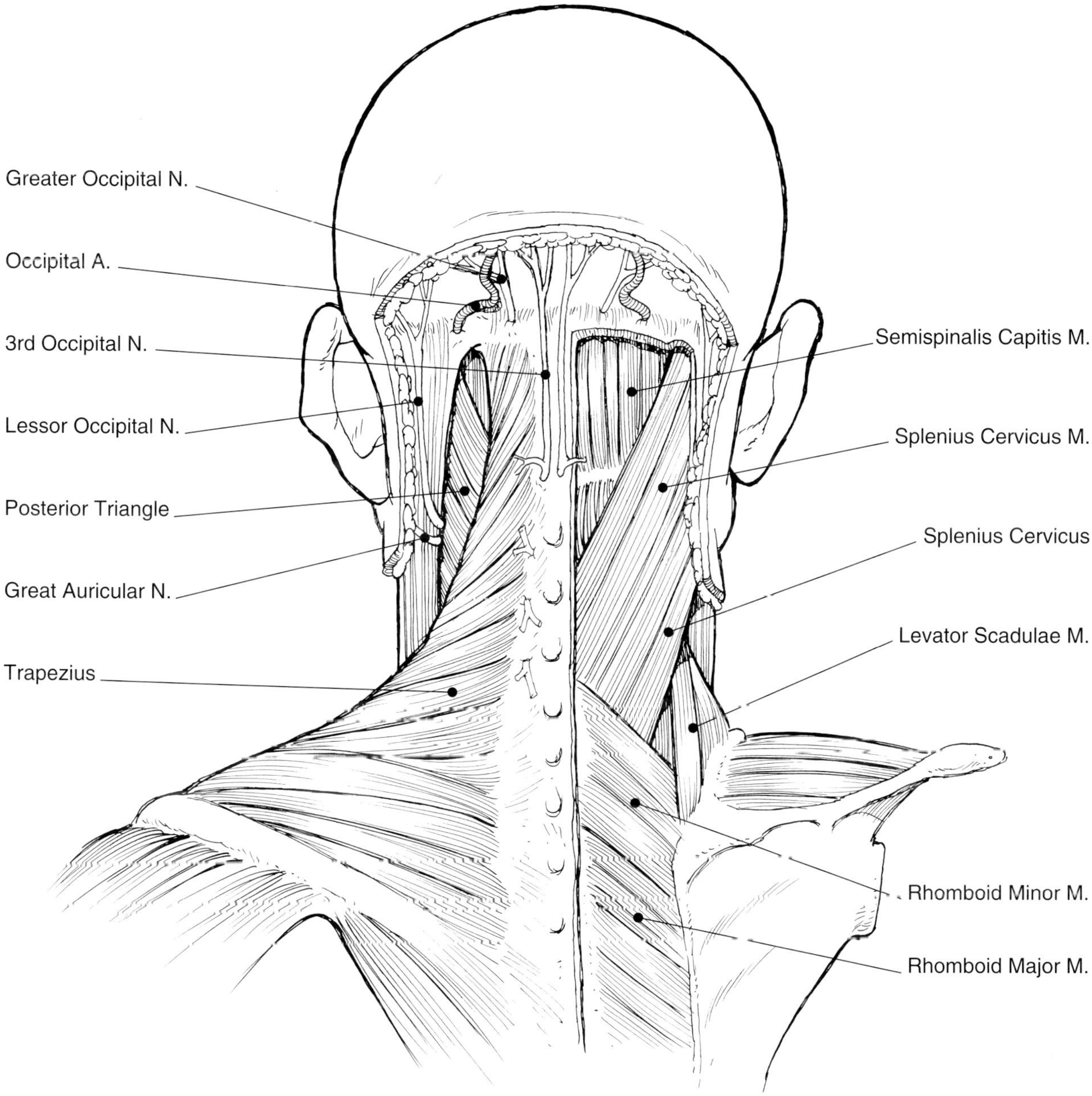


**FIGURE I–7A**

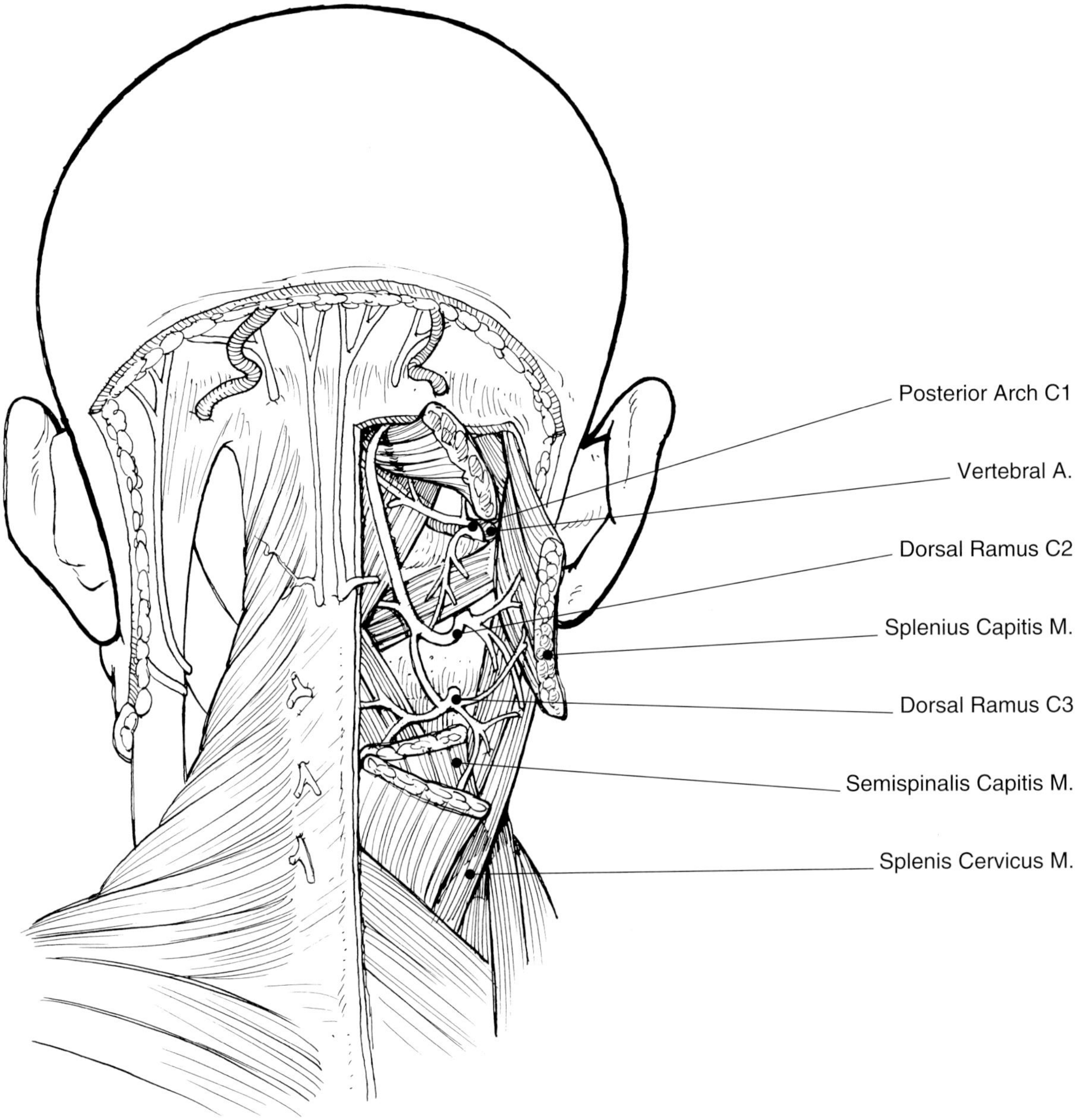
Posterior Arch C1
Vertebral A.
Dorsal Ramus C2
Splenius Capitis M.
Dorsal Ramus C3
Semispinalis Capitis M.
Splenis Cervicus M.

**FIGURE I–7B**

# Anterior Approach to the Base of the Skull and the First Two Cervical Vertebrae

***Applications***

This approach may be used for anterior cervical fusion from the base of the skull through the second cervical vertebral body in the treatment of ligamentous instability associated with rheumatoid arthritis or Down's syndrome. It may also be used to treat unstable odontoid fractures.

***Technique***

The patient is placed supine with the neck extended. Traction halter, Gardner-Wells tongs, or halo traction is applied to the skull for both intraoperative positioning and stabilization. Somatosensory evoked potentials are used to monitor spinal cord function throughout the procedure. Awake fiberoptic nasotracheal intubation should be used if the spine is unstable. The anterior aspect of the base of the skull down to the level of the third cervical vertebra can be most safely approached by the techniques of McAffee et al (2). This approach requires dissection of the subglottic structures medial to the carotid sheath. The dissection can be performed on either the left or right side.

A curved, transverse submandibular incision is placed approximately 2 cm distal to the inferior edge of the mandible (I-8). The platysma muscle is transected parallel to the skin incision, and the soft tissue dissection is expanded deep to the

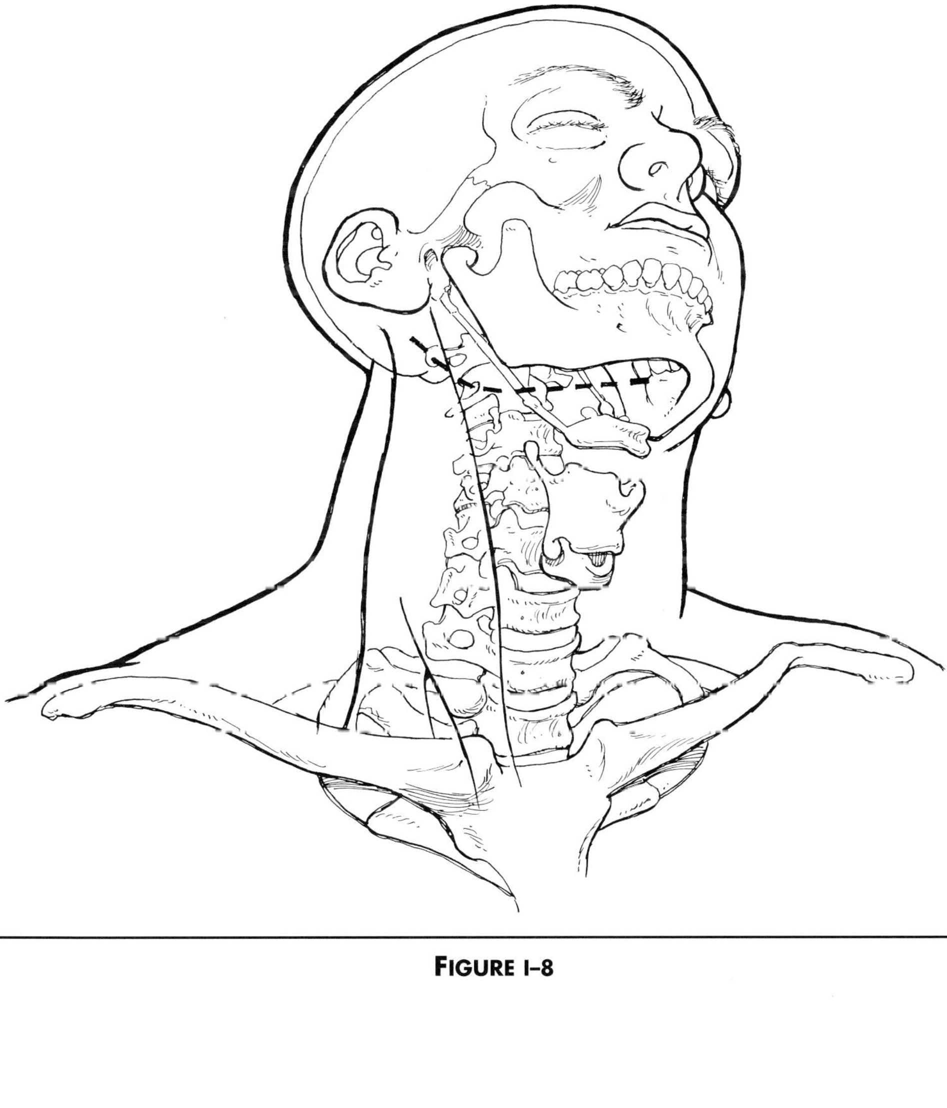

**FIGURE I–8**

superficial fascia. The marginal mandibular branch of the facial nerve should be identified and preserved. The retromandibular veins are transected and ligated near where they empty into the internal jugular vein. The marginal mandibular branch of the facial nerve lies superficial to the retromandibular vein and is protected by this approach (I-9). The deep fascia is then incised longitudinally along the anterior edge of the sternocleidomastoid to expose the muscle belly. Doing this allows palpation of the carotid artery for localization of the carotid sheath. The submandibular salivary gland is then mobilized by freeing its posterior and inferior margins. If necessary, it can be excised and the duct can be ligated. The posterior belly of the digastric and stylohyoid muscles are identified next. The digastric muscle is tagged and divided at the middle tendinous portion. The stylohyoid can be detached from the hyoid and tagged to allow visualization of the hypoglossal nerve on the lateral surface of the hyoglossus muscle. The nerve can then be mobilized posteriorly to the base of the skull and retracted superiorly (I-10). The carotid sheath is retracted laterally and the "visceral compartment" is retracted medially. The interspace will be traversed by branches of the external carotid artery and external jugular vein that must be ligated. These branches are, from inferior to superior: the superior thyroid artery and vein, lingual artery and vein, ascending pharyngeal artery and vein, and facial artery and vein (I-11). The external branch of the superior laryngeal nerve runs adjacent to the superior thyroid artery and should be preserved. Blunt dissection is then used to define the midline of the atlas

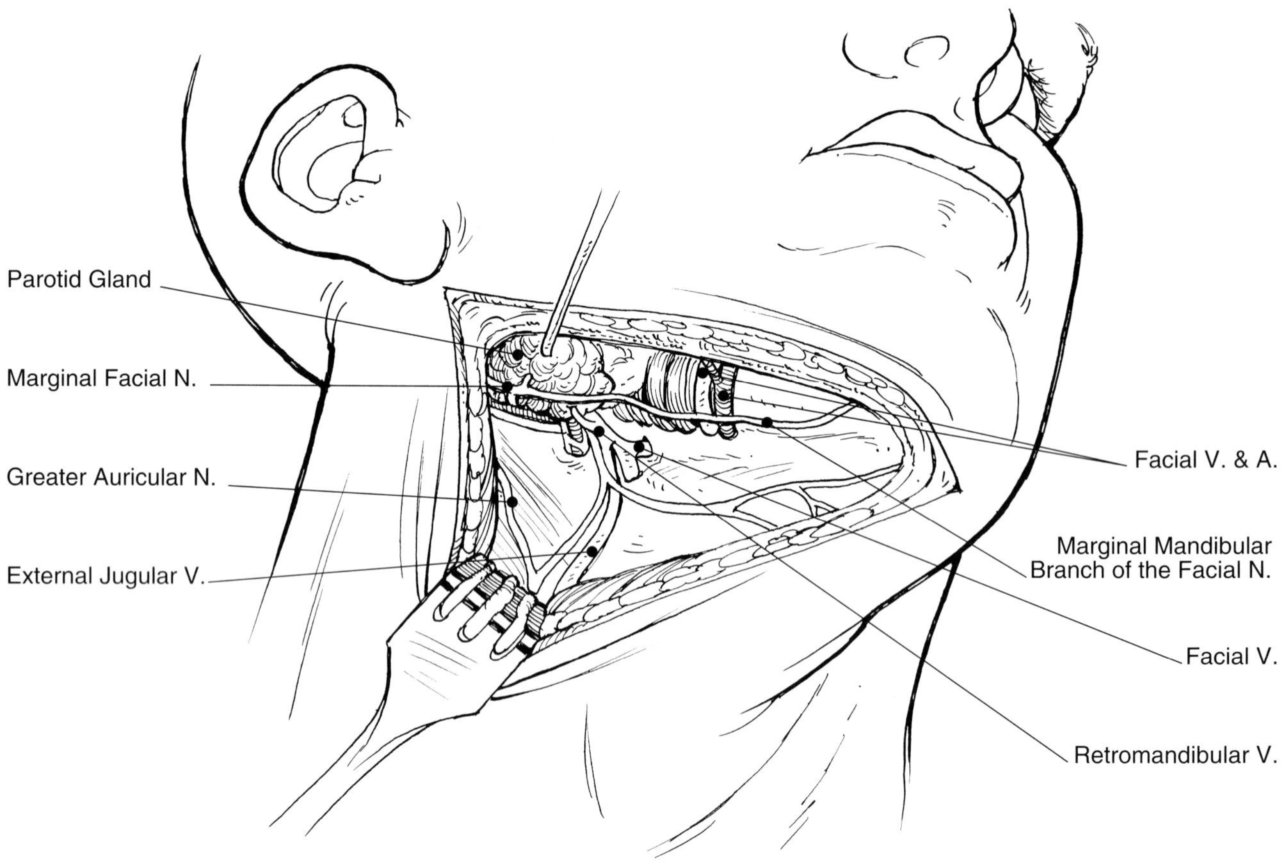


**FIGURE I–9**

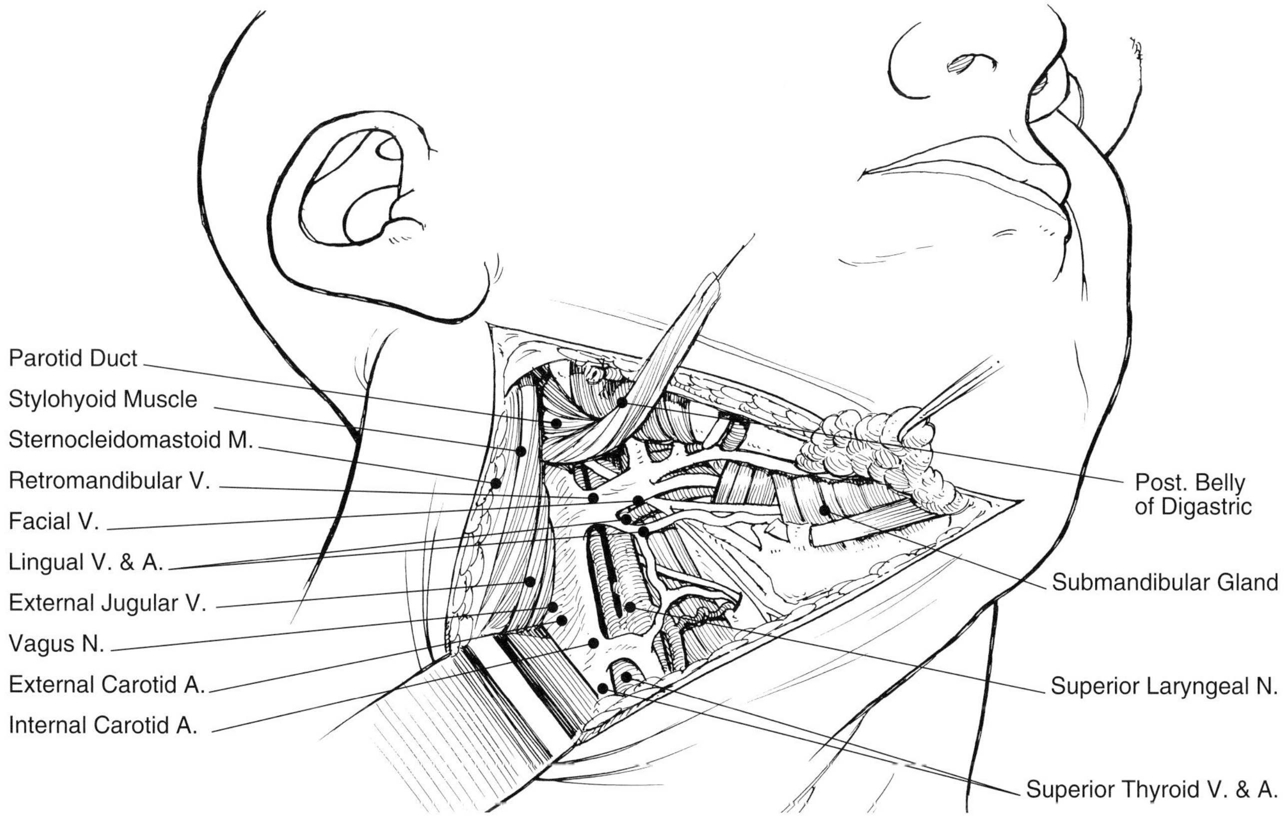


**FIGURE I–10**

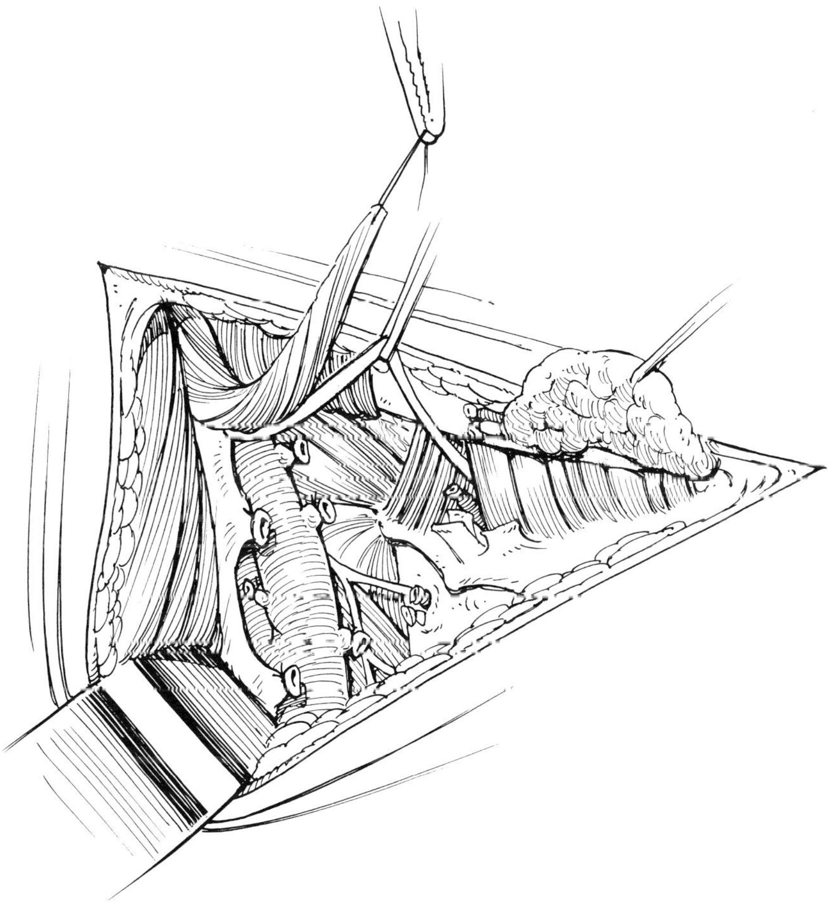

**FIGURE I–11**

and the medial edge of the longus colli muscle. An incision is made longitudinally in the midline from the base of the skull to the base of the second cervical vertebra. The muscles and anterior longitudinal ligament are then mobilized subperiosteally from medial to lateral (I-12A and I-12B).

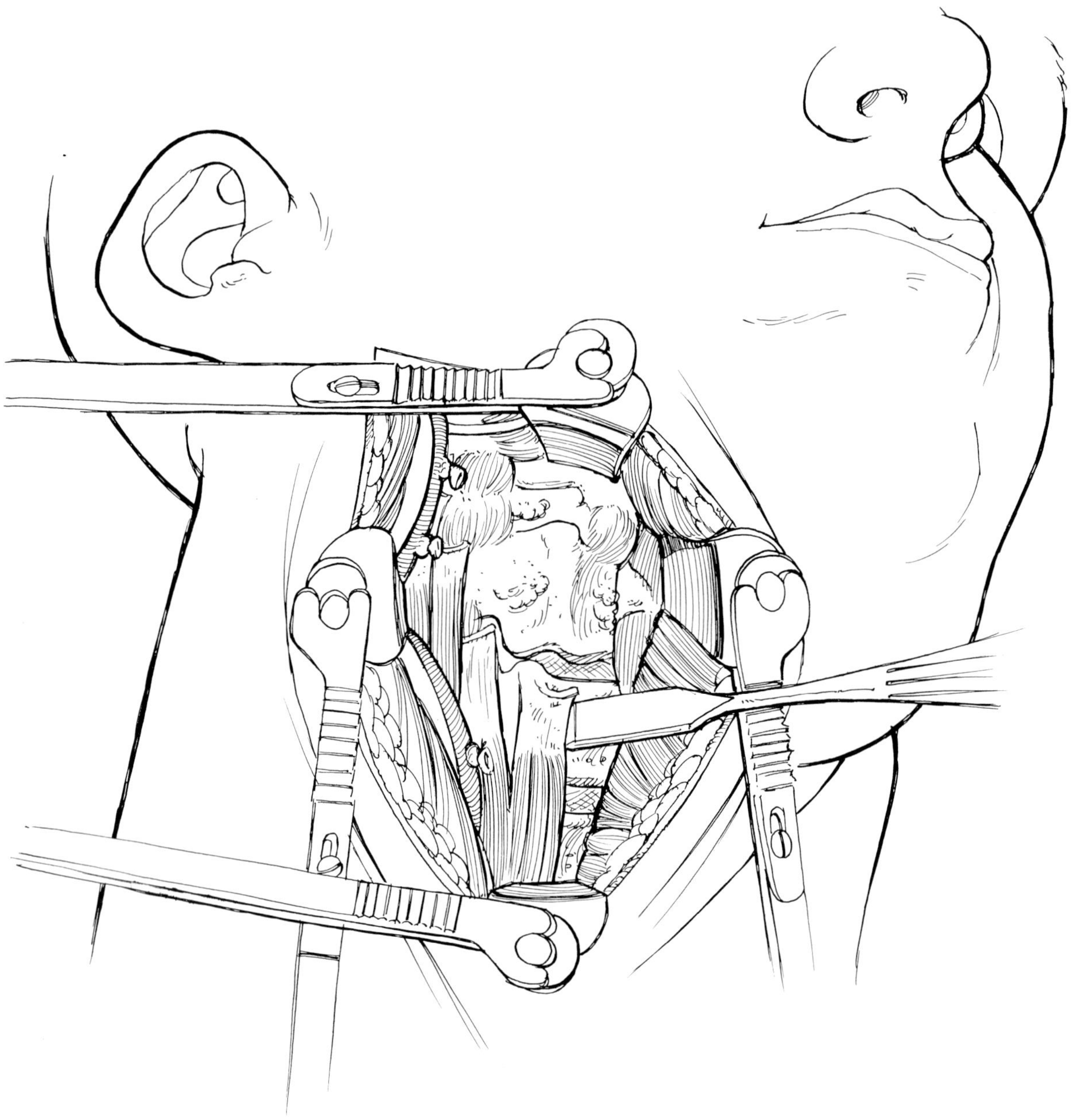

**FIGURE I–12A**

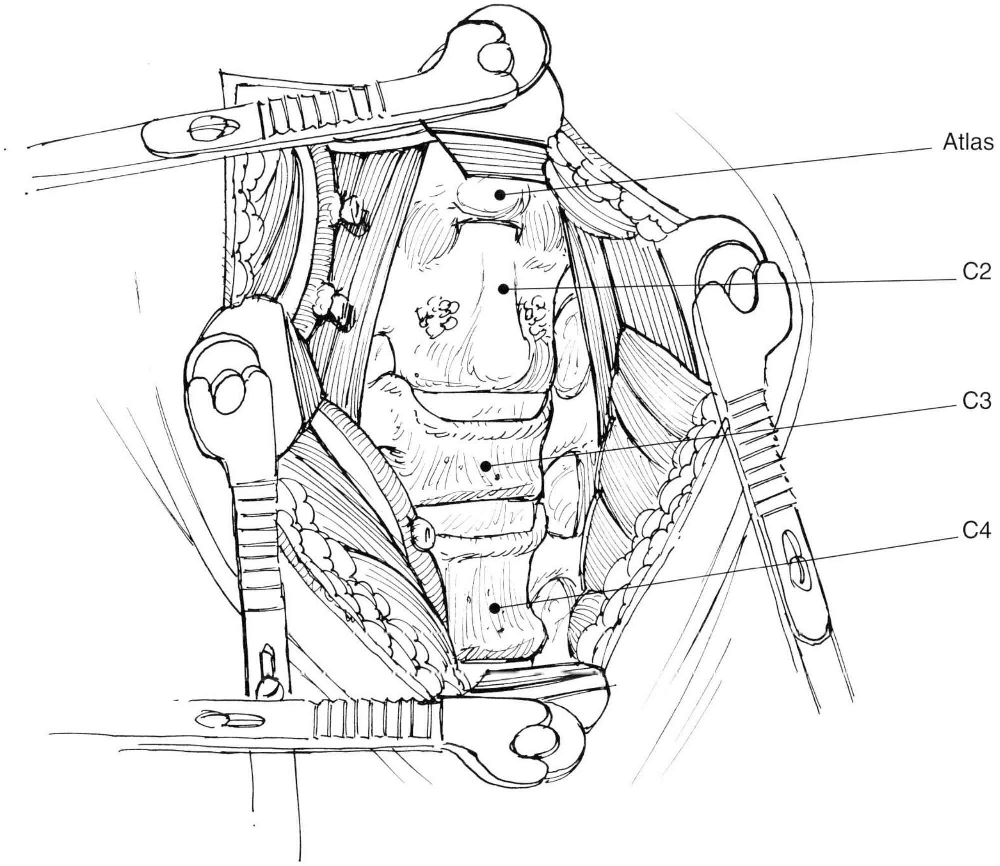


**FIGURE I–12B**

*Dangers*

Dissection into the muscles can result in profuse bleeding from the extensive venous plexus that lies within them. Retropharyngeal swelling or damage to the superior laryngeal nerve can result in upper airway obstruction. The numerous arterial branches must be carefully exposed and preserved or ligated. Damage to the hypoglossal nerve may cause partial paralysis of the tongue with resultant dysphagia or dysarthria.

*Limitations*

This approach is limited to and only necessary for exposure of the base of the skull to the second cervical vertebra. The extensive dissection and major risks of airway obstruction must be weighed against the necessity of an anterior approach because the occiput and upper cervical spine can also be reached by a much simpler posterior approach, particularly if fusion alone is the goal.

# Anterior Approach to the Third through Seventh Cervical Vertebrae

*Applications*

This approach is usually attributed to Robinson and Smith (3). The dissection is caudal to the superior thyroid vessels and the external branch of the superior laryngeal nerve. This is the most commonly used approach to the anterior cervical spine. It may be used for cervical diskectomy (4), removal of osteophytes and fusion, and anterior cervical osteotomy.

### *Technique*

The patient lies supine with the neck extended. Traction is applied to the head and countertraction is applied to the shoulders with wide cotton tape. The preferred dissection is through the left side to avoid injury to a superficially located recurrent laryngeal nerve. The chin is rotated slightly to the right and a roll of towels is placed under the shoulders to support the neck. The skin incision is placed 2 to 4 cm above the clavicles and extends from the midline in a skin crease over the belly of the sternocleidomastoid (I-13). The platysma is divided in the same line as the skin incision (I-14). Deep to the platysma, the dissection is expanded into the space between the sternocleidomastoid and infrahyoid muscles (I-15). The deep fascia is incised longitudinally, medial to the edge of the sternocleidomastoid. This interval is then extended medial to the carotid sheath, lifting the esophagus away from the anterior aspect of the vertebral bodies. The dissection is extended bluntly in this plane to allow exposure of the midline of the vertebral bodies (I-16). The longus colli muscle is elevated subperiosteally from the midline along with the anterior

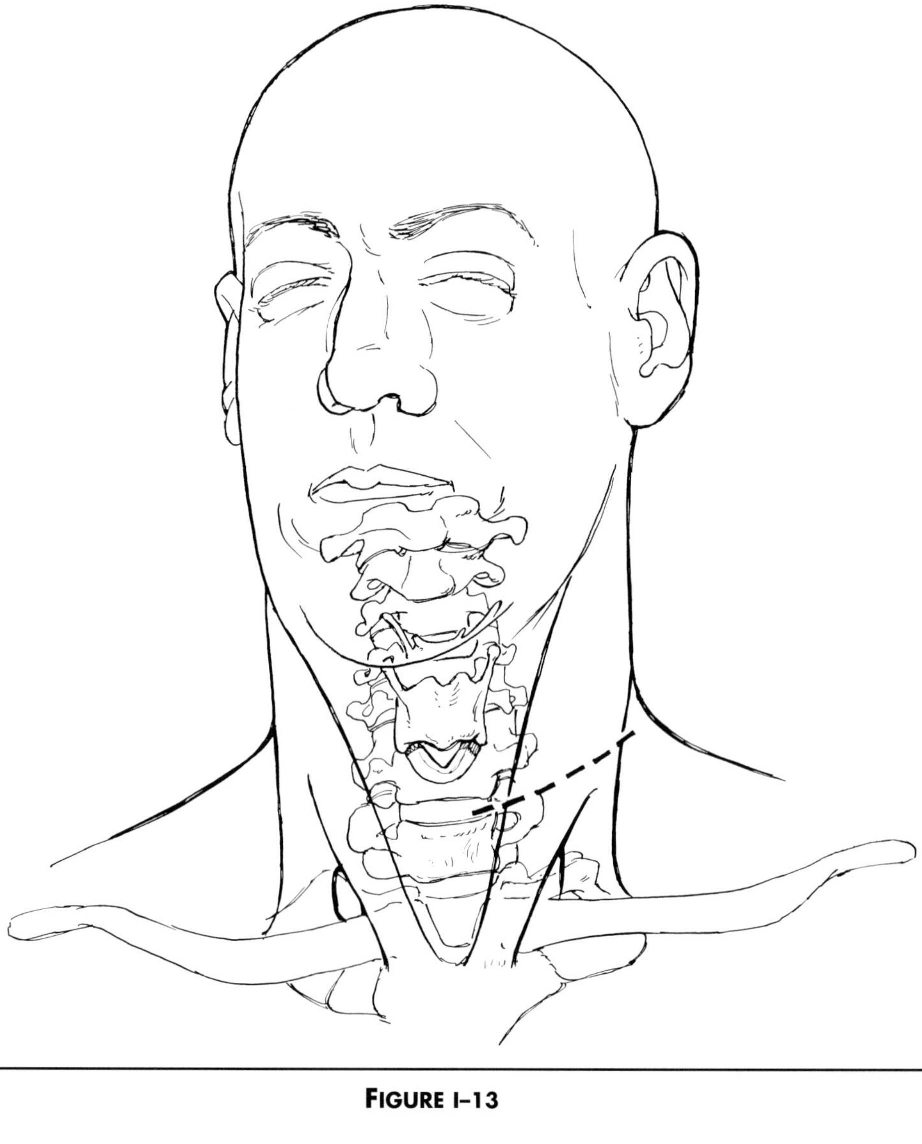

**FIGURE I–13**

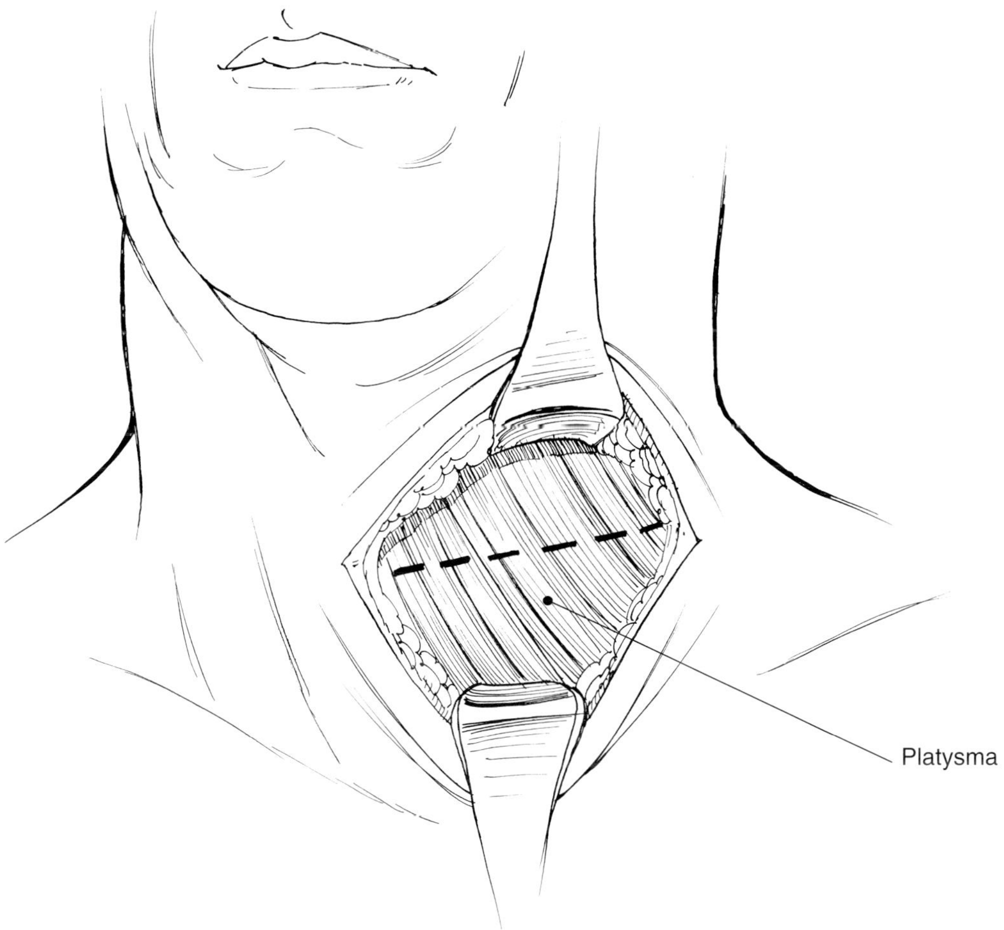


**FIGURE I–14**

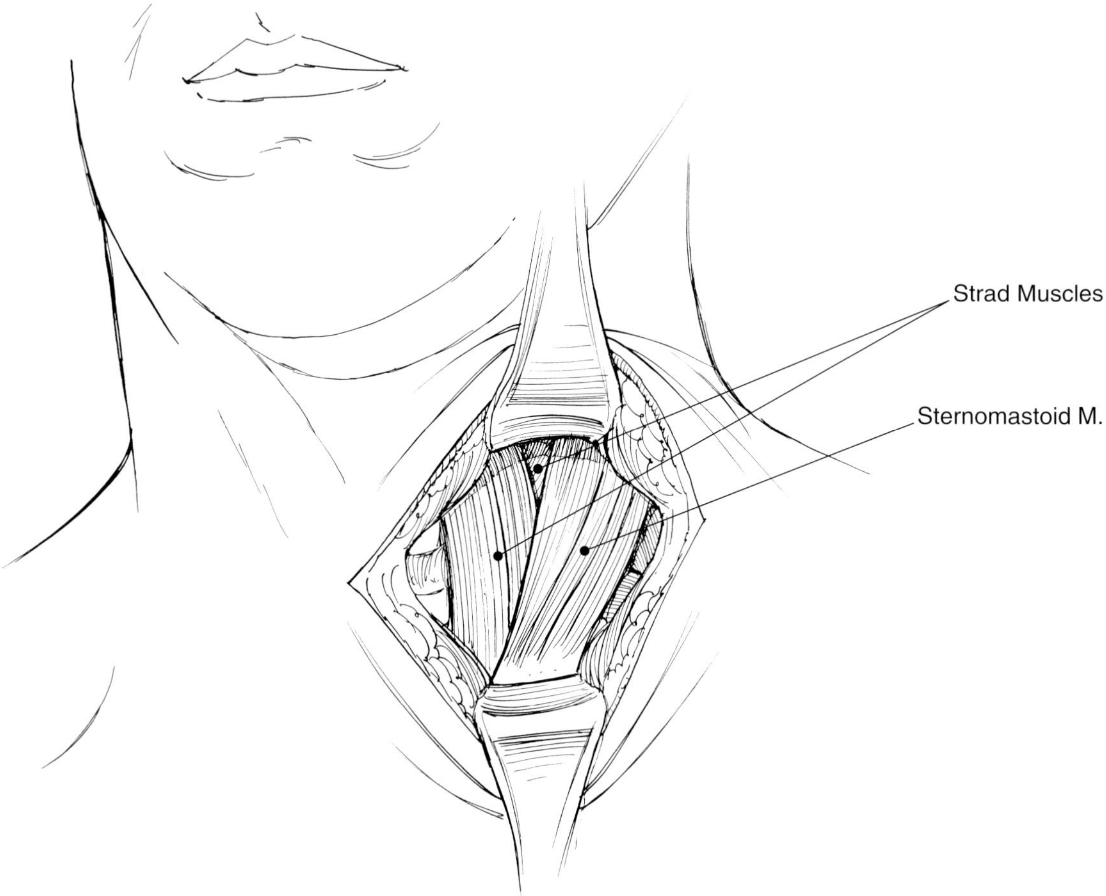


**FIGURE I–15**

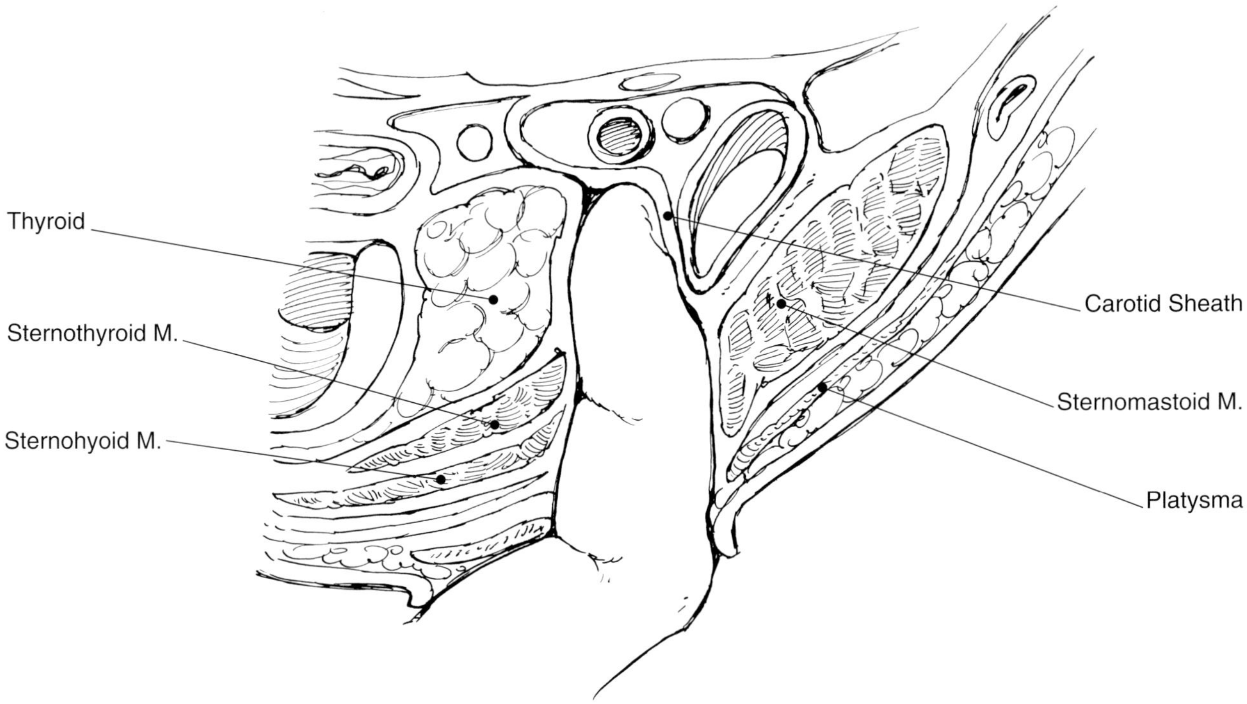


**FIGURE I–16**

longitudinal ligament (I-17). The longus colli muscles cover the transverse processes of the lower cervical vertebrae so dissection should not extend laterally beyond this muscle. To expose C6, C7, and T1, the dissection should be carried out inferior to the level of the omohyoid muscle.

***Dangers***

The hazards of this approach are all outlined at the beginning of this chapter. Risk of hoarseness, Horner's syndrome, or problem bleeding can be minimized by using a careful technique to minimize traction on the nerves and by keeping the exposure of the vertebral bodies in the subperiosteal plane.

***Limitations***

This approach cannot be extended proximally (above the third cervical vertebra) or distally (below T1). It provides exposure to the vertebral bodies, disks, and anterior spinal canal of the third through seventh cervical vertebrae. Lateral extension is prohibited by the vertebral arteries which are anchored in bone.

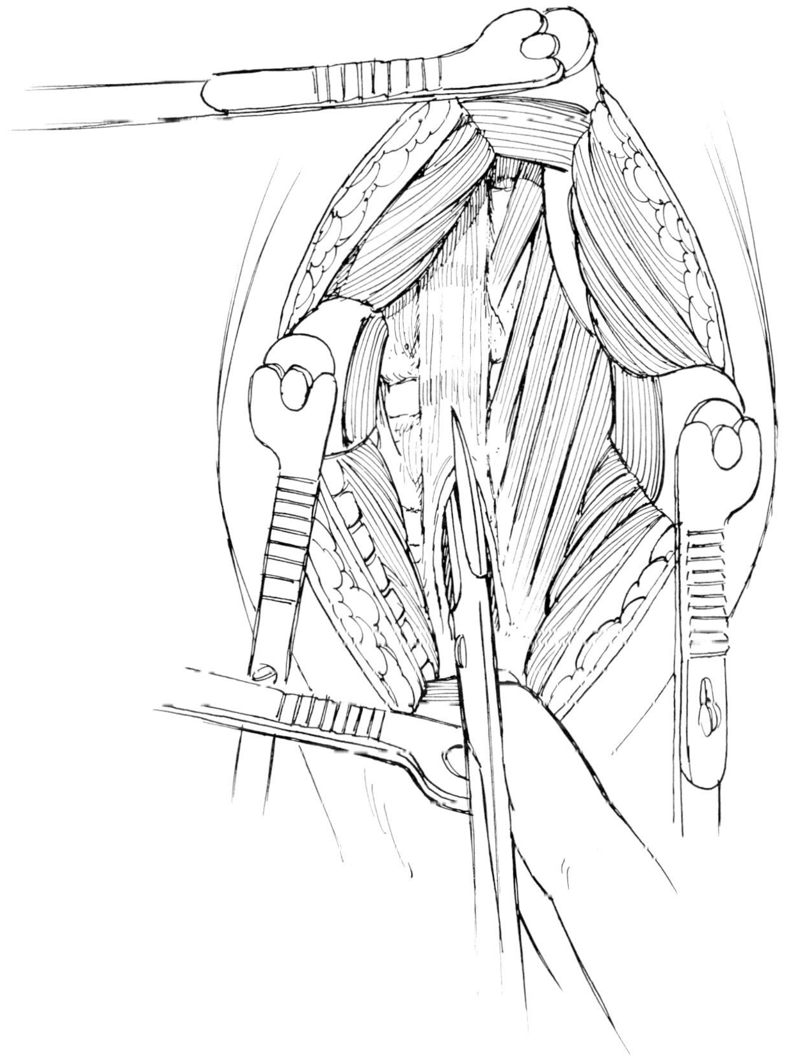

**FIGURE I–17**

# Anterior Approach to the Cervicothoracic Junction

*Applications*

The anterior approach to the cervicothoracic junction can provide reliable access to the seventh cervical and first thoracic vertebrae. This exposure may be necessary for removal of tumors, infection, bone fragments, or disk fragments or for anterior fusion.

*Technique*

This approach may be carried out on either the left or right side, although the right side is preferred to avoid injury to the thoracic duct on the left (5,6). The patient is placed supine with a bolster under the shoulders to allow extension of the neck. The head is rotated away from the surgical side. A long transverse incision is made from the midline of the neck to the lateral edge of the sternocleidomastoid. The incision is 1 cm above and parallel to the clavicle (I-18). The platysma is divided transversely. The external jugular vein and medial supraclavicular nerve

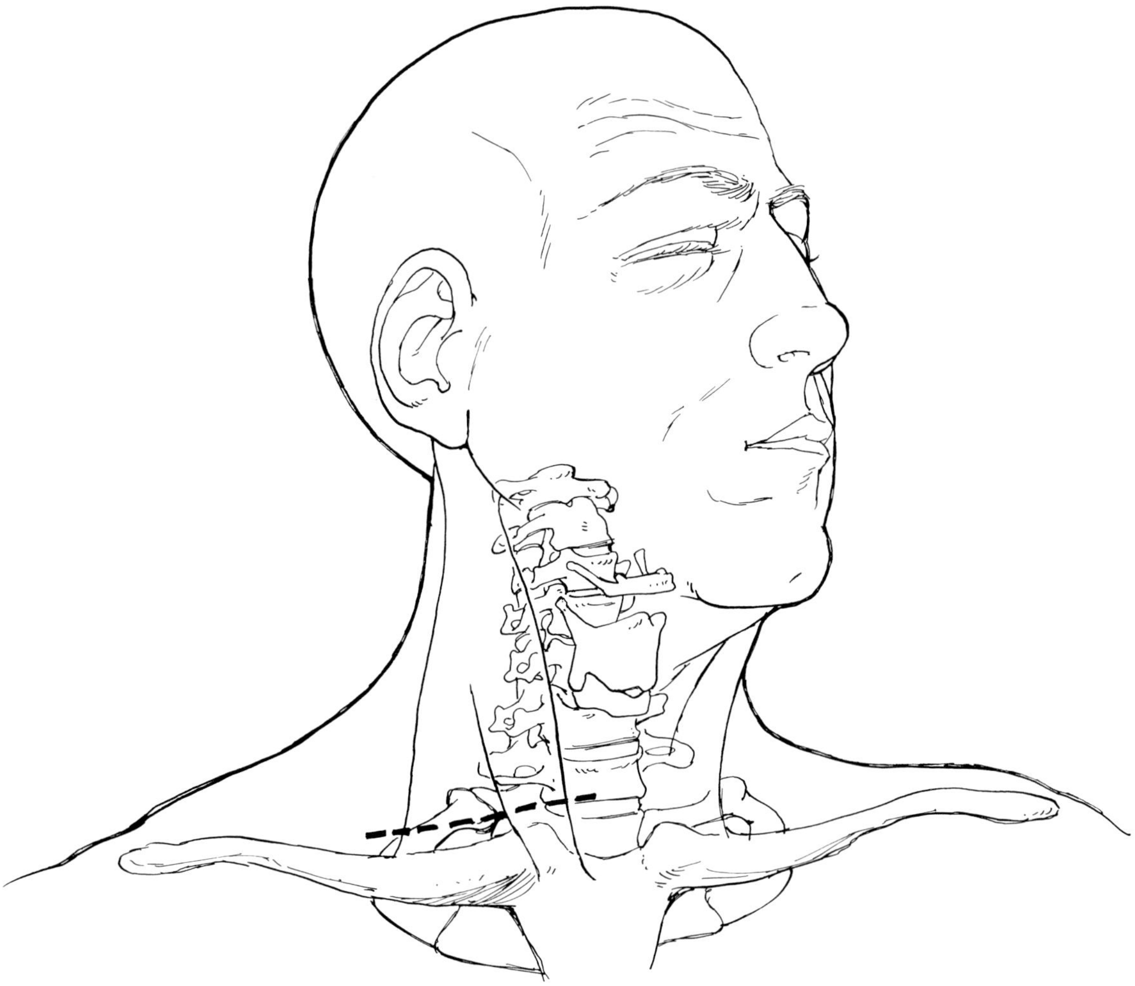

**FIGURE I–18**

will be found just lateral to the platysma and sternocleidomastoid (I-19). Next, the triangular defect between the clavicular and sternal heads of the sternocleidomastoid is opened bluntly. The internal jugular and subclavian veins lie immediately deep to the deep cervical fascia in this space. Therefore, this space should be opened by blunt finger dissection until a finger can be placed deep to the clavicular head of the sternocleidomastoid. The clavicular head is then divided transversely, close to the clavicle (I-20).

The omohyoid crosses the field, descending obliquely from medial to lateral. The fascial pulley of the middle cervical fascia is divided transversely to allow this muscle to be retracted superiorly. The fat pad deep to the fascia contains the thyrocervical trunk. The deep boundary of this space is the anterior scalene muscle. The phrenic nerve lies on the anterior surface of this muscle. The carotid sheath and its contents should be retracted medially to better expose the anterior scalene

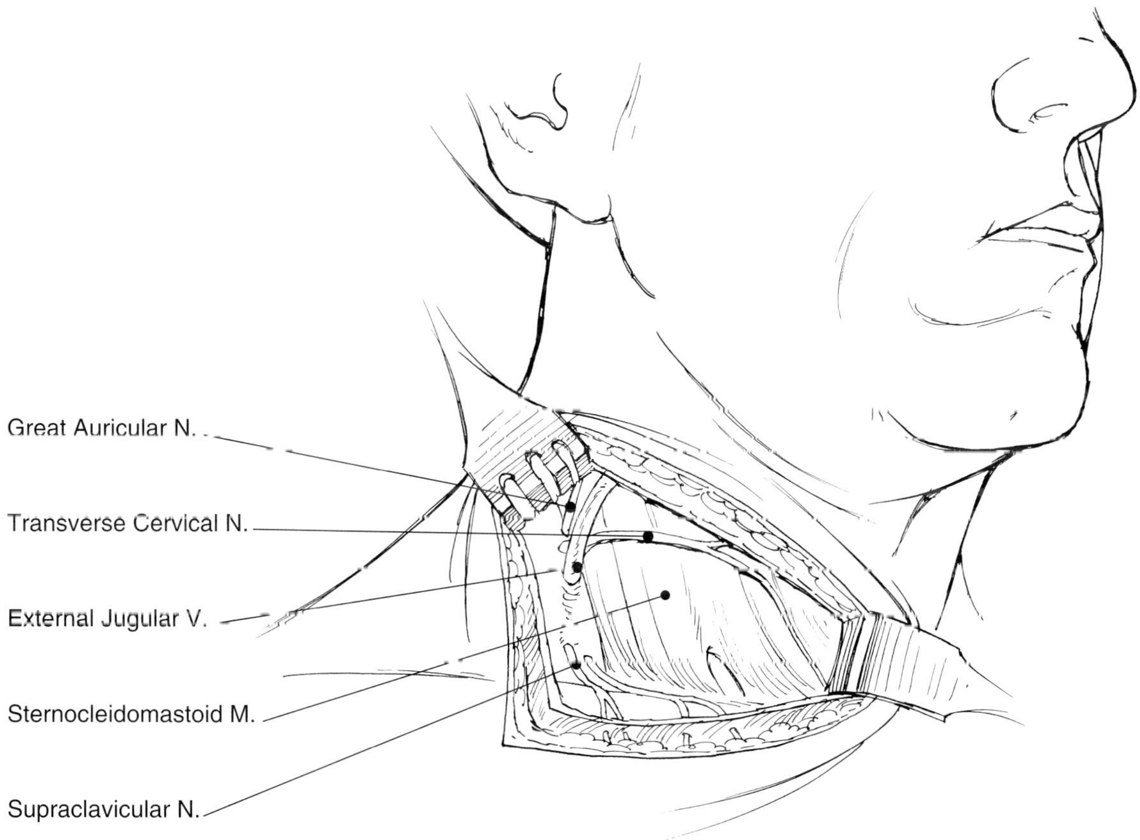


**FIGURE I–19**

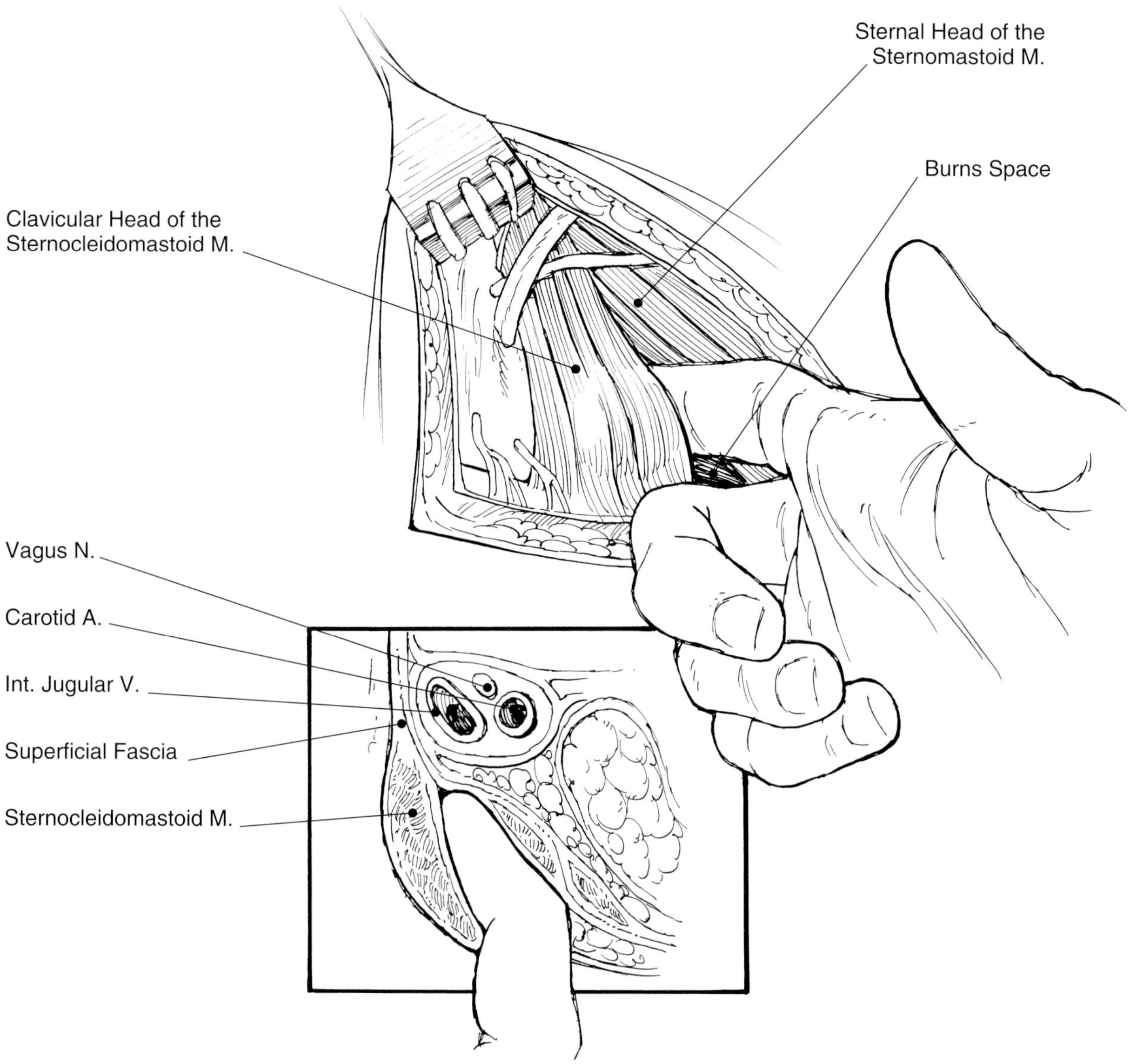
Sternal Head of the
Sternomastoid M.
Burns Space
Clavicular Head of the
Sternocleidomastoid M.
Vagus N.
Carotid A.
Int. Jugular V.
Superficial Fascia
Sternocleidomastoid M.

**FIGURE I–20**

(I-21). The suprascapular artery and transverse cervical artery arise from the thyrocervical trunk and run transversely through the fat pad at the cephalad end of the field. The phrenic nerve is mobilized and retracted medially. The medial and lateral edges of the sternocleidomastoid muscle are defined, a clamp is placed deep to the muscle, and it is divided transversely onto the clamp (I-22). The ascending cervical branch of the subclavian artery can be seen entering this muscle. It should be ligated. The anterior scalene muscle is divided in similar fashion (I-23). In the caudal end of the field, deep to the anterior scalene muscle, the fascia covering the dome of the lung (Sibson's fascia) is encountered. Careful opening of this fascia allows blunt dissection into the thorax with distal and lateral retraction of the lung. Injury to the pleura should be avoided because of the risk of a pneumothorax. The stellate ganglion is found posteriorly, overlying the neck

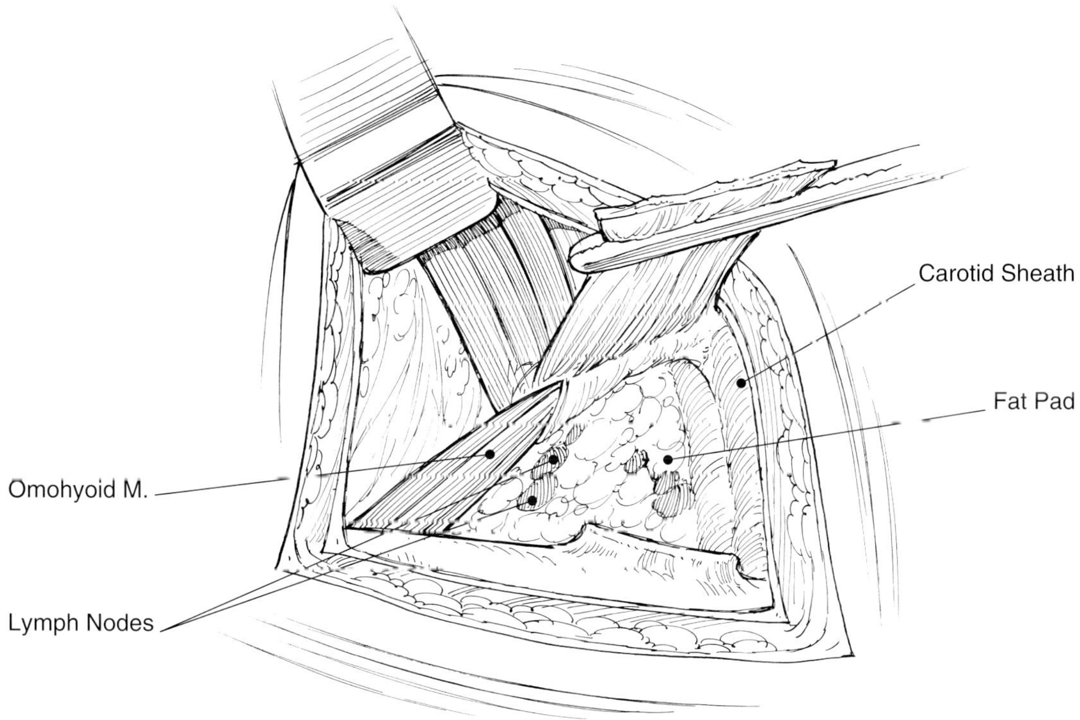


**FIGURE I–21**

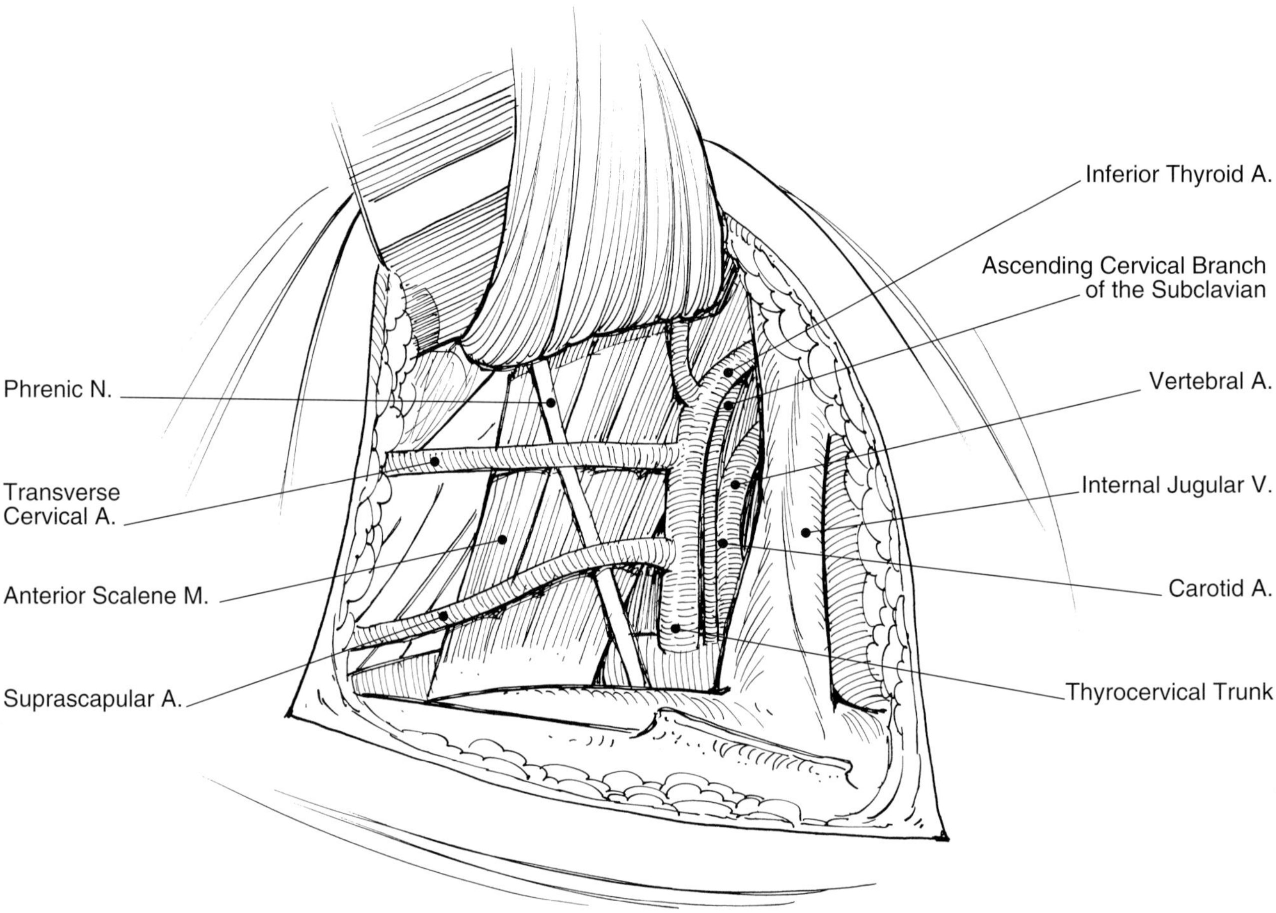
Inferior Thyroid A.
Ascending Cervical Branch of the Subclavian
Phrenic N.
Vertebral A.
Transverse Cervical A.
Internal Jugular V.
Anterior Scalene M.
Carotid A.
Suprascapular A.
Thyrocervical Trunk

**FIGURE I–22**

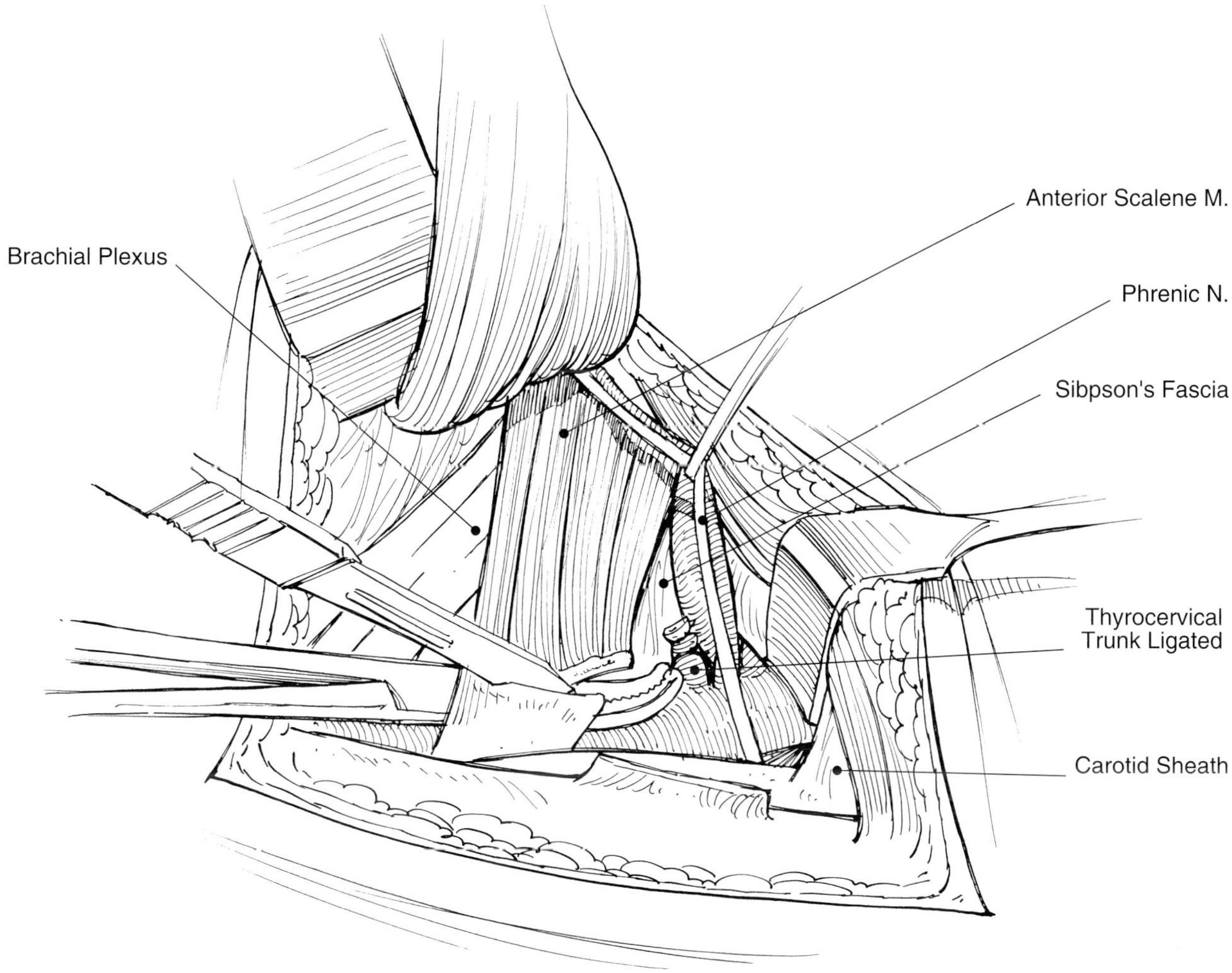
Anterior Scalene M.
Brachial Plexus
Phrenic N.
Sibpson's Fascia
Thyrocervical
Trunk Ligated
Carotid Sheath

**FIGURE I–23**

of the first rib. The first thoracic nerve root will be found just lateral to the ganglion, running on the upper surface of the first rib (I-24). The vertebral bodies lie medial to the ganglion. The first rib articulates with the bodies of C7 and T1. The periosteum of the vertebral bodies is incised in the midline and reflected laterally to expose the vertebrae and disk. At the completion of the procedure, the anterior scalene muscle and sternocleidomastoid should be repaired. Proximal extension of this dissection is limited by the subclavian vessels and the recurrent laryngeal nerve. This approach may be carried medial to the carotid sheath by mobilizing the recurrent laryngeal nerve and retracting it medially along with the esophagus and trachea (7,8).

***Dangers***

A drain should be placed above the dome of the lung to prevent fluid accumulation. While usually encountered on the left, the thoracic duct may be encountered on either side. If it is damaged, it should be carefully ligated to prevent the formation of a chylothorax or a chylous fistula. Damage to the phrenic nerve can result in paralysis of the hemidiaphragm. A chest x-ray should be obtained during wound closure to look for a pneumothorax.

***Limitations***

This approach may be used to reach as far distally as the second or third thoracic vertebra in slender people with small necks, but it is not reliable for wide access to this area.

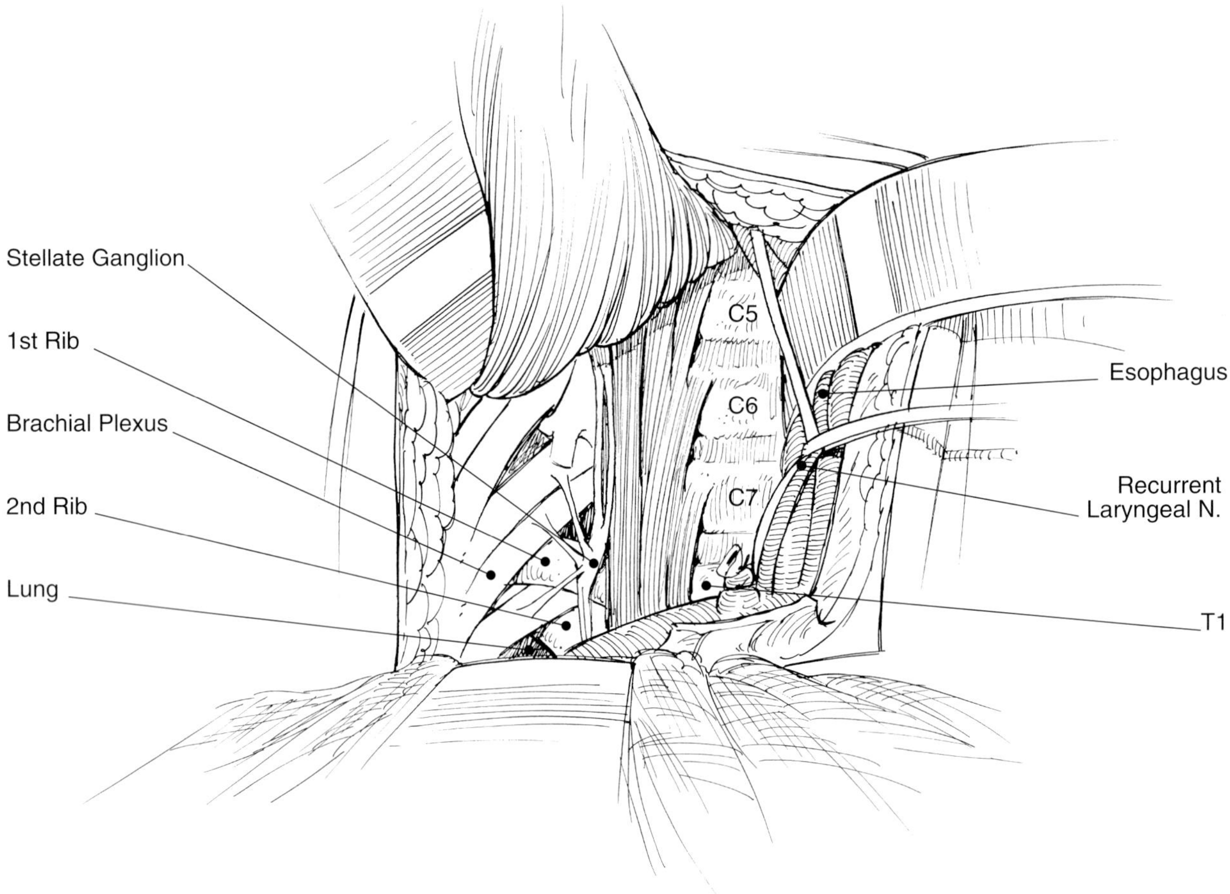


**FIGURE I–24**

# Midline Posterior Approach to the Occiput and Cervical Spine

*Applications*

The midline posterior approach allows safe and quick access to the posterior elements of the cervical spine. It is useful for decompression of the spinal cord, removal of tumors in the spinal cord, and instrumentation and fusion of the cervical spine.

*Technique*

The patient is positioned prone with the neck slightly flexed and the head supported in a head brace or traction ring. The incision is made in the midline, longitudinally over the area of interest (I-25). A midline approach through the ligamentum nuchae causes minimal bleeding (I-26). The paraspinal muscles are elevated subperiosteally from the spinous processes as far laterally as the transverse processes (I-27). The vertebral artery runs through the foramina of the transverse process and is vulnerable to injury in the interspace between the vertebrae. At C1, it passes through the transverse foramen of C1, then turns medially deep to the posterior atlantooccipital membrane to run along the posterior arch of C1. It is vulnerable to injury during mobilization of the atlantooccipital membrane from C1. The spinous processes, laminae, and small transverse process are widely exposed by retraction of the paraspinal muscles.

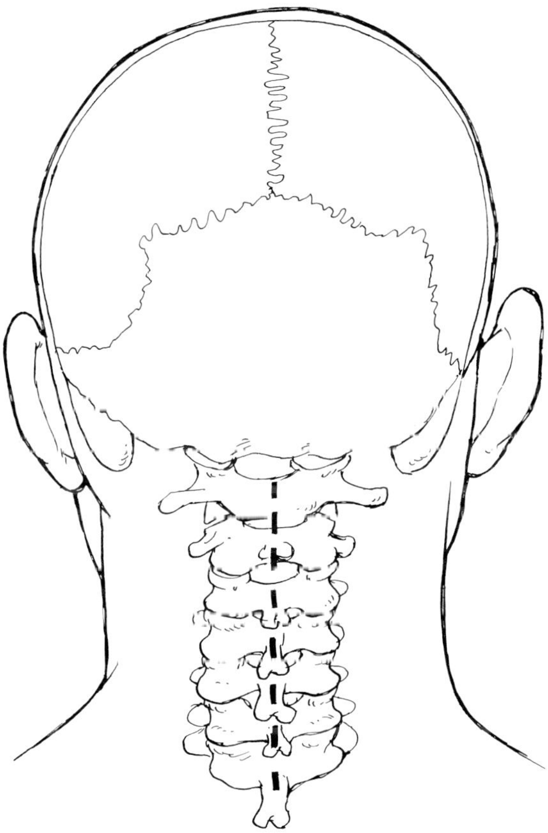

**FIGURE I–25**

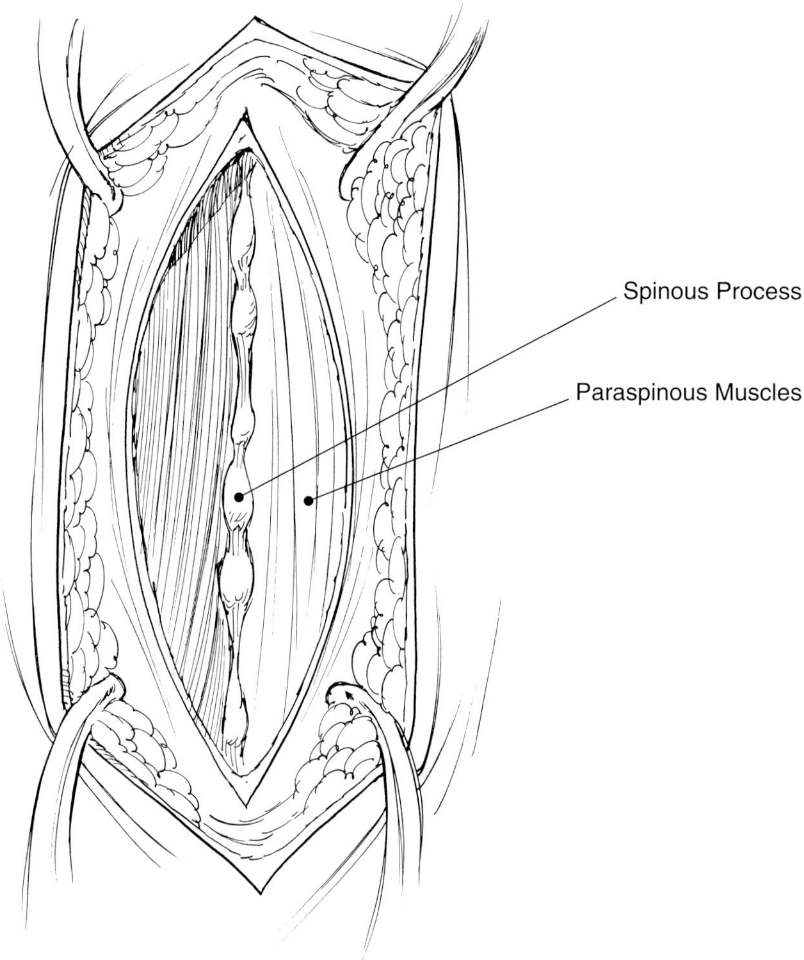


**FIGURE I–26**

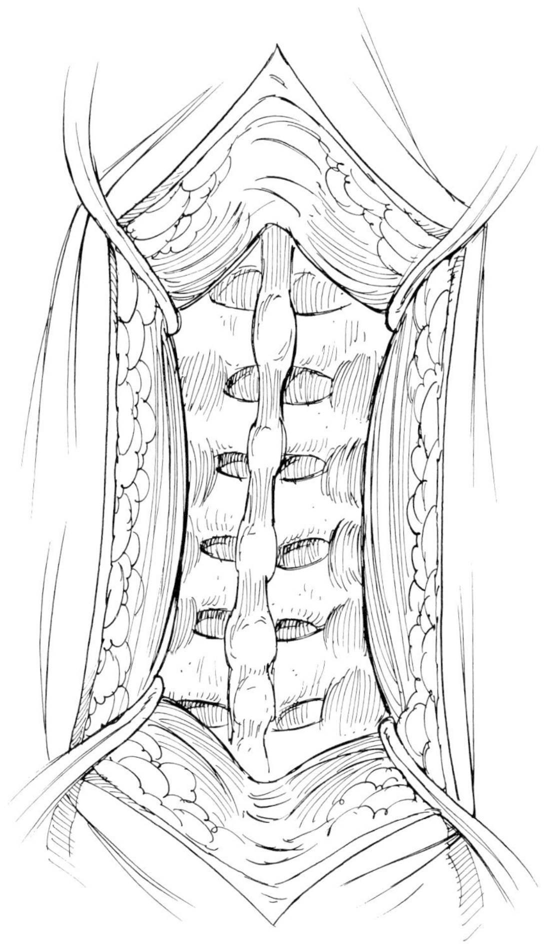

**FIGURE I–27**

*Dangers*

The major hazard of this approach is injury to the vertebral artery. Lateral dissection should be kept on the dorsal surface of the bone to prevent inadvertent injury to the vessels in the interspace between the transverse processes.

*Limitations*

This approach can be extended as far longitudinally as necessary. The lateral limit is the posterior surface of the transverse processes. Laminectomy exposes the dura and nerve roots. Careful dissection and gentle retraction of the spinal cord allows removal of osteophytes from the anterior floor of the spinal canal.

# References

1. Johnson RM, Murphy MJ, Southwick WO. Surgical approaches to the spine. In: Rathman RH, Simeon FA, eds. The Spine, 3rd ed. Philadelphia: W.B. Saunders, 43:1607–1696, 1992.
2. McAffee PC, Bohlman HH, Riley LH, et al. The anterior retropharyngeal approach to the upper part of the cervical spine. J Bone Joint Surg 69A:1371–1383, 1987.
3. Robinson RA, Smith GW. Anterolateral cervical disc removal and interbody fusion for cervical disc syndrome. Bull Johns Hopkins Hosp 96:223, 1955.

4. Cloward RB. The anterior approach for removal of ruptured cervical disks. J Neurosurg 15:402, 1958.
5. Kurz LT, Persch SE, Herkowitz HN. Modified anterior approach to the cervicothoracic junction. Spine 16(10):S542–S547, 1991.
6. Micheli LJ, Horel RW. Anterior exposure of the cervicothoracic spine using a combined cervical and thoracic approach. J Bone Joint Surg 65:992–997, 1983.
7. Birch R, Bonney G, Marshall R. A surgical approach to the cervicothoracic spine. J Bone Joint Surg Br 72(5):904–907, 1990.
8. Charles R, Govender S. Anterior approach to the upper thoracic vertebrae. J Bone Joint Surg 71(1):81–84, 1989.

# II

# SURGICAL APPROACHES TO THE THORACIC SPINE

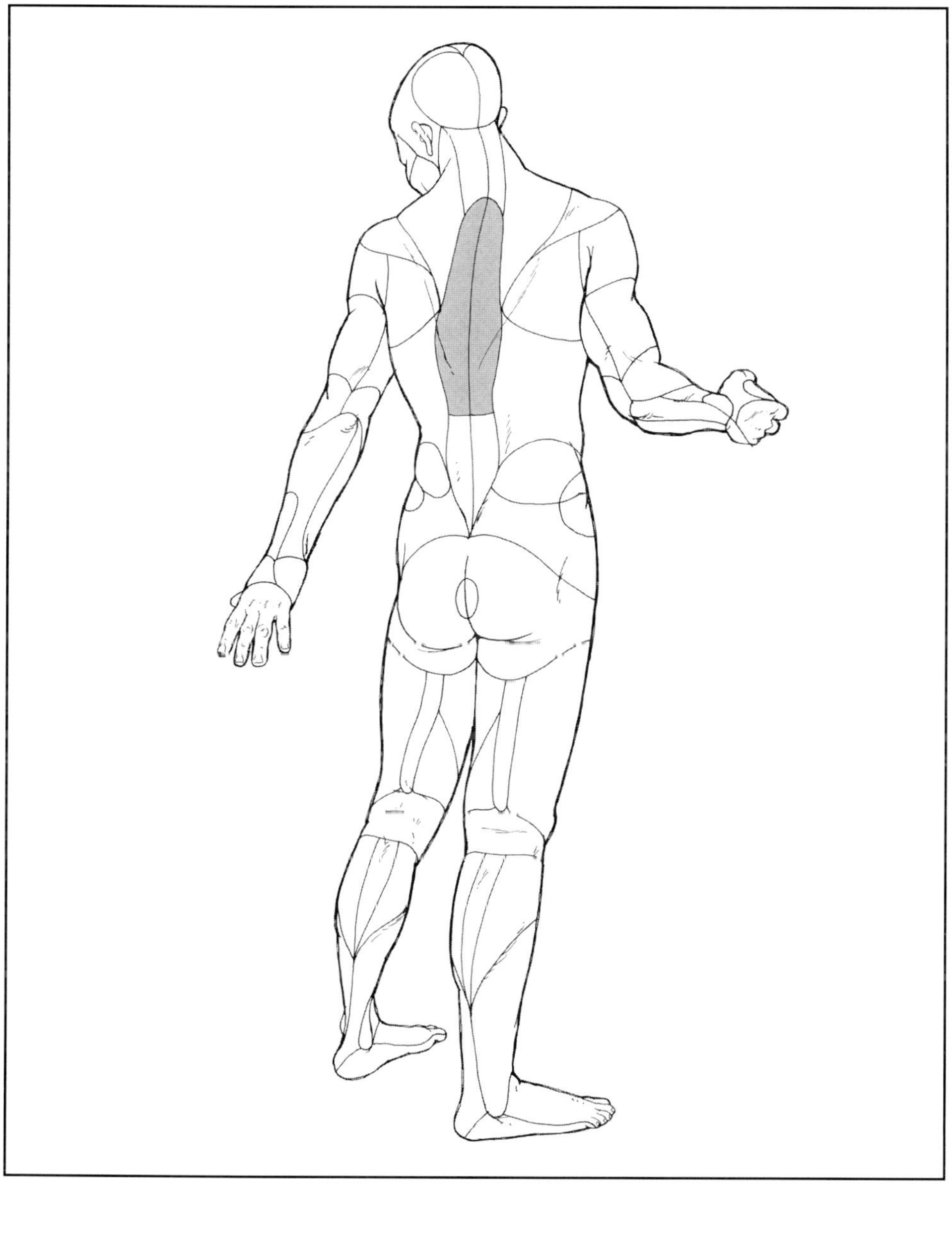

## General Principles and Complications

The selection of a surgical approach to the thoracic spine is dictated primarily by the location of the disease process. Access to the vertebral bodies, especially at more than one or two levels, requires an anterior transthoracic approach. The pedicles and transverse processes for two to three levels can be exposed through a posterolateral costotransversectomy. The posterior elements can be easily reached by a posterior midline approach. A thoracotomy can create significant morbidity for the patient such as major fluid shifts, atelectasis, pulmonary edema, and pneumonia. The patient must have adequate cardiac and pulmonary reserves to tolerate this procedure. The thoracic spinal cord has a relatively sparse collateral blood supply. Therefore, extensive dissection in this area increases the risk of anterior cord syndrome or paraplegia. Prolonged problems such as persistent pneumothorax, chylothorax, or esophageal fistula are also possible (1).

## Surgical Anatomy

The thoracic inlet severely narrows the space above the third rib, making approaches to the vertebrae in this area impossible from inside the chest. The approach through the cervicothoracic junction to the first two thoracic vertebrae has been previously described. The third through last thoracic vertebrae can be reached with ease through the thoracic approach. If the lower thoracic and upper two lumbar vertebrae must be accessed together, then a combined thoracoabdominal approach will be necessary.

The posterior thorax is shrouded by the trapezius and latissimus dorsi muscles. The first five ribs are also covered by the scapula. The approach to the upper chest at this level requires detachment of the rhomboid muscles from the medial edge of the scapula. The aortic arch is tightly adherent to the fourth thoracic vertebra, then it descends along the left side of the vertebral column. Above the aortic arch, the esophagus, the thoracic duct, and the subclavian artery lie intimately adjacent to the anterior aspect of the vertebral bodies (II-1). In the lower thorax, the azygos vein and thoracic duct run along the right side of the vertebral bodies. The sympathetic trunks run along the lateral vertebral bodies throughout the thorax. On the right side, the liver fills the space below the diaphragm, making exposure of the lower thoracic vertebrae difficult. The diaphragm originates from the cartilaginous segment of the lower six ribs and the xiphoid. Posteriorly, the diaphragm projects onto the upper two lumbar vertebrae through the crura. The diaphragm bridges the psoas and quadratus lumborum muscles through the medial and lateral arcuate ligaments (II-2). The arcuate ligaments attach to the tips of the transverse processes of the first lumbar vertebra and onto the tips of the twelfth ribs.

The segmental arteries leave the aorta and run laterally along the body of each thoracic vertebra. Just lateral to the vertebral body, the arteries bifurcate into the dorsal ramus and intercostal artery. The dorsal ramus passes medial to the superior costotransverse ligament to ascend into the erector spinae muscles. The intercostal nerve, artery, and vein run anterior to the costotransverse ligament to reach the inferior margin of the rib (II-3). The costotransverse ligament anchors the ribs to the vertebrae. The *posterior* and *superior* costotransverse ligaments extend from the inferior aspect of one transverse process to the inferior aspect of the underlying rib.

The capsular ligament secures the rib to the facet on the ventral surface of the transverse process. The *lateral* costotransverse ligament extends from the tip of the transverse process to the posterior tubercle of the same rib. The pedicle of the thoracic vertebra lies directly ventral to the base of the transverse process (II-4).

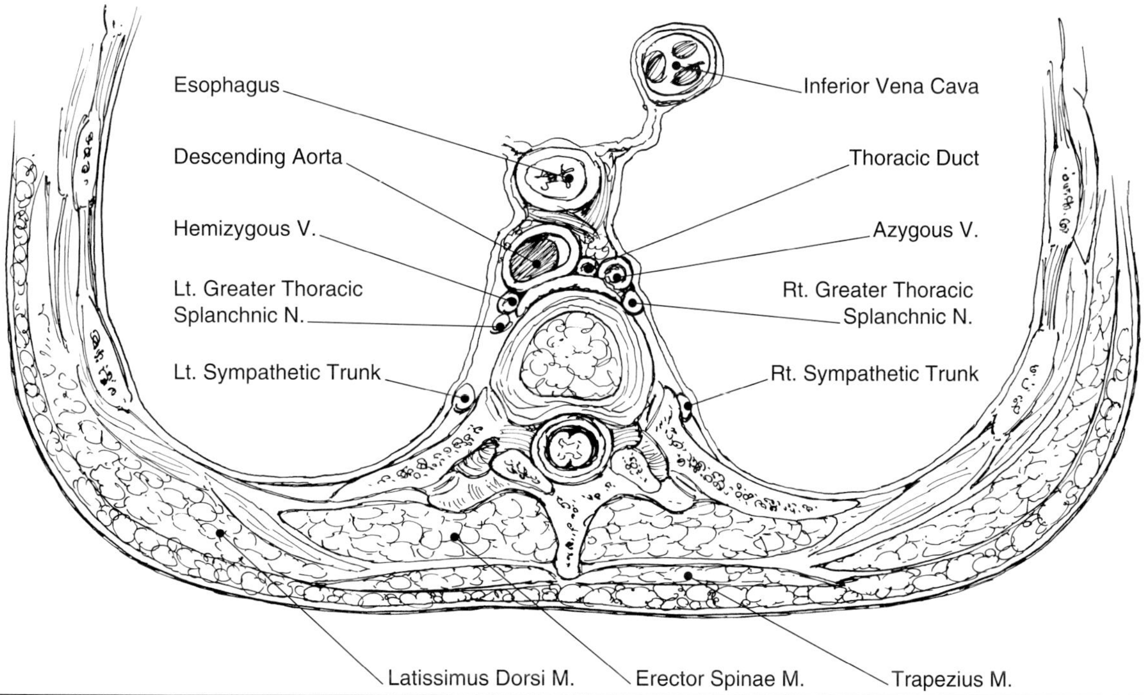


**FIGURE II–1**

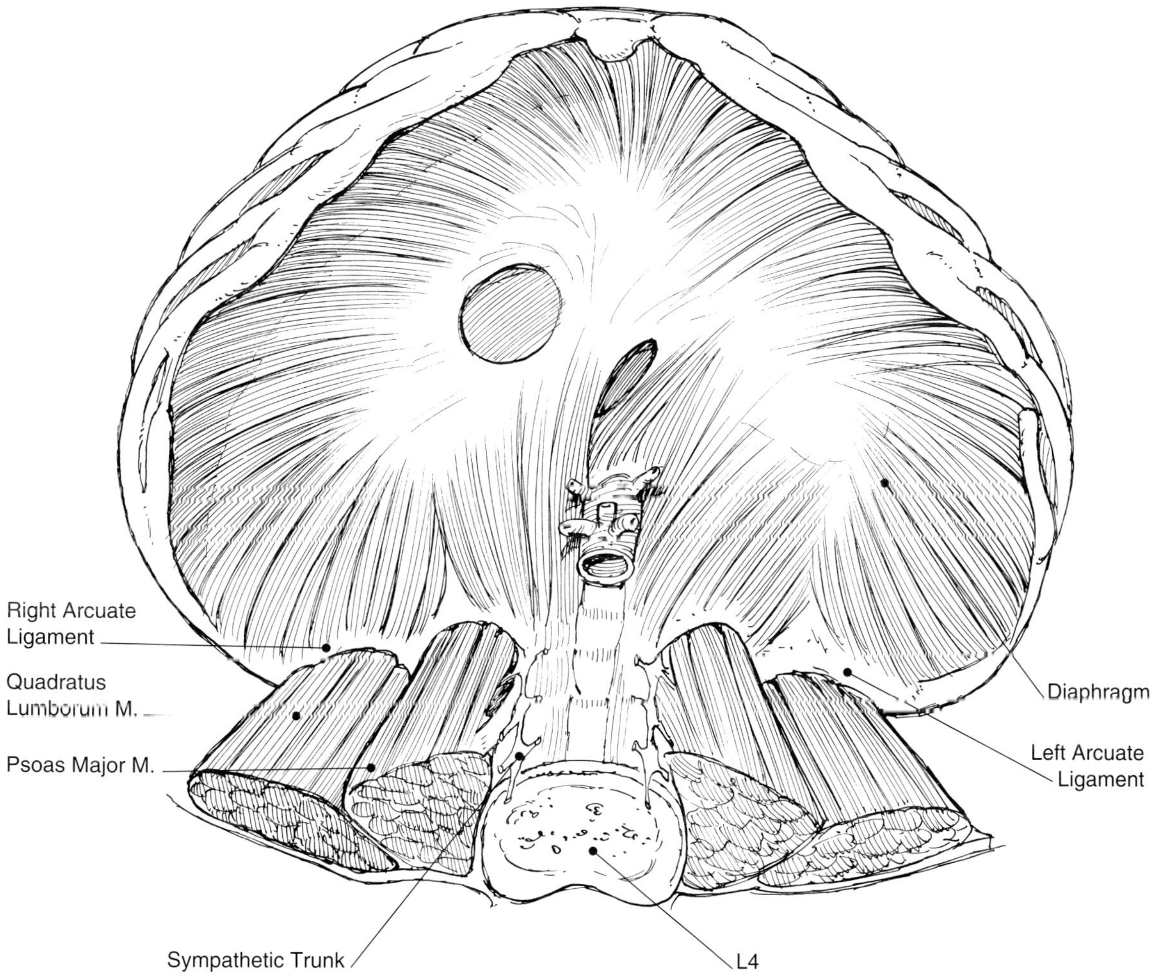


**FIGURE II–2**

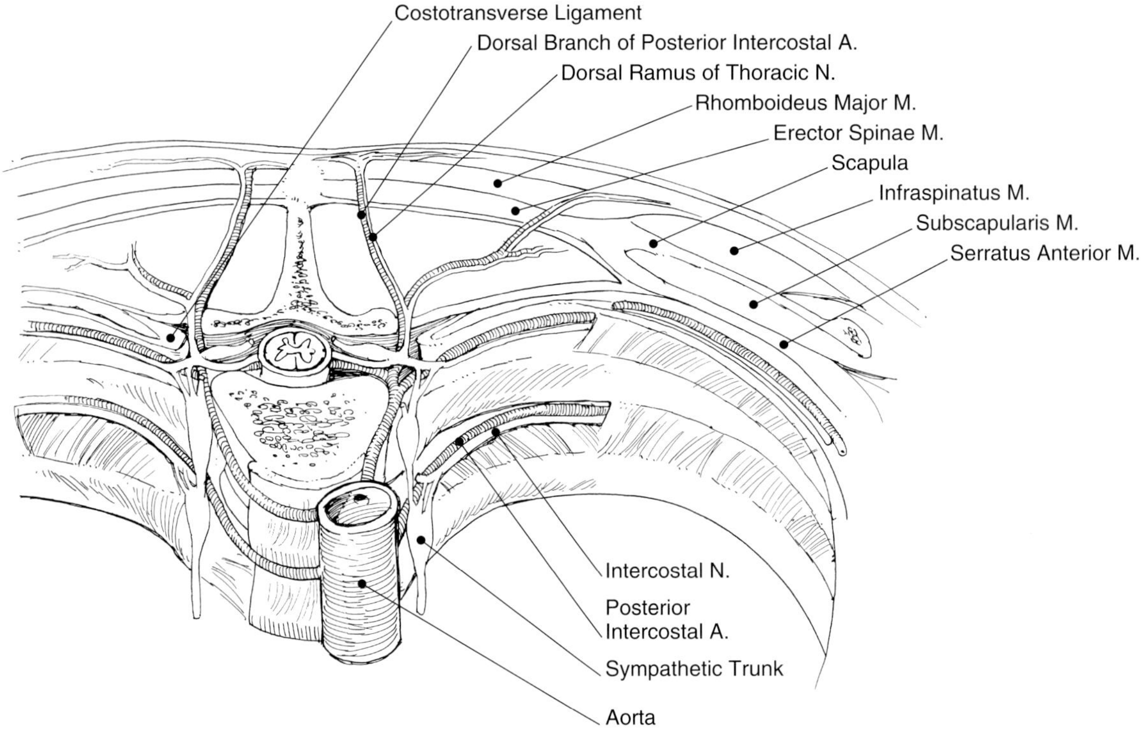


**FIGURE II–3**

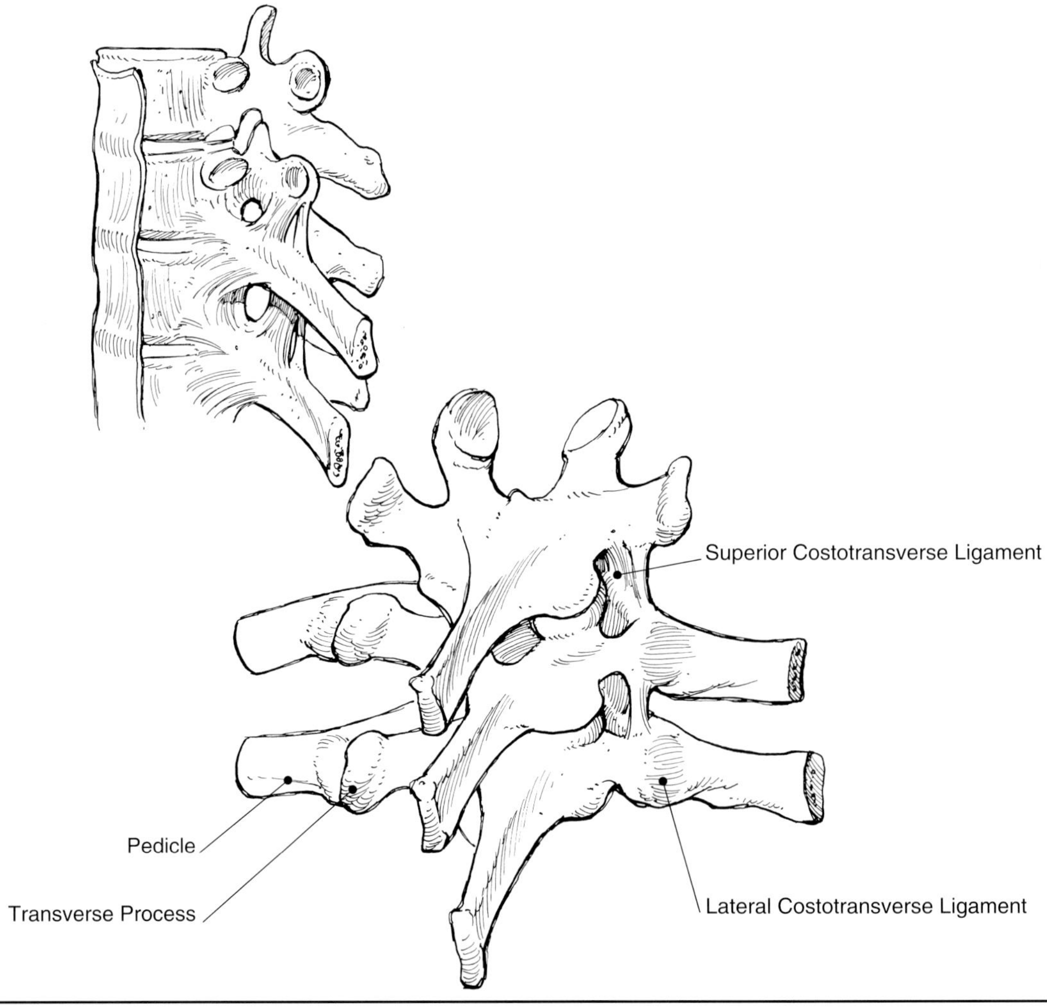


**FIGURE II–4**

# Anterior Transthoracic Approach to the Thoracic Spine

***Applications***

The left posterolateral thoracotomy provides access to the third through twelfth thoracic vertebrae. This approach may be used for anterior release of fixed kyphotic deformities, spinal instrumentation and fusion for scoliosis (especially if the posterior elements are deficient as in myelomeningocele), debridement of vertebral osteomyelitis or a disk space infection, or removal of a tumor of the vertebral body.

***Technique***

The patient is placed in the right lateral decubitus position. The left arm is suspended overhead and an axillary roll is placed on the right. Adequate exposure can be achieved only by resecting one rib. The rib to be resected is usually the one that articulates with the vertebral body to be exposed or the one immediately caudal to it. An arcuate incision is made over the rib to be resected from the anterior axillary line to the lateral border of the paraspinal muscles (II-5A). The latissimus

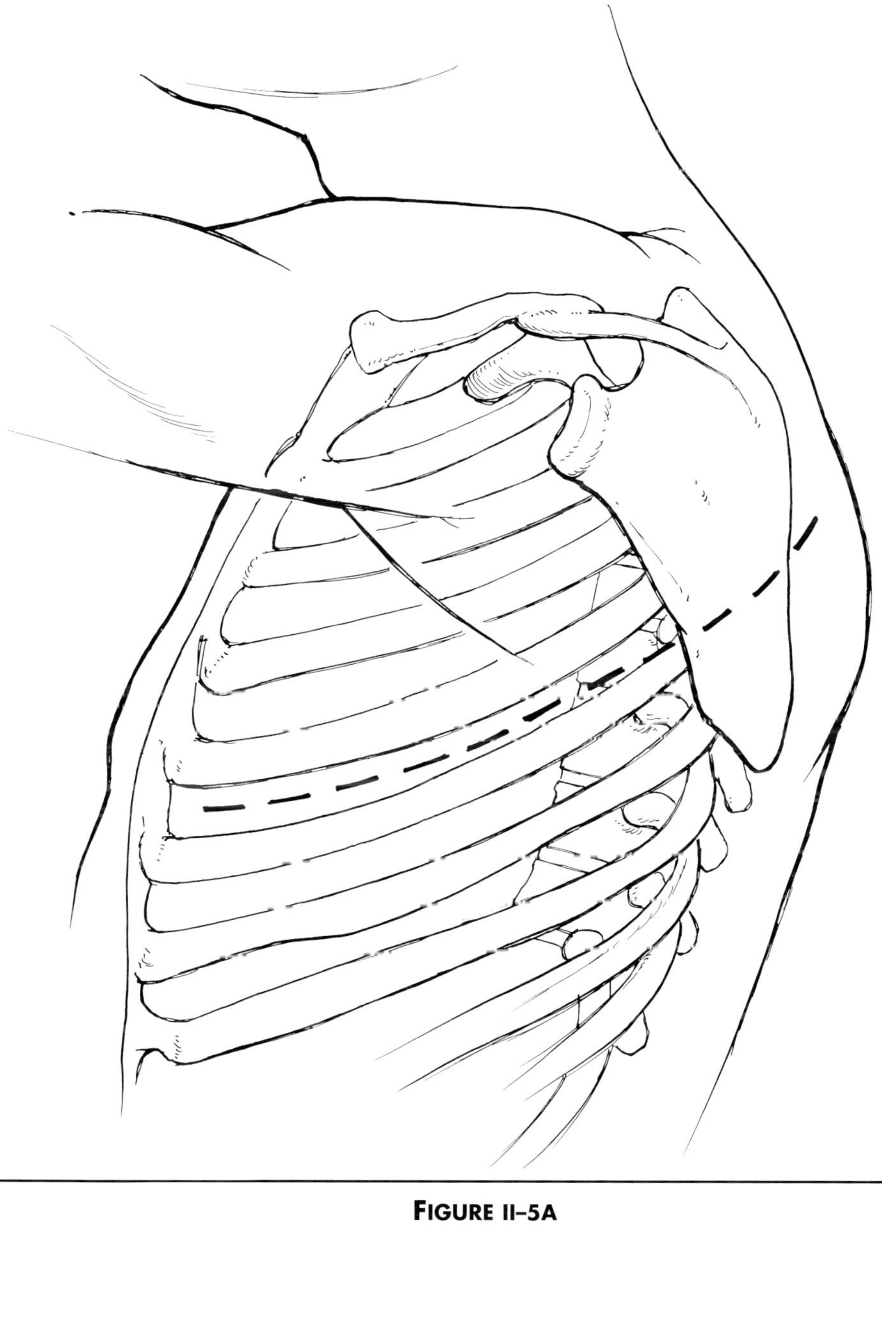

**FIGURE II–5A**

dorsi is mobilized by blunt dissection and transected in line with the incision. The serratus anterior is then elevated from the chest wall to expose the ribs. The lateral margin of the trapezius is identified and transected as needed to fully expose the rib. If the third, fourth, or fifth rib is to be excised, the rhomboid major and minor may be detached from the medial edge of the scapula to allow elevation of the scapula from the chest wall. The appropriate rib level should be confirmed by radiographic control. The periosteum over the rib is then incised (II-5B). The rib is mobilized by careful subperiosteal dissection to avoid an intercostal vessel injury. The rib should be resected from the costochondral junction to its posterior angle (II-6). The endothoracic fascia and parietal pleura are then opened with scissors. The ribs are spread with a self-retaining retractor, and the lung is deflated and

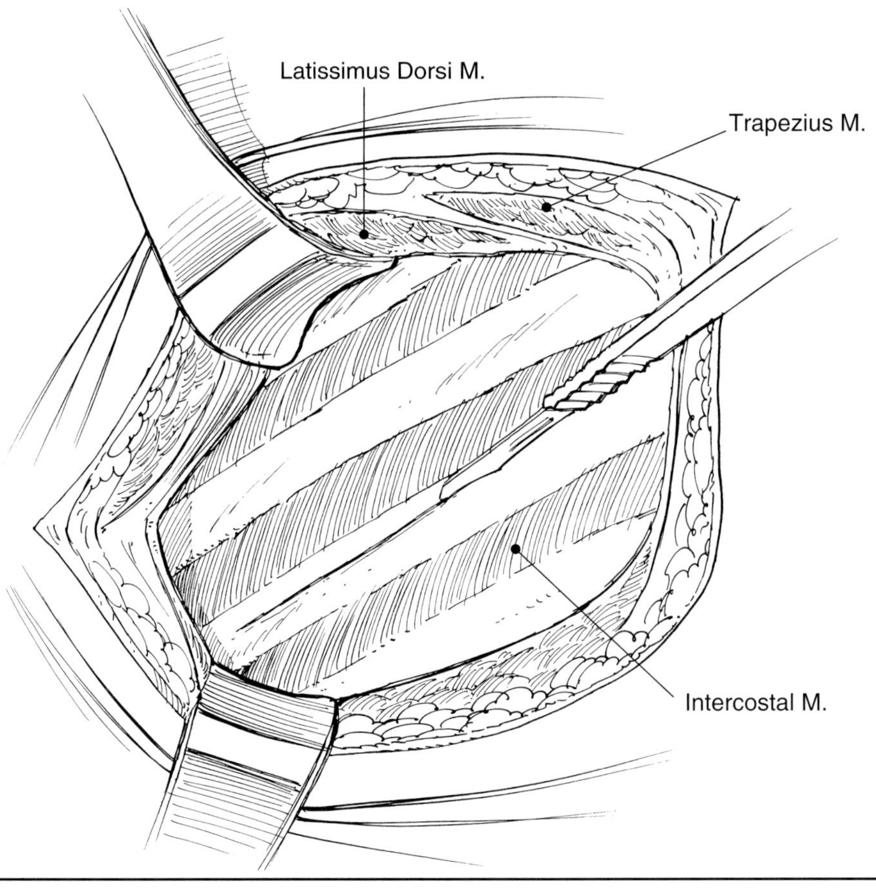


**FIGURE II–5B**

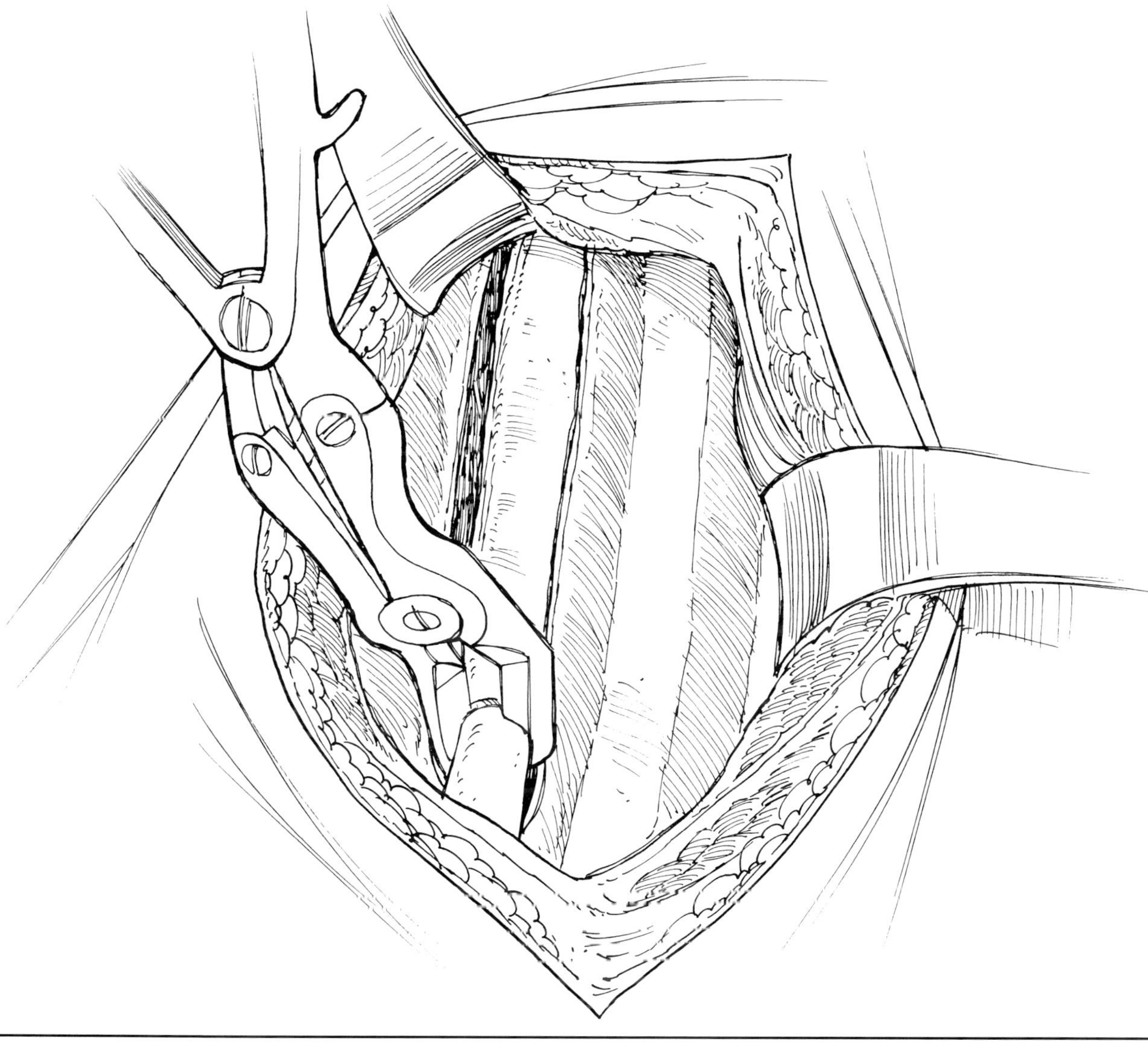

**FIGURE II–6**

retracted anteriorly (II-7A). The parietal pleura is cleared from the vertebral bodies by blunt dissection, sparing the intercostal vessels and the sympathetic trunk. If necessary, the intercostal vessels may be ligated and transected (II-7B).

For closure, two chest tubes should be placed, one above the incision into the upper chest, and the second below the incision into the posterior angle of the diaphragm. The chest wall must be closed airtight, and the transected latissimus dorsi, trapezius, rhomboids, and serratus anterior should each be repaired.

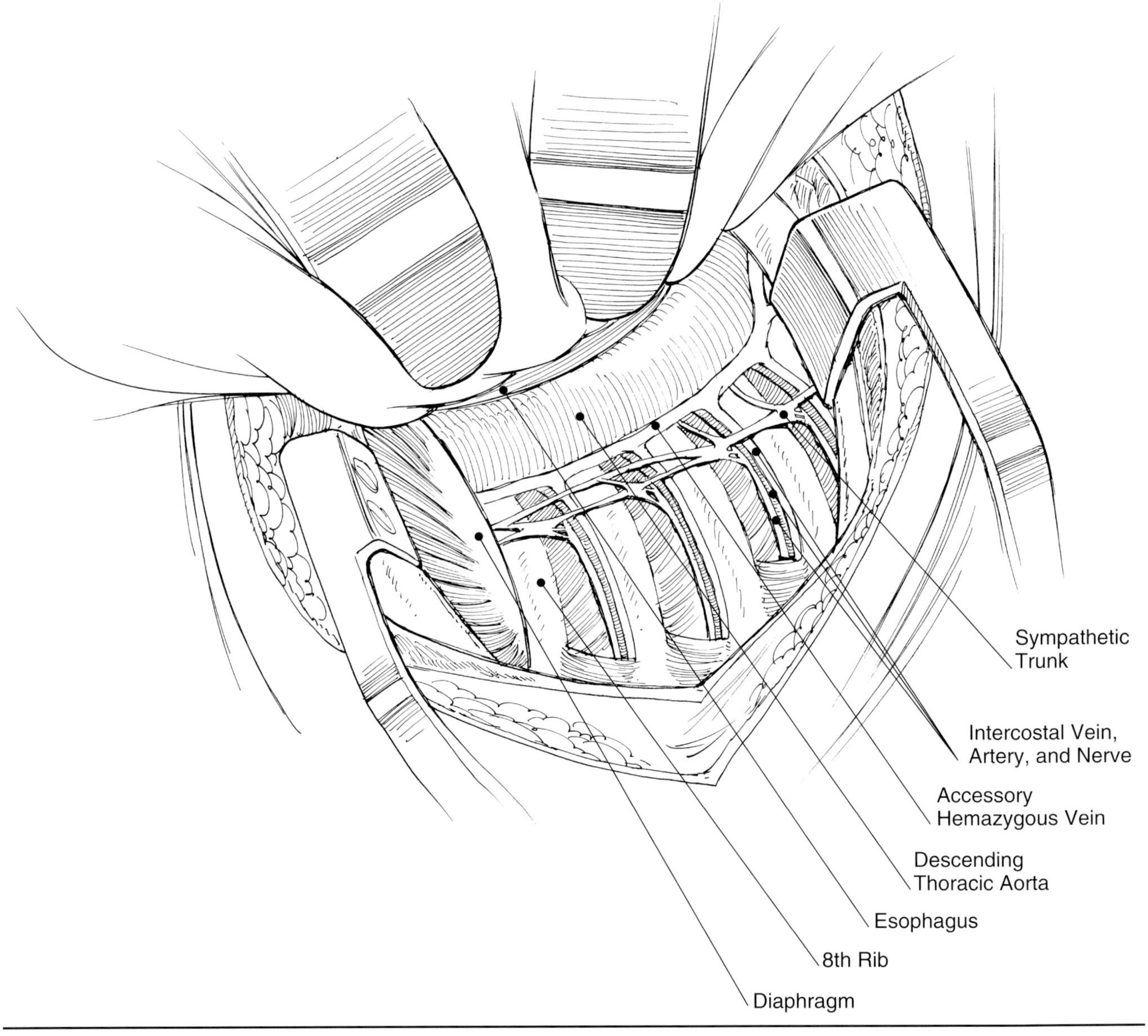


**FIGURE II–7A**

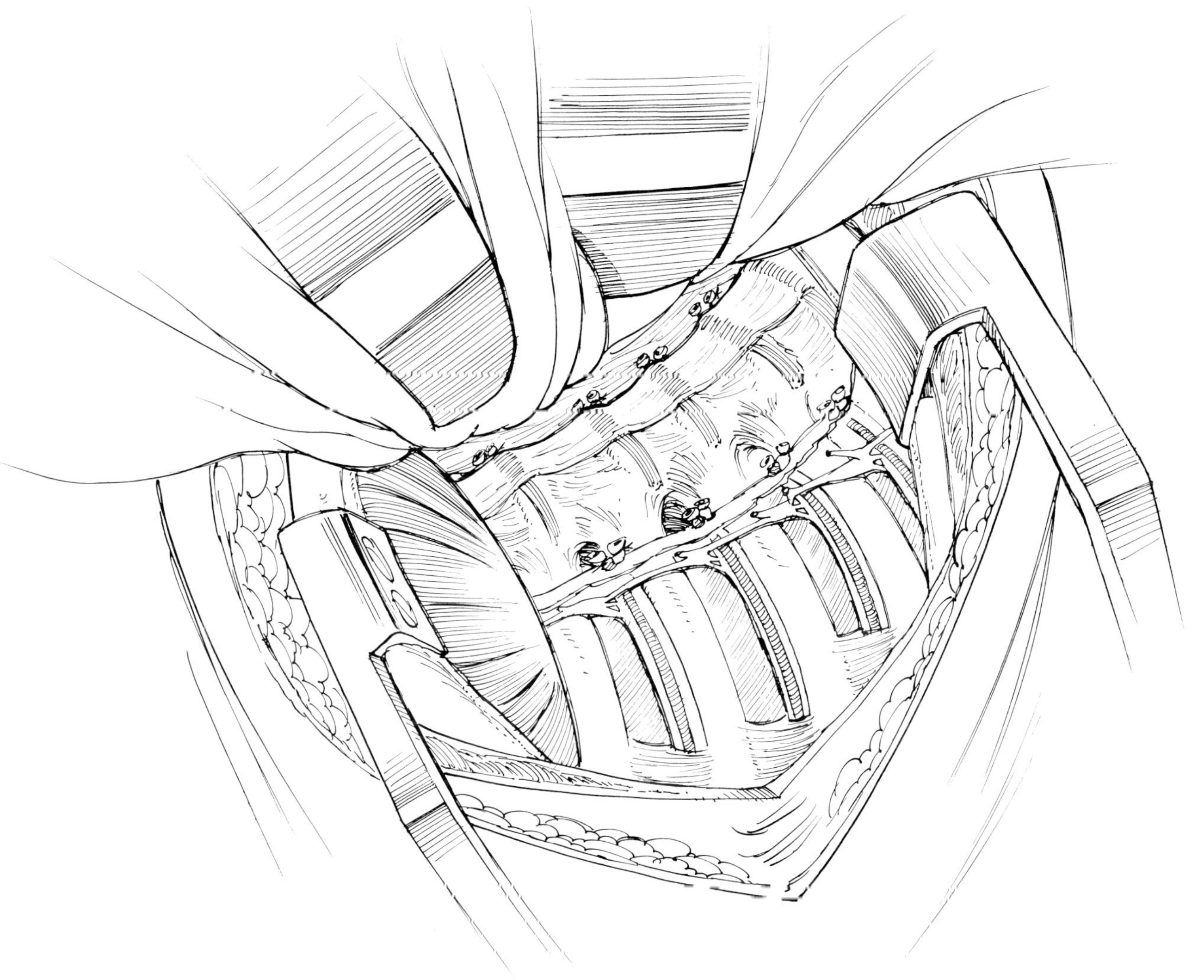

**FIGURE II–7B**

***Dangers***

The hazards of thoracotomy have been previously outlined. The thoracic vertebrae are relatively small and damage to the spinal cord or nerve roots is possible when dissecting in this limited area. Substantial bleeding can be encountered when dissecting into the vertebral bodies, especially when treating metastatic carcinoma. Spinal cord ischemia caused by segmental vessel ligation can result in paraplegia or anterior cord syndrome.

***Limitations***

The upper two thoracic vertebrae cannot be reached safely by a transthoracic approach. The crus of the diaphragm prevents wide exposure of the vertebrae below the twelfth thoracic.

## Thoracoabdominal Approach to the Thoracolumbar Junction

***Applications***

This approach is most likely to be used for anterior release and fusion of severe thoracolumbar scoliosis, tumors of the vertebral bodies of the twelfth thoracic or first lumbar vertebra, or unstable fractures at the thoracolumbar junction. It is necessary only if wide exposure is needed to at least three vertebral levels at the thoracolumbar junction (2).

***Technique***

The patient is placed in the right lateral decubitus position. The use of a kidney rest and flexion of the table at the level of the lower chest may be helpful. A posterolateral incision is made parallel to the level of planned rib resection. This can vary from the seventh to the eleventh rib, depending on the level of the vertebra to be exposed. The incision extends from the lateral edge of the paraspinal muscles to the anterior edge of the rib cage (II-8). The latissimus dorsi and serratus anterior muscles are divided. A rib may be removed or the intercostal muscles may be divided. The ribs are spread with a self-retaining rib retractor. The lung is deflated and retracted anteriorly. An incision is then made along the circumference of the muscular portion of the diaphragm and carried posteriorly to the lateral arcuate ligament (II-9). The peritoneum is usually entered to expose the contents of the left upper quadrant of the abdomen (II-10). The parietal peritoneum is then bluntly mobilized behind the spleen to open the retroperitoneal space. The dissection is carried bluntly posterior to the renal fascia. The spleen and kidney are retracted medially, and the dissection is expanded to expose the aorta and vertebral bodies (II-11). The left crus of the diaphragm is reflected off the anterior longitudinal ligament to expose the upper lumbar vertebral bodies (II-12). The attachment of the arcuate ligament to the transverse process of the first lumbar vertebra is detached, and the original diaphragm incision is carried down through the lateral arcuate ligament (II-13). The anterior longitudinal ligament can then be elevated from the vertebrae as needed.

On closure, the peritoneum is repaired. The crus of the diaphragm is repaired to the anterior longitudinal ligament to tightly close the aortic hiatus. The arcuate ligament is repaired, and the diaphragm is closed in layers. Chest tubes are inserted and the chest wall is tightly repaired. The serratus anterior and latissimus dorsi muscles are individually repaired.

***Dangers***

This approach carries with it all of the morbidity and risks associated with a thoracotomy. In addition, it has the morbidity of a wide retroperitoneal dissection. Major problems with fluid shifts, ileus, atelectasis, and respiratory dysfunction can be expected. The dangers of operating around the thoracic spinal cord and aorta have been previously outlined. Finally, injury to the spleen, kidney, or ureters is possible.

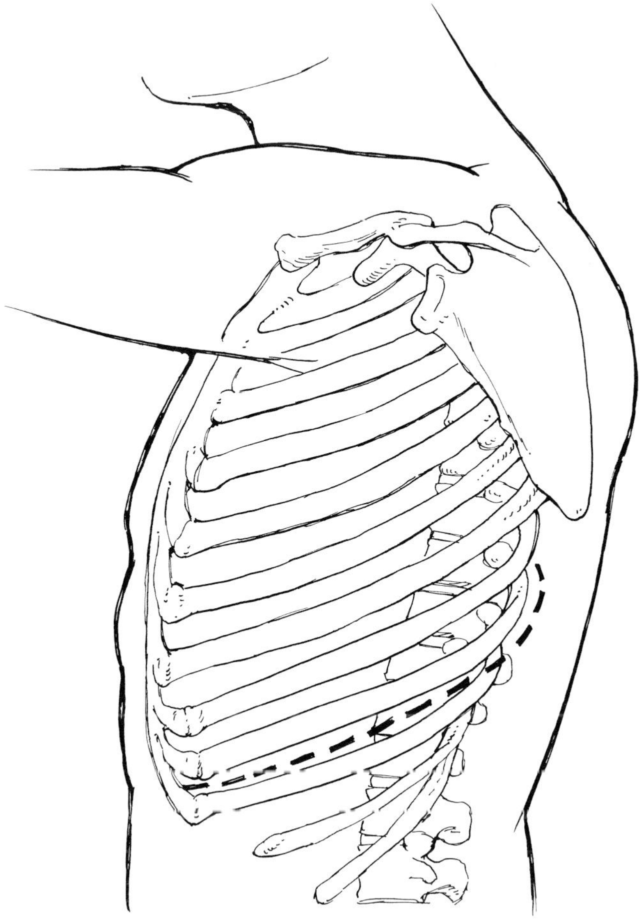

**FIGURE II–8**

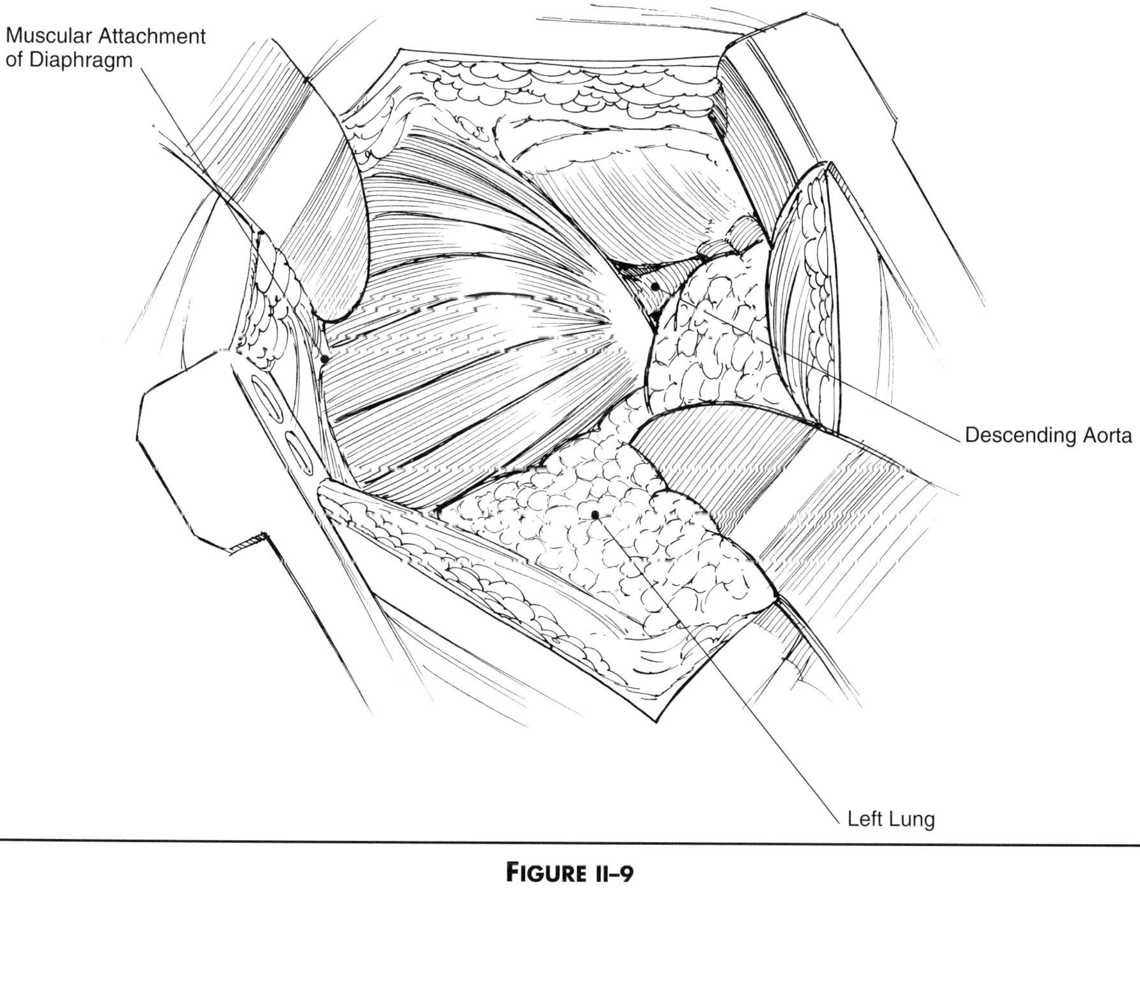


**FIGURE II–9**

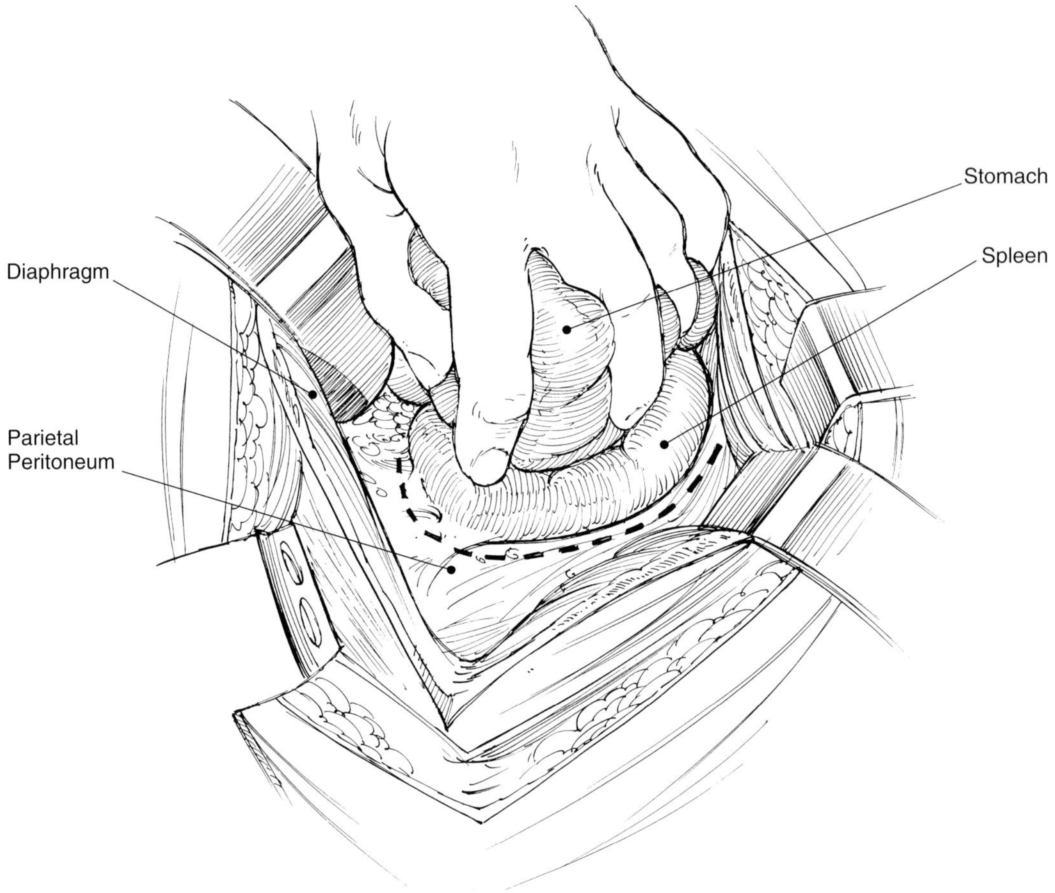


**FIGURE II–10**

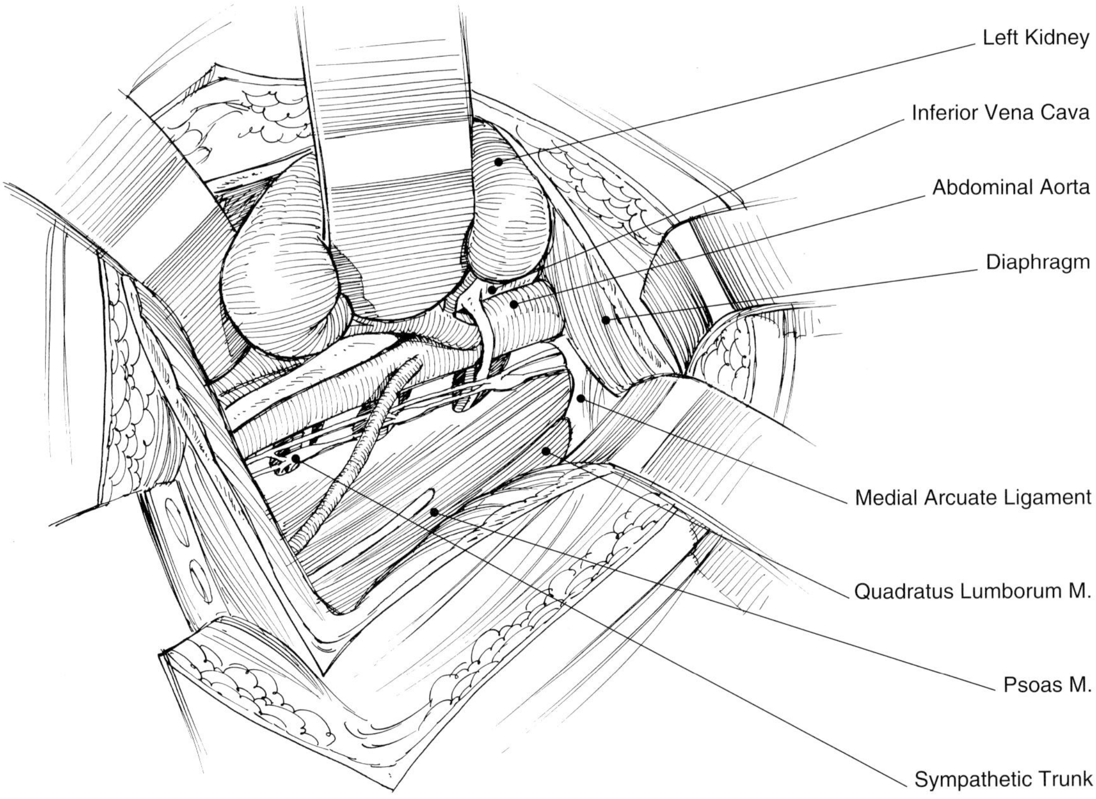


**FIGURE II–11**

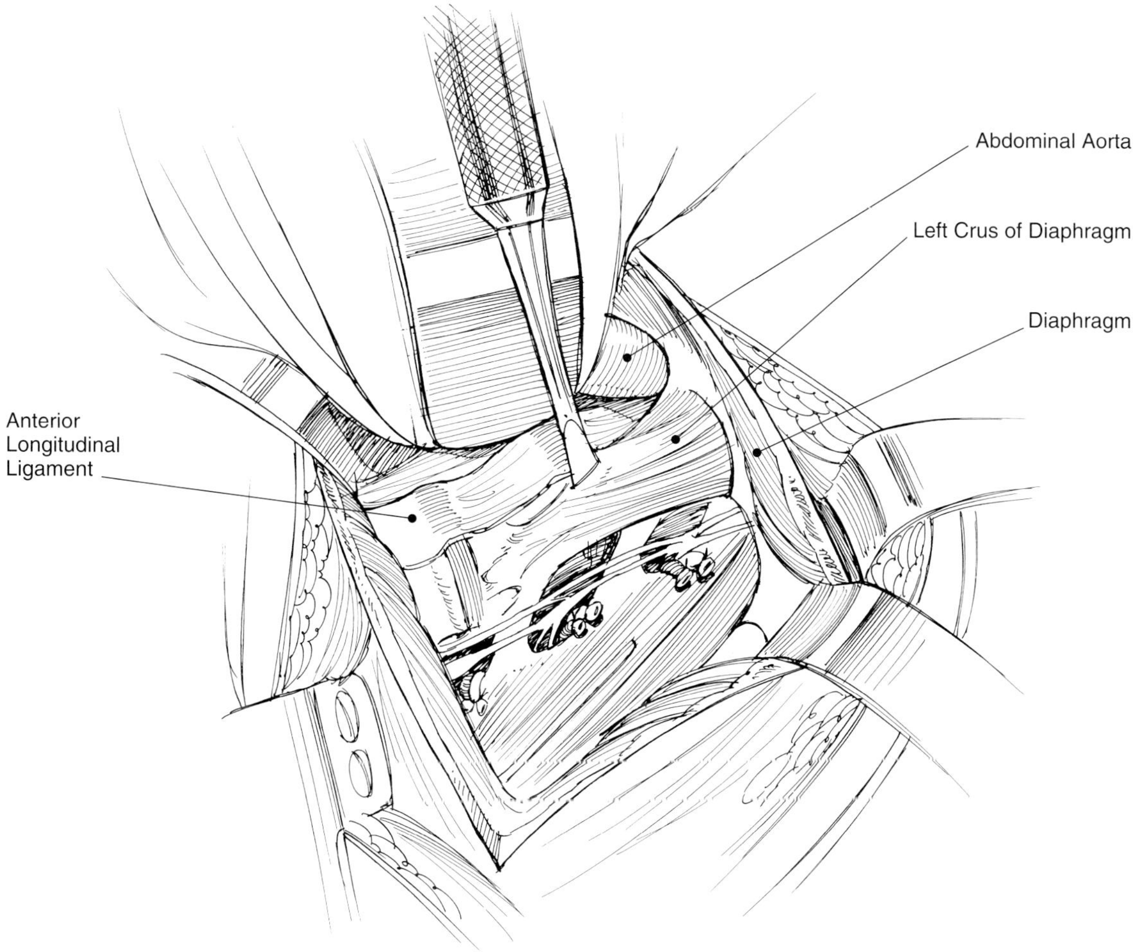


**FIGURE II–12**

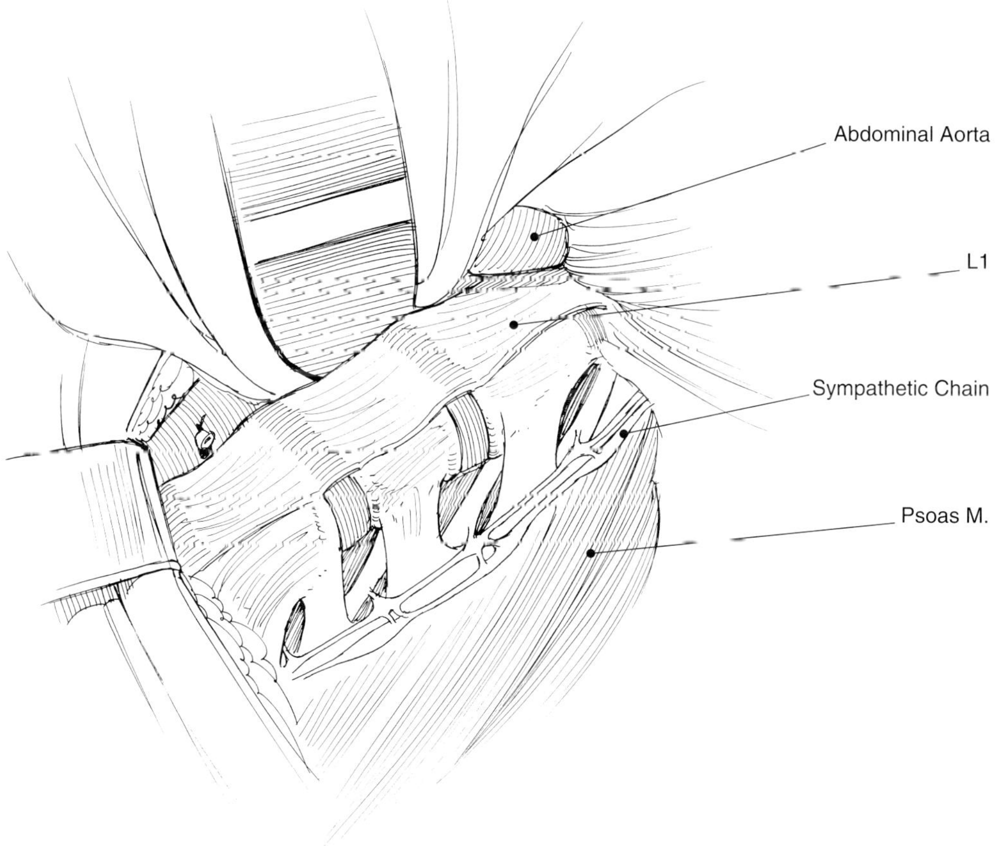


**FIGURE II–13**

*Limitations*

This approach provides wide exposure to the thoracolumbar junction; however, because of the morbidity associated with this procedure, it should be restricted to relatively healthy patients and used only when access to three or more vertebral levels at the thoracolumbar junction is needed.

## Posterolateral Costotransversectomy Approach to the Thoracic Spine

*Applications*

This approach provides access to the dorsal aspect of the vertebral bodies and pedicles without entering the pleural cavity. It is ideal for biopsy of the vertebral bodies or for drainage of an abscess or infected disk space, especially in a debilitated patient who cannot tolerate a thoracotomy. This approach was classically described for drainage of tubercular abscesses (3).

*Technique*

The patient is placed in either a lateral or prone position. A longitudinal incision is made, centered over the desired level, approximately 5 cm lateral to the spinous process and just medial to the palpable prominence of the posterior angle of the rib (II-14). The trapezius and latissimus dorsi are divided longitudinally. The paraspinal muscles are elevated from the ribs and transverse processes and retracted medially. The proper spinal level should be confirmed by radiograph. The costo-

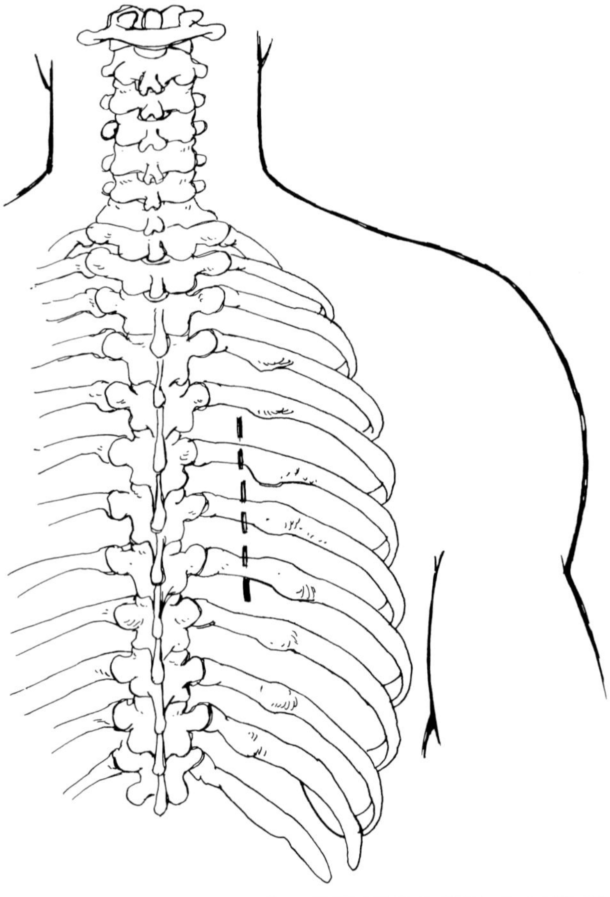

**FIGURE II–14**

transverse ligaments are transected sharply, and the transverse process is transected at its base, adjacent to the pedicle (II-15). The periosteum of the rib is incised from the tip of the transverse process to the angle of the rib. The medial segment of rib is then mobilized subperiosteally. The rib is then transected at the angle and the segment is removed. The pedicle, adjacent intercostal nerve, and spinal foramen should be identified. A Cobb elevator can then be used to elevate the sympa-

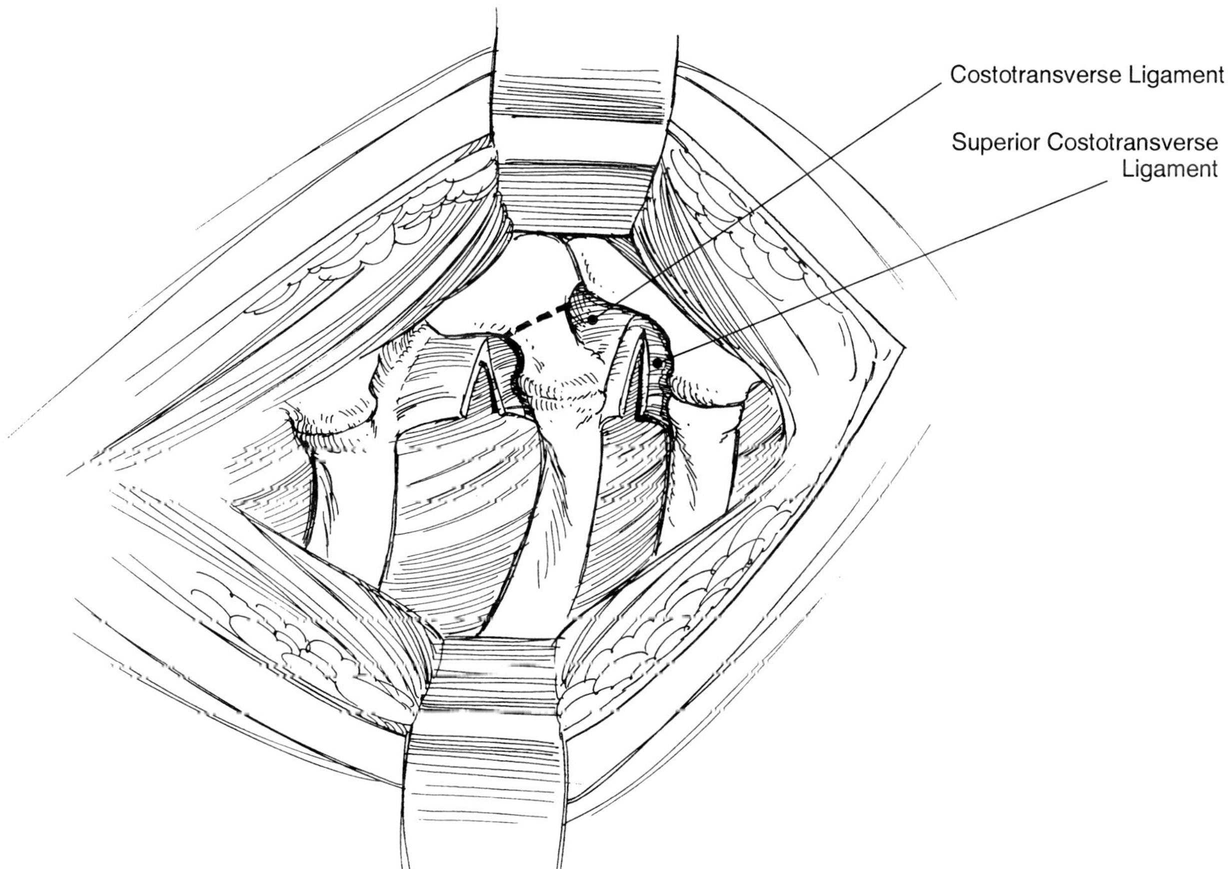


**FIGURE II-15**

thetic trunk and parietal pleura from the lateral vertebral body (II-16). The dissection can then be extended proximally and distally to expose the vertebral bodies and disk space. The parietal pleura can be mobilized by finger dissection from the side of the vertebral body. This exposure may be carried out at three to four adjacent levels if necessary.

***Dangers*** The neural foramina are directly exposed. The dura can be torn, leading to a cerebrospinal fluid fistula. The wound must be carefully explored for signs of pneumothorax before closure.

***Limitations*** This approach does not allow complete exposure for a wide vertebrectomy. The maximal extent of exposure is three to four levels because a more extensive resection might create a flail chest segment.

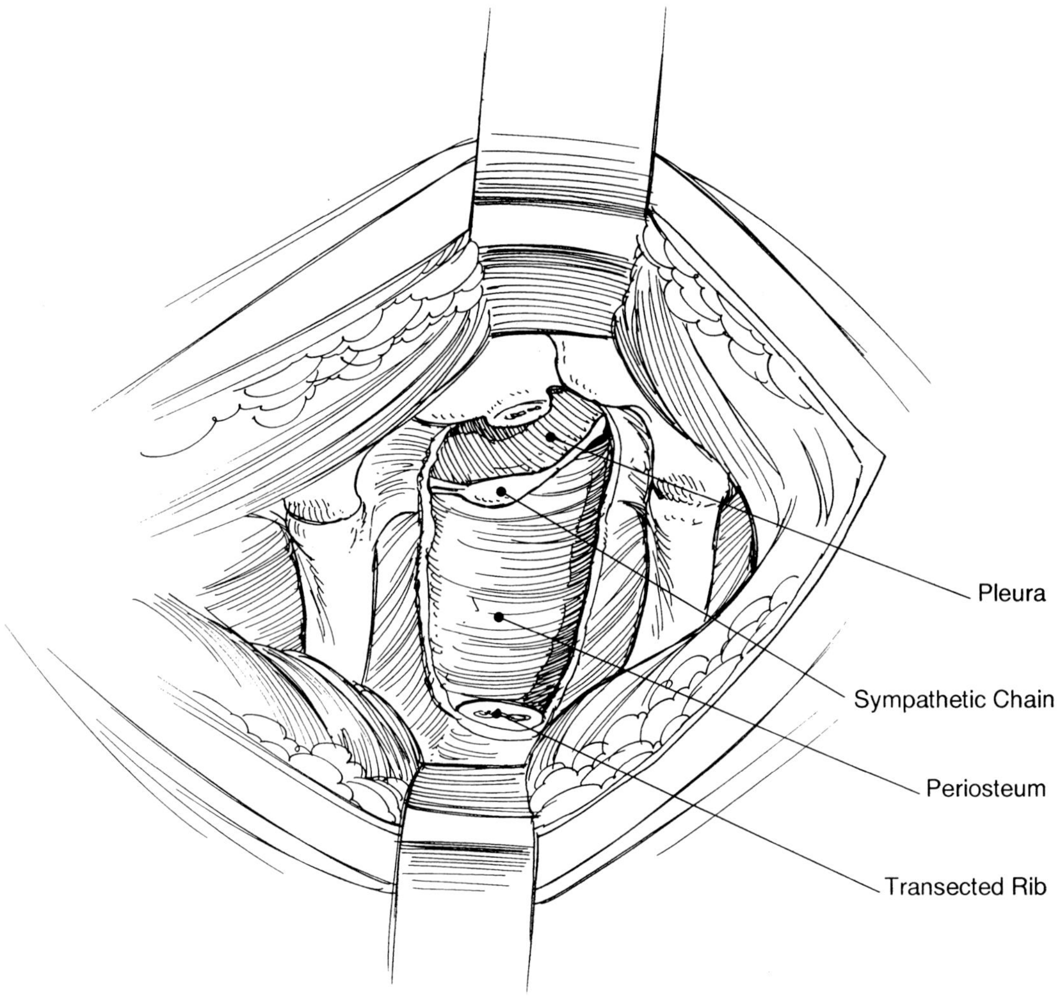


**FIGURE II-16**

# Midline Posterior Approach to the Thoracic Spine

### *Applications*

This is the most common approach to the thoracic spine and is used for spinal instrumentation for scoliosis, decompressive laminectomy, tumor resection, and fractures.

### *Technique*

The patient is placed prone and the level of the approach is confirmed by radiograph. A midline incision is made longitudinally and carried down to the tips of the spinous processes. The paraspinal muscles are then elevated subperiosteally to expose the laminae, ligamentum flavum, and transverse processes (II-17).

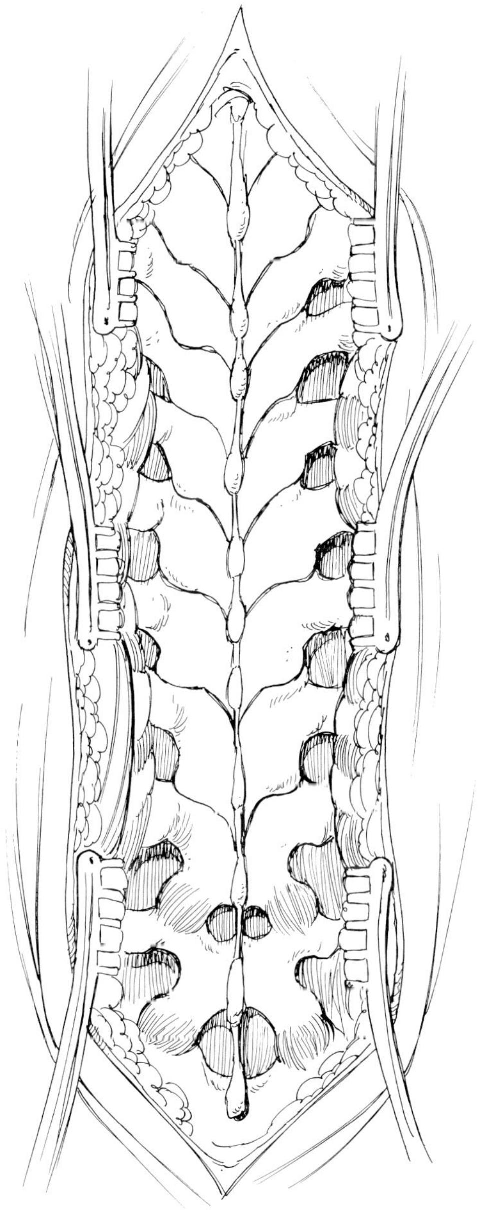

**FIGURE II–17**

*Dangers*

The dissection should not be carried laterally beyond the tips of the transverse processes. Careless dissection in this area may cause an incidental pneumothorax or disruption of an intercostal vessel which can produce vigorous bleeding.

*Limitations*

There is no longitudinal limitation to this approach. The spinal canal can only be reached by dorsal laminectomy through this approach. The vertebral body and disk can be reached through the canal, but only by retracting the spinal cord, which should be kept to a minimum to prevent ischemic injury.

## References

1. Johnson RM, Murphy MJ, Southwick WO. Surgical approaches to the spine. In: Rathman RH, Simeone FA, eds. The Spine, 3rd ed. Philadelphia: W.B. Saunders, 43:1696–1720, 1992.
2. Heitmiller RF. The left thoracoabdominal incision. Ann Thorac Surg 46:250–253, 1988.
3. Ménard V. Causes de la paraplégie dans le maladie de Pott, son traitment chirurgical por l'ouverture directe du foyer tuberculeux des vertébres. Rev Orthop 5:47–64, 1894.

# III

# SURGICAL APPROACHES TO THE LUMBAR SPINE

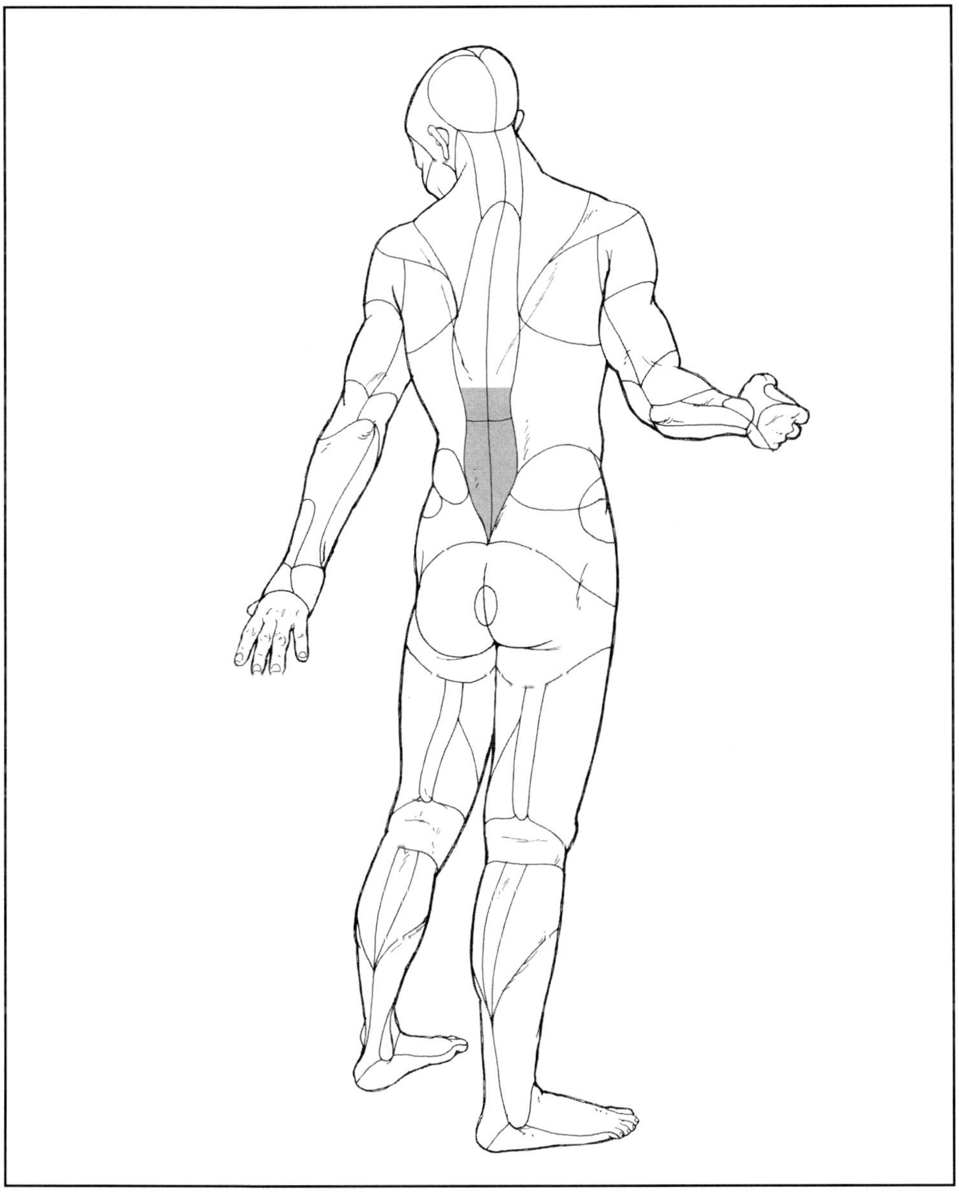

## General Principles and Complications

The lumbar spine can be readily exposed by an anterolateral or posterior approach. The anterolateral approach provides access to the vertebral bodies, pedicles, and paraspinal region. The posterior approach provides access to the lamina, facets, and transverse processes. By laminectomy, the spinal canal can be explored and the disk space can be debrided. Complications to these approaches are primarily due to inadvertent injury to nerve roots or adjacent structures, especially in the anterolateral approach (1).

## Surgical Anatomy

The left side is preferred for the anterolateral approach. The liver is on the right and is large and difficult to retract. The inferior vena cava is also on the right and is susceptible to injury that can lead to serious bleeding that can be difficult to control. The plane of approach to the anterior lumbar spine is external to the transversalis fascia. This fascia engulfs the descending colon, kidney, and ureter (III-1). As long as this fascia is intact, the visceral organs can be safely retracted without

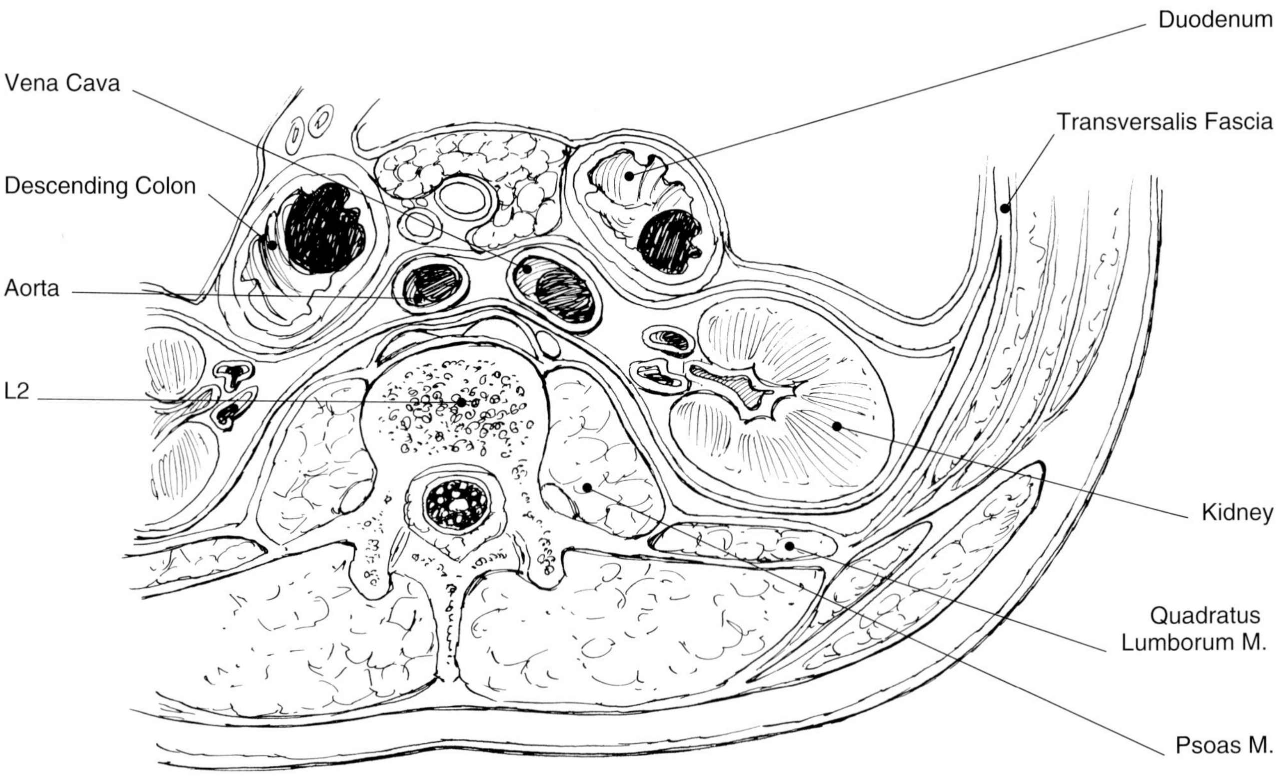


**FIGURE III–1**

exposure. The left crus of the diaphragm extends to the second lumbar vertebra and attaches to the anterior longitudinal ligament. The diaphragm bridges over the psoas and quadratus lumborum by the arcuate ligaments (III-2). The psoas fills most of the space adjacent to the lumbar vertebral bodies and is intimately related to branches of the lumbosacral plexus. The genitofemoral nerve lies on the ventral surface of the psoas belly. The nerve roots giving rise to the femoral nerve are found in the substance of the muscle with the nerve running along its lateral edge

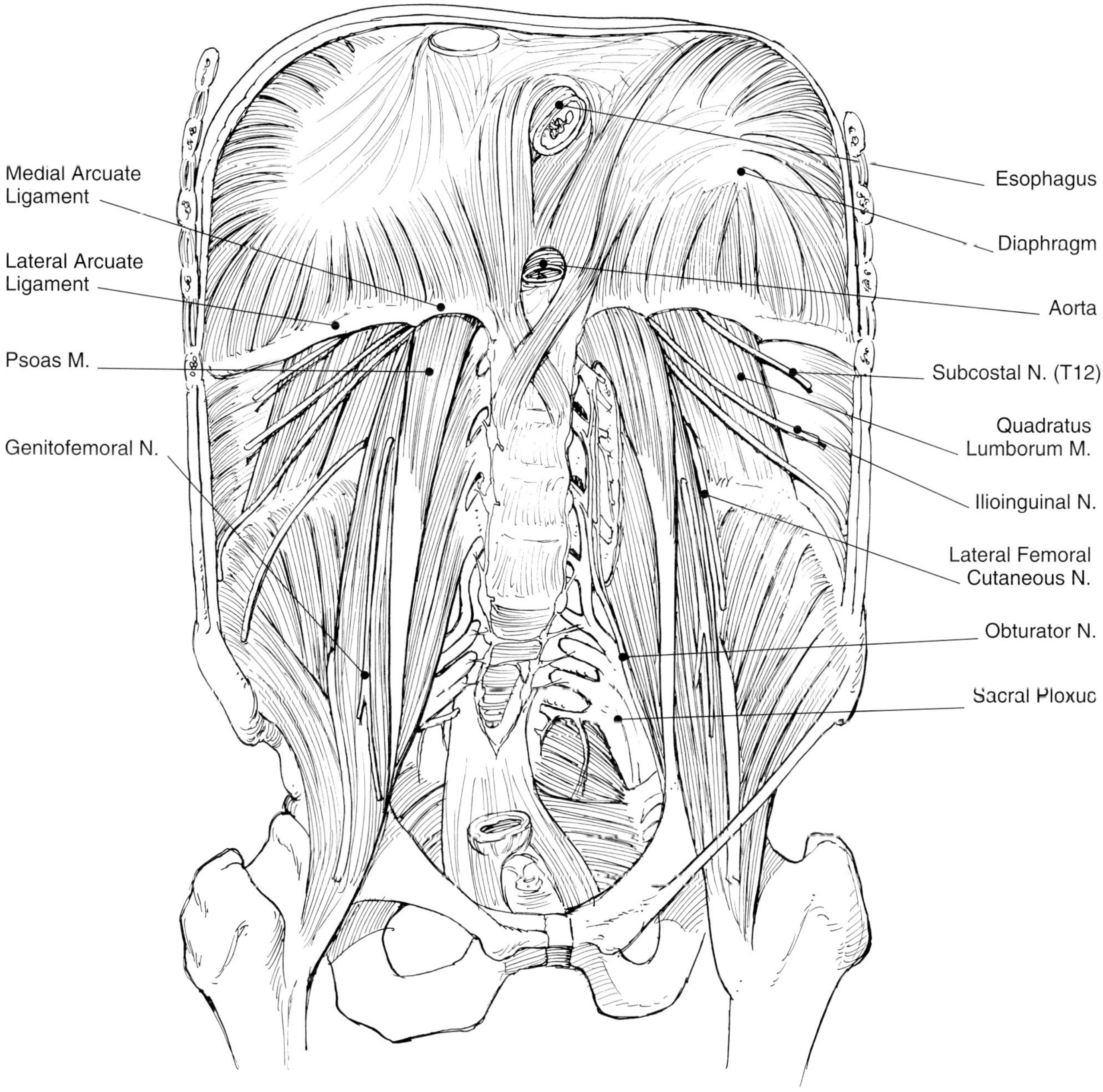


**FIGURE III–2**

in the lower lumbar region. The obturator nerve will be found along the medial edge of the psoas. The lateral femoral cutaneous nerve will exit the upper edge of the psoas and can be seen passing into the pelvis. Segmental vessels pass around each vertebral body intimately over the periosteum (III-3). The aorta and inferior vena cava bifurcate over the fourth lumbar vertebra. Therefore, the common iliac artery and vein will be encountered in an attempt to reach the fifth lumbar vertebra.

## Anterolateral Approach to the Lumbar Spine

***Technique***

A preoperative bowel prep is recommended to decompress the colon. The patient is placed at a 60° incline to the right, supported by bolsters under the hip and shoulder. The table is flexed at the thoracolumbar junction. The incision begins at

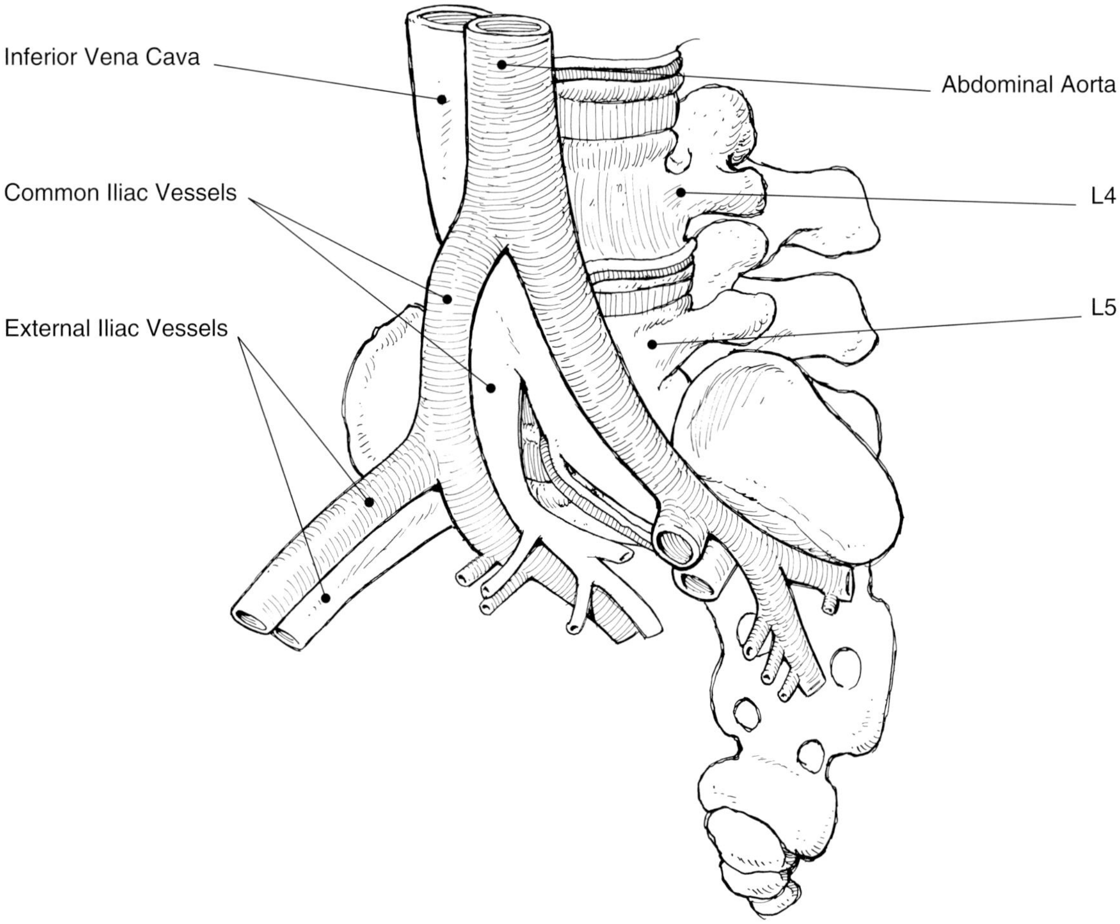


**FIGURE III–3**

the lateral edge of the paraspinal muscles and follows the twelfth rib anteriorly. It then follows an arc above the iliac crest to a point midway between the pubic symphysis and umbilicus. The incision is carried anteriorly to the lateral edge of the rectus abdominous sheath (III-4). The twelfth rib is excised subperiosteally. The external abdominal oblique muscle fibers are split parallel to the incision. The

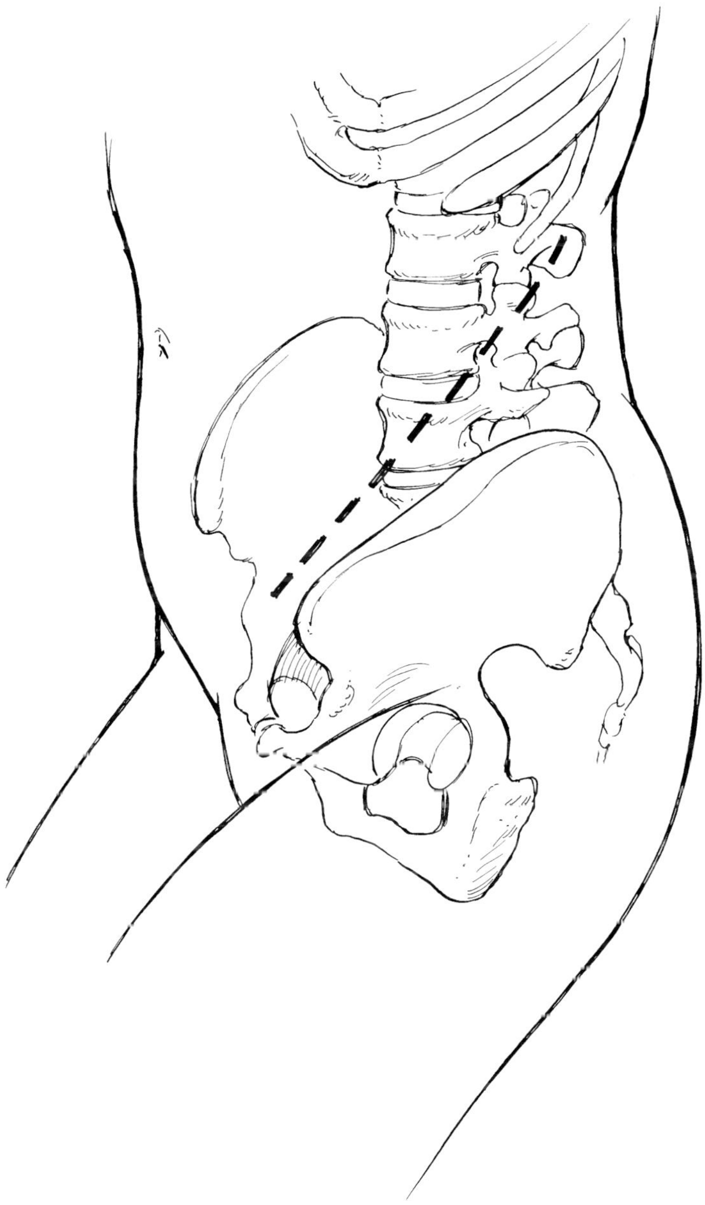

**FIGURE III–4**

internal abdominal oblique and transverse abdominal muscles are elevated by finger dissection and transected in line with the skin incision (III-5). The parietal peritoneum is encountered deep to the transverse abdominals. It is followed posteriorly in the fascia overlying the quadratus lumborum and psoas.

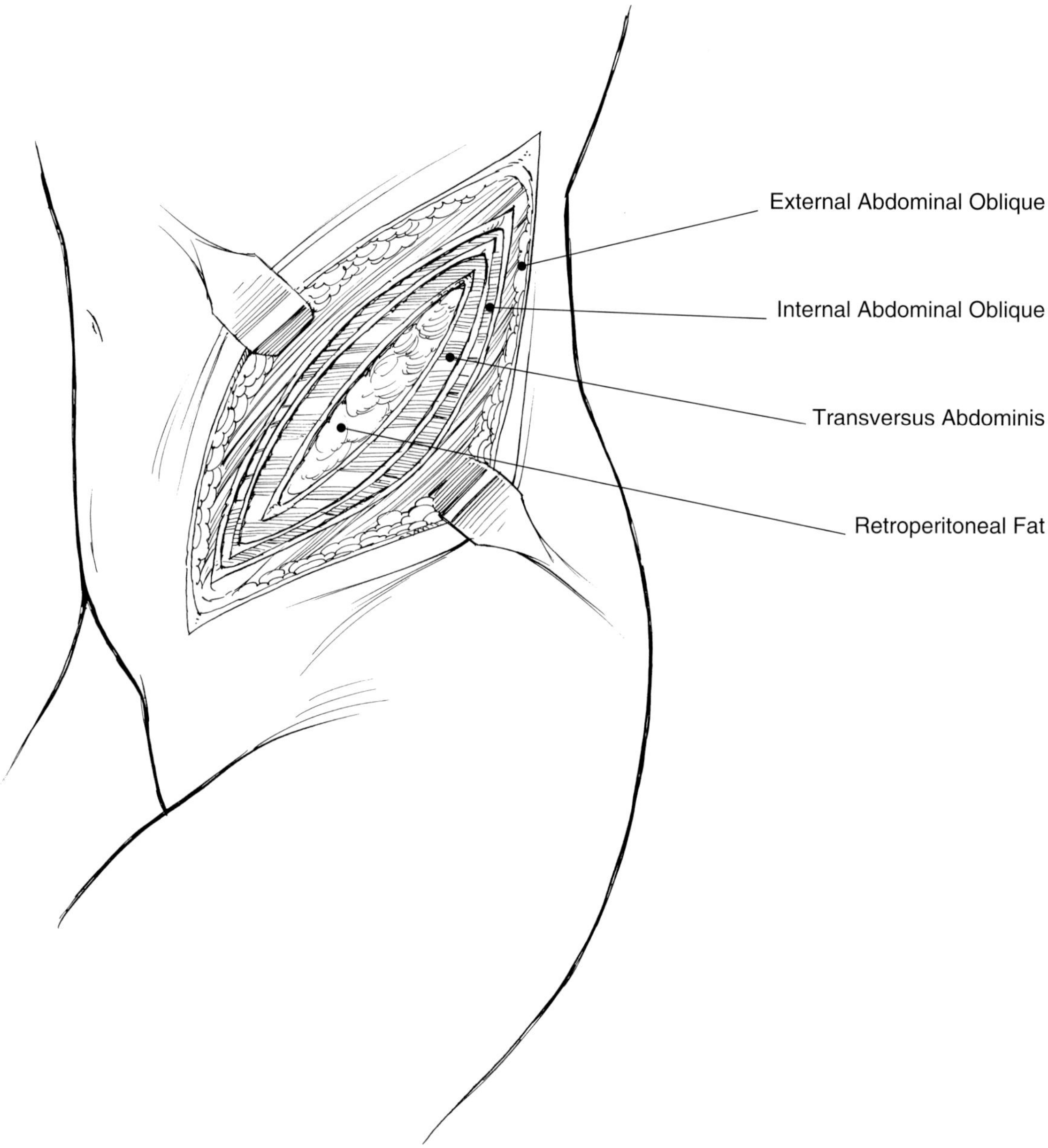


**FIGURE III-5**

A self-retaining retractor is then placed to retract the abdominal wall (III-6). Blunt retraction is used to retract the abdominal viscera. The quadratus lumborum and psoas muscles should be fully visualized. To approach the vertebral bodies, the psoas is carefully elevated from the lateral surface, exposing the segmental vessels.

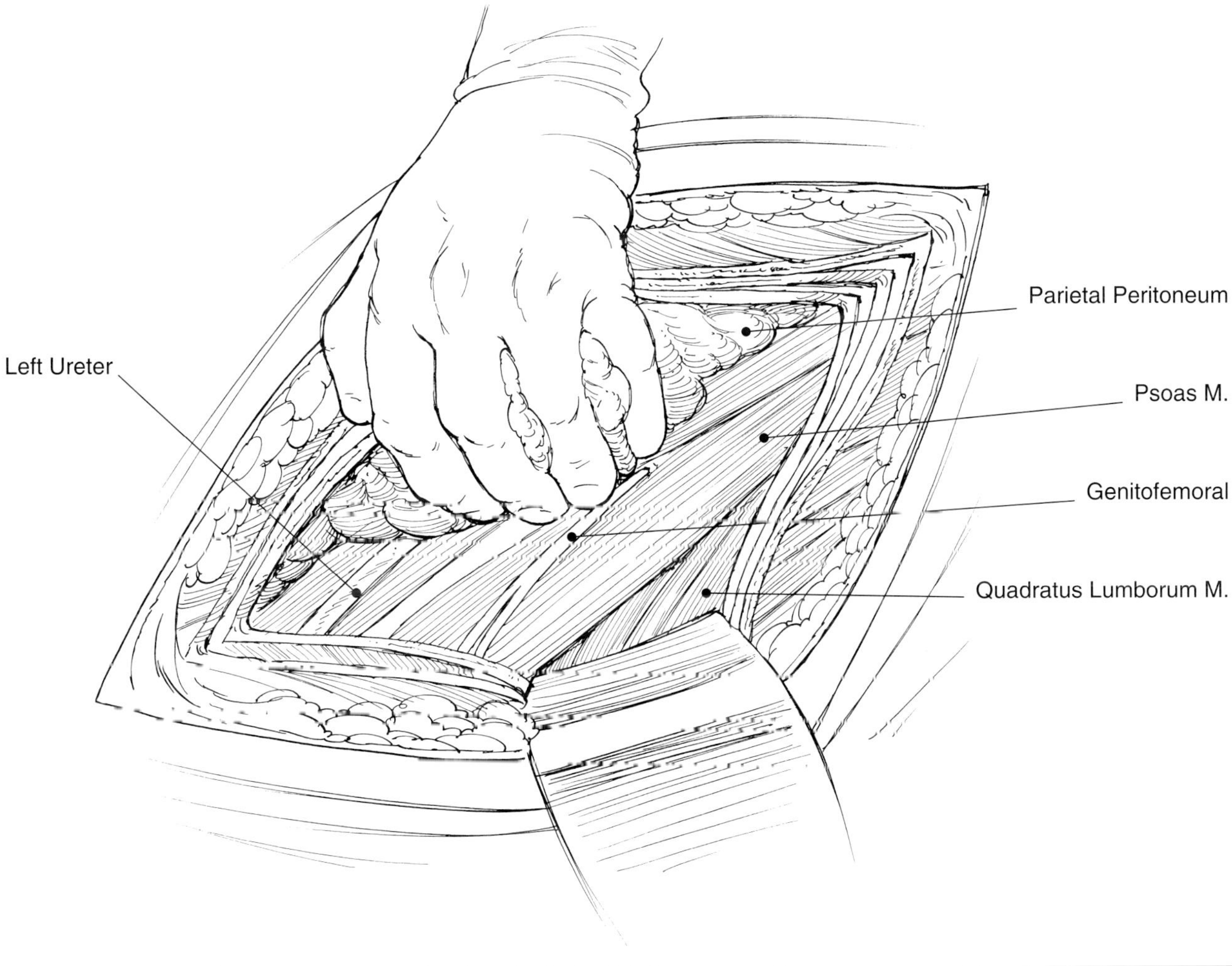


**FIGURE III–6**

These may be ligated and transected as necessary (III-7). The periosteum is split longitudinally and a Cobb elevator is used to elevate the anterior longitudinal ligament (III-8). Staying deep to the ligament avoids disruption of the aorta or inferior vena cava. At the cephalad end, the crus of the diaphragm attaches to the anterior longitudinal ligament and must be elevated for exposure of the twelfth thoracic and first two lumbar vertebrae. The caudal end of the sympathetic chain will

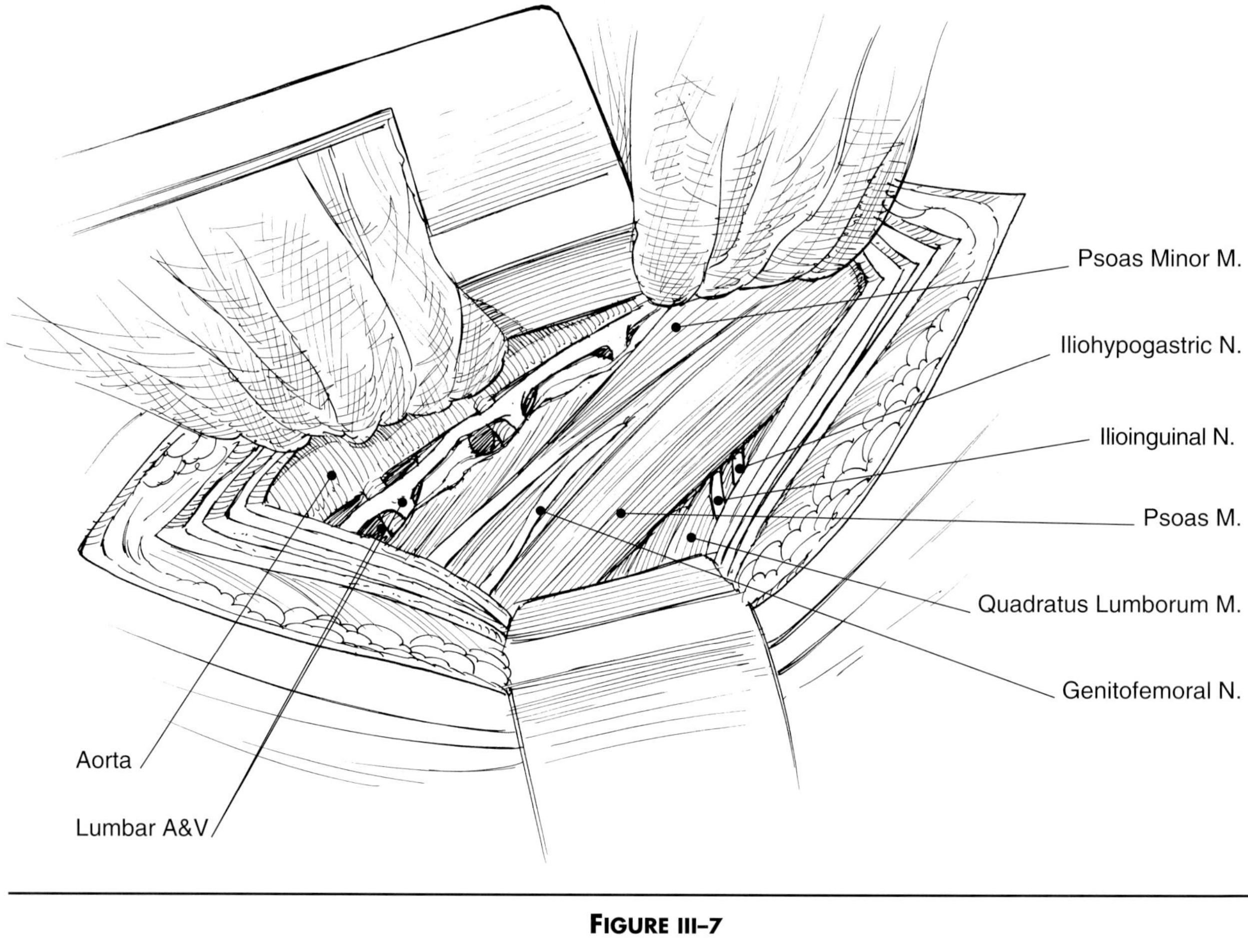


**FIGURE III–7**

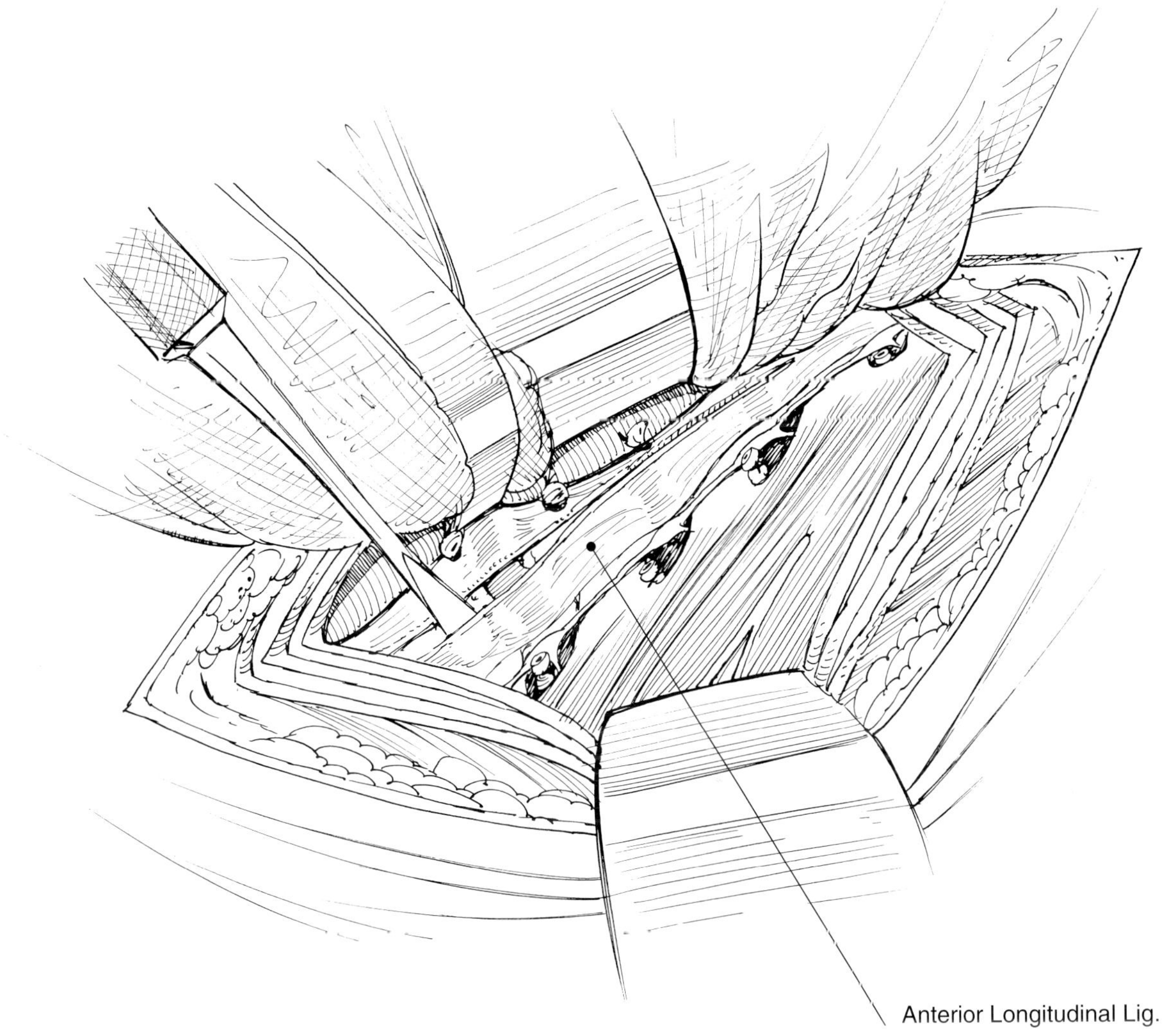


**FIGURE III–8**

be found here, medial to the psoas belly (III-9). The psoas may be retracted laterally to expose the lumbar nerve roots.

The muscles of the abdominal wall should be repaired in layers during closure to prevent an abdominal hernia.

### *Dangers*

The major hazards in this approach are injury to the adjacent structures. These include the kidney, spleen, ureter, and inferior vena cava. A postoperative ileus is relatively common. Rare complications include an anterior cord syndrome or sexual dysfunction in males, usually impotence or retrograde ejaculation.

### *Limitations*

The eleventh and twelfth thoracic vertebrae can be reached by this approach. However, extensive dissection at these levels is prohibited through this approach. The thoracolumbar approach is necessary for more extensive procedures above the first lumbar vertebra. The fifth lumbar vertebra can be seen and exposed on the left side. However, the lumbosacral disk and first sacral vertebra are difficult to

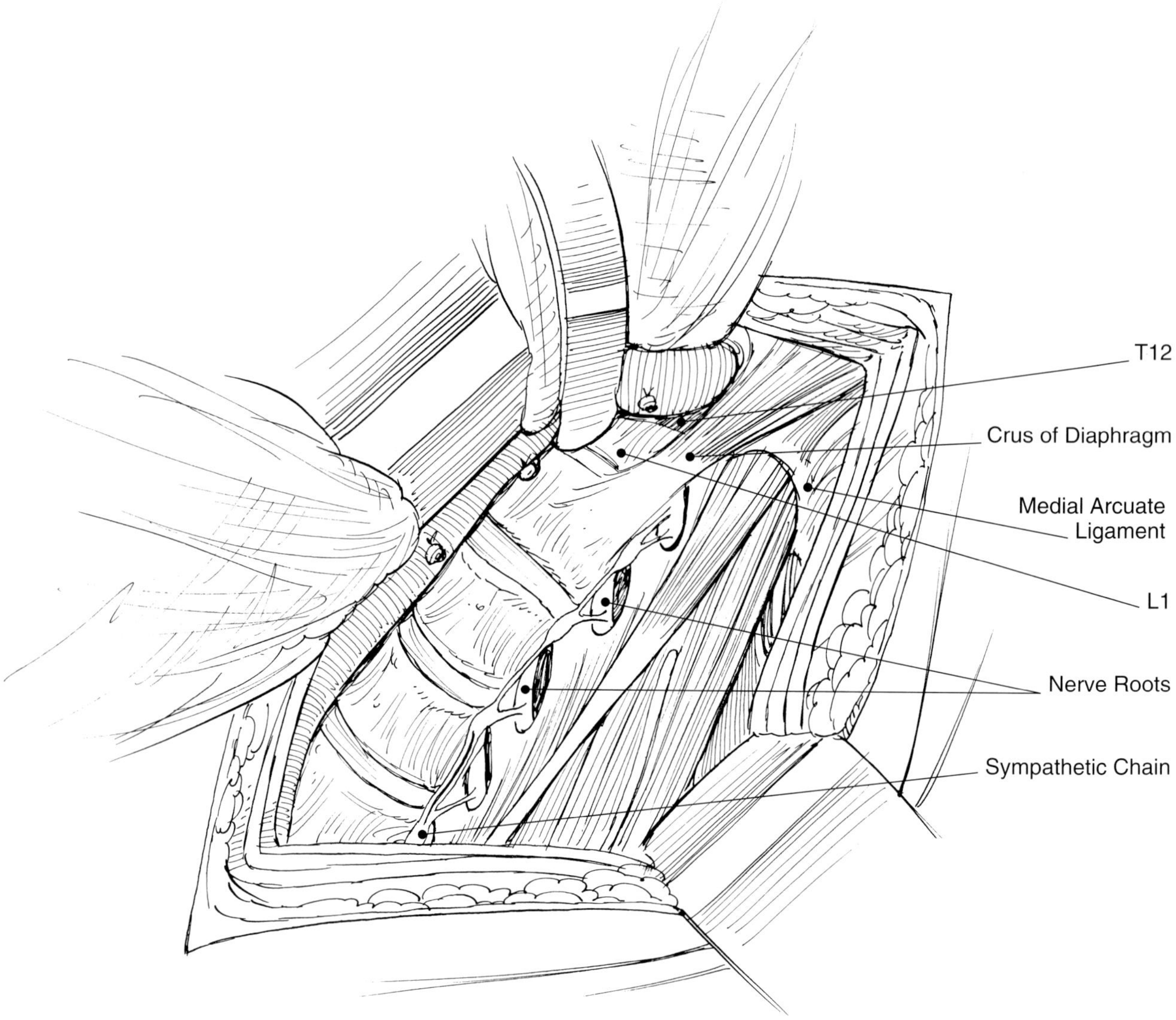


**FIGURE III-9**

reach. The overlying left common iliac vein limits this exposure. The hazard of injury to that vessel makes placement of instruments in this area dangerous. The incision described can be extended distally along the edge of the rectus sheath for better exposure of the lumbosacral junction.

## Posterior Approach to the Lumbar Spine

***Applications***

This is the common route for laminectomy for fractures, diskectomy, decompression of stenosis, or instrumentation of scoliosis.

***Technique***

The patient is placed in the prone position with the chest supported. The abdomen should be as free as possible to minimize abdominal pressure and thus decrease bleeding in the epidural veins. An incision is made longitudinally in the midline to the tips of the spinous processes (III-10A and III-10B). The level should

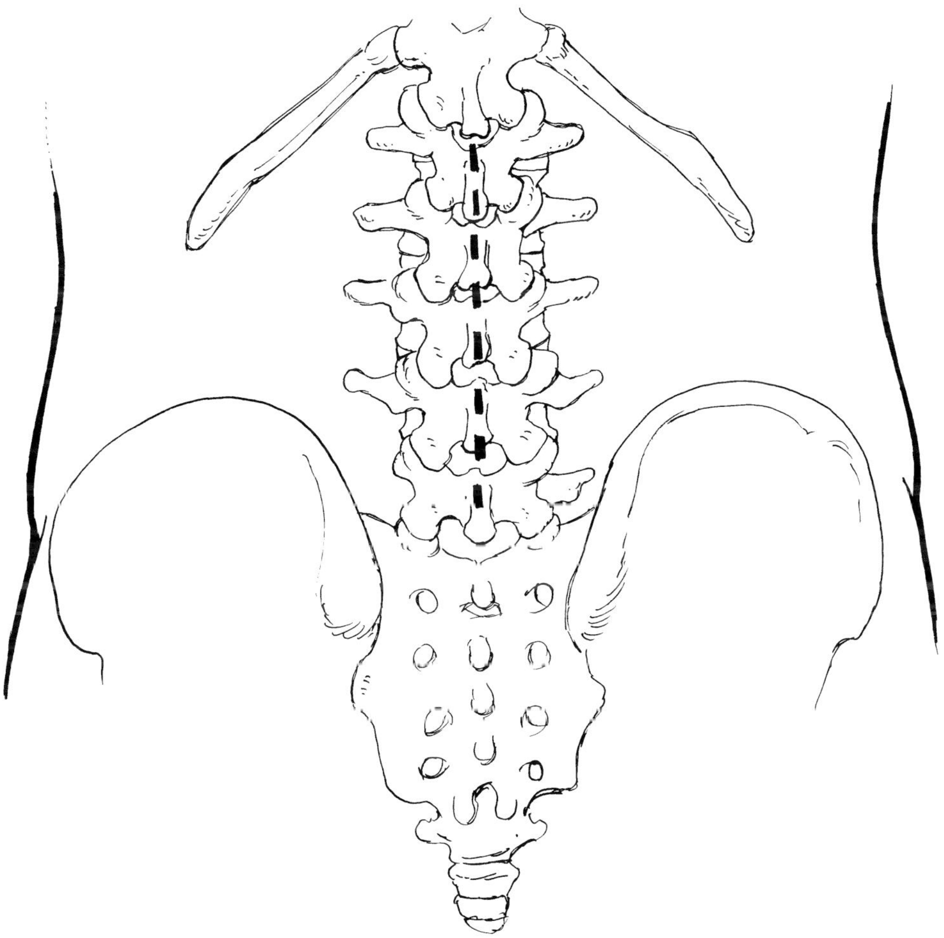

**FIGURE III-10A**

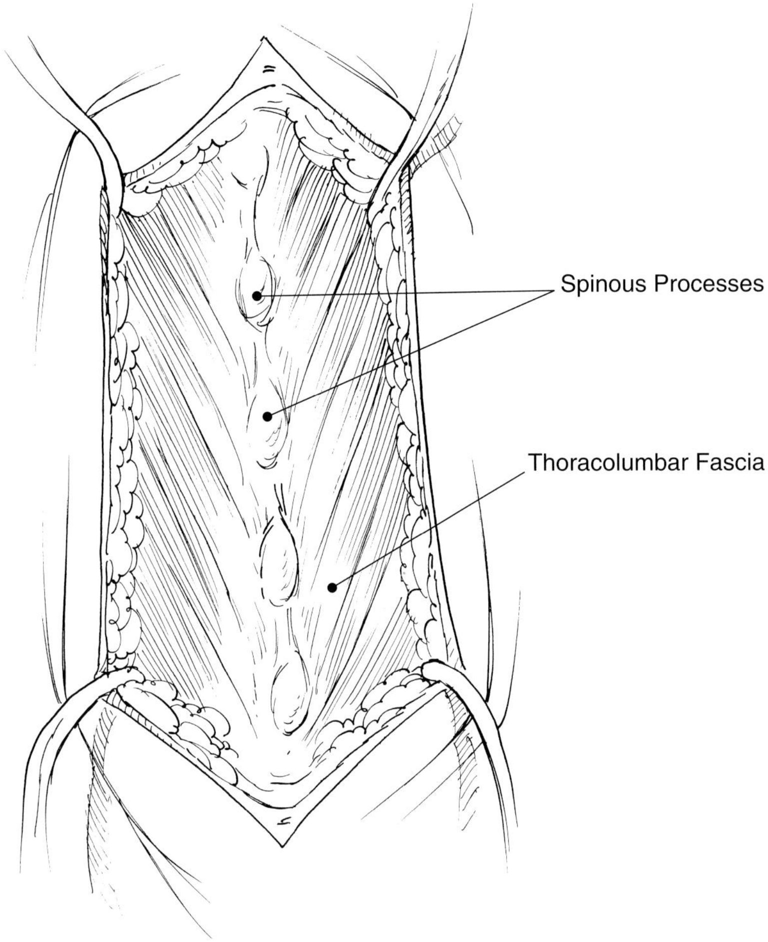


**FIGURE III–10B**

be confirmed by radiograph. The erector spinae muscles are then elevated subperiosteally from the spinous processes and laminae (III-11). This exposure can be extended laterally beyond the facets to the tips of the transverse processes for lateral fusion (III-12). The capsule of the vertebral facet should be left intact unless the spine is to be fused.

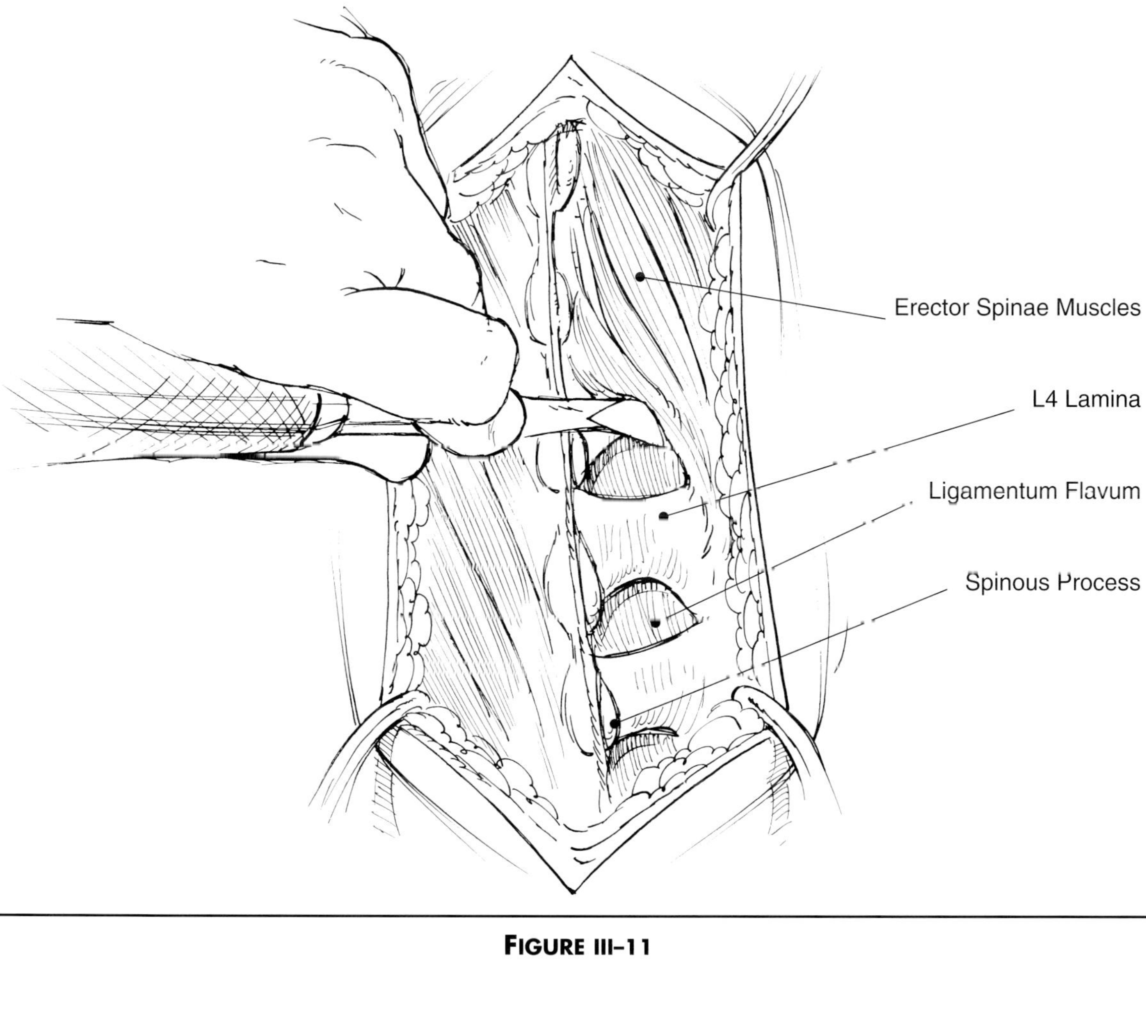


**FIGURE III–11**

***Dangers*** The further laterally this dissection is carried, the more likely the surgeon will run into the nerve roots. During laminectomy, the dura or nerve root may also be damaged. Bleeding from the epidural veins can make visualization within the spinal canal difficult.

***Limitations*** This approach gives wide exposure to the dorsal elements of the spine. Exposure to the disk is through the spinal canal by retraction of the dura and nerve roots and, therefore, is limited. The pedicles can be visualized along the edge of the canal, but their orientation for transpedicular hardware placement is difficult to visualize.

# References

1. Johnson RM, Murphy MJ, Southwick WO. Surgical approaches to the spine. In: Rathman RH, Simeone FA, eds. The Spine, 3rd ed. Philadelphia: W.B. Saunders, 43:1720–1738, 1992.

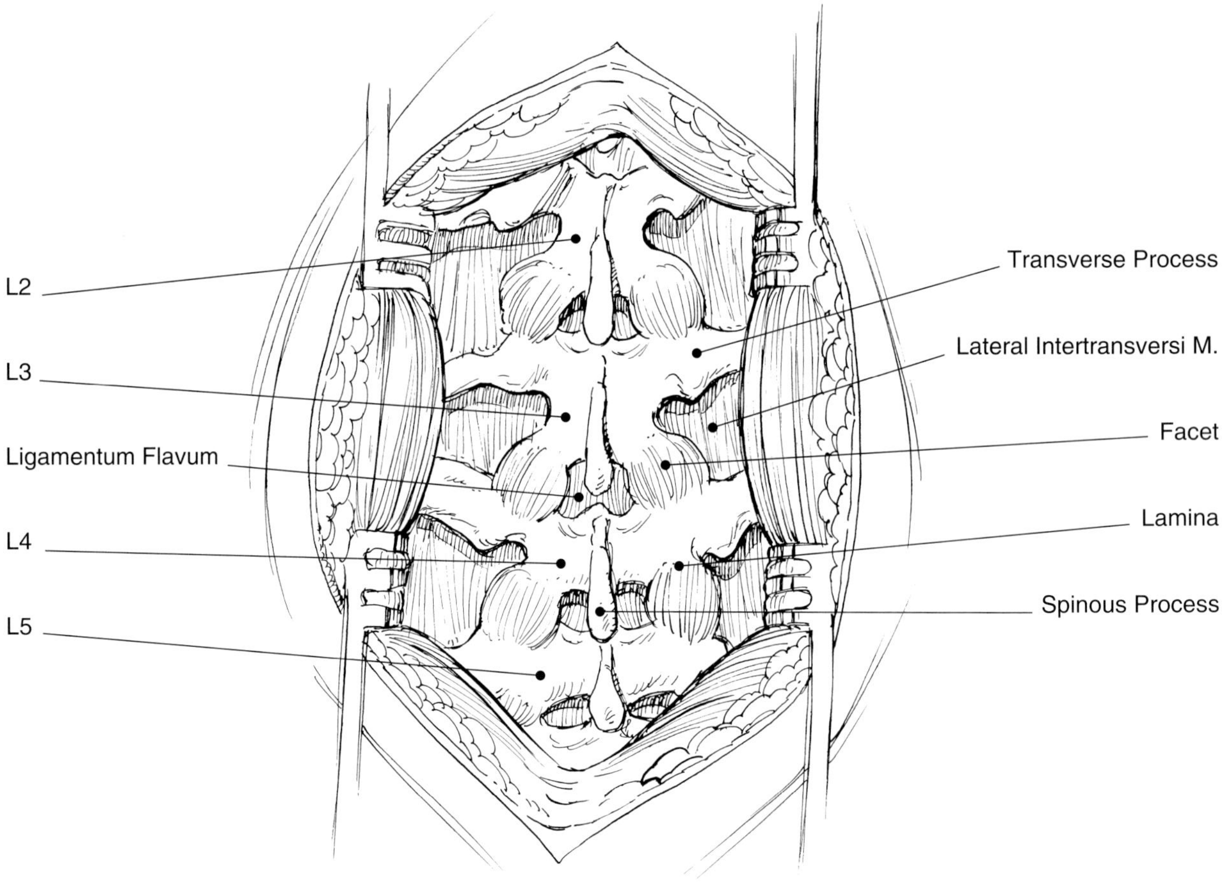


**FIGURE III–12**

# IV

# SURGICAL APPROACHES TO THE SHOULDER

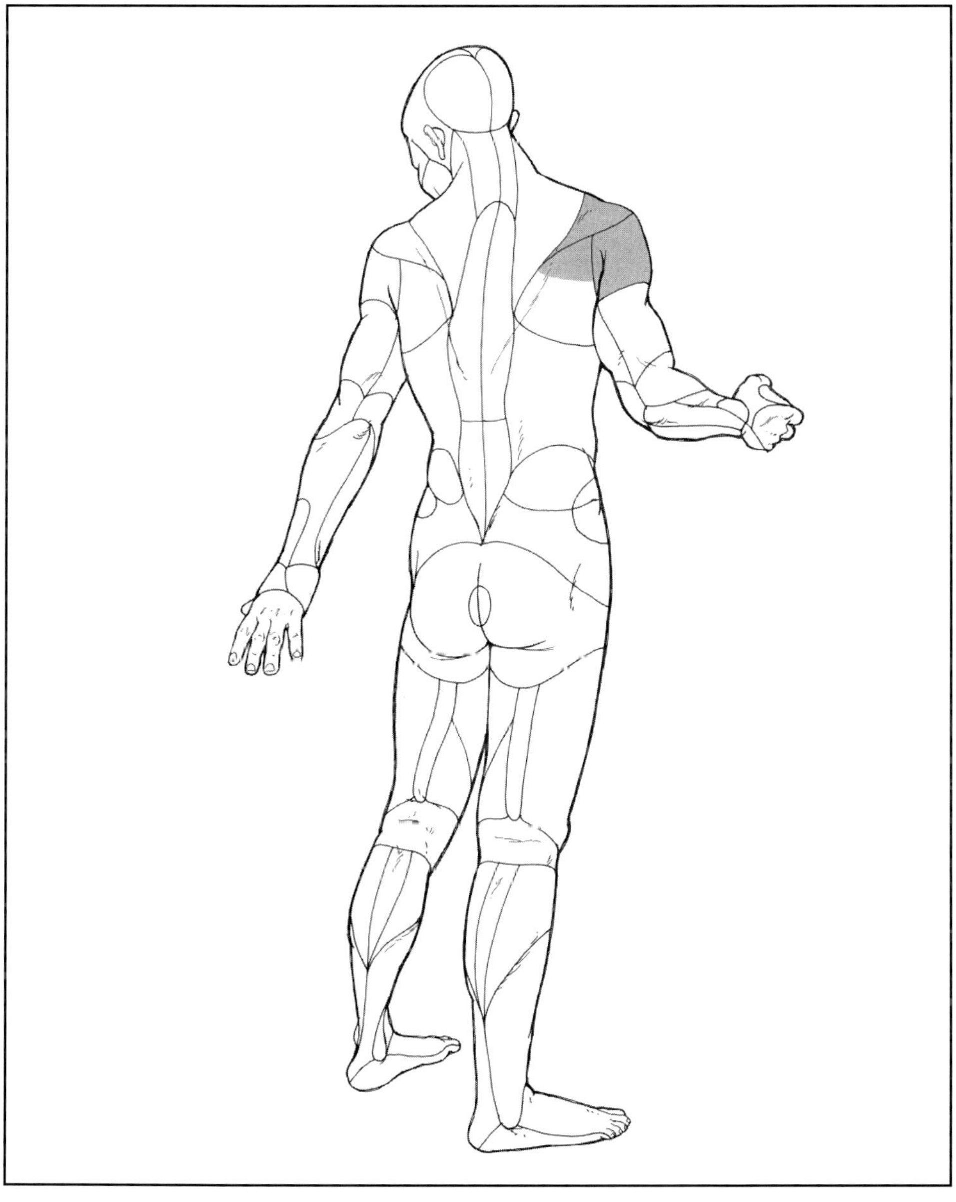

## General Principles and Complications

The shoulder is an extremely mobile joint, designed to allow positioning of the hand in space. The normal motion of this joint requires the concerted action of the deltoid and rotator cuff muscles. The vast majority of surgery on the shoulder is done for degenerative lesions of the rotator cuff or for instability. Restoring function of the shoulder following surgery requires aggressive rehabilitation. Therefore, the surgical approaches to the shoulder for these problems should minimize disruption of the muscular sleeve. Tumors of the scapula or proximal humerus that require extensive resection can be excised by combining the techniques of the anterior and posterior approaches (1).

The major problem faced in shoulder surgery is allowing adequate exposure for the intended procedure without injuring the neurovascular plexus.

The brachial plexus and axillary artery pass medial to the shoulder, giving off numerous branches around the shoulder. The skin of the shoulder has a generous blood supply and can tolerate the creation of large fasciocutaneous flaps. Skin cleavage lines tend to run axially around the shoulder so that longitudinally-oriented incisions can create unsightly scars; however, transverse incisions limit the longitudinal exposure needed to retract the shoulder muscles. As a result, the surgeon will need to decide preoperatively which incision orientation to use for each patient based on the extent of the planned procedure and the importance of cosmesis to the patient.

## Surgical Anatomy

The shoulder is enshrouded by the broad expanse of the deltoid muscle. The deltoid originates from the lateral clavicle, the acromion, and the scapular spine and descends onto the deltoid tuberosity of the humerus. It is divided anatomically and functionally into posterior, lateral, and anterior components (IV-1). There are more or less distinct cleavage planes dividing these muscle segments. The pectoralis major arises from the clavicle and chest wall to cover the medial aspect of the anterior shoulder. It is encapsulated in the tough fibrous clavipectoral fascia. The coracoid process of the scapula can be palpated roughly at the interval between the deltoid and the pectoralis major. It serves as the origin of the short head of the biceps and the coracobrachialis and as the insertion of the pectoralis minor (IV-2). Immediately medial to the coracoid and deep to the pectoralis minor are the axillary artery, axillary vein, and brachial plexus (IV-3). This area is not entered during most procedures on the shoulder joint, but the surgeon must always be aware of its contents. The axillary nerve exits the anterior shoulder between the subscapularis and teres major muscles. It passes through the quadrangular space along with the posterior humeral circumflex artery to innervate the teres minor and the deltoid. It runs along the deep surface of the deltoid, roughly 7 cm distal to the acromion, to distribute to the anterior portion of the deltoid (IV-3). The musculocutaneous nerve passes just below the coracoid process to run through the coracobrachialis muscle. The suprascapular nerve enters the posterior shoulder through the suprascapular notch to distribute to the supraspinatus and infraspinatus muscles. It wraps around the base of the acromion to pass from the supraspinous fossa to the infraspinous fossa (IV-4).

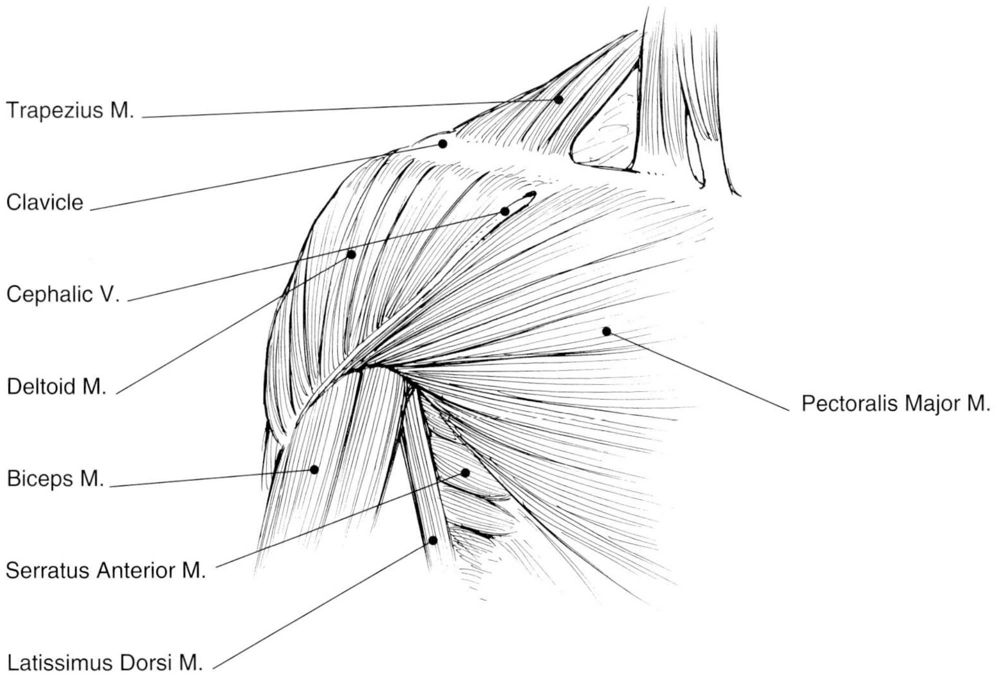


**FIGURE IV–1**

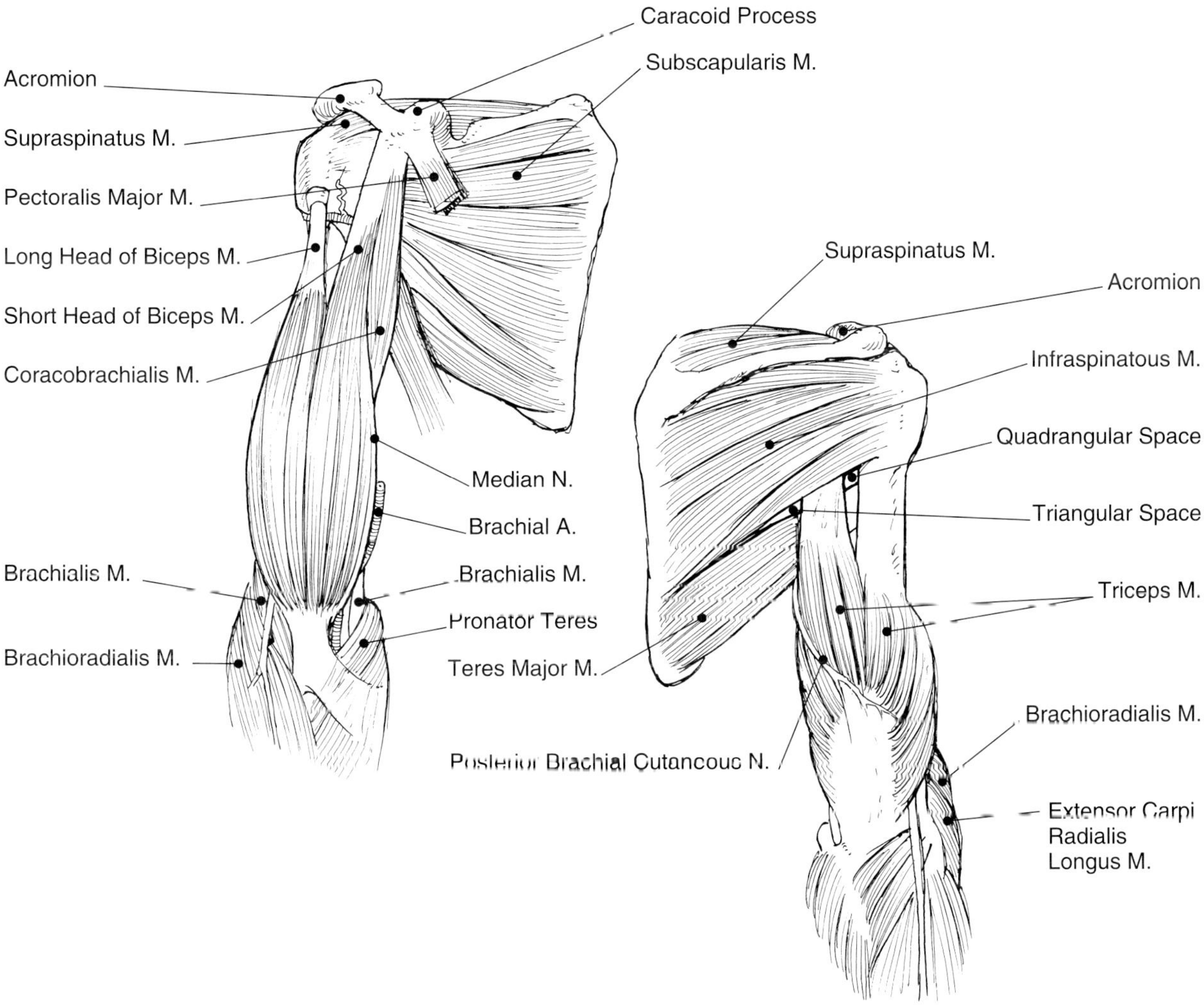


**FIGURE IV–2**

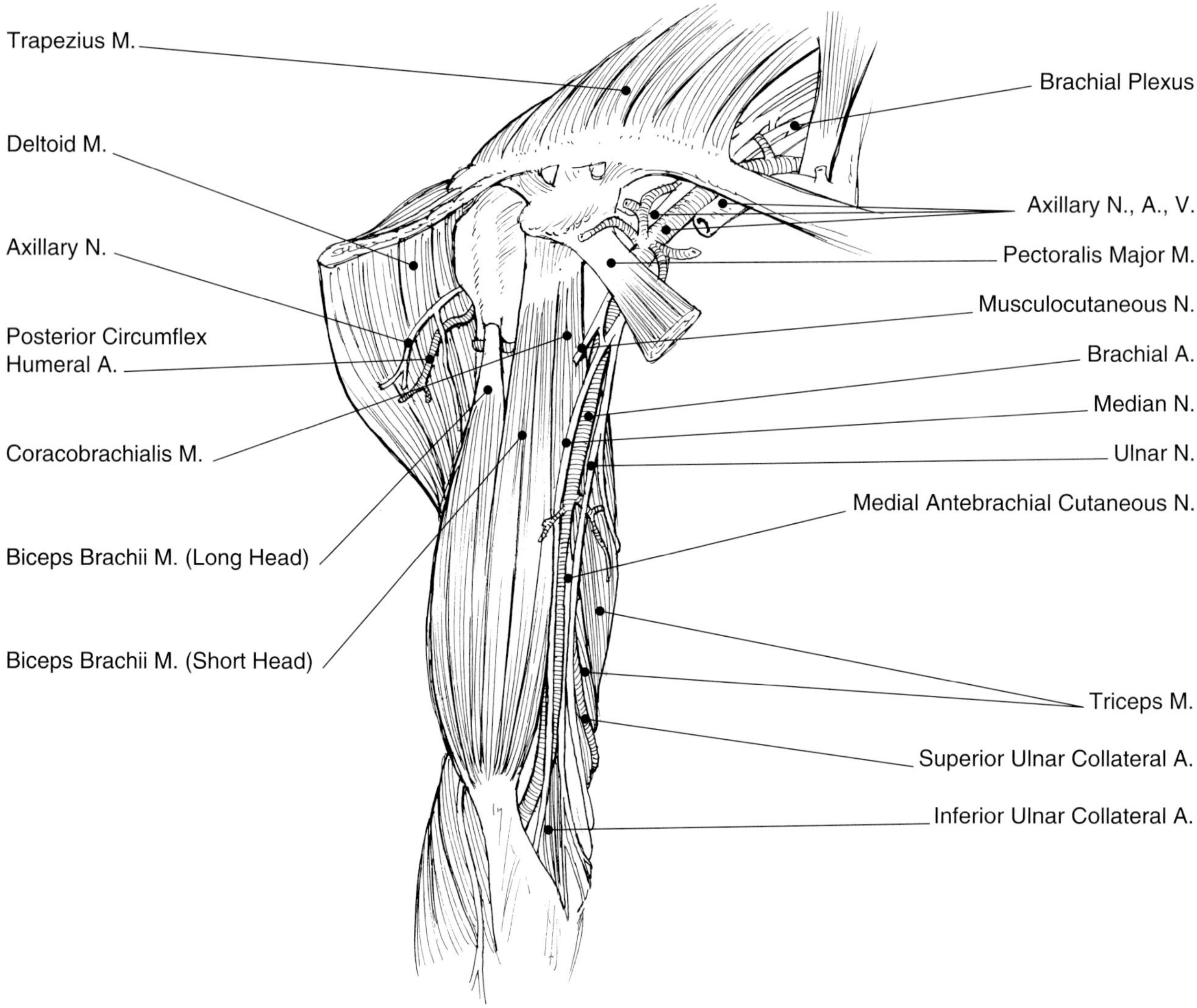


**FIGURE IV–3**

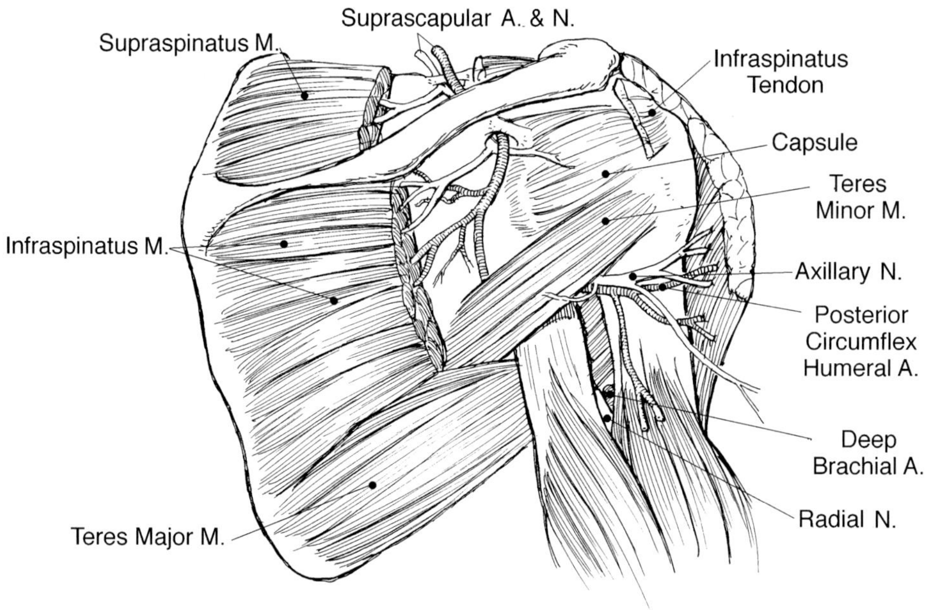


**FIGURE IV–4**

# Anterior Approach to the Shoulder

***Applications***

The anterior approach can be used for shoulder arthroplasty (2,3), fracture fixation, anterior reconstruction for instability, and proximal humeral replacement. It can also be used for reconstruction of the brachial plexus or axillary artery.

***Technique***

The patient is placed in the "beach chair" position with the face turned away from the operated side. The entire upper extremity is draped free. The skin incision is on a line from the middle of the clavicle to the deltoid tuberosity. It should pass directly over the coracoid process. The incision begins approximately 1 cm below the clavicle and is carried as far distally as necessary; for exposure of the proximal half of the humerus, the incision can be carried just distal to the deltoid tuberosity (IV-5). The cephalic vein is located by blunt dissection and is reflected laterally along with the deltoid muscle (IV-6). The deltopectoral interval is then opened and the deltoid is retracted laterally to expose the shoulder, pectoralis major tendon, and coracoid (IV-6). Keeping the arm in a slightly flexed and abducted position allows the deltoid to be retracted with minimal tension. Internal rotation of the shoulder allows access to the greater tuberosity while external rotation brings the subscapularis tendon into view. The anterior deltoid fibers can be elevated from the tuberosity if necessary for better exposure, but they should not be detached from the clavicle.

The conjoined tendon of the short head of the biceps and coracobrachialis is exposed and the coracoid is clearly identified. For procedures on the shoulder joint, the dissection remains lateral and superior to the coracoid. If the brachial plexus or axillary artery are to be included in the procedure, the margins of the

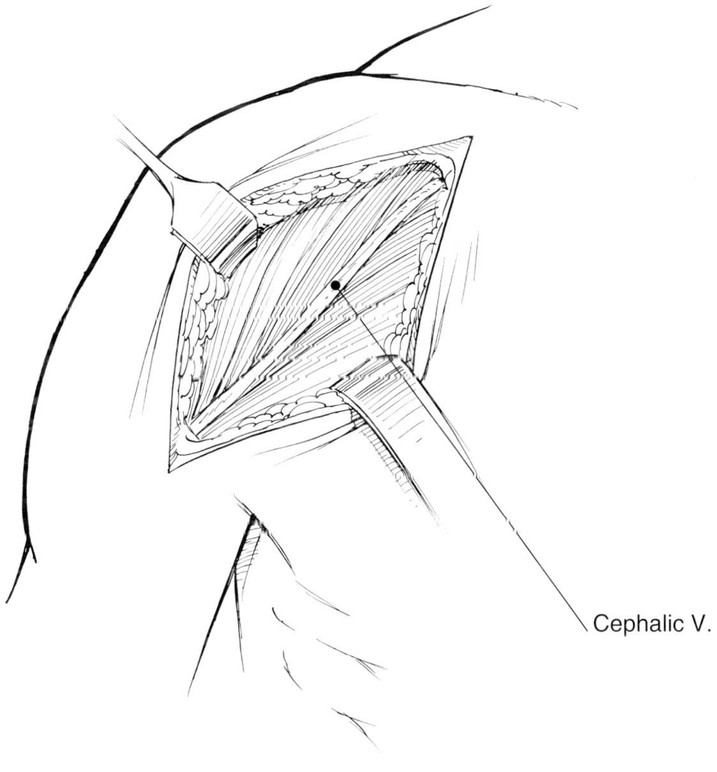


**FIGURE IV-5**

pectoralis minor are defined and the tendon is tagged and then detached from the coracoid (IV-7). Release of the superior 1 cm of the pectoralis major in its tendinous portion near the humerus can facilitate exposure of the shoulder.

To enter the shoulder joint, the tendon of the subscapularis is defined superiorly and inferiorly. A hemostat can be placed bluntly deep to the tendon. The tendon is then tagged and transected (IV-8). The shoulder capsule is then opened at the humeral edge for exposure of the humeral head and glenoid (IV-9A and IV-9B).

***Dangers***

The brachial plexus, axillary artery and vein, axillary nerve, and musculocutaneous nerve are all in the immediate vicinity of this approach. They are most likely to be injured by excessive retraction of the medial edge of the wound.

***Limitations***

This approach can be extended over the scapula to communicate with the posterior incision for complete excision of the scapula and proximal humerus. Distally, it can be continued down the lateral arm to the elbow. It does not provide ready access to the subacromial space which is more easily reached by the lateral deltoid splitting approach, nor does it provide direct access to the posterior rotator cuff tendons. The skin incision does not follow the skin cleavage lines and may leave an unsightly scar.

## Lateral Subacromial Approach to the Shoulder

***Applications***

This approach is ideal for decompression of the subacromial space and acromioplasty, for rotator cuff repair, and for fixation of fractures of the greater tuberosity.

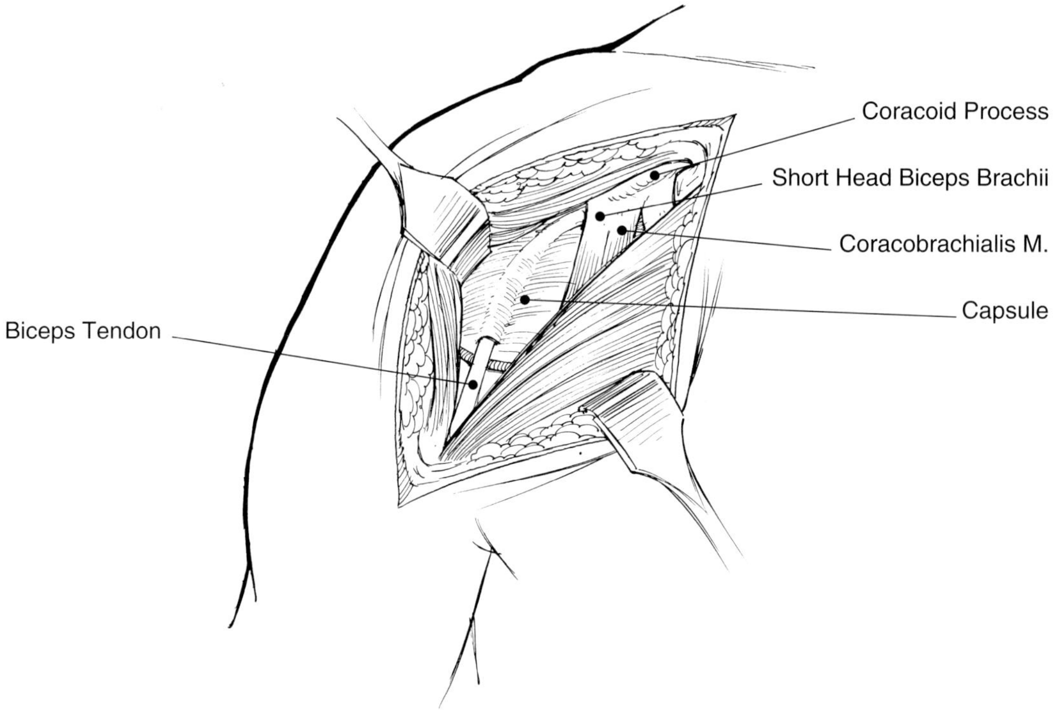


**FIGURE IV-6**

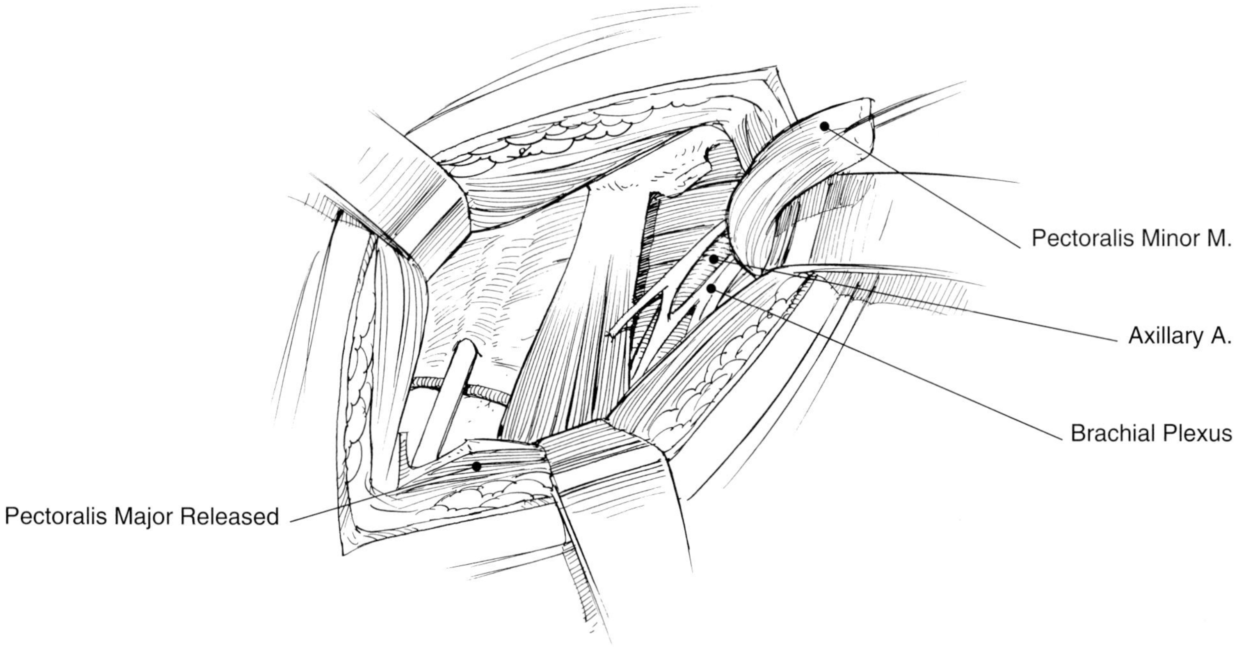


**FIGURE IV-7**

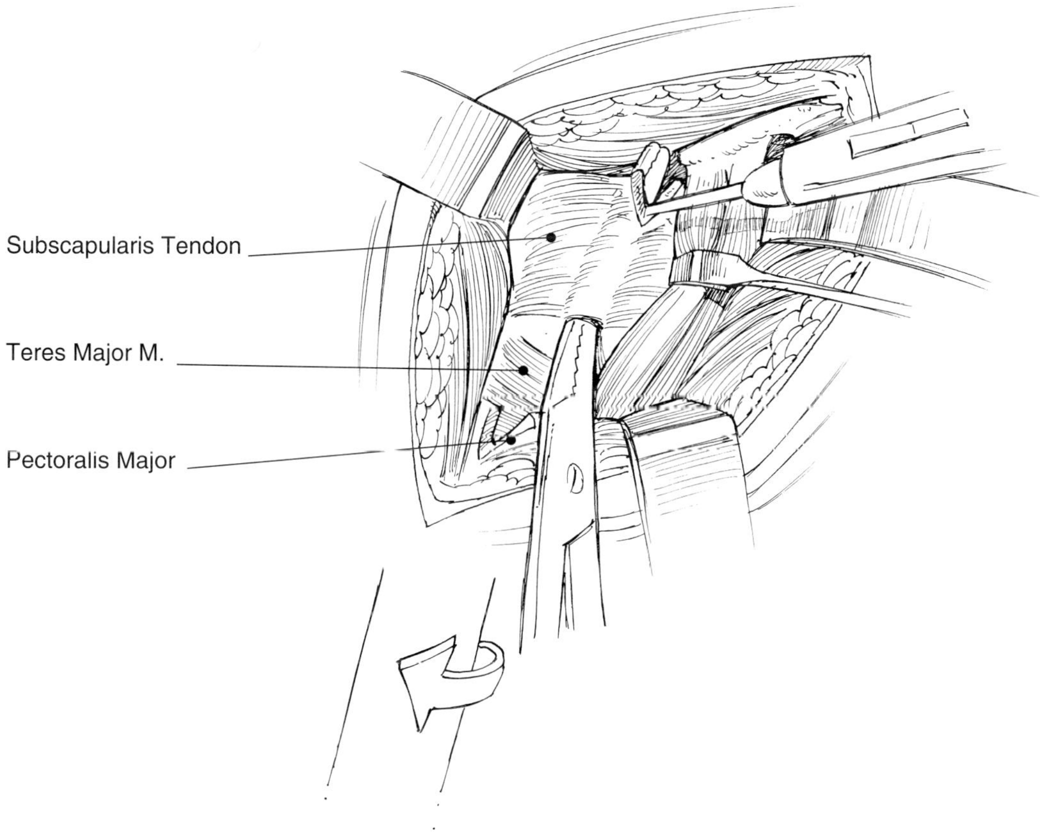


**FIGURE IV-8**

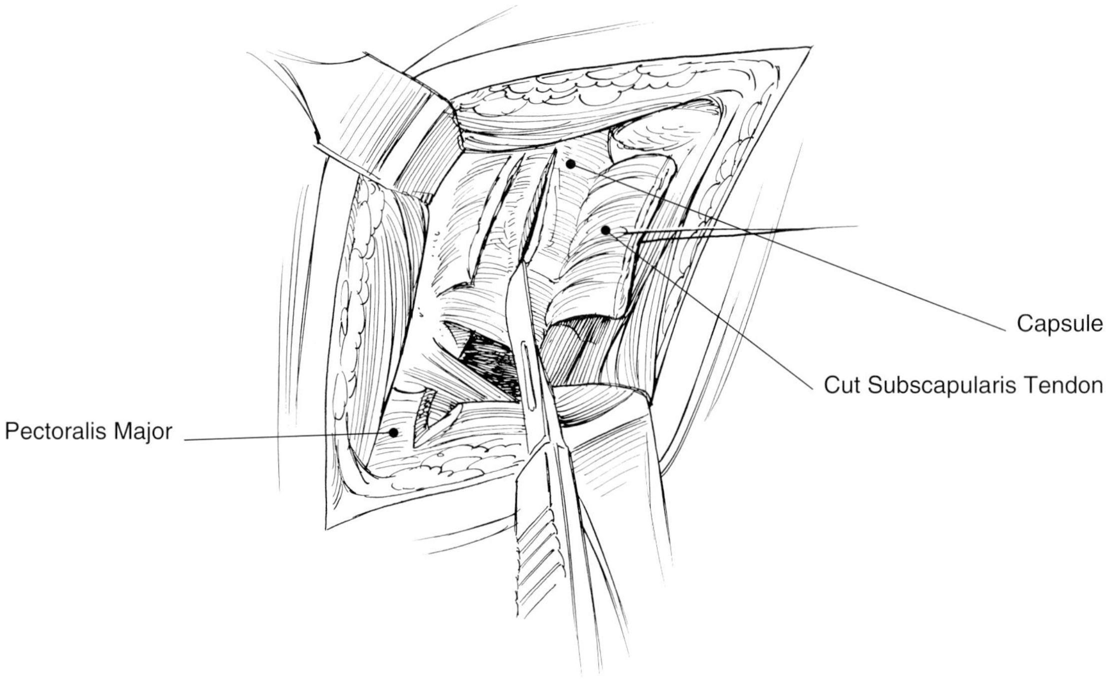


**FIGURE IV–9A**

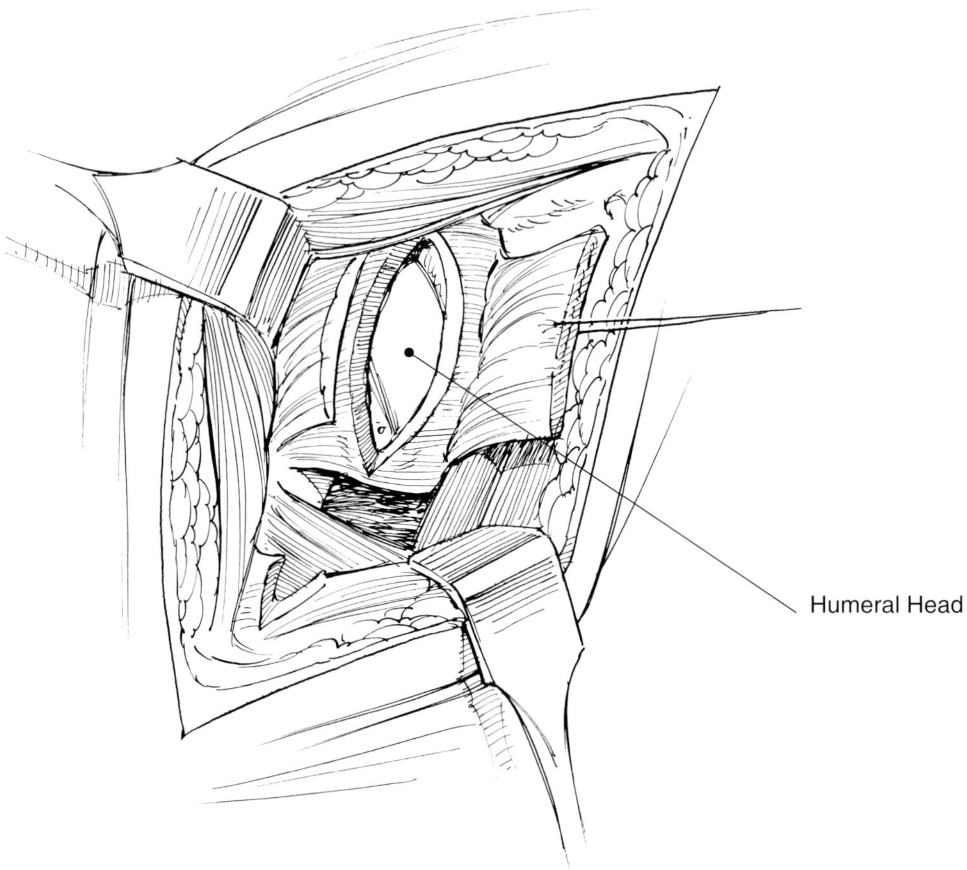


**FIGURE IV–9B**

***Technique***

The patient is in the "beach chair" position. The skin incision can be either transversely or longitudinally oriented. The transverse incision is more in line with the skin cleavage planes and more likely to produce a cosmetically acceptable scar. However, for biopsy of a potentially malignant tumor of the humeral head or shoulder, a longitudinal skin incision is preferable as it facilitates excision later. The transverse incision is placed just lateral to the lateral edge of the acromion. It extends along the breadth of the lateral acromion edge and then distally and anteriorly for an additional 2 cm (IV-10A). The incision is taken down to the deltoid fascia and the superior flap is retracted to expose the acromion. The longitudinal incision begins over the roof of the acromion and is carried distally over the interval between the anterior and lateral portions of the deltoid for approximately 3 cm (IV-10B). For biopsy of a tumor of the humeral head, a shorter incision is made over only the deltoid muscle to prevent contamination of the acromion and the subacromial space.

The fibrous capsule between the anterior and lateral deltoid is split by finger dissection to expose the greater tuberosity. The dissection is then carried up to the acromion, splitting the periosteum over the roof of the acromion. With subperiosteal dissection, the anterior and lateral acromion are exposed by elevation of the deltoid muscle. The greater tuberosity, supraspinatus tendon, and anterior inferior surface of the acromion can be well exposed (IV-11).

***Dangers***

The serious danger of this approach is an excessive distal extension of the dissection which can transect the axillary nerve. As long as the dissection is kept within 3 cm of the acromion, this risk should be minimal. Care also must be taken to neatly elevate the periosteum of the acromion to prevent damage to the fibers of the deltoid.

***Limitations***

The approach provides access to the greater tuberosity and supraspinatus tendons. There is limited access to the shoulder joint and the anterior or posterior aspects of the rotator cuff. The superior flap of the transverse incision can be retracted to expose the acromioclavicular joint and the distal clavicle can be excised through this approach.

## Axillary Approach to the Shoulder

***Application***

The axillary incision is placed posterior to the anterior axillary fold and parallel to the skin cleavage lines and creates, cosmetically, the best incision about the shoulder. It provides adequate access to the shoulder for anterior instability repairs, capsular release, tendon lengthening, and synovial debridement or biopsy(4).

***Technique***

The skin incision begins just posterior to the anterior axillary fold under the palpable tendon of the pectoralis major. It is carried posteriorly for 4 to 6 cm along the skin cleavage lines in the axilla (IV-12). The clavipectoral fascia around the pectoralis major is dissected to allow mobility of the muscle. The skin incision is then retracted anteriorly and superiorly to allow opening of the deltopectoral interval. By palpating the coracoid, the interval is easily identified and opened. The anterior shoulder exposure is then the same as in the anterior approach (IV-13). The subscapularis muscle can be elevated with blunt dissection, with care to avoid the anterior humeral circumflex vessels adjacent to its caudal edge (IV-14).

***Dangers***

The surgeon must use the pectoralis major tendon and coracoid as landmarks and continue the dissection anteriorly. A posterior dissection leads into the axillary vessels and the brachial plexus. The axillary nerve can be encountered along the cau-

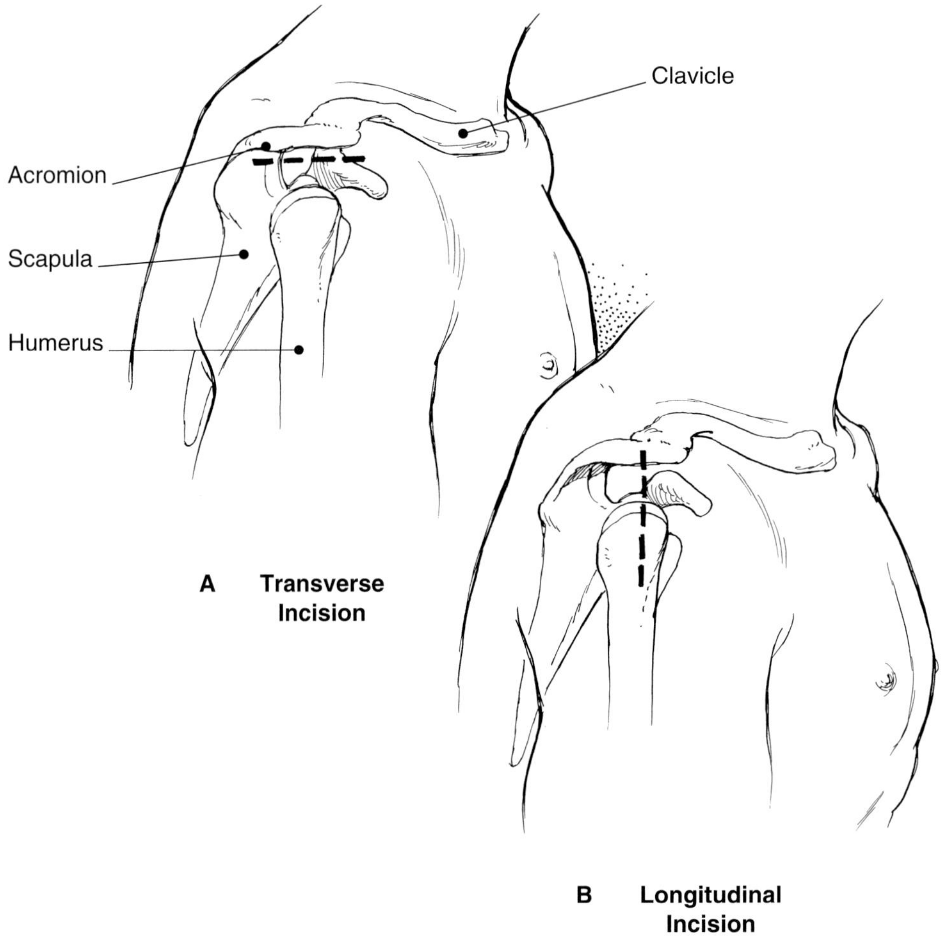


**FIGURE IV–10 A & B**

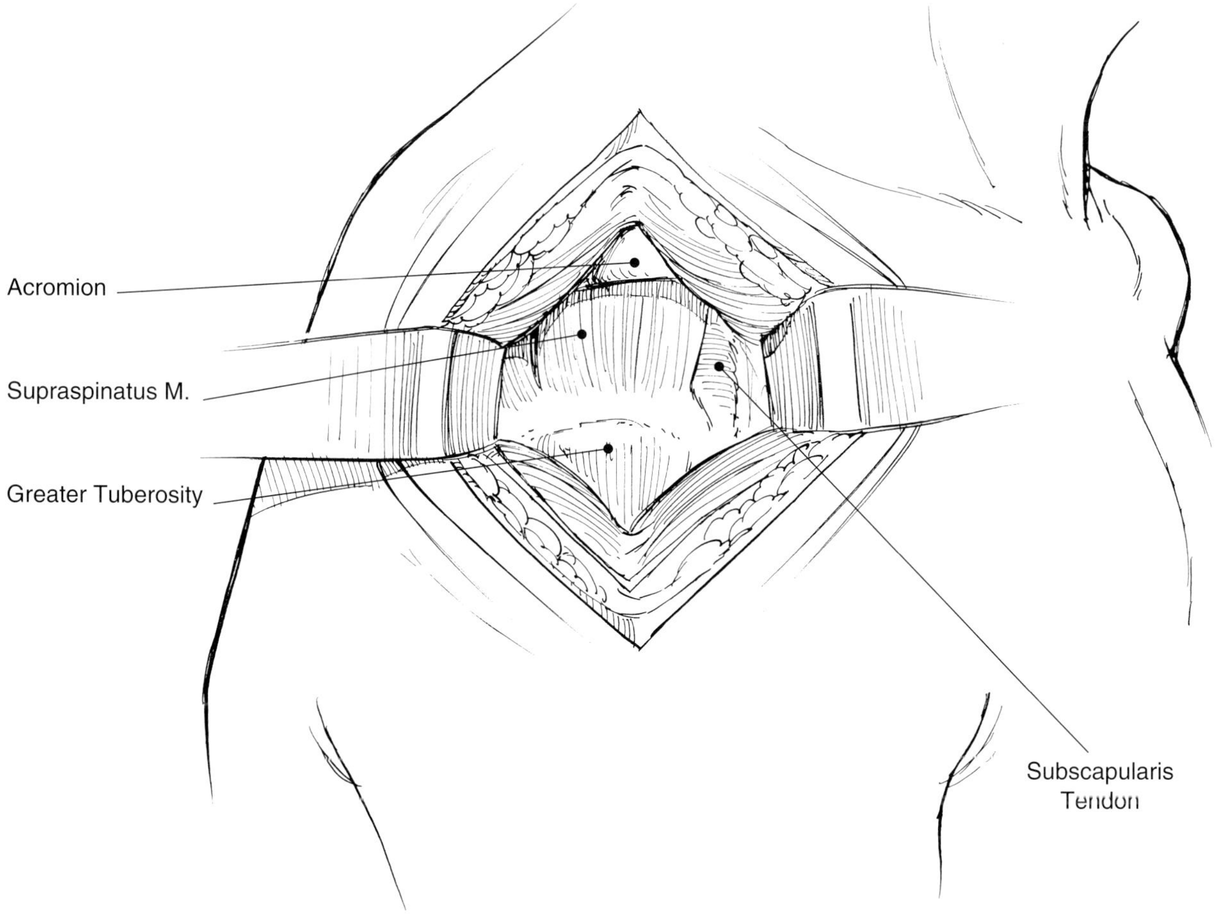


**FIGURE IV–11**

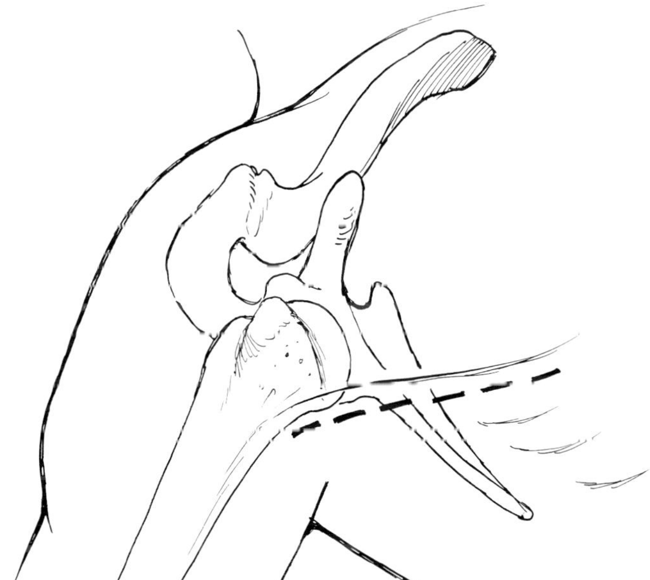

**FIGURE IV–12**

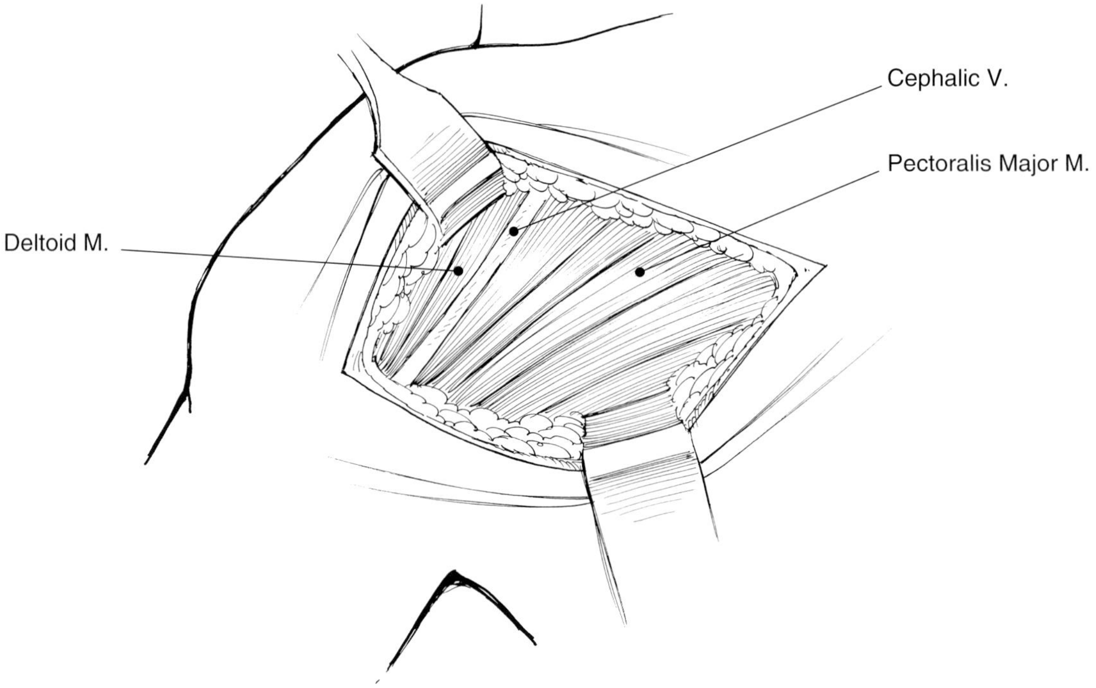


**FIGURE IV–13**

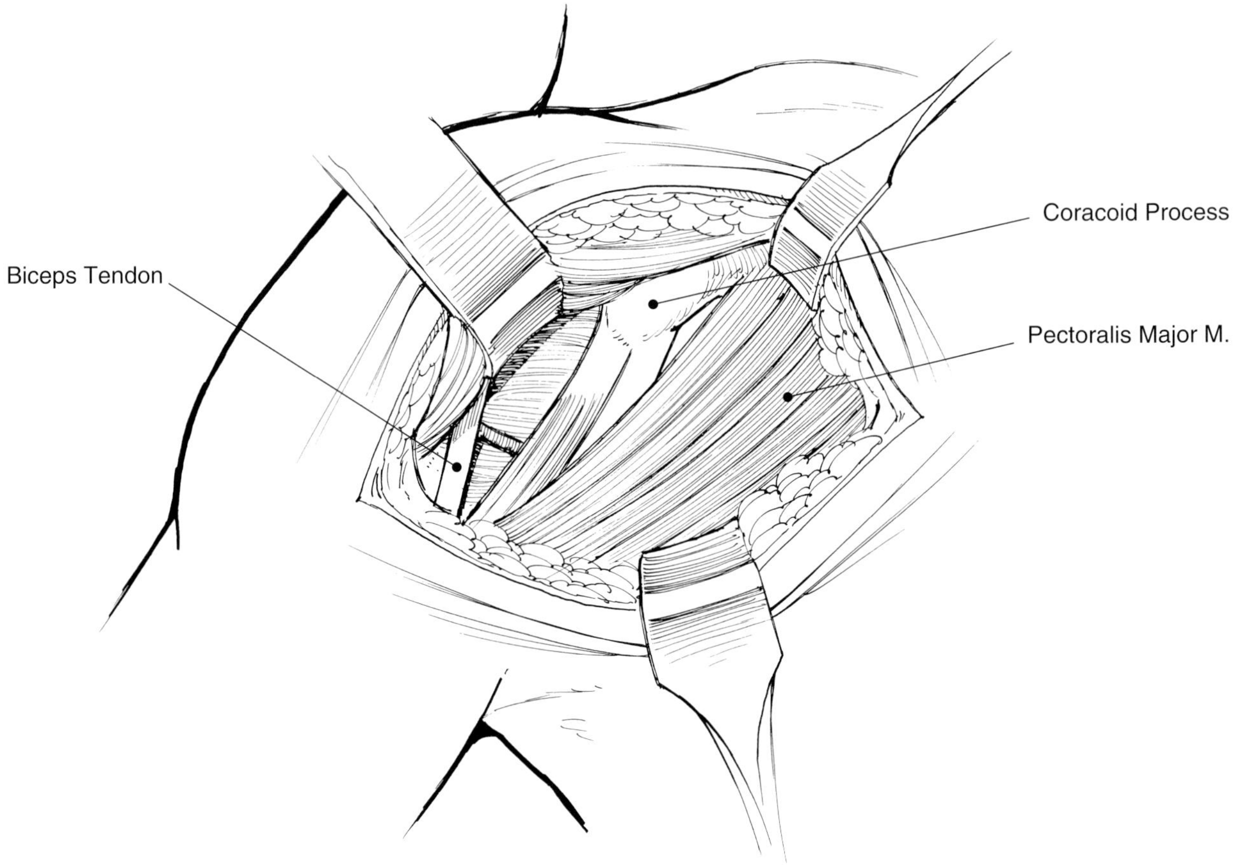


**FIGURE IV–14**

dal edge of the subscapularis muscle as it runs obliquely across the medial edge of the field.

*Limitations*

This approach provides access to the anterior and inferior aspects of the shoulder joint. It is a poor choice for tumor biopsy because of its proximity to the major neurovascular trunks. It can be extended anteriorly over the anterior axillary fold, but then the scar will be visible anteriorly, defeating the major purpose of this approach.

## Posterior Approach to the Shoulder

*Applications*

The posterior approach is especially useful for drainage of a septic shoulder, posterior capsular repair, glenoid osteotomy, fixation of scapular neck fractures (5), or resection of all or part of the scapula for tumors.

*Technique*

The patient is placed in the lateral decubitus position and the forequadrant draped free. A vertical incision is made beginning at the inferior lateral edge of the acromion and extending distally for 6 cm to just above the posterior axillary fold (IV 15). The fibers of the deltoid are split in the interval between the posterior and lateral segments (IV-16). Using the scapular spine as a guide, the interval between

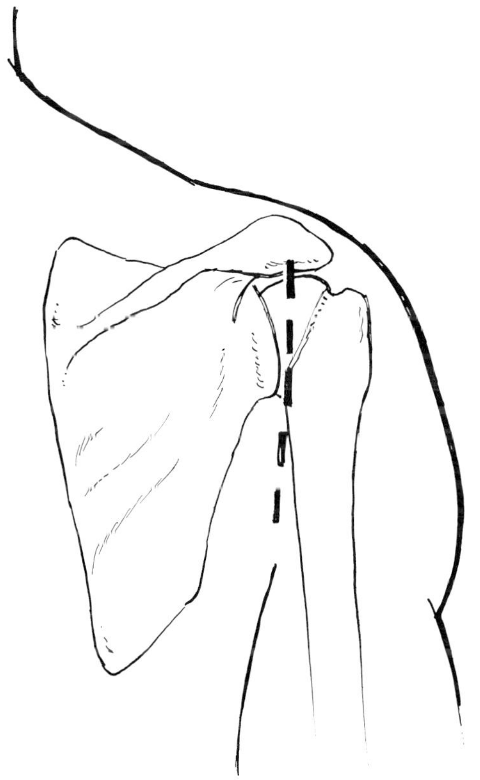

**FIGURE IV–15**

the infraspinatus and the teres minor is identified and opened. The infraspinatus can be elevated from the posterior capsule and retracted cephalad to expose the glenoid neck and posterior capsule (IV-17). For wider exposure of the joint or for capsular repair, the tendons of the infraspinatus and teres minor can be elevated and transected (IV-18).

Alternatively, for excision of all or part of the scapula, an S-shaped incision is made. This incision begins at the inferior medial angle of the scapular body and extends in an arc to the scapular spine. The incision then follows the spine to the medial edge of the acromion and turns to ascend over the shoulder, parallel to the

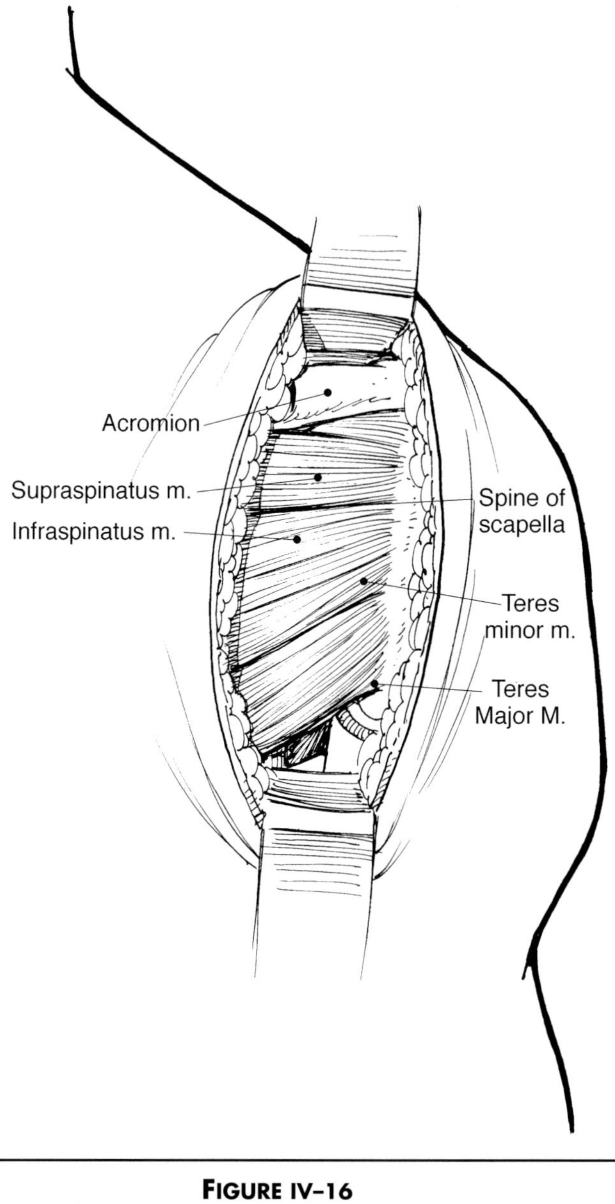


**FIGURE IV–16**

medial acromial edge (IV-19). For resection of the entire shoulder and scapula, this incision is then carried anteriorly over the clavicle to continue with the anterior deltopectoral approach, creating large flaps over the scapula. The trapezius and posterior deltoid are detached from the scapular spine and the dissection stays deep to these muscles to preserve the blood supply to the skin (IV-20). For complete excision of the scapula, the medial edge can be freed by detaching the rhomboids, levator scapula, and serratus anterior, allowing the scapula to be elevated and rotated anteriorly for exposure of the axillary vessels and brachial plexus (IV-21).

***Dangers***

The vertical posterior incision is centered over the intermuscular plane between the subscapularis and teres minor. Misidentification of this interval can result in an approach caudal to the teres minor into the quadrangular space, putting the axillary nerve and posterior humeral circumflex vessel in jeopardy. Vigorous retraction on the teres minor can produce damage to the suprascapular nerve.

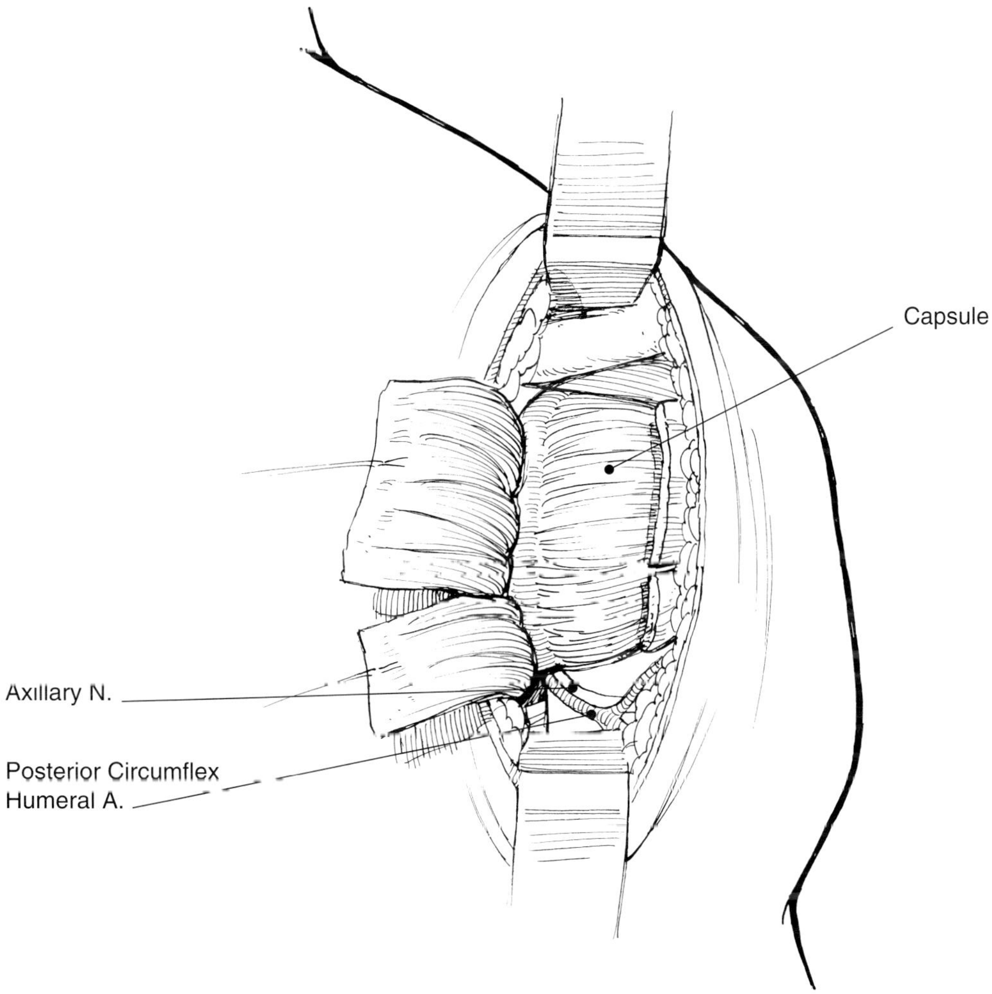


**FIGURE IV-17**

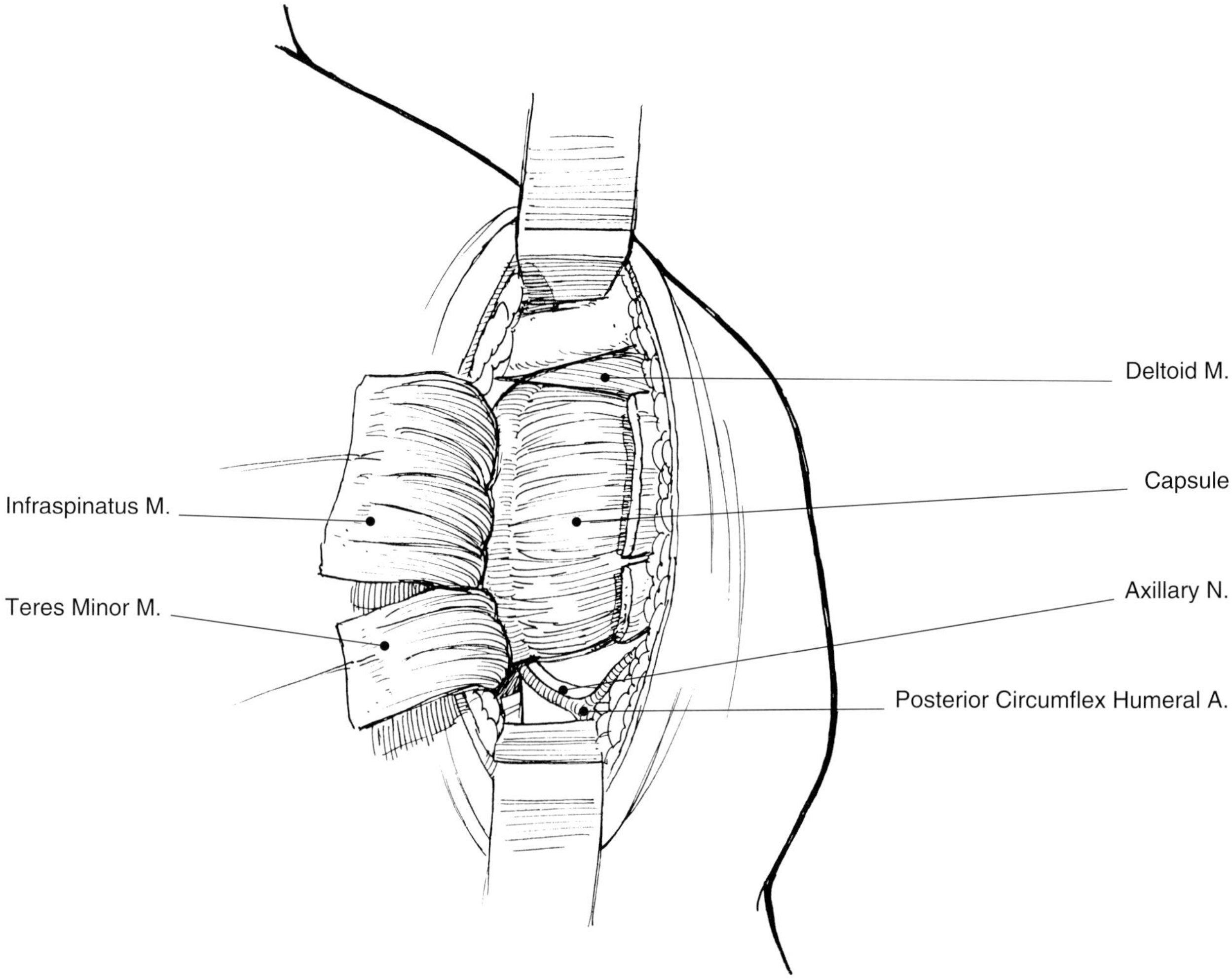
Deltoid M.
Capsule
Infraspinatus M.
Axillary N.
Teres Minor M.
Posterior Circumflex Humeral A.

**FIGURE IV–18**

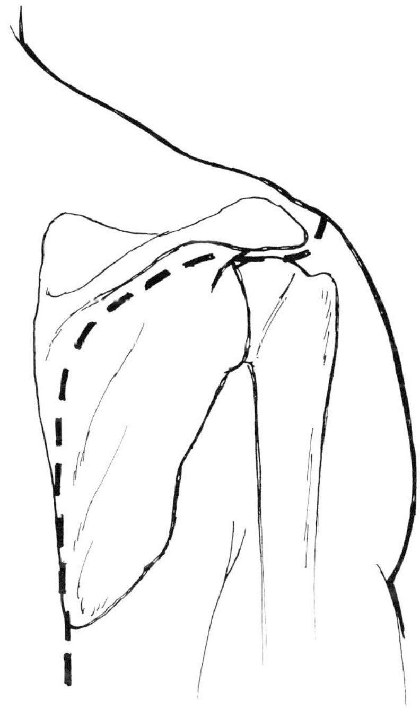

**FIGURE IV–19**

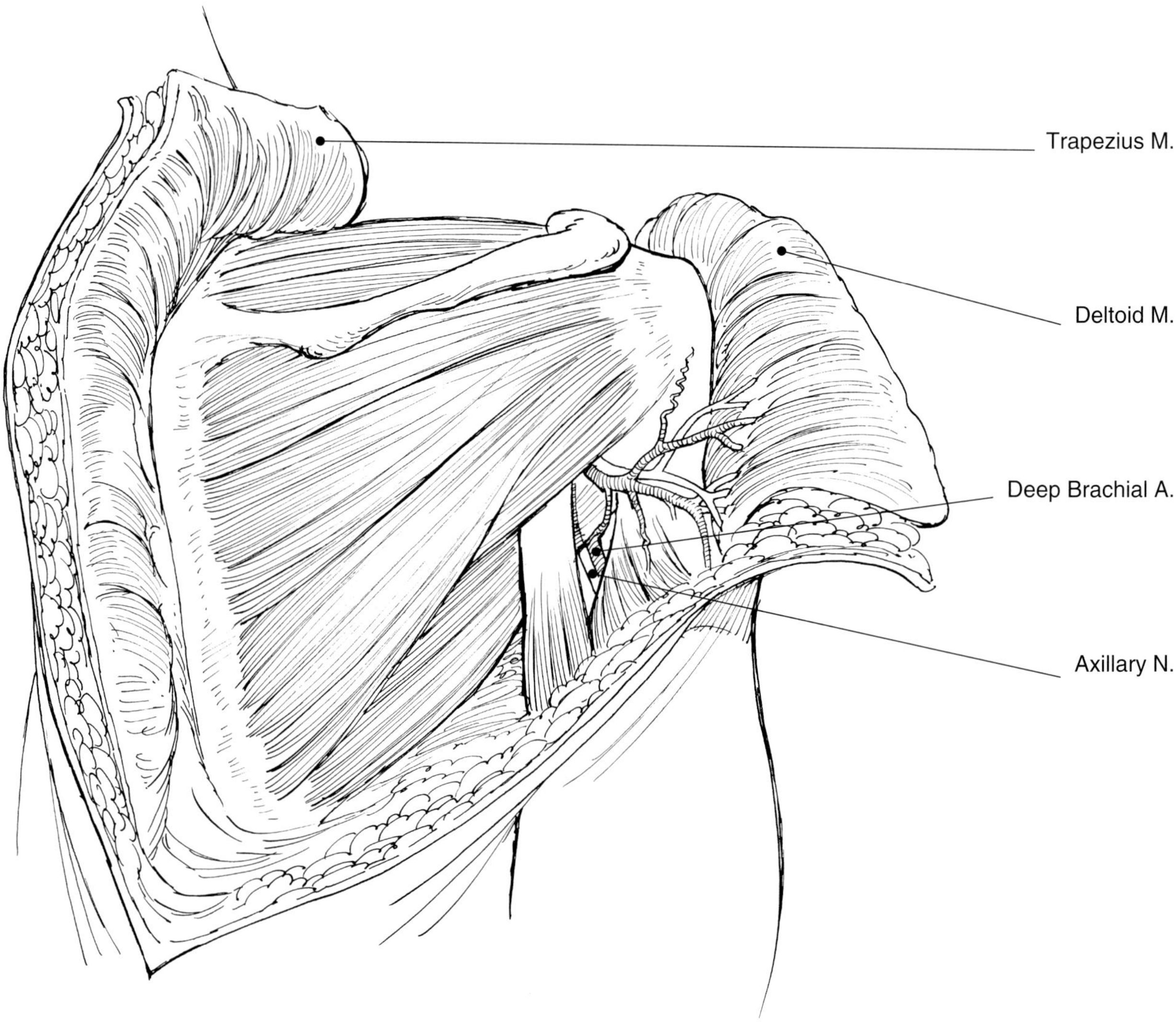


**FIGURE IV–20**

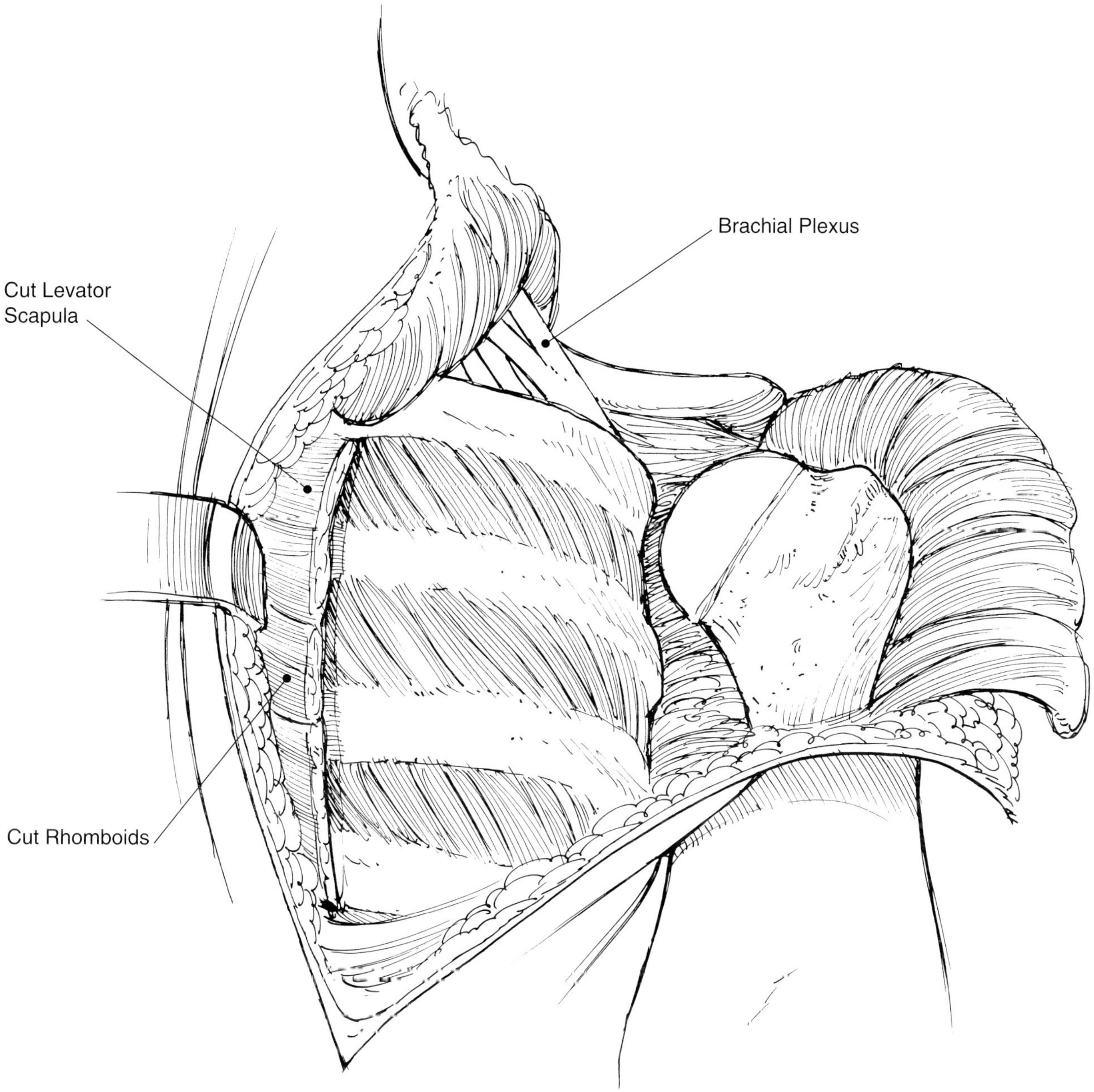


**FIGURE IV–21**

***Limitations***

Through the vertical posterior incision, access is limited to the glenoid neck and the posterior aspect of the joint. The longitudinal incision can be carried as far as necessary for any extensive procedure around the scapula and proximal humerus. Keeping the dissection deep to the enveloping muscles (trapezius and deltoid) allows extensive flaps to be retracted to expose the lateral neck and chest wall as necessary while preserving a reliable blood supply to the skin. With total scapulectomy, these sheets of muscle can be reapproximated to aid in suspending the extremity.

# References


1. Malawer MM. Tumors of the shoulder girdle. Technique of resection and description of a surgical classification. Orthop Clin North Am 22(1):7–35, 1991.
2. Harryman DT. Common surgical approaches to the shoulder. Instructional Course Lecture 41:3–11, 1992.
3. Neer CS. Prosthetic replacement of the humeral head: indications and operative technique. Surg Clin North Am 43:1581, 1963.
4. Leslie JT Jr, Ryan TJ. The anterior axillary incision to approach the shoulder joint. J Bone Joint Surg 44:1193, 1962.
5. Rowe K, Vee LBK. A posterior approach to the shoulder joint. J Bone Joint Surg 26:580, 1944.

# V

# SURGICAL APPROACHES TO THE HUMERUS

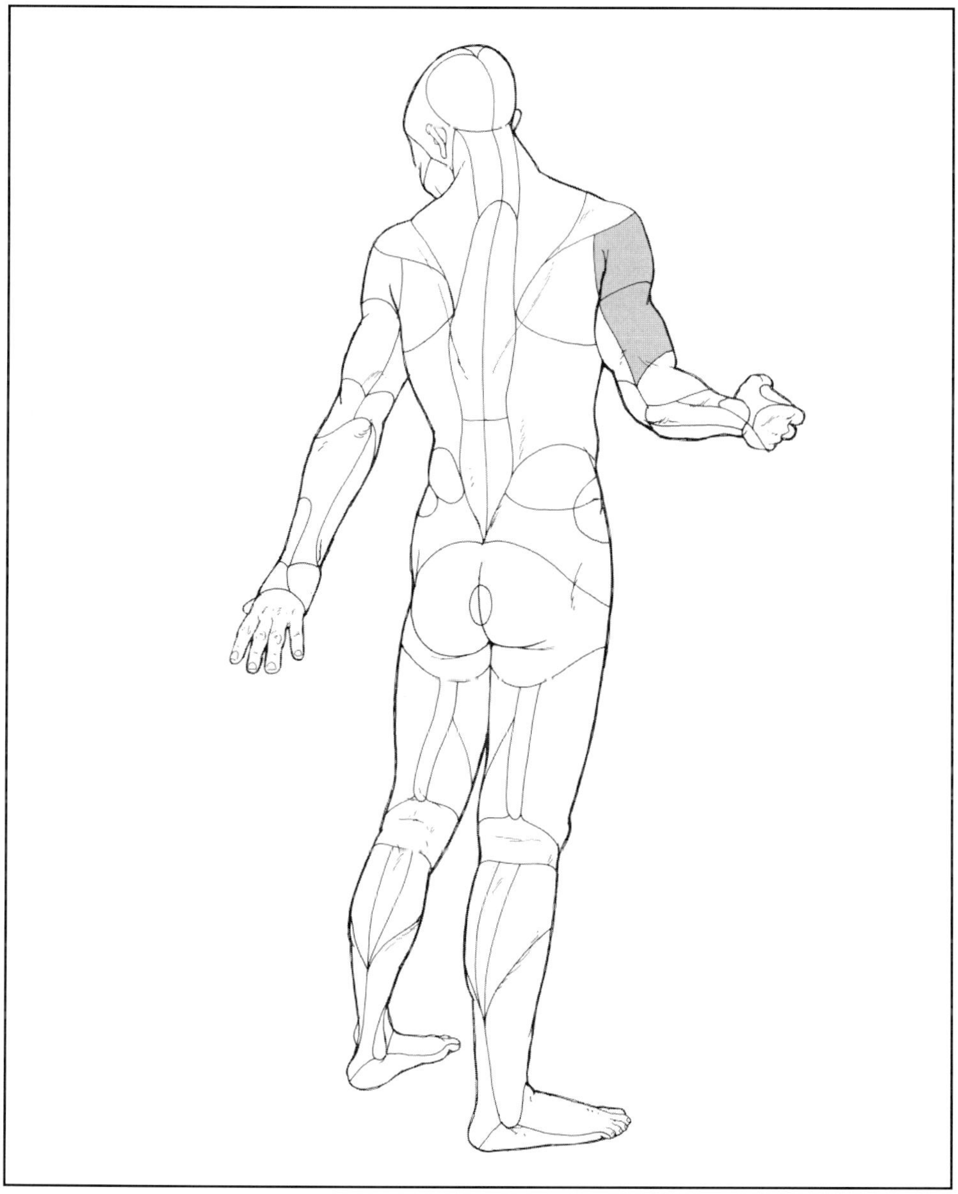

# General Principles and Complications

Surgical exposure of the humerus is relatively simple and has been well described by Henry (1). The most common complication is injury to the radial nerve. The radial nerve is intimately attached to the humerus as it spirals around the diaphysis. Therefore, most surgery on the humerus begins by identifying and mobilizing this nerve. A medial approach requires dissection of the axillary vessels as well as the median and ulnar nerves. Posterior approaches are rarely used because of the loss of elbow extension caused by disruption of the triceps muscle.

# Surgical Anatomy

The arm is divided into anterior (flexor) and posterior (extensor) compartments. The anterior compartment consists of the coracobrachialis, biceps, and brachialis (V-1). The musculocutaneous nerve supplies and traverses the anterior compartment, passing between the biceps and brachialis. The brachial artery runs in the anterior compartment, medial to the humerus, until it reaches the distal third. Here it passes laterally to run down the anterior surface to the elbow (V-2). The ulnar nerve runs posterior to the brachial artery in the anterior compartment until it reaches the distal third of the arm where it pierces the medial intermuscular septum to pass posterior to the medial epicondyle.

The posterior compartment consists of the triceps brachii and is supplied by the radial nerve (V-3). The radial nerve passes along the posterior wall of the axilla to run anterior to the long head of the triceps and the teres major against the posterior shaft of the humerus. The nerve then runs in the spiral groove beneath the lateral and medial heads of the triceps. After providing motor branches to the triceps, the radial nerve pierces the lateral intermuscular septum to enter the anterior compartment where it lies between the brachioradialis and the brachialis (V-4). It is tethered in the spiral groove and also as it passes through the lateral intermuscular septum. The profunda brachii artery follows the radial nerve to supply the posterior compartment.

## Anterolateral Approach to the Humerus

***Applications***

This extensile approach allows access to the entire length of the humeral shaft along its anterior surface. It can be continued proximally as the anterior approach to the shoulder and distally as the anterolateral approach to the elbow. It is most commonly used for fixation of fractures of the humerus, but it can also be used for tumor resection in the anterior compartment or to explore the radial nerve in the middle and distal arm.

***Technique***

The patient is placed in the lateral decubitus position or supine with the extremity on an arm board. A longitudinal incision is made, beginning at the coracoid and extending distally and laterally to follow the contour of the anterior deltoid. The incision is then carried distally along the posterior lateral edge of the biceps (V-5). The incision may be carried distally into the depression between the biceps and the brachioradialis. The fascia is opened and the cephalic vein is reflected laterally (V-6). The deltoid is retracted laterally and the biceps medially to expose the proximal humeral shaft (V-7). The radial nerve should be identified and protected as it enters the anterior compartment in the distal arm (V-8). The brachialis muscle can then be elevated from the midhumerus (V-9). The radial nerve is

*(continued on page 97)*

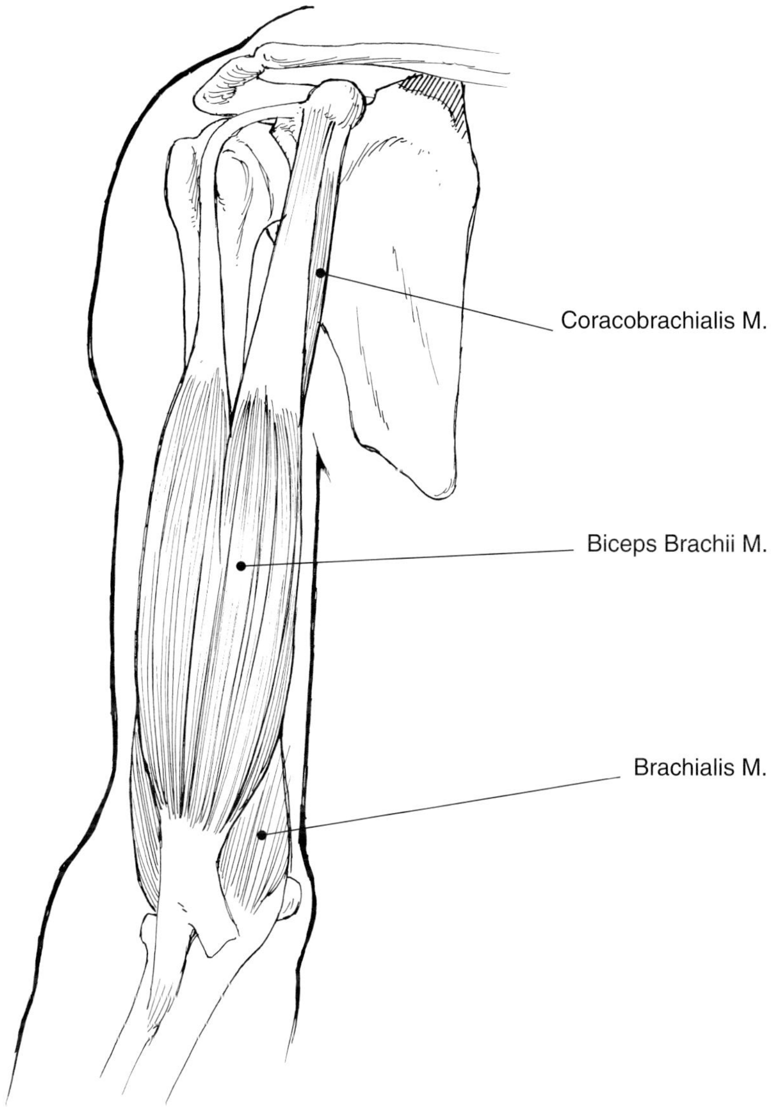


**FIGURE V–1**

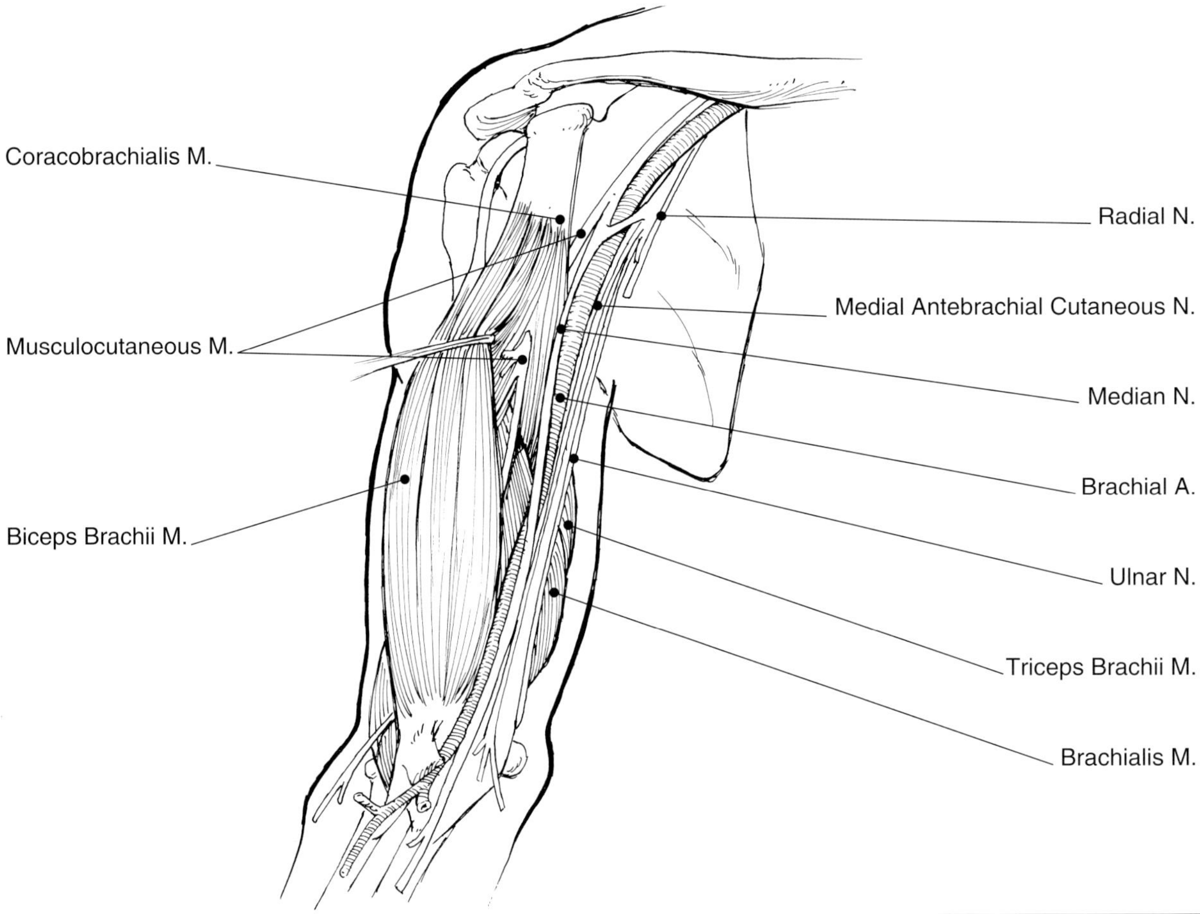
Coracobrachialis M.
Musculocutaneous M.
Biceps Brachii M.
Radial N.
Medial Antebrachial Cutaneous N.
Median N.
Brachial A.
Ulnar N.
Triceps Brachii M.
Brachialis M.

**FIGURE V-2**

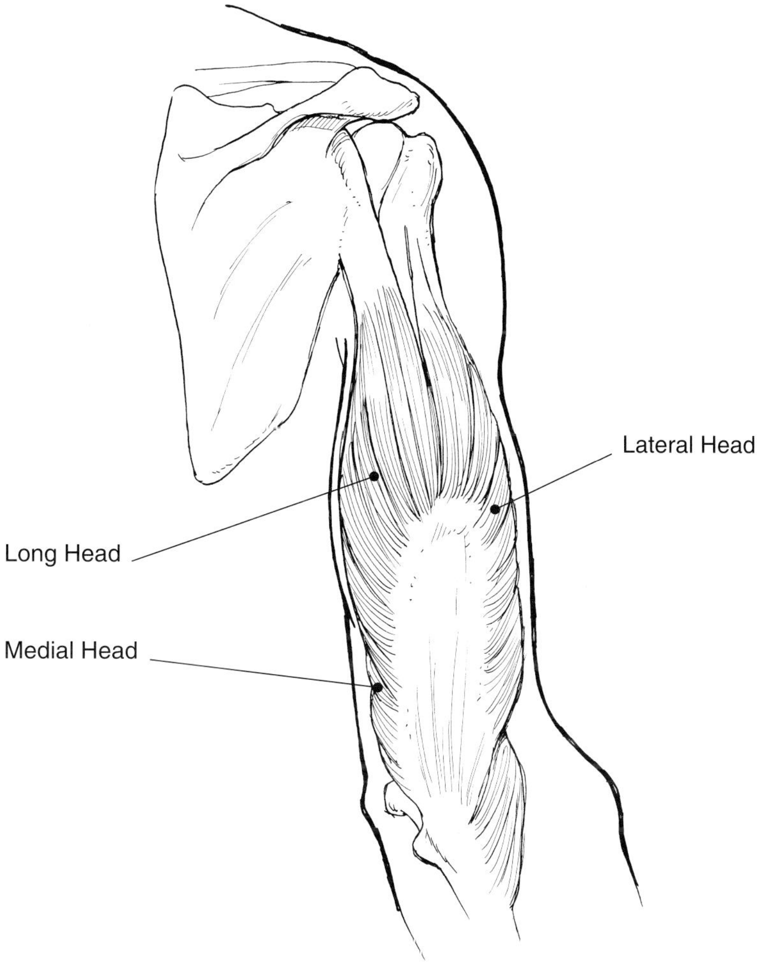


**FIGURE V-3**

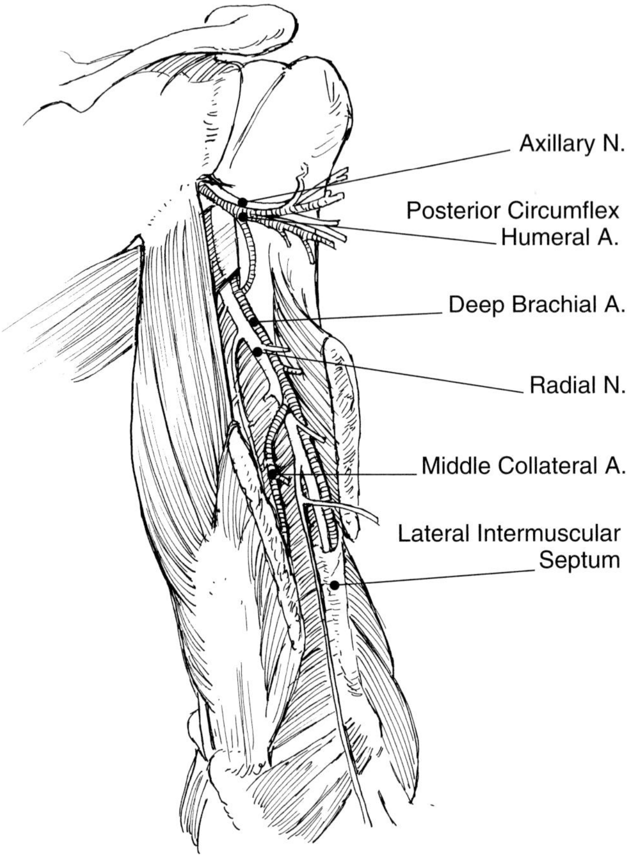


**FIGURE V-4**

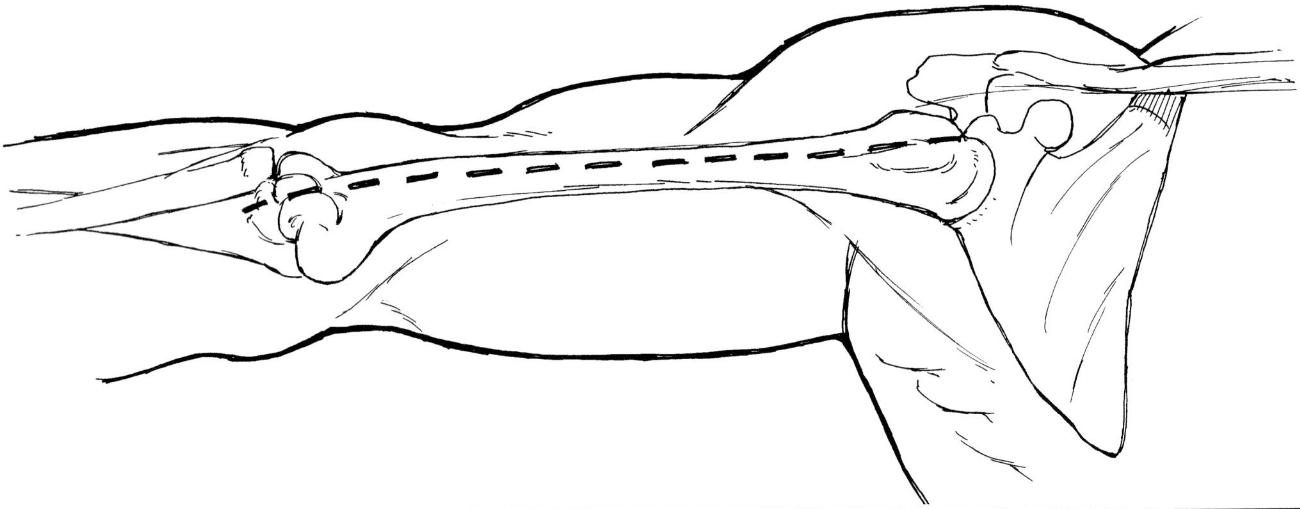

**FIGURE V-5**

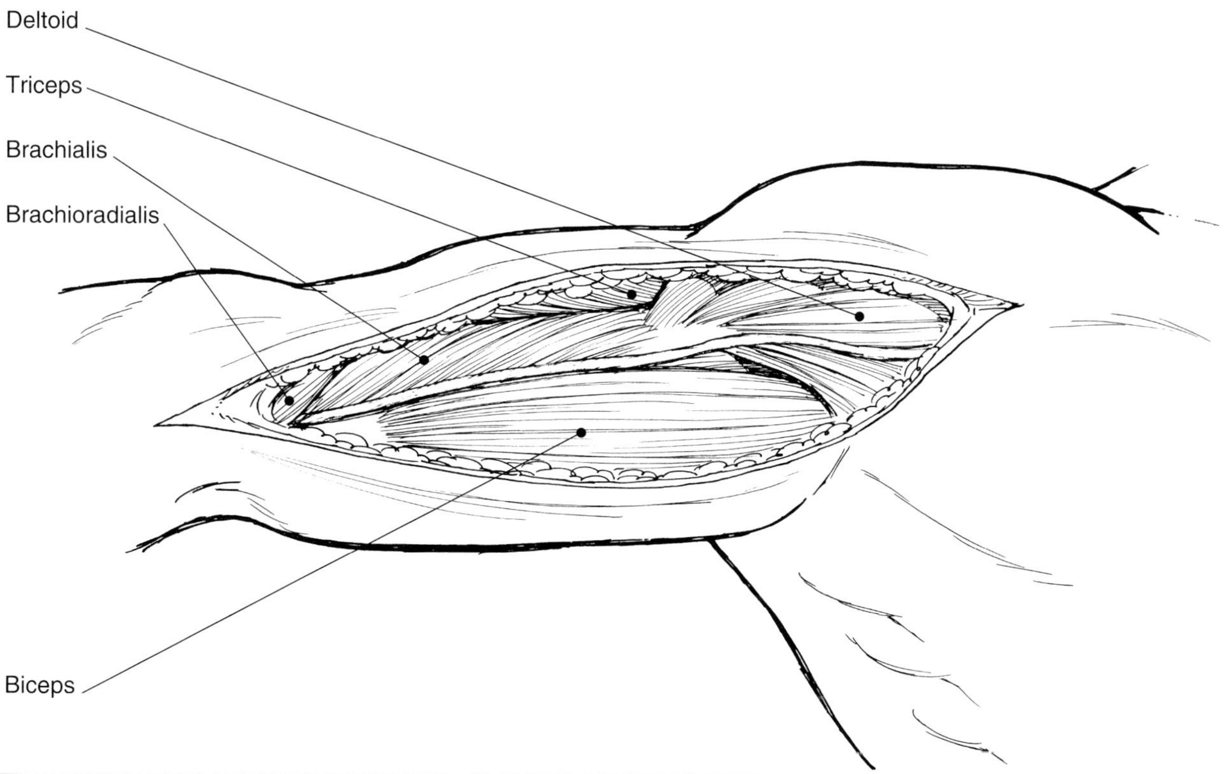


**FIGURE V-6**

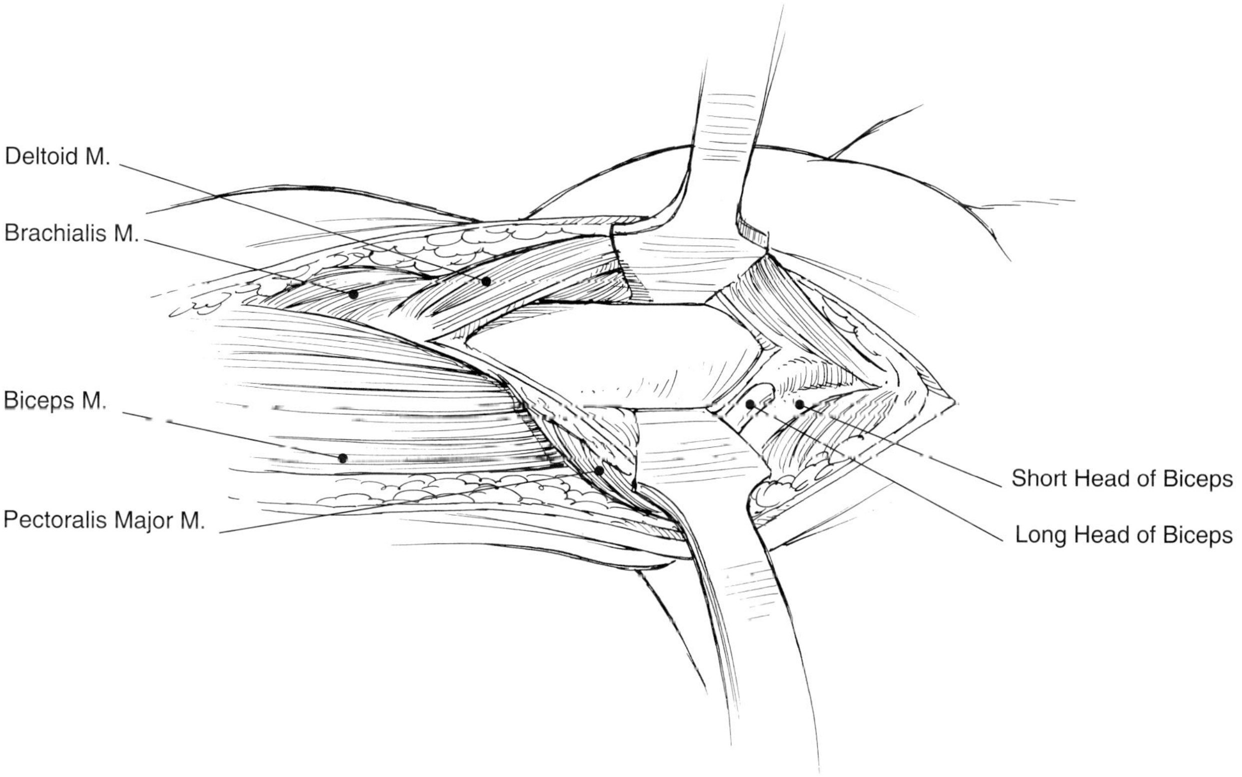


**FIGURE V-7**

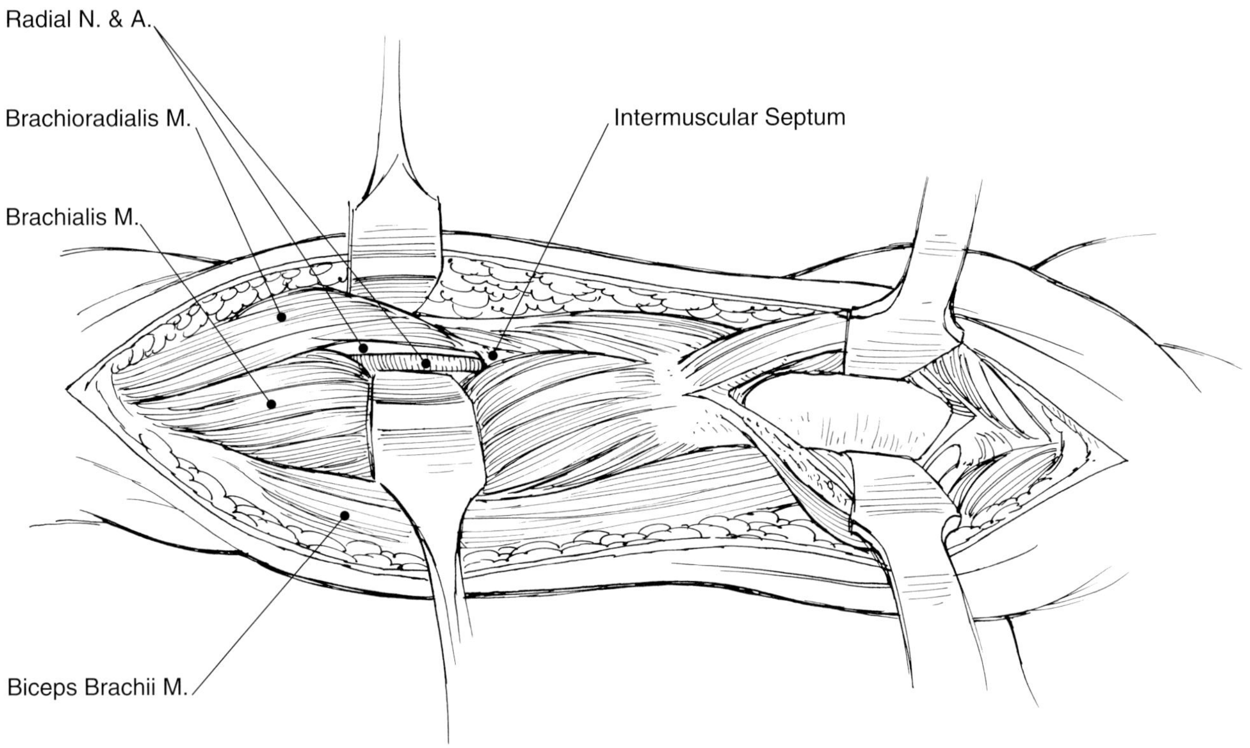


**FIGURE V–8**

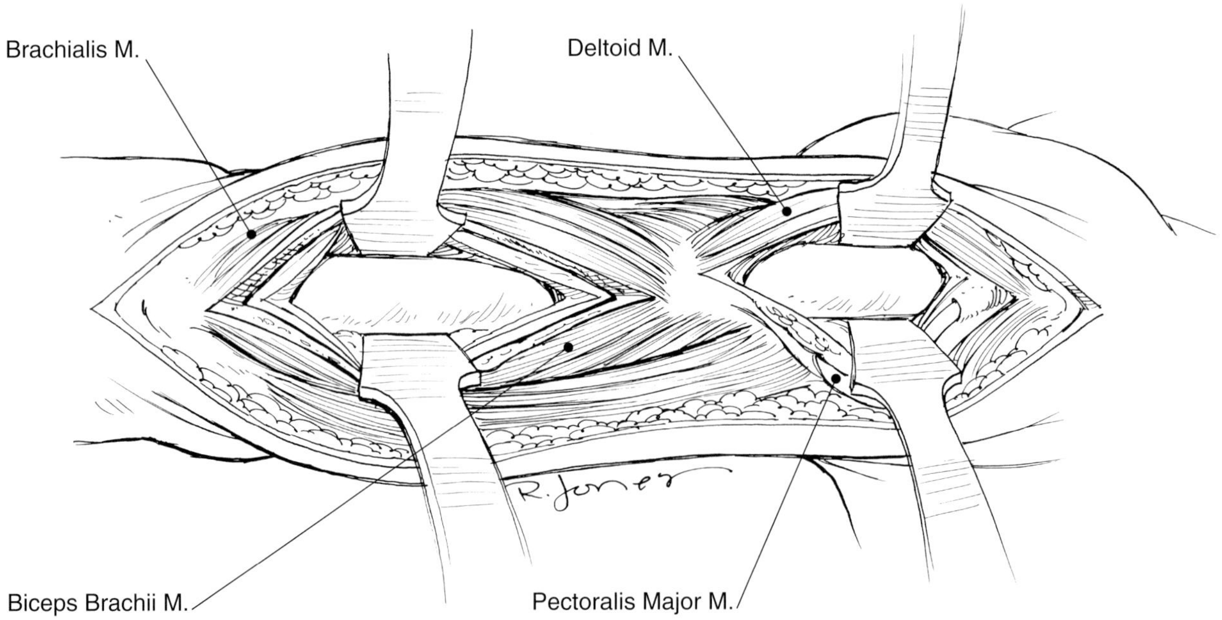


**FIGURE V–9**

traced into the distal forearm between the brachioradialis and the brachialis. The nerve is mobilized and retracted gently to allow subperiosteal elevation of the brachialis to expose the anterior shaft of the humerus.

*Dangers*

The critical part of this dissection is preservation of the radial nerve. The musculocutaneous nerve lies between the biceps and brachialis and is not likely to be damaged as long as the dissection stays deep to the brachialis.

*Limitations*

The entire extent of this approach is rarely needed. In most cases, only a portion is necessary. When more extensive exposure is needed, for example during radial nerve exploration, the incision can be carried distally into the anterior elbow and forearm.

## Posterior Approach to the Proximal Humerus

*Applications*

This approach is rarely necessary, but it can be useful for excision of a tumor of the proximal part of the posterior compartment of the arm or the posterior humerus. It allows direct exposure of the posterior surface of the proximal third of the humerus (2).

*Technique*

The patient is placed in the lateral decubitus position. The incision begins approximately 3 cm distal to the base of the acromion in the interval between the posterior deltoid and the lateral head of the triceps. It extends to the level of the deltoid tuberosity (V-10). The fascia is opened and the interval between the deltoid and the lateral head of the triceps is opened onto the periosteum. The periosteum is incised and the lateral triceps is elevated subperiosteally and retracted laterally (V-11). The radial nerve and profunda brachii artery are defined as they pass through the triceps to enter the spiral groove just proximal to the deltoid tuberosity (V-12). The lateral head of the triceps originates distally along the lateral edge of the spiral groove. The deltoid can be retracted laterally and mobilized proximally until the axillary nerve and the posterior humeral circumflex vessels are encountered.

*Dangers*

The danger of this approach is the proximity to the radial and axillary nerves. There should be minimal medial retraction of the triceps to decrease the risk of injury to these structures.

*Limitations*

This approach is limited proximally by the axillary nerve and posterior humeral circumflex vessels and distally by the radial nerve.

## Posterior Approach to the Distal Humerus

*Applications*

This approach provides access to the distal two-thirds of the humerus. It is useful for fracture fixation, debridement of infection, or excision of tumors.

*Technique*

The patient is placed in the lateral decubitus position. The incision is made in the midline of the posterior arm from the level of the deltoid tuberosity to the olecranon fossa (V-13). The fascia is incised, and the long and lateral heads of the triceps are split from proximal to distal, incising the aponeurosis longitudinally (V-14). The radial nerve will be found in the spiral groove in the proximal end of the dissection, at the proximal origin of the medial (deep) head of the triceps (V-15).

*(continued on page 103)*

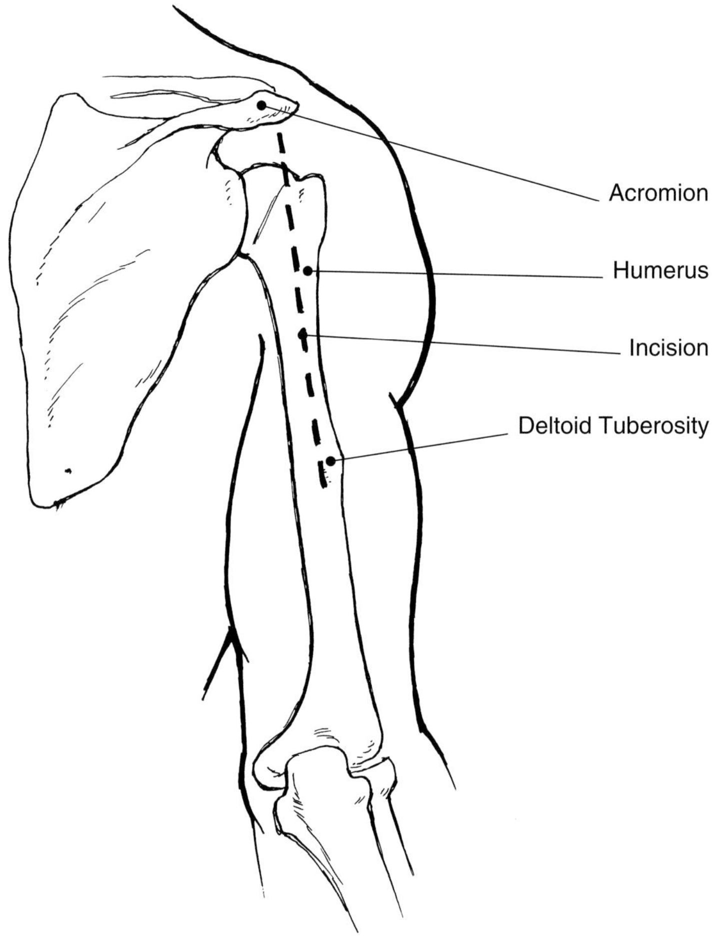


**FIGURE V–10**

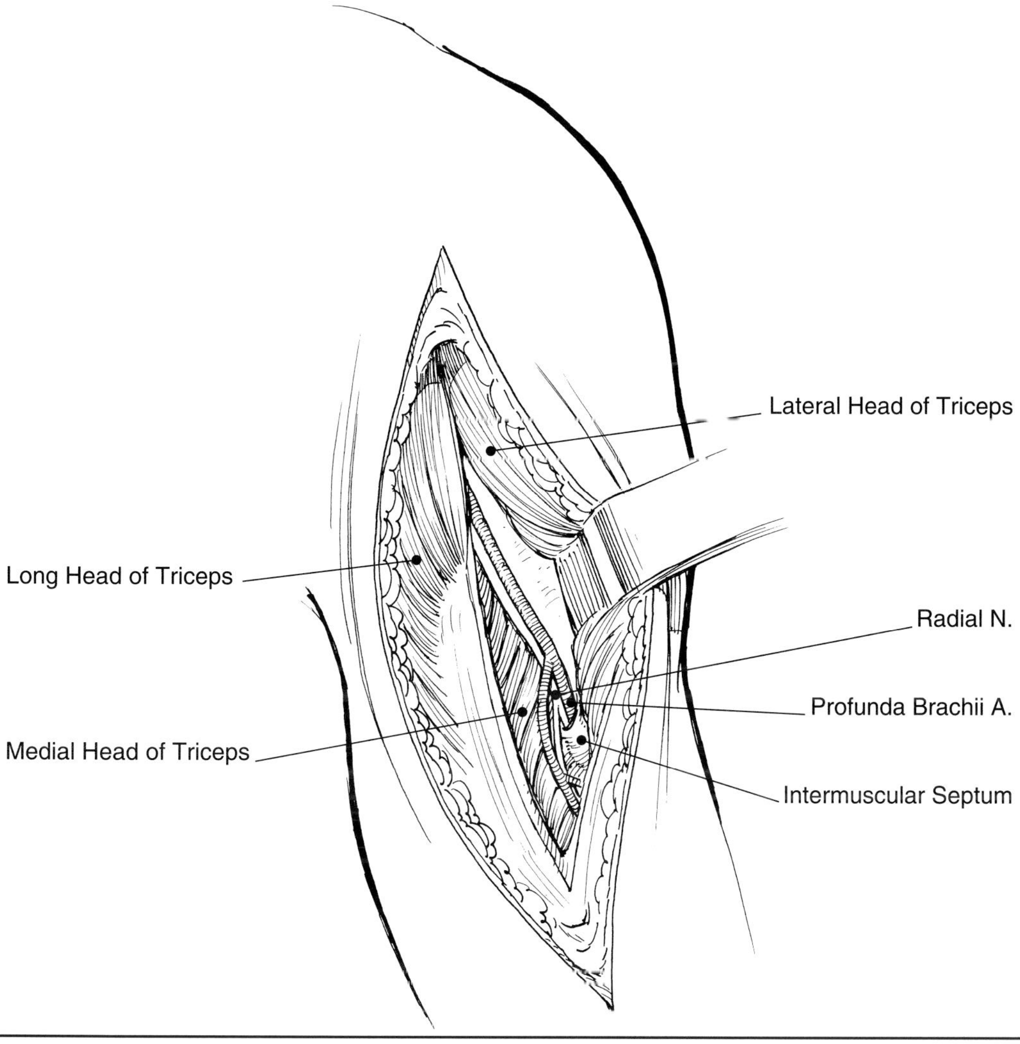
Lateral Head of Triceps
Long Head of Triceps
Radial N.
Profunda Brachii A.
Medial Head of Triceps
Intermuscular Septum

**FIGURE V–11**

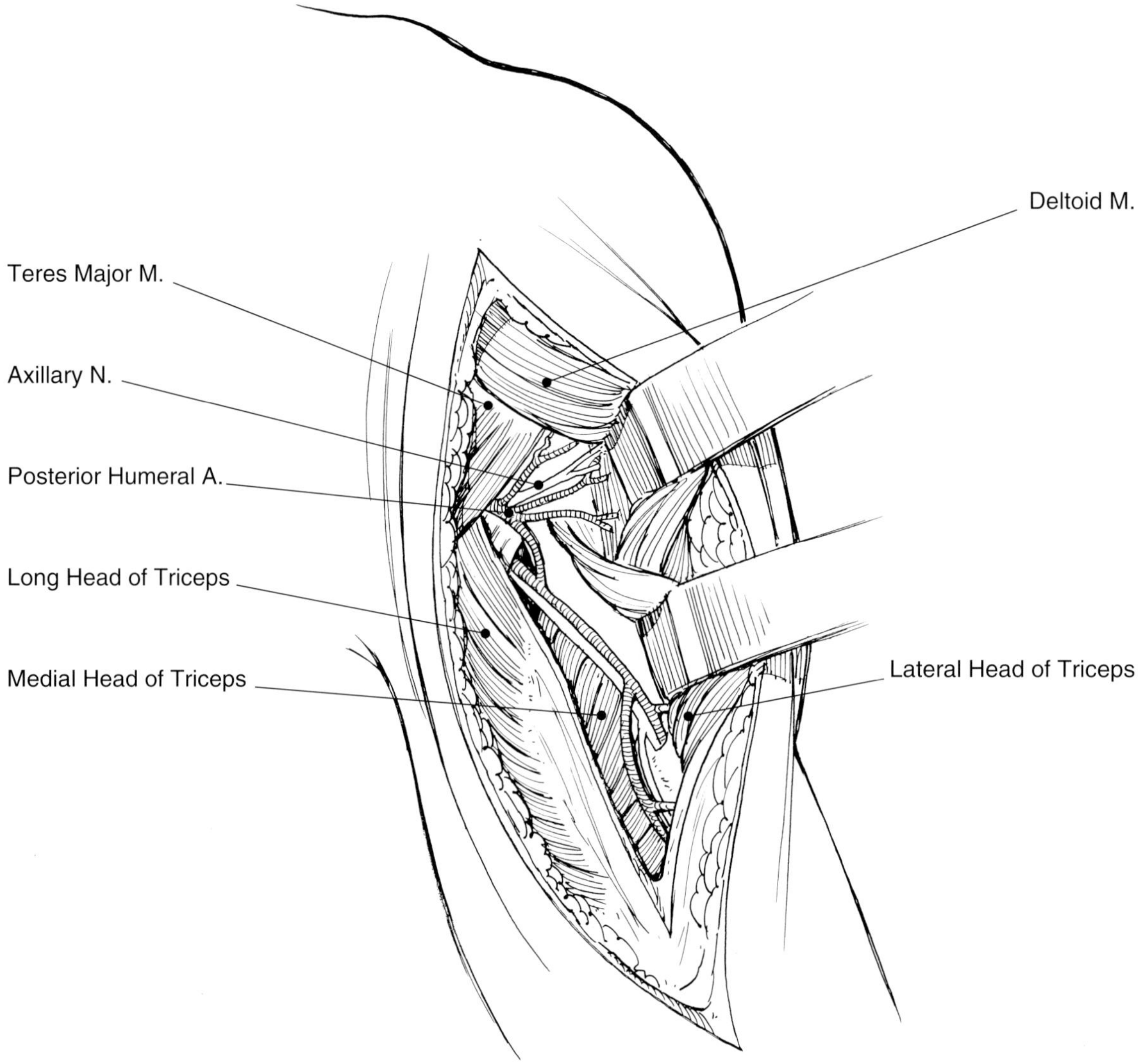
Deltoid M.
Teres Major M.
Axillary N.
Posterior Humeral A.
Long Head of Triceps
Medial Head of Triceps
Lateral Head of Triceps

**FIGURE V–12**

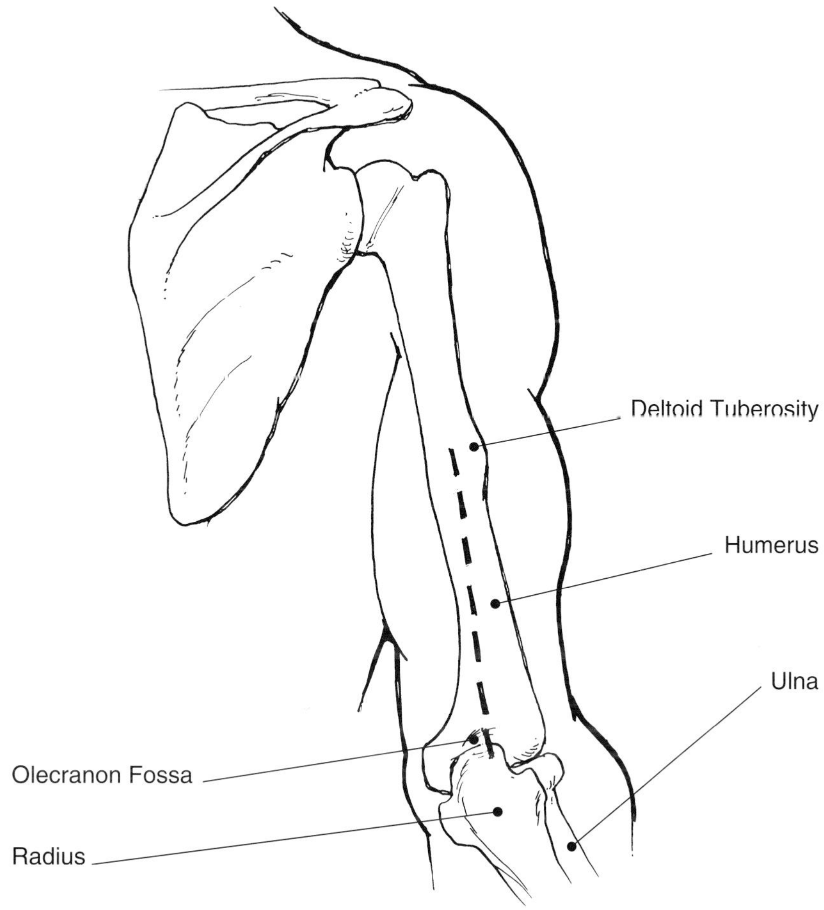


**FIGURE V–13**

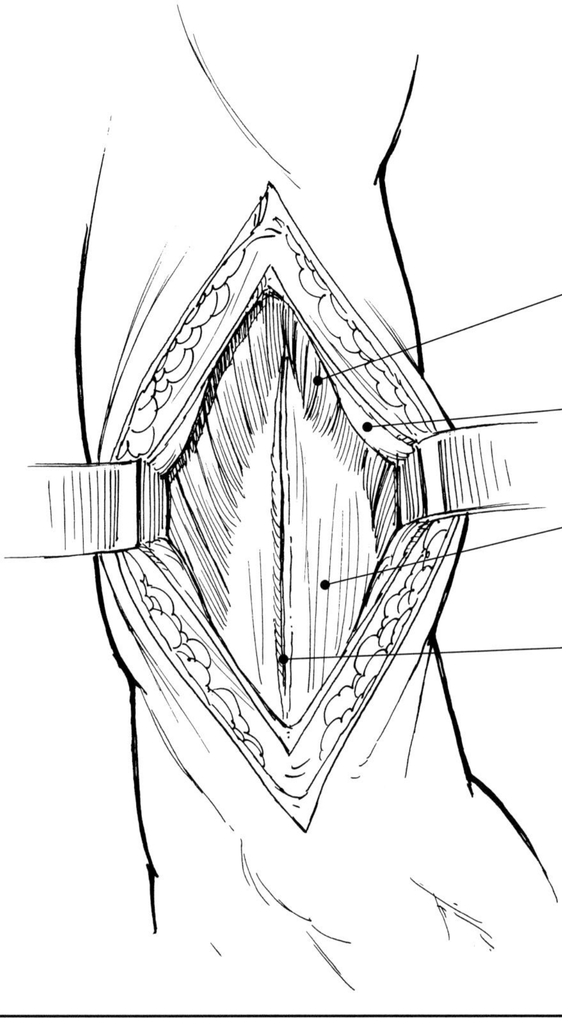


**FIGURE V–14**

Once the nerve is identified, the belly of the medial head can be split longitudinally and elevated from the posterior humerus (V-16).

***Dangers***

The major risks in this dissection are injury to the radial nerve or the ulnar nerve. The ulnar nerve is protected by avoiding excision or retraction of the medial head of the triceps.

***Limitations***

This approach is limited proximally by the radial nerve. Distally, the incision can be carried into the elbow; however, this is infrequently done because splitting the triceps leads to elbow stiffness.

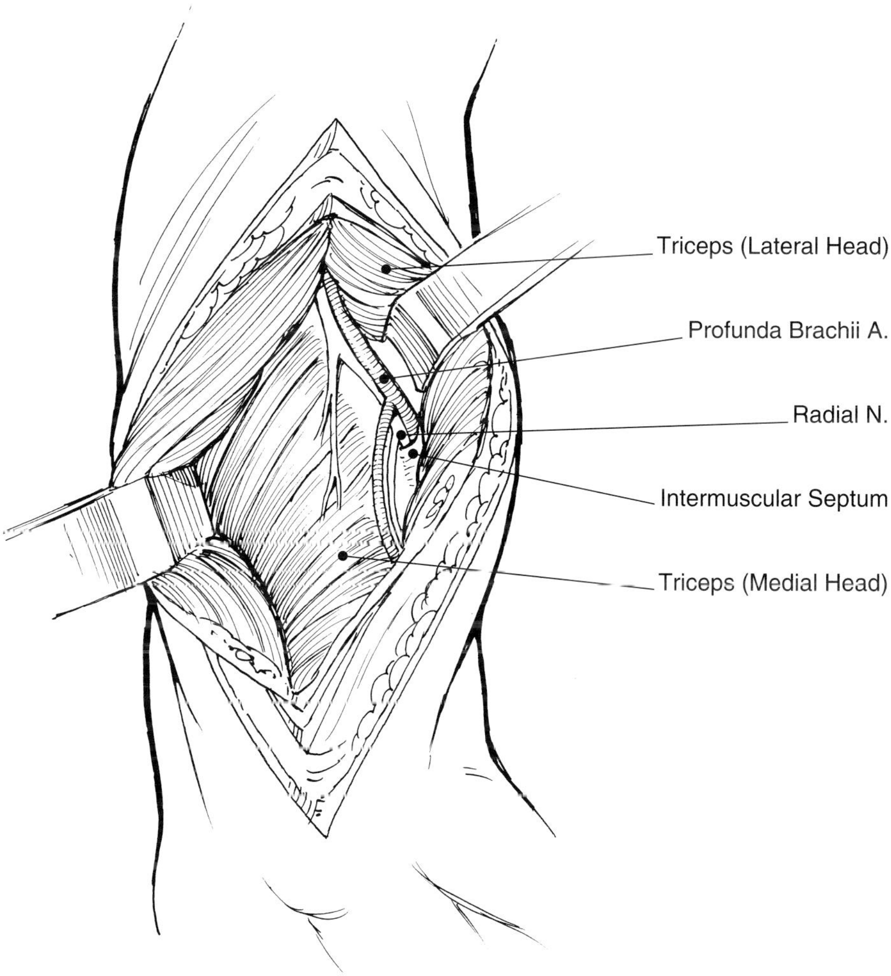


**FIGURE V–15**

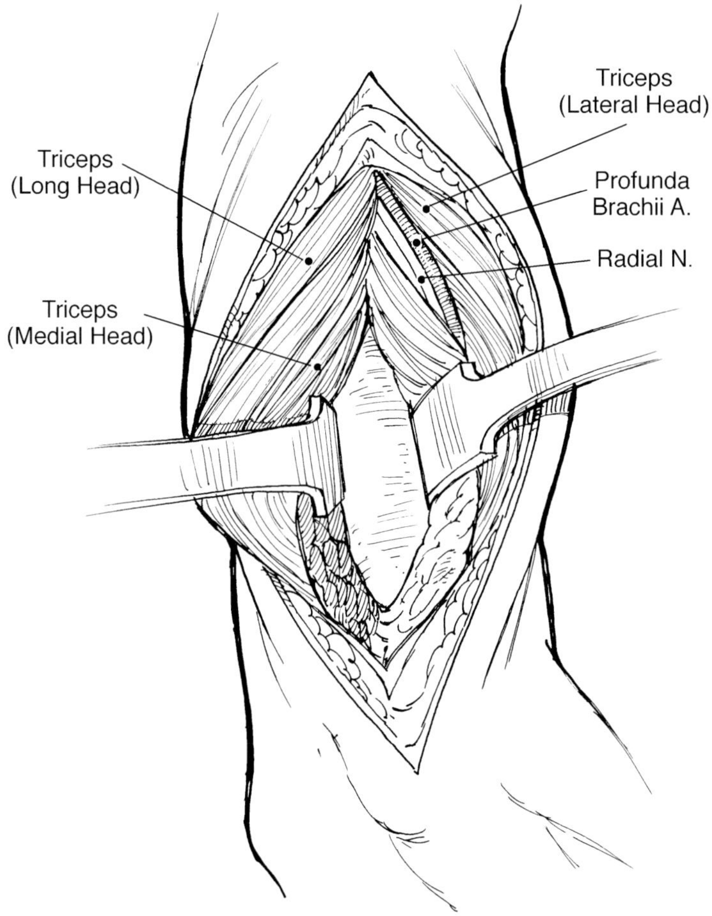
Triceps
(Lateral Head)
Triceps
(Long Head)
Profunda
Brachii A.
Radial N.
Triceps
(Medial Head)

**FIGURE V–16**

# Medial Approach to the Humerus

*Applications*

This approach was described for vascularized bone transfer to the humerus for nonunions (3). Its obvious use is for any procedure requiring access to the brachial artery or the median or ulnar nerves in the arm.

*Technique*

The patient is supine with the arm supported on an arm board. The incision is in the midline of the medial arm, beginning 5 cm distal to the axilla, and is carried distally to arc across the antecubital fossa from medial to lateral (V-17). The fascia is incised with scissors to expose the brachial artery, its venae comitantes, and the median nerve (V-18). The musculocutaneous nerve is identified as it enters the coracobrachialis. The coracobrachialis and brachialis can then be elevated subperiosteally from the anterior surface of the humerus (V-19).

*Dangers*

The brachial vessels and musculocutaneous, median, and ulnar nerves are all in the immediate vicinity of this approach and must be protected.

*Limitations*

This approach allows exposure from the distal end of the pectoralis major insertion to the coronoid fossa.

# Compartment Resection in the Arm

Either the anterior compartment or the posterior compartment of the arm can be completely excised to remove malignant tumors, with or without removal of an adjacent segment of the humerus. A defect in the humerus can be reconstructed with an autologous fibular transfer (3). Excision of either compartment begins with a gentle S-shaped incision placed longitudinally over the middle of the compartment throughout its length. The fascia is incised in line with the skin incision without any subcutaneous dissection. Large flaps can be created deep to the fascia as far as the medial and lateral intermuscular septa. The muscles can then be ele-

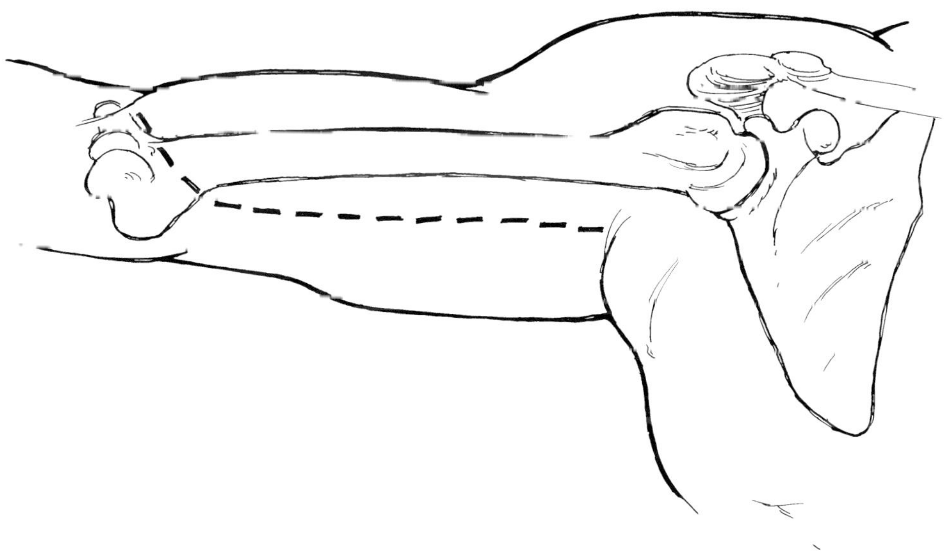

**FIGURE V–17**

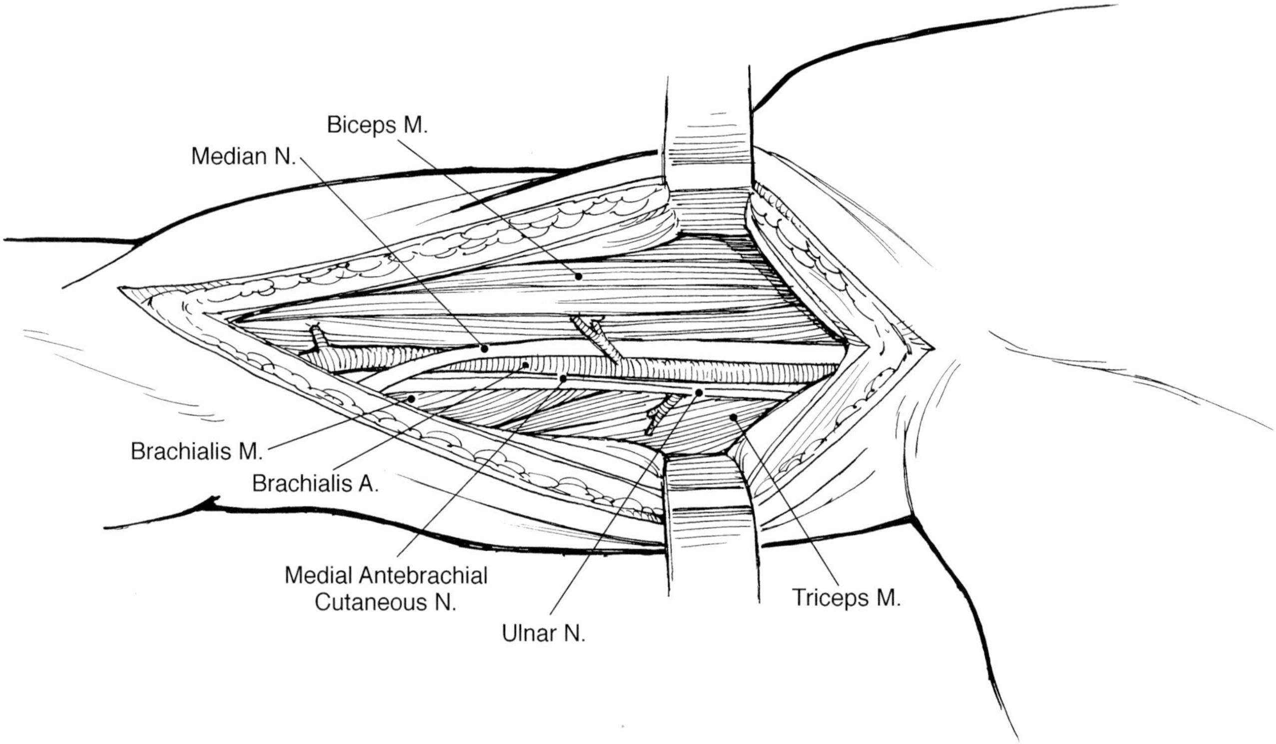


**FIGURE V–18**

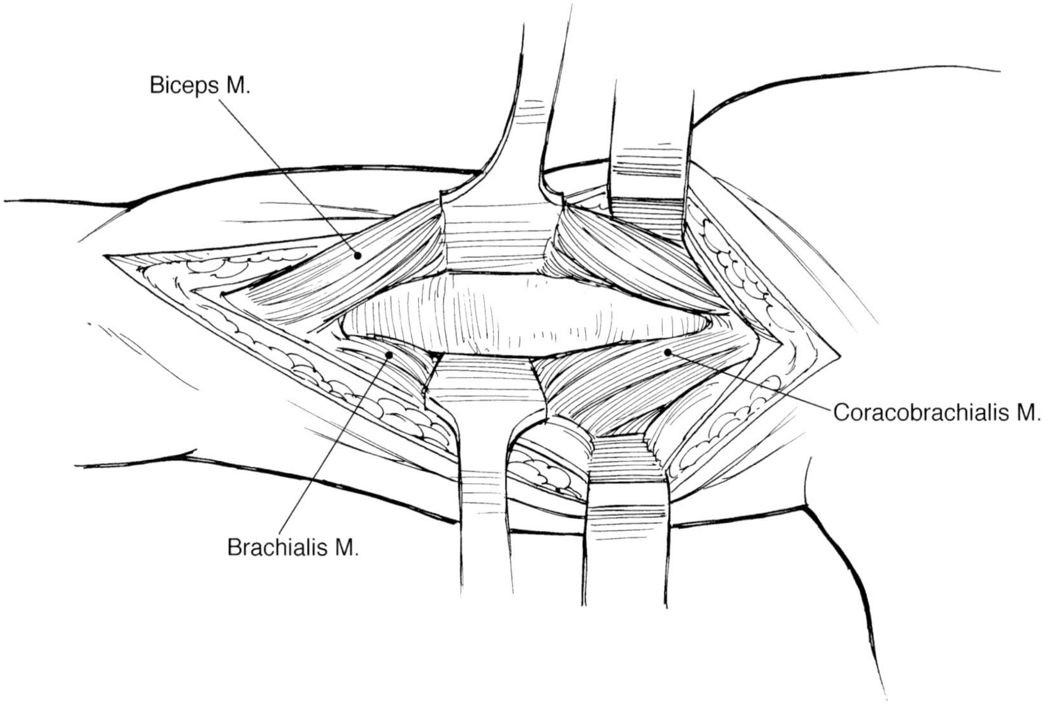


**FIGURE V–19**

vated from the bone and reflected from proximal to distal. The major compartment vessels should be ligated as they are encountered. If the radial nerve is excised, then tendon transfers will be necessary to obtain extension of the elbow, wrist, fingers, and thumb. Excision of the musculocutaneous nerve requires no reconstruction since elbow flexion will be preserved by the function of the brachioradialis. The median and ulnar nerves should be preserved in the arm. If both are excised, then the hand will be severely limited in function. A segmental reconstruction of the axillary or radial artery is usually feasible. The blood supply to the soft tissues of the arm without the axillary artery, however, is usually satisfactory because of the extensive collateral flow about the shoulder.

## References

1. Henry AK. Extensile Exposure, 2nd ed. Edinburgh: C&S Livingston, 1966.
2. Berger RA, Buckwalter JA. A posterior surgical approach to the proximal part of the humerus. J Bone Joint Surg 71(3):407–410, 1989.
3. Jupiter JB. Complex nonunion of the humeral diaphysis. Treatment with a medial approach, an anterior plate, and a vascularized fibular graft. J Bone Joint Surg 72(5):701–707, 1990.

# VI

# SURGICAL APPROACHES TO THE ELBOW

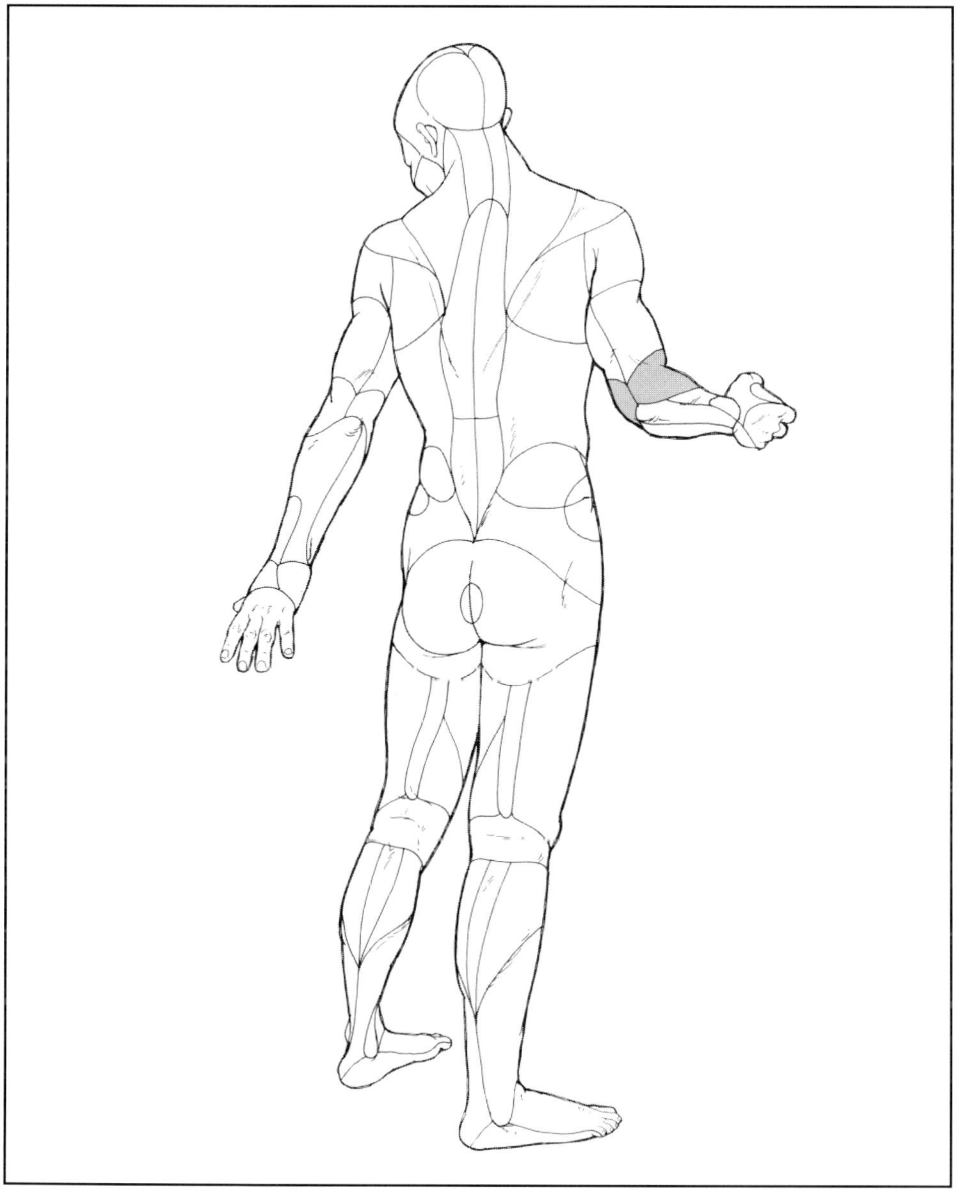

## General Principles and Complications

The elbow is a hinge joint comprised of a tongue-in-groove arrangement between the humerus and the ulna that is supported by strong medial and lateral collateral ligaments. Because of this arrangement, it is difficult to expose the entire joint through any one approach. The widest exposure of the joint can be obtained through a posterior approach. Contemporary surgical approaches to the elbow are designed to minimize disruption of the extensor mechanism and the collateral ligaments to facilitate early motion and rehabilitation of the joint (1). The elbow is surrounded by the radial, median, and ulnar nerves, each of which can be injured by direct manipulation or excessive retraction during surgery. The brachial artery passes anteriorly over the joint where it is also susceptible to damage (VI-1, VI-3). For internal fixation of comminuted intraarticular distal humerus fractures, the surgeon must have adequate exposure to reduce the fragments with minimal disruption of the soft tissue attachments to these fragments to preserve their viability. The posterior approach is usually the most useful for this procedure. Conversely, for release of contractures of the elbow, extensive dissection of the joint capsule and muscles may be necessary to restore joint motion. The anterior approach usually serves this purpose best. The medial collateral ligament is especially crucial to preserving the stability of the joint. If it is released or damaged during the operation, it should be carefully repaired.

## Surgical Anatomy

The elbow is encapsulated by four groups of muscles: anteriorly by the flexors of the elbow, especially the biceps tendon and its aponeurosis; medially by the flexor/pronator group arising from the medial epicondylar ridge of the humerus (VI-1); posteriorly by the aponeurosis of the triceps covering the elbow; and laterally by the extensor/supinator group arising from the lateral epicondylar ridge (VI-2). The median nerve crosses the elbow anteriorly and medially, deep to the bicipital aponeurosis, to pass between the two heads of the pronator teres. The radial nerve crosses the elbow anteriorly and laterally between the brachialis and brachioradialis. It divides at the level of the radiohumeral joint into the posterior interosseous nerve and the superficial radial nerve (VI-3). The ulnar nerve crosses the elbow in the groove in the posterior medial epicondyle to pass into the forearm between the heads of the flexor carpi ulnaris (VI-4). The brachial artery enters the antecubital fossa lateral to the median nerve, passes deep to the bicipital aponeurosis, and bifurcates at this point into the radial and ulnar arteries. The radial artery exits the cubital fossa by passing medial to the biceps tendon and then distally, anterior to the pronator teres. The ulnar artery exits by passing deep to the deep head of the pronator teres.

## Posterior Approach to the Elbow

*Applications*

The posterior approach is most frequently used for fixation of intraarticular distal humerus fractures, elbow arthroplasty, and open reduction of old posterior elbow dislocations and humerus fractures.

*Technique*

The preferred posterior approach is a combination of the principles described by Bryan and Morrey (1) and by Müller et al (2). The transolecranon approach as described by MacAusland (3) provides the same wide exposure as this approach,

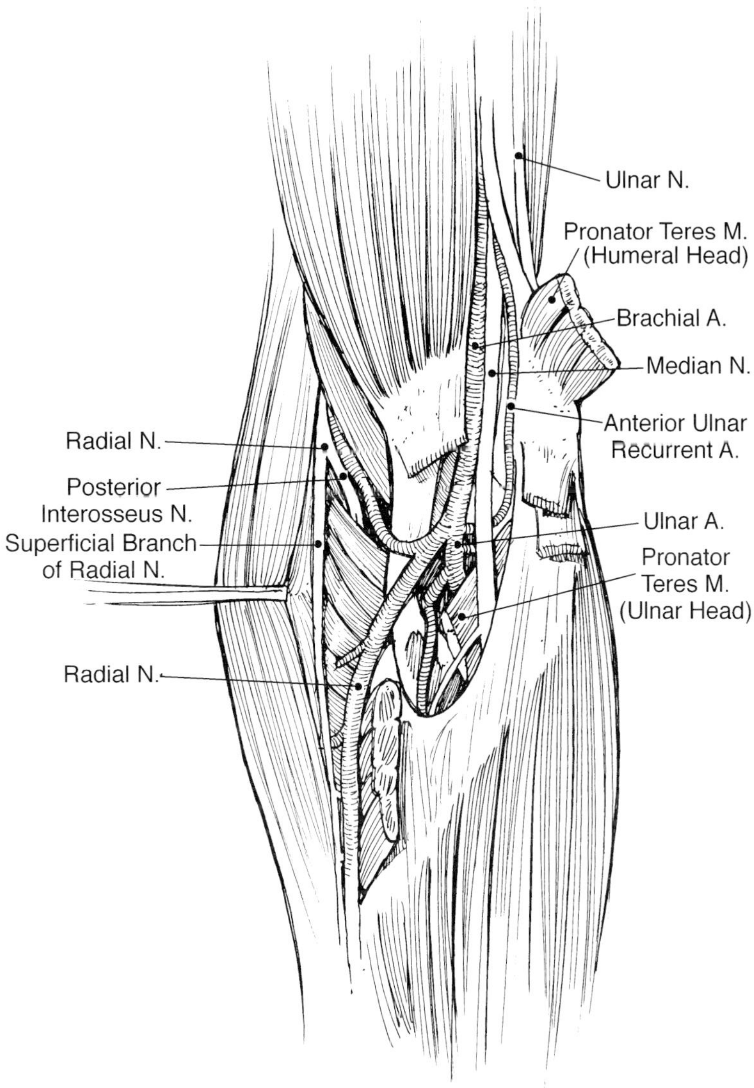
Ulnar N.
Pronator Teres M.
(Humeral Head)
Brachial A.
Median N.
Anterior Ulnar
Recurrent A.
Radial N.
Posterior
Interosseus N.
Superficial Branch
of Radial N.
Ulnar A.
Pronator
Teres M.
(Ulnar Head)
Radial N.

**FIGURE VI-3**

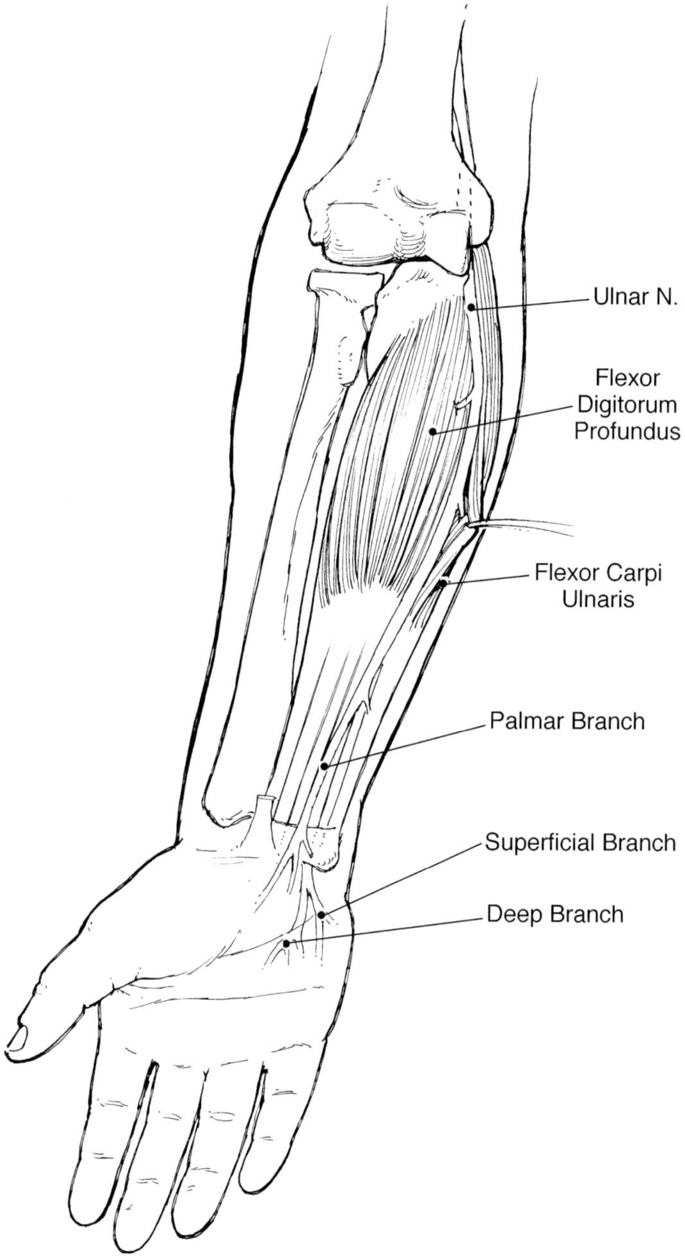
Ulnar N.
Flexor Digitorum Profundus
Flexor Carpi Ulnaris
Palmar Branch
Superficial Branch
Deep Branch

**FIGURE VI-4**

but requires an intraarticular olecranon osteotomy which carries with it a risk of nonunion or avulsion of the extensor mechanism. The posterior approach is usually performed along the medial side of the olecranon, reflecting the triceps laterally. This incision allows mobilization and protection of the ulnar nerve. This approach may be also carried out from the lateral side, retracting the triceps medially, if wider exposure of the lateral condyle is needed.

The patient is placed in the lateral decubitus position. A longitudinal midline posterior incision is made, beginning at the proximal extent of the supracondylar ridges, continuing medial to the apex of the olecranon along the medial edge of the ulna for a distance of 8 cm (VI-5). The ulnar nerve is mobilized from the triceps and freed through its course into the flexor carpi ulnaris. The fascia and joint capsule are incised along the medial border of the ulna, opening the joint capsule (VI-6). This allows visualization of the medial side of the ulna (VI-7). A narrow

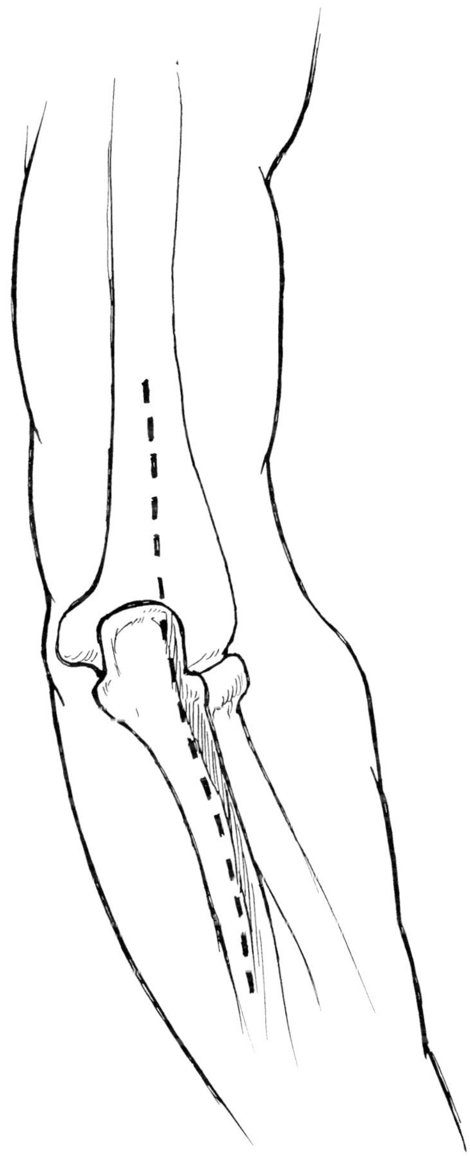

**FIGURE VI-5**

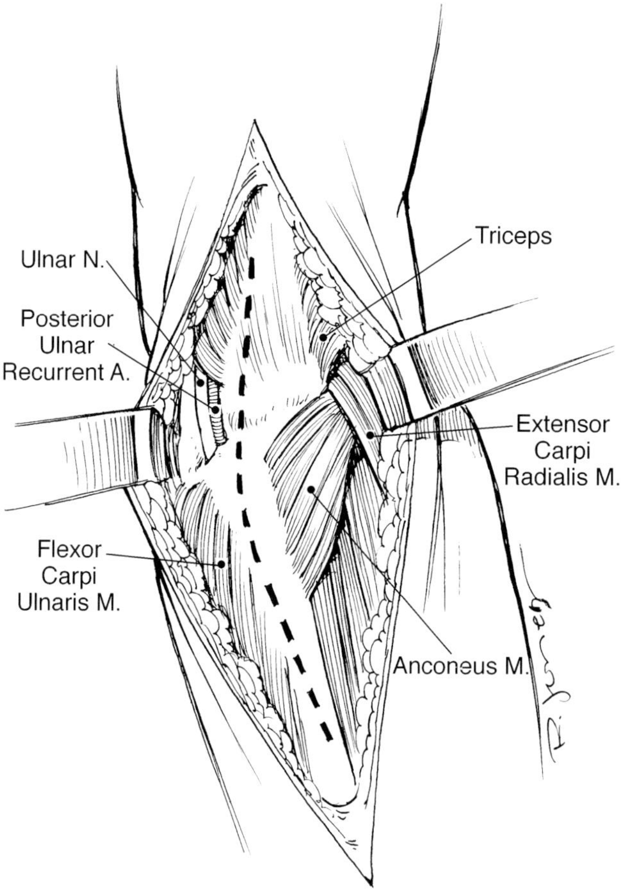


**FIGURE VI-6**

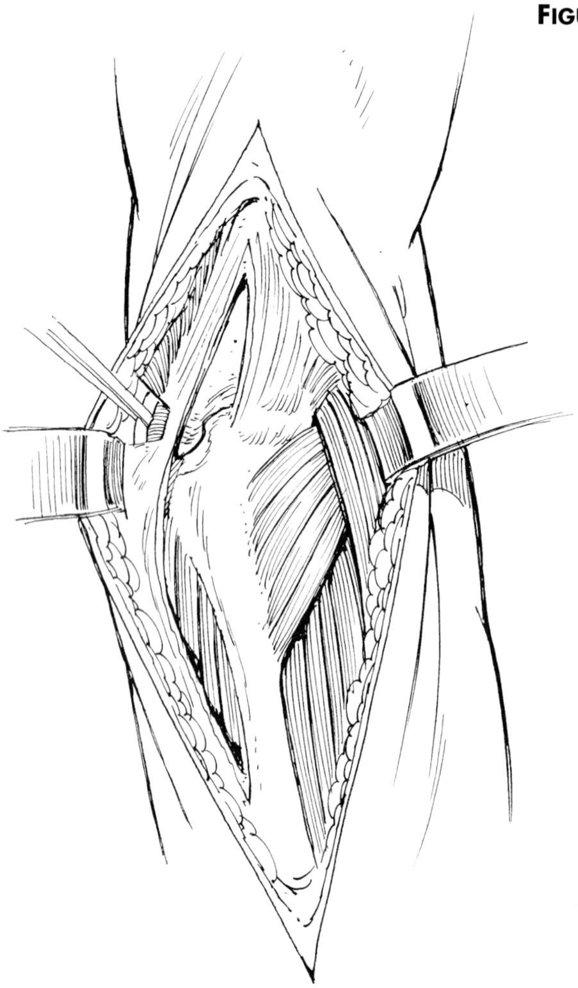

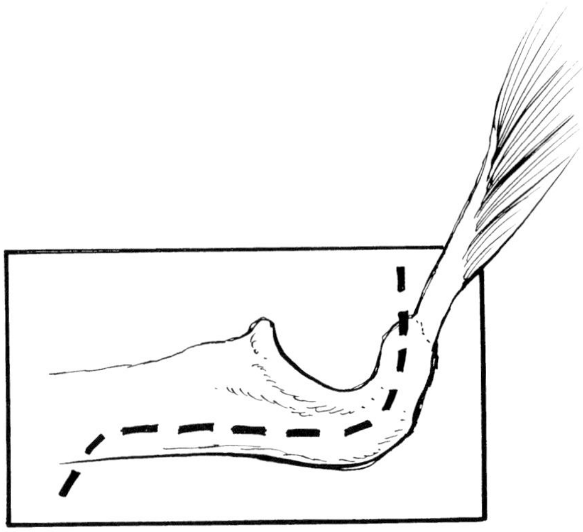

**FIGURE VI-7, VI-8**

(½-inch) curved osteotome is then used to create an osteotomy of the ulna that curves around the tip of the olecranon to preserve the triceps tendon attachment and then continues along the dorsal surface of the ulna for 5 cm (VI-8). Care is taken to complete the osteotomy through the lateral edge of the ulna without disrupting the lateral periosteum or forearm fascia. The flap of bone and periosteum with the triceps tendon attached is then inverted and retracted laterally. The triceps can be elevated from the posterior humerus as necessary to visualize the joint and the distal humerus (VI-9). A retractor can then be placed on the lateral edge of the humerus to provide wide exposure of the joint. Holding the joint in extension relaxes the triceps to facilitate exposure. For closure, the triceps and osseous sleeve are placed back in anatomic position and reattached with sutures placed through drill holes in the ulna, incorporating the periosteum and the forearm fascia (VI-10).

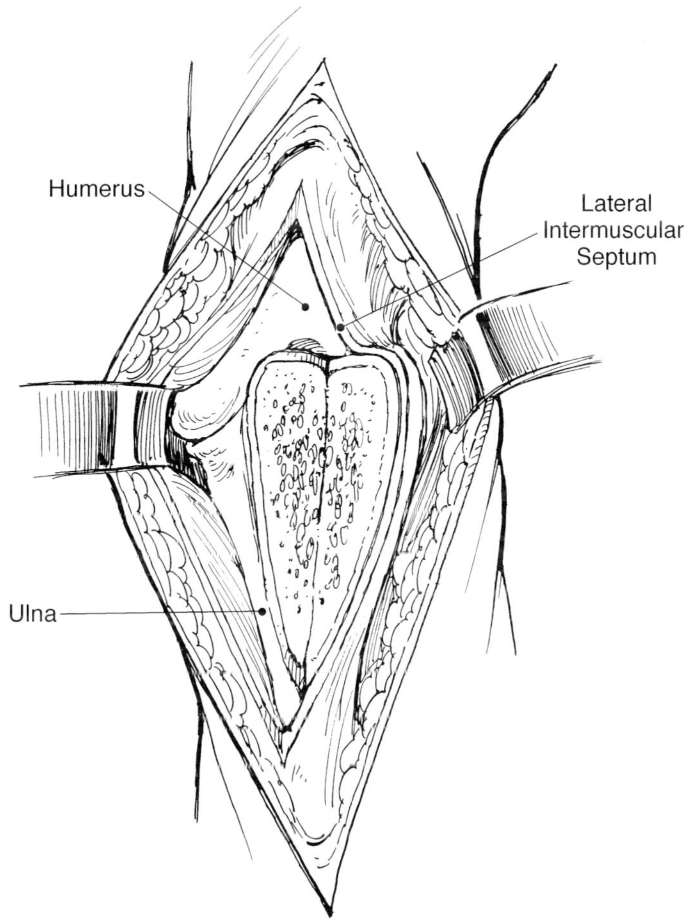


**FIGURE VI–9**

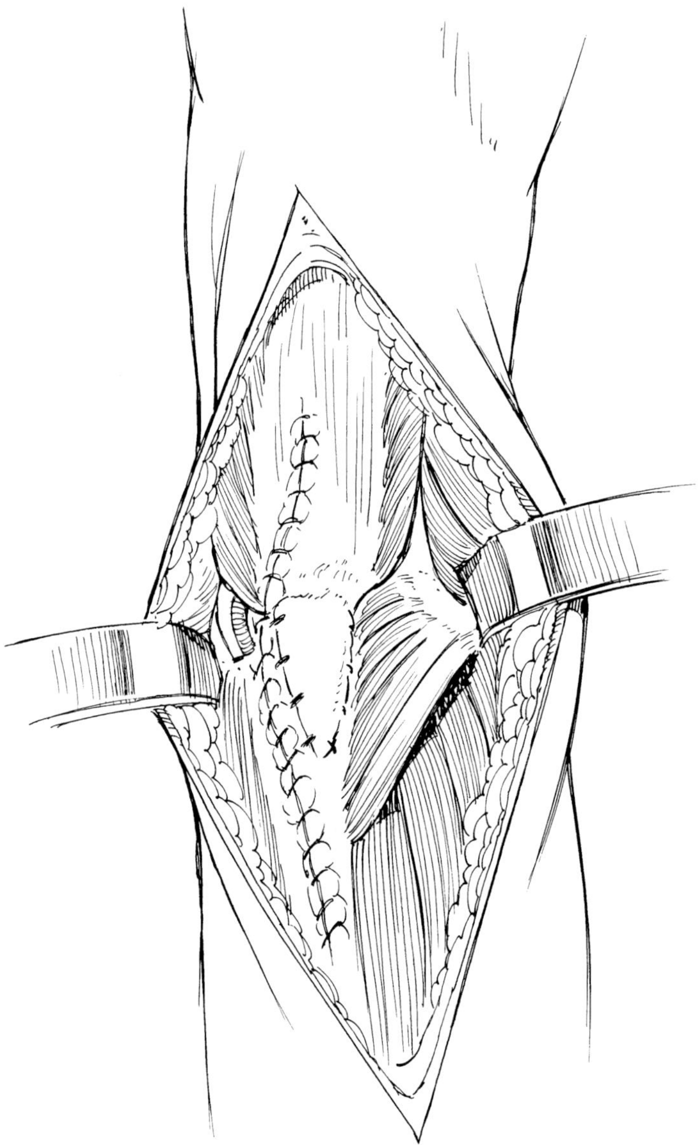

**FIGURE VI–10**

*Dangers*

The ulnar nerve must be carefully mobilized and retracted. Any time the retractor is placed laterally, it should be directly on the bone to avoid injury to the radial nerve. The surgeon must carefully appreciate the attachment of the triceps to the olecranon and create a wide bone flap curving around the apex of the olecranon to preserve the integrity of the triceps mechanism.

*Limitations*

This approach provides a wide exposure of the posterior elbow and distal humerus, but access to the radial head is limited if the capitellum is intact. Exposure of the radial head and neck can be improved by elevating the extensor muscles subperiosteally from the lateral side of the ulna.

## Medial Approach to the Elbow

*Applications*

The medial approach exposes the medial joint and medial humeral condyle. It is most often used for open reduction and internal fixation of the medial condyle. It may also be used for reconstruction or repair of the medial collateral ligament or removal of loose bodies from the anterior aspect of the joint.

*Technique*

The patient is placed supine with the arm on an arm board. The incision is centered over the medial epicondyle and carried in an arc proximally along the medial edge of the humerus and distally over the flexor muscles anterior to the ulnar nerve (VI-11). The ulnar nerve is palpable behind the medial epicondyle. The fascia overlying the ulnar nerve is incised longitudinally from proximal to distal, releasing the nerve into the forearm. The pronator teres is retracted medially and the brachialis is retracted laterally to expose the anterior surface of the medial epicondyle. The ulnar nerve is retracted posteriorly (VI-12). The medial epicondyle is detached with an osteotome and, along with the attached flexor muscles, is then reflected distally (VI-13). The joint capsule can then be elevated from the anterior humerus as needed. If necessary, the joint capsule can be elevated further through the interval between the triceps and the brachialis and the elbow dislocated laterally.

*Dangers*

The ulnar nerve must be meticulously protected. As the median nerve passes through the pronator teres, it can be easily damaged by excessive distal traction on the flexor mass.

*Limitations*

Proximal exposure can be extended to the anterior humerus. Exposure to the lateral elbow is limited unless the elbow is dislocated. Distal exposure is limited by the median nerve.

## Posterolateral (Kocher) Approach to the Elbow

*Applications*

This approach provides direct access to the radial head and the capitellum (4). It is useful for excision or prosthetic replacement of the radial head, or for open reduction and internal fixation of the radial head or capitellum. It is also useful for removal of loose bodies or drainage of a septic elbow joint.

*Technique*

The patient is placed supine with the limb on an arm board. The incision begins immediately posterior to the lateral epicondyle and is carried in a line distally and obliquely toward the ulna for a distance of 6 cm. The fascia is incised in line with the skin to expose the anconeus and extensor carpi ulnaris (VI-14A and VI-14B).

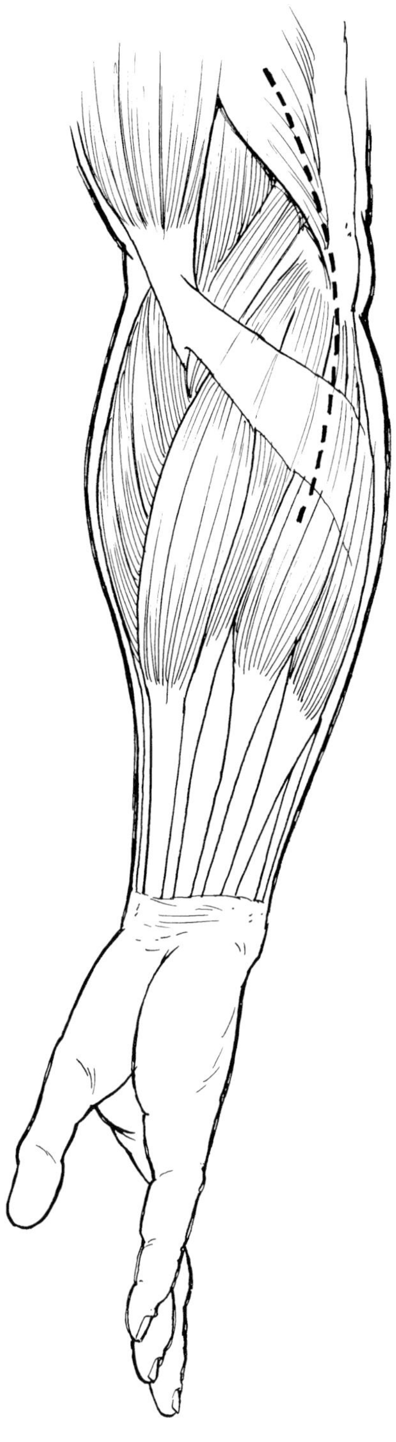

**FIGURE VI–11**

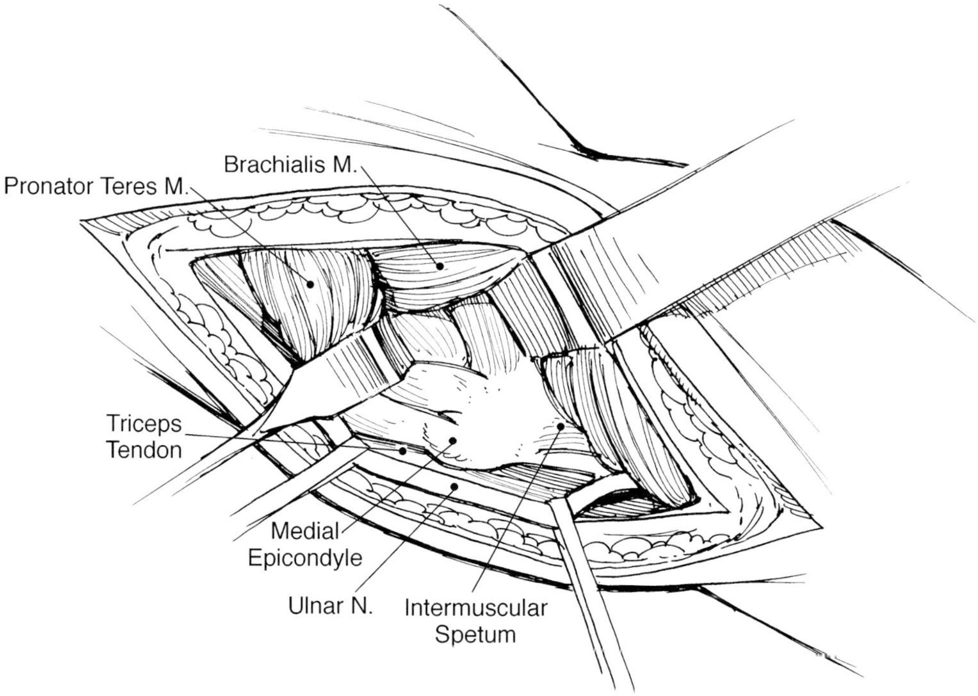


**FIGURE VI–12**

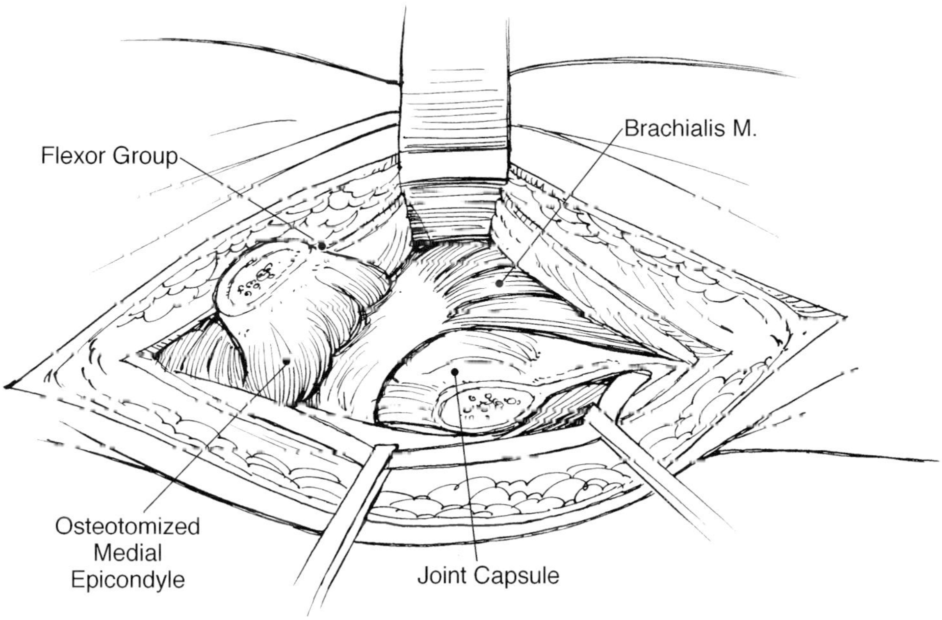


**FIGURE VI–13**

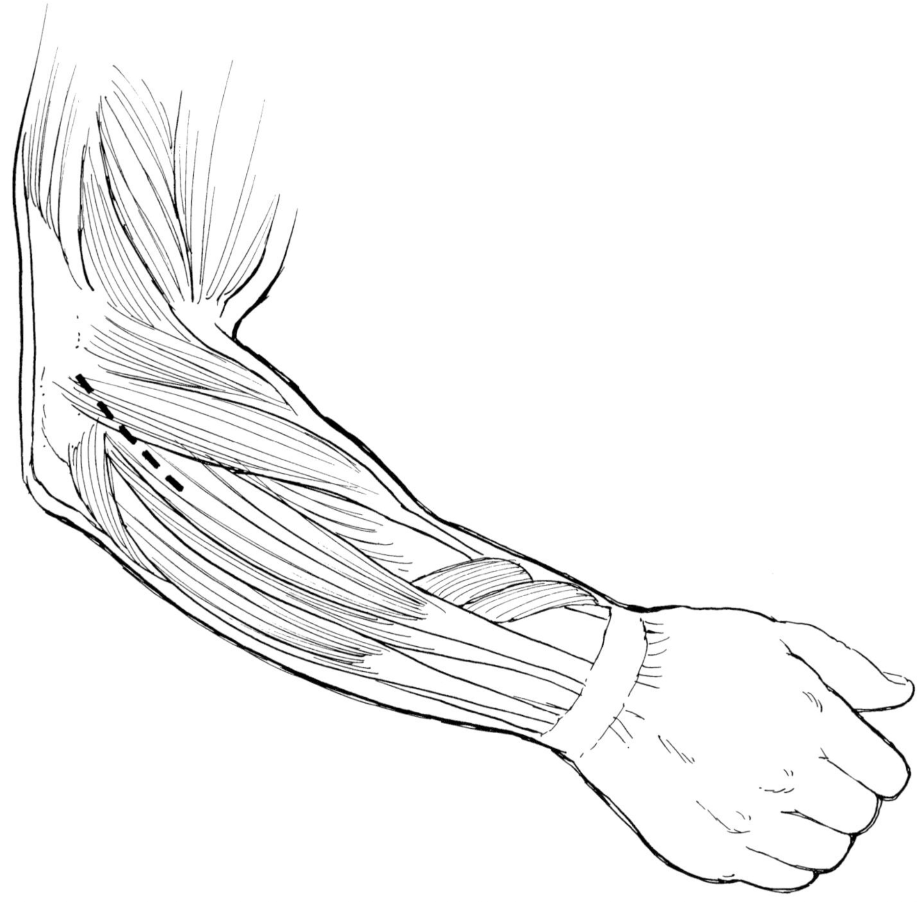

**FIGURE VI–14A**

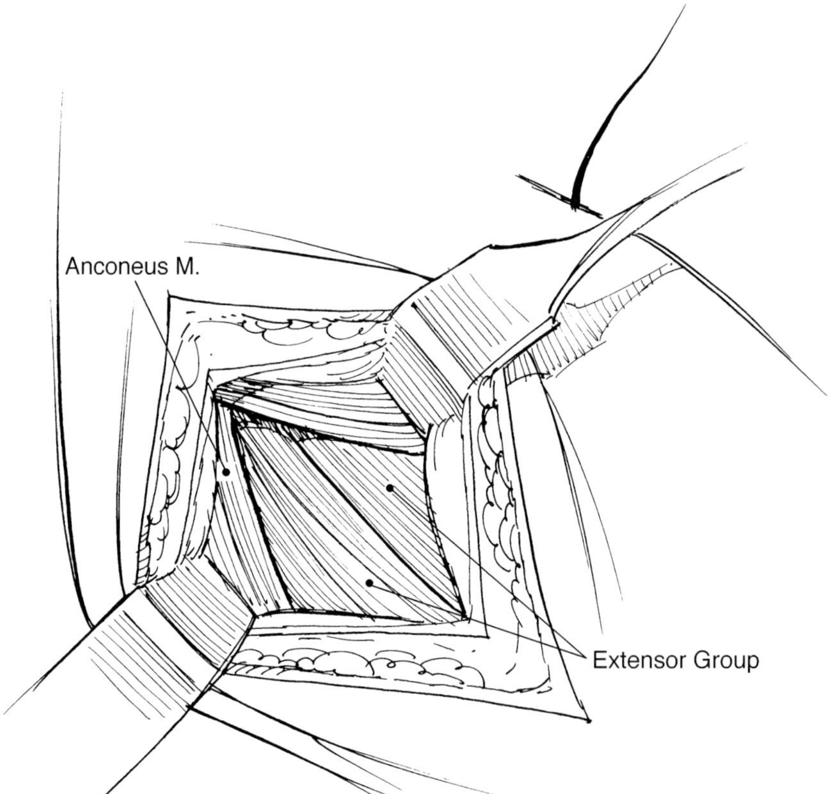


**FIGURE VI–14B**

The forearm is pronated and the anconeus is elevated from the lateral epicondyle to expose the joint capsule (VI-15). The capsule is opened at the edge of the lateral epicondyle to expose the capitellum and radial head (VI-16). The capsule may be incised as far distally as the annular ligament.

*Dangers*

The radial nerve lies on the joint capsule just anterior to this approach and the anterior interosseus nerve lies in the supinator adjacent to the distal end of this exposure. Retractors placed around the radial neck may compress these nerves.

*Limitations*

This approach can be extended proximally by continuing to elevate the muscles of the lateral supracondylar ridge and thus provide access to the distal humerus and allow release of the anterior capsule. The dissection should not be extended distally because of the risk to the posterior interosseous nerve.

# Anterolateral Approach to the Elbow

*Applications*

This approach exposes the anterior lateral half of the elbow joint, specifically the capitellum and the proximal third of the radius. It is useful for open reduction of fractures of the capitellum, excision of tumors of the proximal radius, exploration of the radial and posterior interosseous nerves, and repair of biceps tendon avulsions.

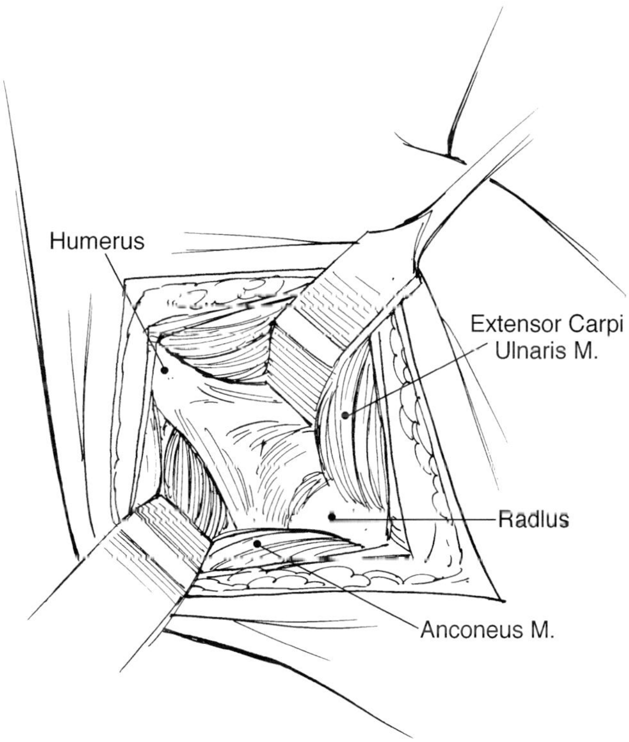


**FIGURE VI-15**

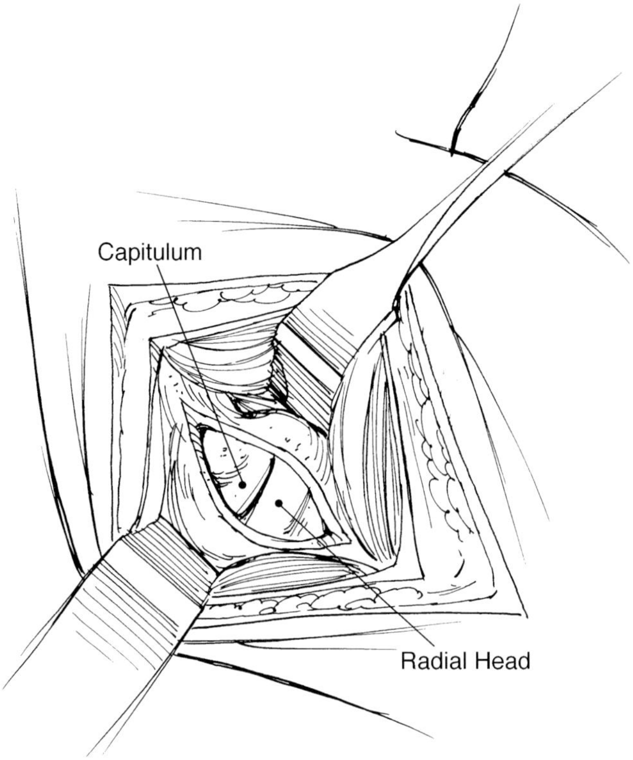


**FIGURE VI–16**

*Technique*

The patient is placed supine with the arm on an arm board. The incision begins 5 cm proximal to the flexor crease of the elbow and runs along the lateral edge of the biceps. At the flexor crease, it curves medially along the crease then curves distally along the medial edge of the brachioradialis for 5 cm or more (VI-17). The lateral antebrachial cutaneous nerve will be found in the subcutaneous tissue and should be preserved (VI-18). The fascia is split medial to the brachioradialis and incised proximally in the interval between the brachialis and the brachioradialis. The brachioradialis is retracted laterally and the brachialis and biceps are retracted medially to expose the radial nerve (VI-19). The radial nerve winds distally until it terminates in the posterior interosseous nerve (which enters the supinator), the superficial radial nerve, and the motor branch to the extensor carpi radialis brevis.

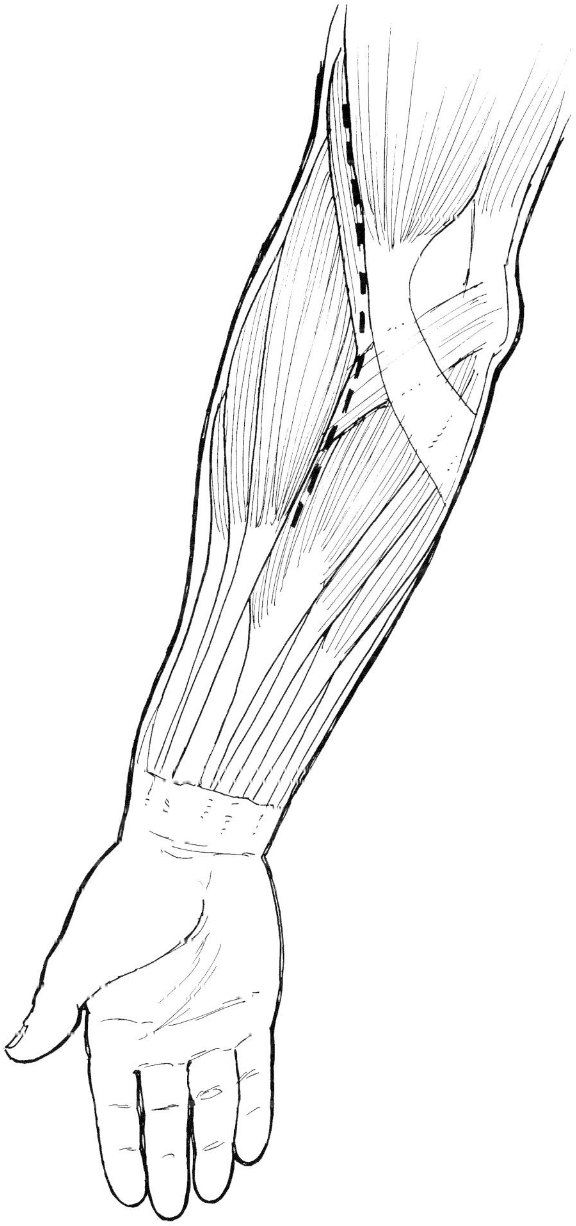

**FIGURE VI-17**

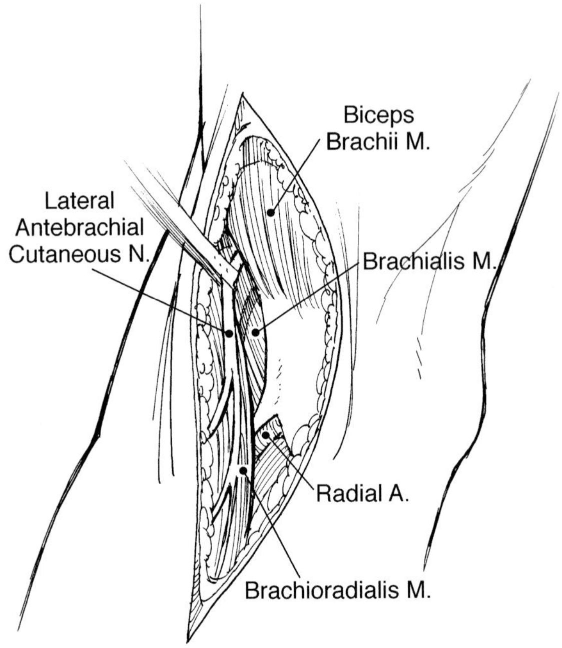


**FIGURE VI-18**

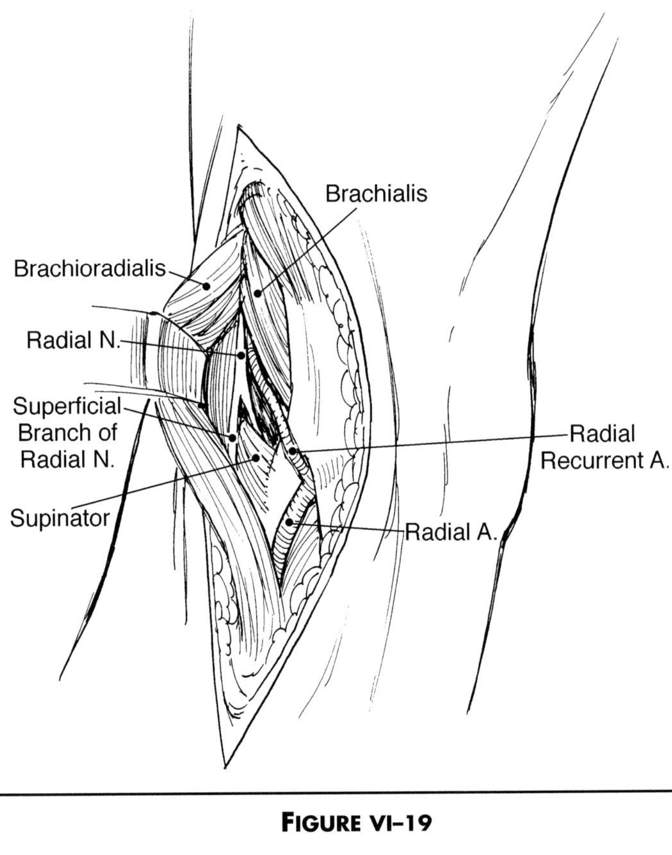


**FIGURE VI-19**

The forearm is fully supinated, bringing the bicipital tuberosity into view (VI-20). The recurrent branch of the radial artery will cross the field close to the proximal end of the supinator and should be ligated to allow the radial artery to retract safely. Muscular arterial branches to the brachialis muscle may also need to be ligated. The origin of the supinator is found on the ulnar side of the radius, adjacent to the belly of the pronator teres. The supinator origin is incised longitudinally so that the supinator can be elevated subperiosteally from the radius. The longitudinal dissection is carried proximally through the anterior joint capsule, just lateral to the brachialis. The capsule is then elevated anteriorly to expose the capitellum and the distal radius (VI-21).

***Dangers***

The radial nerve and posterior interosseus nerve are susceptible to injury. The recurrent branch of the radial artery can produce troublesome bleeding if not controlled.

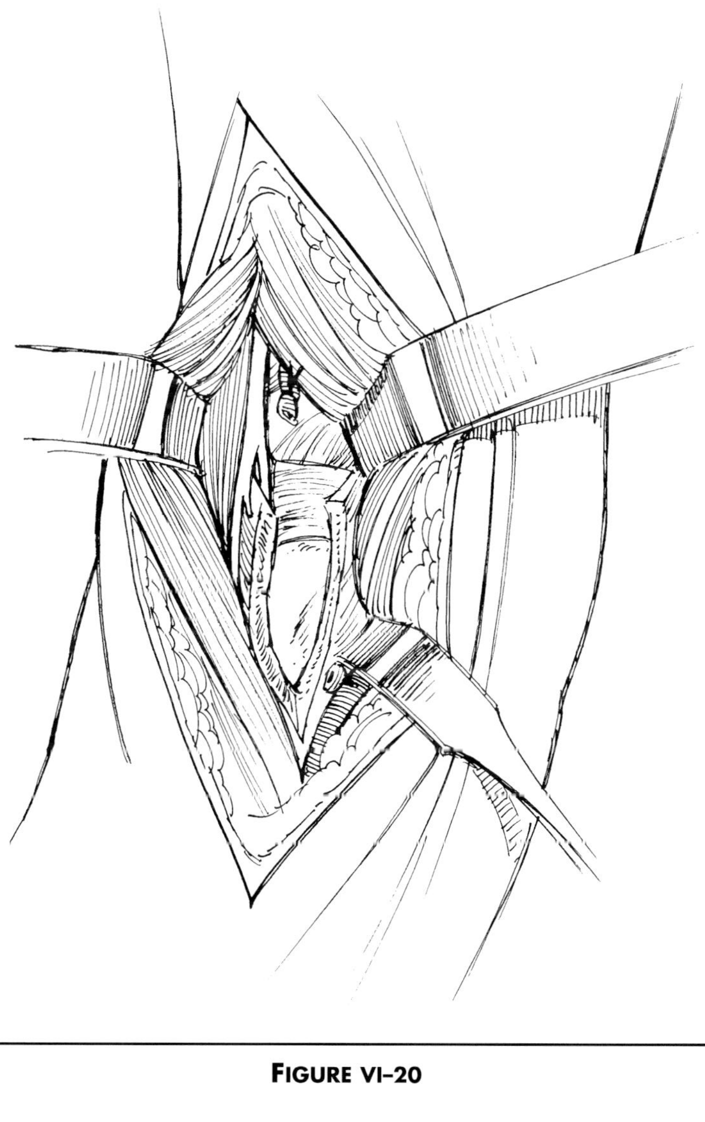

**FIGURE VI–20**

***Limitations***

Proximally, there is no limitation as this exposure can be extended into the anterolateral approach to the humerus. Distally, the anterior surface of the proximal half of the radius can be exposed by developing the plane between the brachioradialis and the pronator teres.

## Anterior Approach to the Elbow

***Applications***

This approach is used primarily for repair or exploration of the neurovascular structures in the cubital fossa: the median nerve, the brachial artery, and the radial nerve. This approach is also used for repair or reattachment of the biceps tendon.

***Technique***

The patient is placed supine with the arm extended on an arm board. The incision begins medially 5 cm proximal to the elbow flexor crease and is carried down to the crease, curved across the antecubital fossa in the crease, then extended distally for 5 cm along the ulnar border of the brachioradialis (VI-22). The fascia is incised in line with the skin incision and proximal, lateral, and distal medial flaps are elevated deep to the fascia. The bicipital aponeurosis is located and transected at its origin from the biceps tendon and retracted. The radial artery lies immediately deep to the aponeurosis. It is traced proximally to its origin from the brachial artery (VI-23). The brachial artery and median nerve are medial to the tendon.

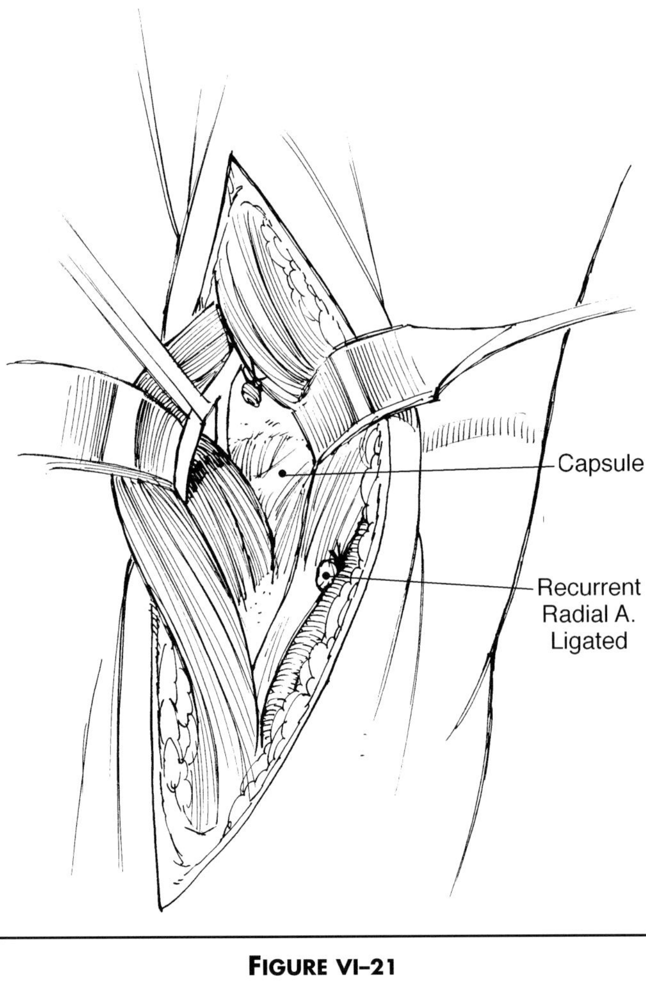


**FIGURE VI–21**

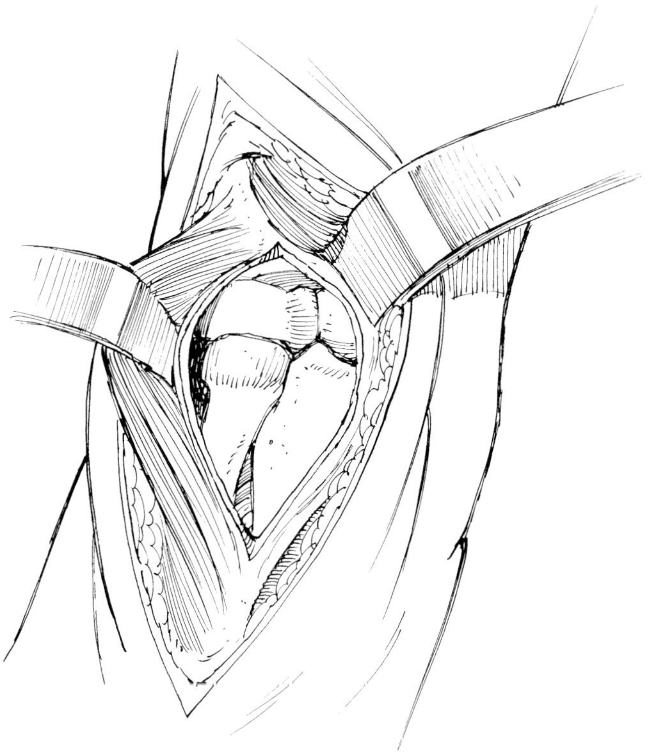

**FIGURE VI–22**

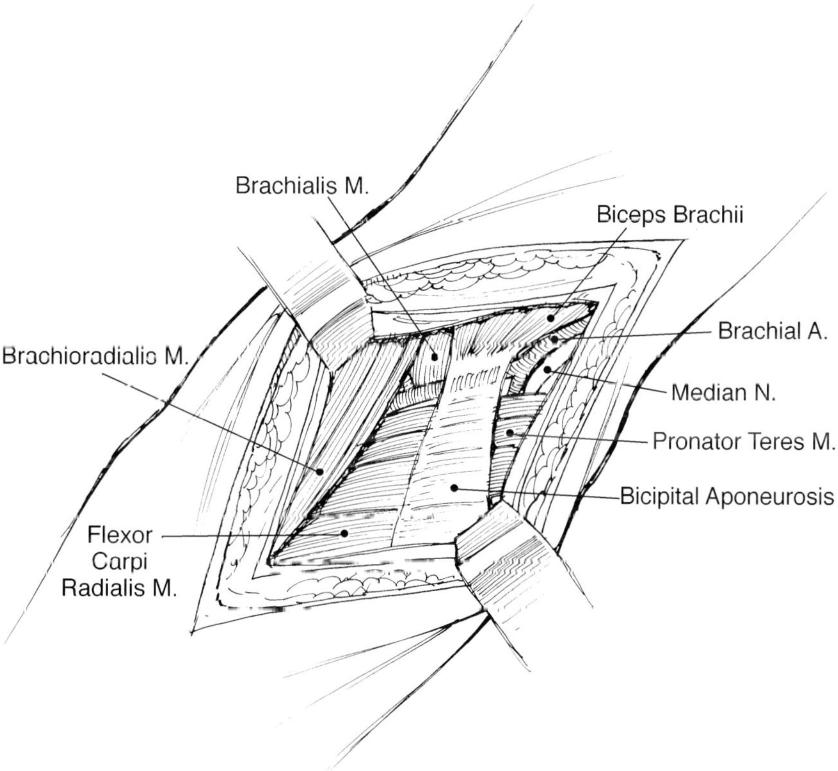


**FIGURE VI–23**

The brachioradialis is retracted laterally to expose the radial nerve, which lies between it and the brachialis muscle (VI-24). The neurovascular structures can be retracted to expose the bicipital tuberosity which is easily palpable when the forearm is supinated (VI-25).

***Dangers***

The lateral anterobrachial cutaneous nerve, radial nerve, radial artery, and median nerve are all susceptible to injury in this approach.

***Limitations***

This exposure is useful for direct access to the major nerves and vessels. It is not ideal for exposure of the joint because of the dissection and retraction of the nerves and vessels that is necessary. The incision may be carried medially to continue as the medial approach to the humerus. It can be extended distally to expose the anterior radius as discussed above in the anterolateral approach to the elbow.

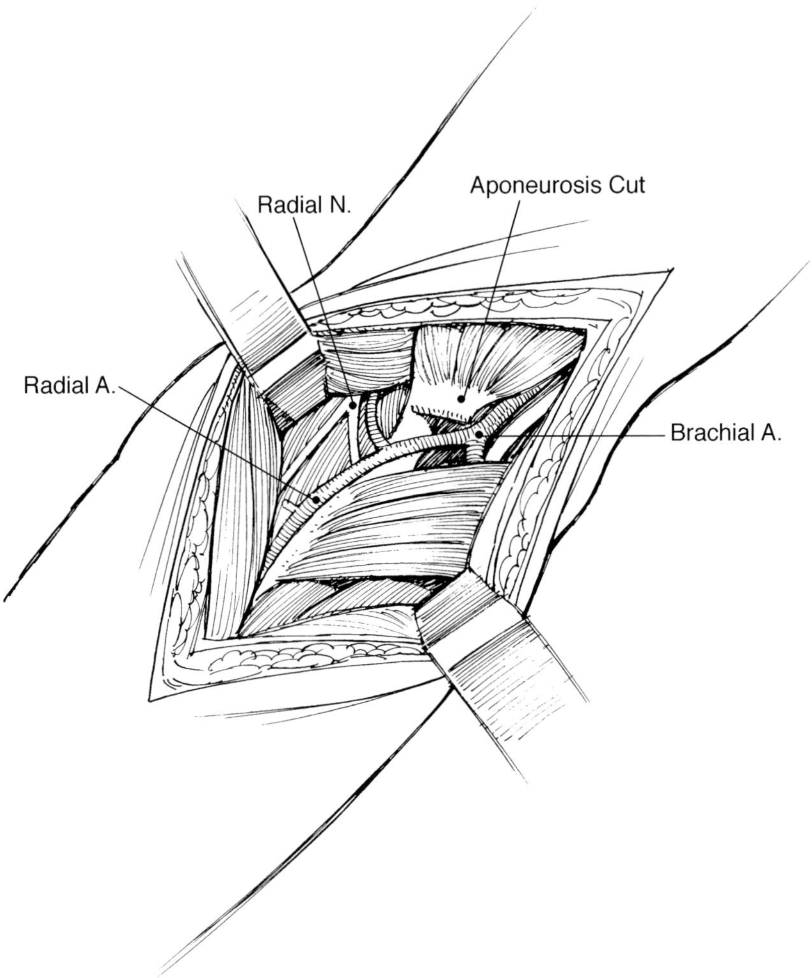


**FIGURE VI–24**

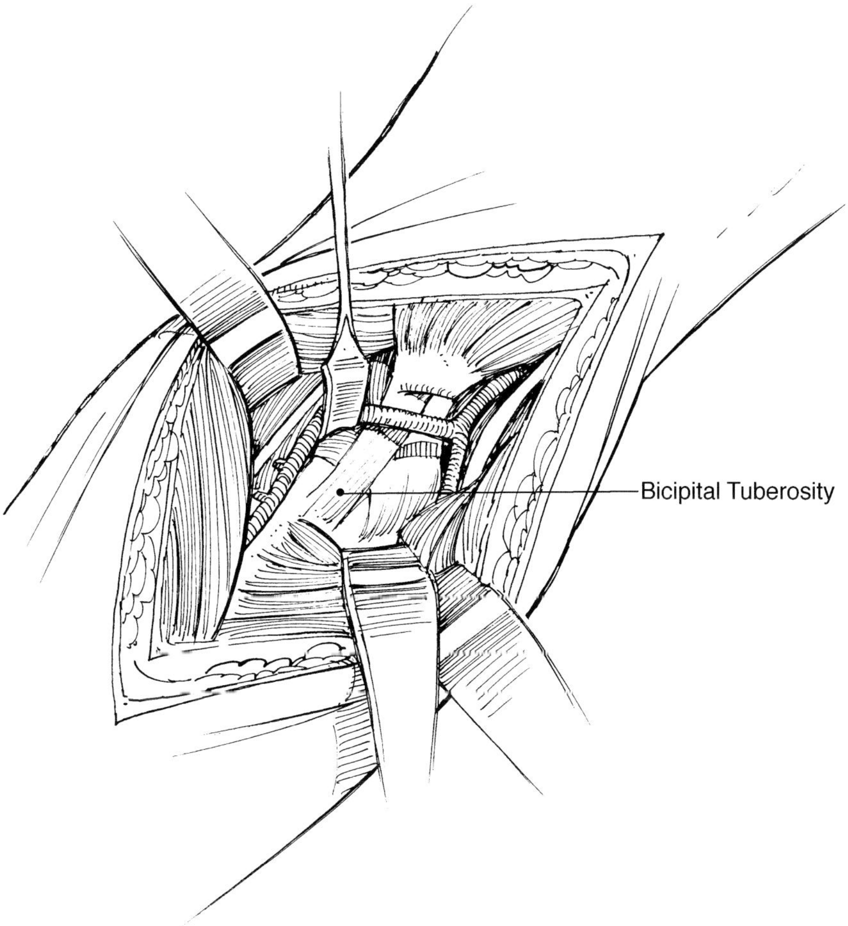


**FIGURE VI-25**

# References


1. Bryan RS, Morrey BF. Extensive posterior exposure of the elbow. A triceps-sparing approach. Clin Orthop 166:188–192, 1982.
2. Müller ME, Allgower M, Willenegger H. Manual of Internal Fixation. New York: Springer-Verlag, 1970.
3. MacAusland WR. Ankylosis of the elbow: with report of four cases treated by arthroplasty. JAMA 64:312, 1915.
4. Kocker T; Stiled HJ, Paul LB, trans. Textbook of Operative Surgery, 3rd ed. London: Adam and Charles Black, 1911.

# VII

# SURGICAL APPROACHES TO THE FOREARM

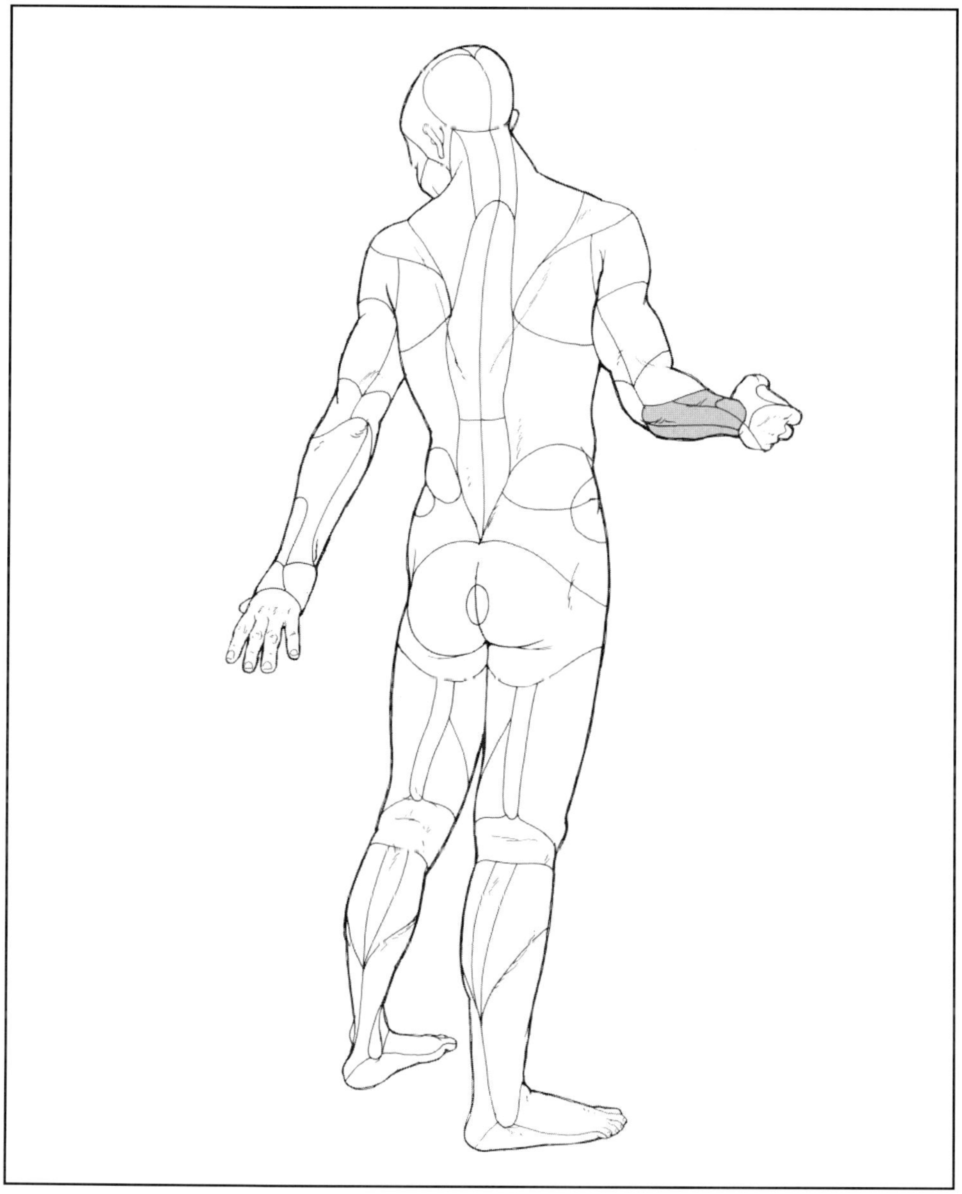

## General Principles and Complications

Trauma is the most common reason for surgery of the forearm. The loss of function of a hand is such a serious disability that elaborate, staged reconstructions of the forearm may be warranted to preserve the function of the hand. Early rehabilitation to preserve motion is critical to restoring hand function. Anatomic alignment of the radius and ulna is necessary to preserve pronation, supination, and normal wrist motion. Therefore, almost all adult radius fractures require internal fixation. Malignant tumors that require wide excision may necessitate the use of a combination of the surgical exposures presented here.

Complications of surgery in the forearm are primarily related to nerve or vessel injury. As the dissection proceeds distally in the extremity, the collateral circulation diminishes and more vessels become terminal branches that must be preserved. Therefore, surgical dissections are almost always carried longitudinally to preserve nerve and vascular supply. Furthermore, the distal aspects of the extremities have a relative paucity of soft tissue in proportion to bone. Preservation of the soft tissues thus becomes a progressively more critical concern as dissection progresses distally. In general, skin incisions should not be placed directly over bony prominences. The loss of overlying skin and muscle can result in serious problems such as osteomyelitis and infected nonunions. An incision placed over the muscle allows the fascia to be opened and the dissection to proceed deep to the fascia to preserve the blood supply to the skin. Careful dissection with a minimal amount of soft tissue disruption is crucial in the forearm and hand to maintain the dexterity of the hand and fingers.

## Surgical Anatomy

The flexor-pronator muscles fill the anterior compartment of the forearm. They are arranged in three layers. The most superficial group includes the pronator teres, flexor carpi radialis, palmaris longus, and flexor carpi ulnaris (VII-1). The middle layer consists of the flexor digitorum superficialis. The deep layer consists of the flexor digitorum profundus, flexor pollicis longus, and pronator quadratus (VII-2). The lateral boundary of the forearm consists of the "mobile wad of three" muscles: brachioradialis, extensor carpi radialis longus, and extensor carpi radialis brevis. The extensor compartment consists of the "mobile wad of three," the superficial extensors (anconeus, extensor carpi ulnaris, extensor digiti minimi, and extensor digitorum communis [VII-3]), and the deep extensors (the abductor pollicis longus, extensor pollicis brevis, extensor pollicis longus, and supinator [VII-4]). The superficial radial nerve and radial artery lie on the radial side of the forearm under the brachioradialis. The median nerve lies in the volar midforearm, between the middle and deep layers. The ulnar nerve and artery lie in the ulnar forearm, deep to the flexor carpi ulnaris (VII-5). The anterior interosseous nerve and artery lie on the interosseous membrane, deep to the flexor digitorum profundus (VII-6). The posterior interosseous nerve descends through the supinator to distribute to the muscles of the extensor supinator compartment. The posterior interosseous artery runs on the interosseous membrane to join the posterior interosseous nerve distal to the supinator (VII-7). A significant portion of the blood supply to the extensor compartment arises from perforators of the anterior interosseous artery.

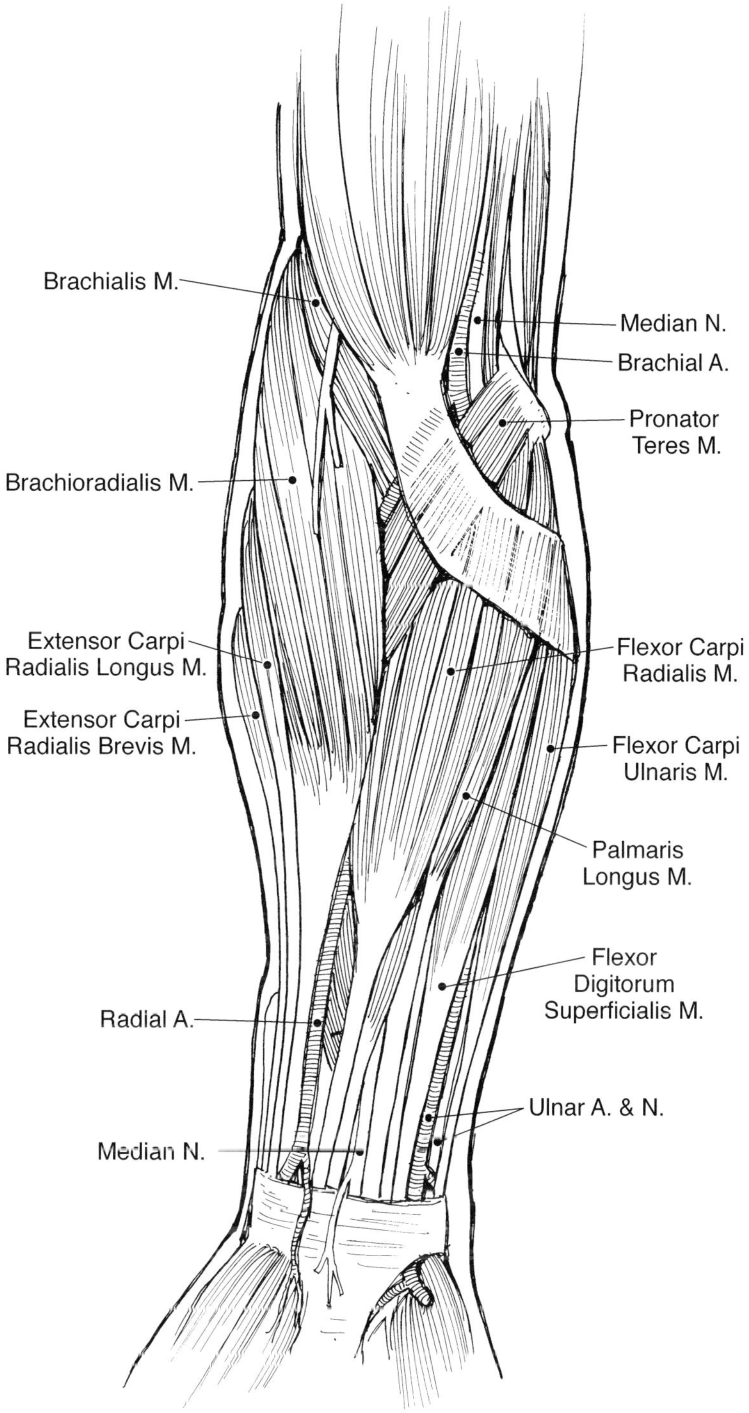
Brachialis M.
Median N.
Brachial A.
Pronator Teres M.
Brachioradialis M.
Extensor Carpi Radialis Longus M.
Flexor Carpi Radialis M.
Extensor Carpi Radialis Brevis M.
Flexor Carpi Ulnaris M.
Palmaris Longus M.
Flexor Digitorum Superficialis M.
Radial A.
Ulnar A. & N.
Median N.

**FIGURE VII–1**

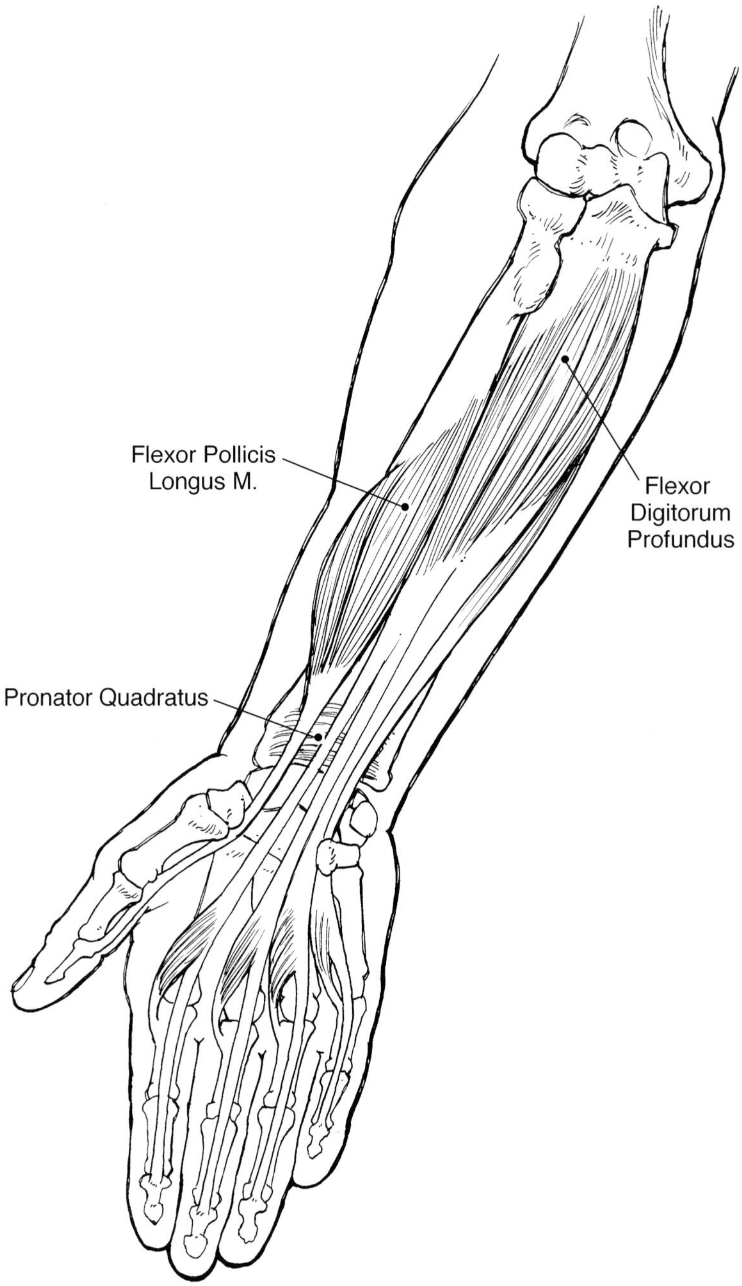
Flexor Pollicis Longus M.
Flexor Digitorum Profundus
Pronator Quadratus

**FIGURE VII–2**

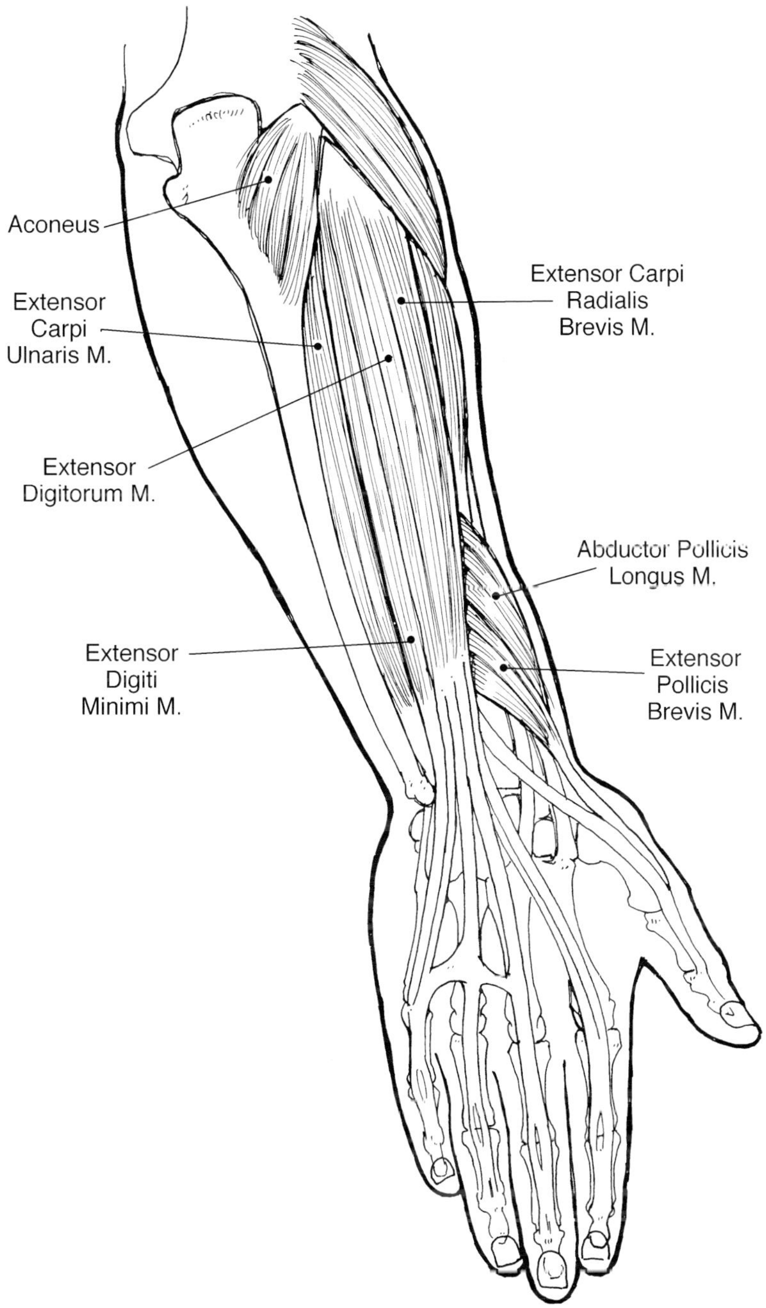
Aconeus
Extensor Carpi Ulnaris M.
Extensor Digitorum M.
Extensor Digiti Minimi M.
Extensor Carpi Radialis Brevis M.
Abductor Pollicis Longus M.
Extensor Pollicis Brevis M.

**FIGURE VII–3**

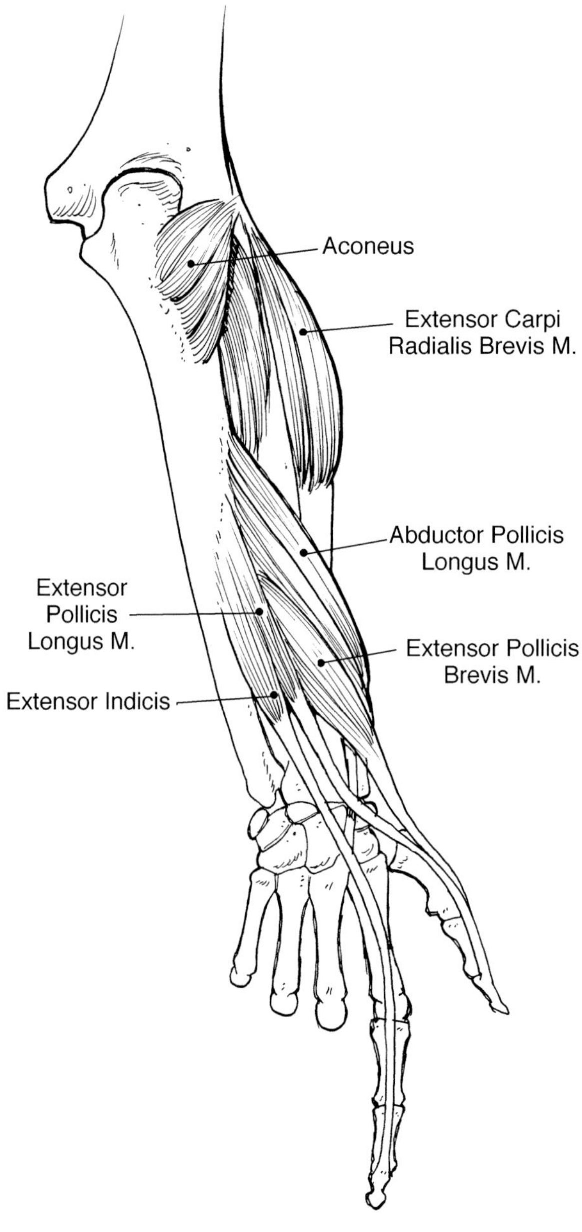
Aconeus
Extensor Carpi Radialis Brevis M.
Abductor Pollicis Longus M.
Extensor Pollicis Longus M.
Extensor Pollicis Brevis M.
Extensor Indicis

**FIGURE VII-4**

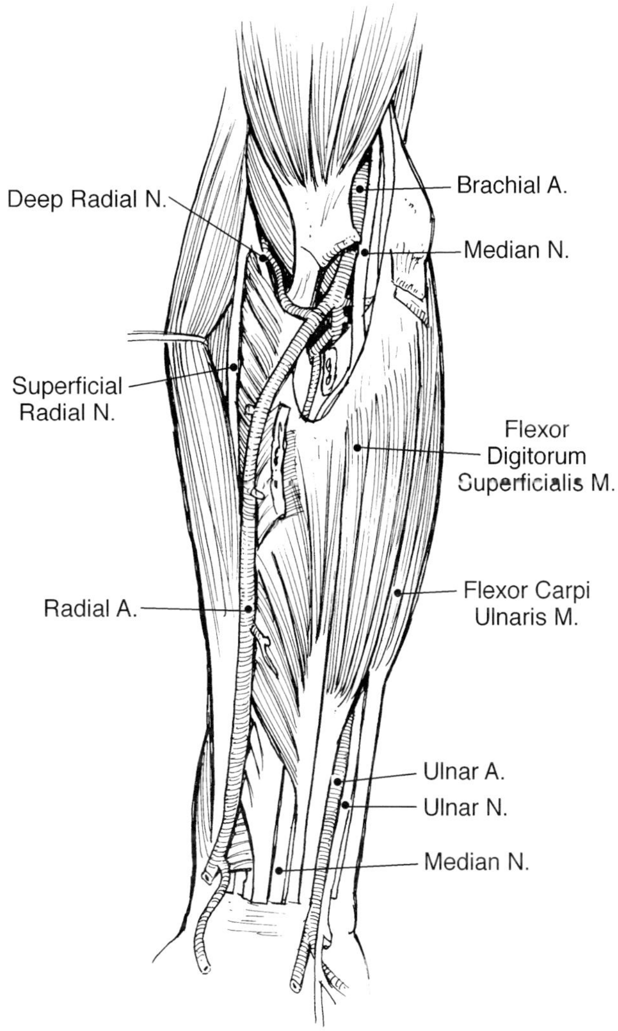
Deep Radial N.
Brachial A.
Median N.
Superficial Radial N.
Flexor Digitorum Superficialis M.
Radial A.
Flexor Carpi Ulnaris M.
Ulnar A.
Ulnar N.
Median N.

**FIGURE VII-5**

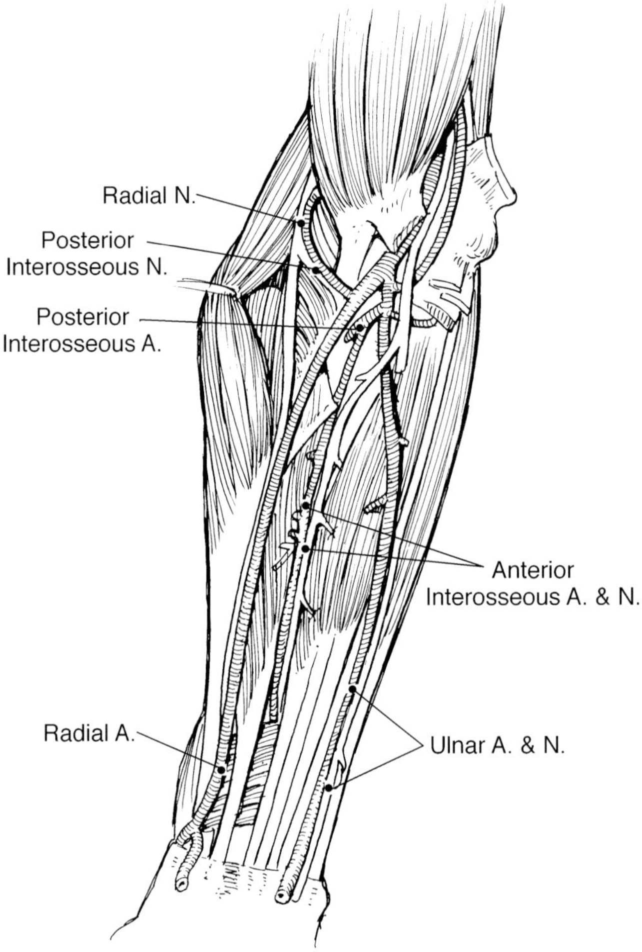
Radial N.
Posterior Interosseous N.
Posterior Interosseous A.
Anterior Interosseous A. & N.
Radial A.
Ulnar A. & N.

**FIGURE VII–6**

## Dorsal (Boyd) Approach to the Ulna and Proximal Radius

***Applications***

This approach was described by Boyd (1) in 1940. It provides wide exposure to the proximal third of the radius and the entire length of the ulna. Its major application is for open reduction and internal fixation of Monteggia-type fractures. This approach has the advantage of providing access to the elbow joint during open reduction of the ulna.

***Technique***

The patient may be in the lateral decubitus position or lying supine with the limb on an arm board. The incision begins 1 cm proximal to the tip of the olecranon, just lateral to the edge of the triceps tendon. It is carried across the elbow in a

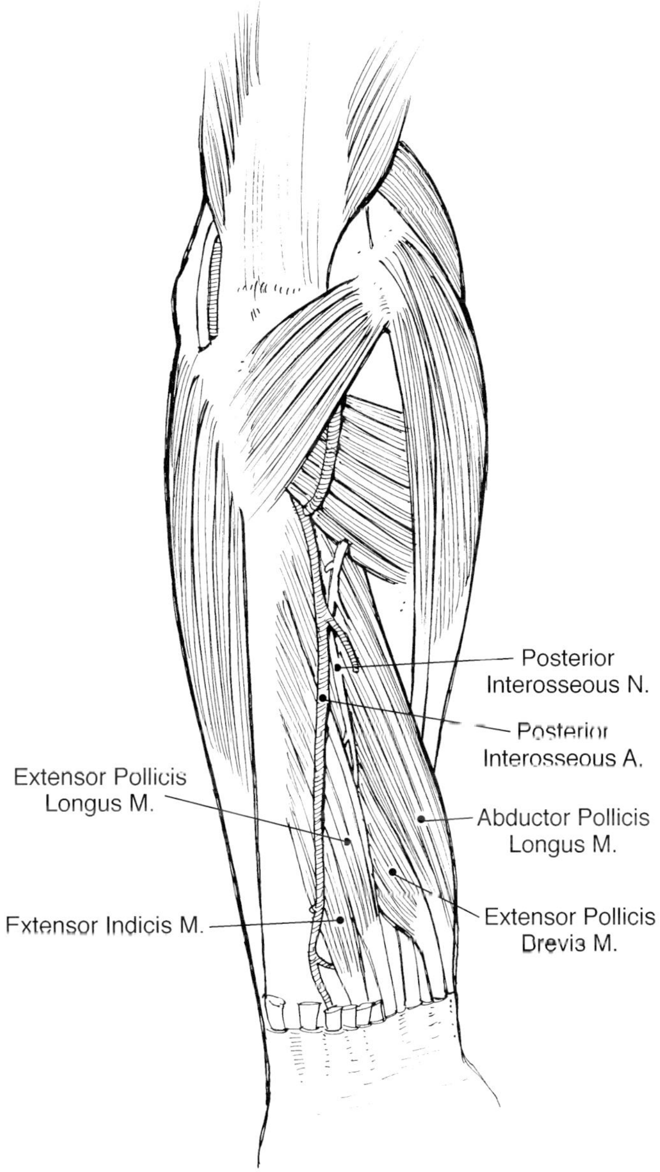


**FIGURE VII–7**

straight line along the lateral edge of the ulna, as far distally as necessary (VII-8). The anconeus and supinator are elevated subperiosteally from the ulna and retracted laterally (VII-9). As the dissection is extended distally, the origins of the abductor pollicis longus, extensor carpi ulnaris, and extensor pollicis longus are elevated (VII-10). The extensor muscles are retracted to expose the radial head and neck and the shaft proximal to the interosseous membrane. The posterior interosseous artery may be ligated as it enters the extensor compartment to facilitate mobilization of the muscles. The muscles are then elevated off of the interosseous membrane to expose the dorsal, medial surface of the radius (VII-11). This exposure can be extended distally to the distal edge of the supinator. The posterior interosseous nerve lies in the substance of the supinator and is retracted with the muscle mass.

***Dangers***

The critical structure in this dissection is the posterior interosseous nerve. The muscle elevation must be kept on the interosseous membrane to protect the nerve.

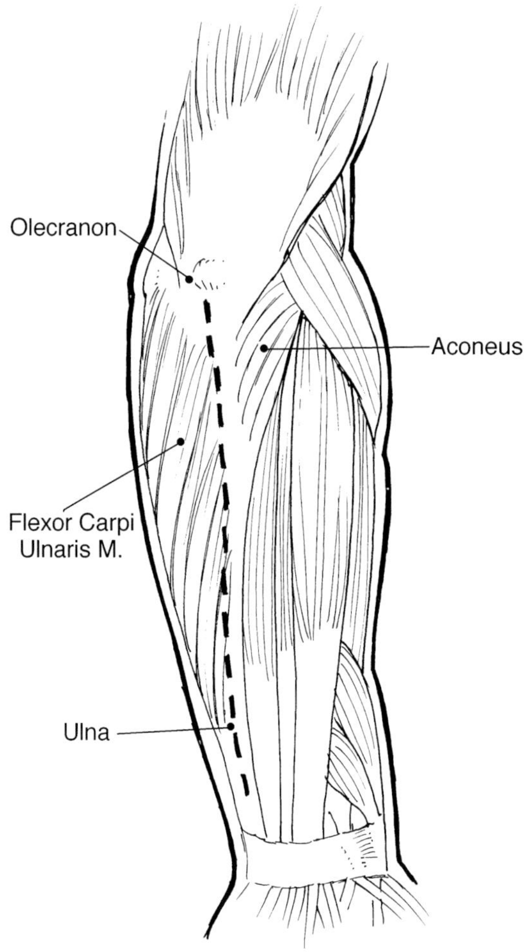


**FIGURE VII–8**

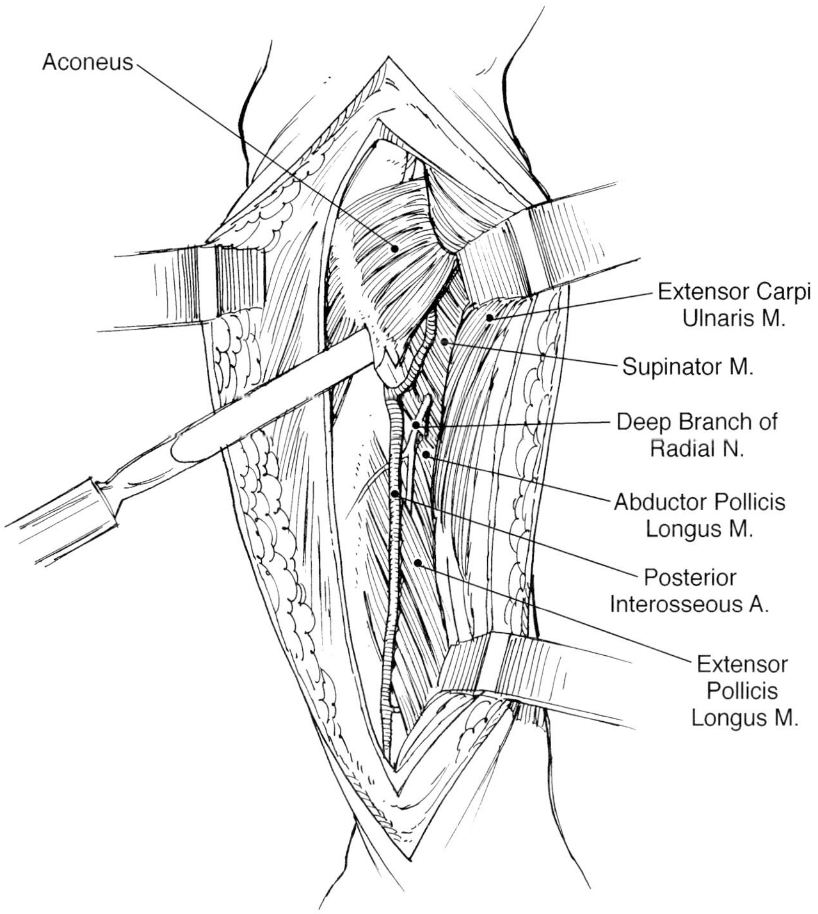
Aconeus
Extensor Carpi Ulnaris M.
Supinator M.
Deep Branch of Radial N.
Abductor Pollicis Longus M.
Posterior Interosseous A.
Extensor Pollicis Longus M.

**FIGURE VII–9**

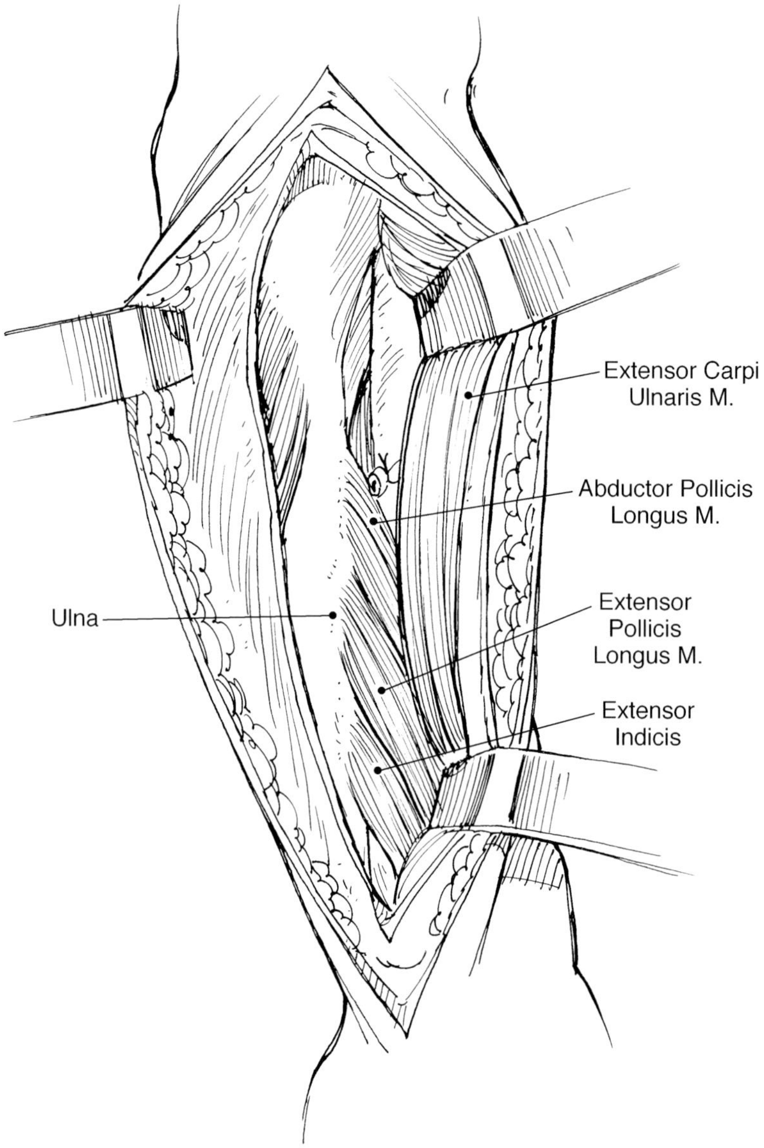


**FIGURE VII–10**

*Limitations*

Exposure to the radius is limited to the proximal third. This approach can be extended proximally as a posterior approach to the elbow and distal humerus by medial reflection of the triceps.

# Subcutaneous Approach to the Ulna

*Applications*

The ulna lies subcutaneously throughout its length and is simple to expose. This approach may be used for open reduction and internal fixation of fractures and nonunion, treatment of osteomyelitis, release of ulnar club hand, or ulnar lengthening or shortening for wrist problems.

*Technique*

The patient lies supine with the arm on an arm board. A longitudinal incision is made anterior and parallel to the subcutaneous edge of the ulna (VII-12). The periosteum is then incised longitudinally along the ulna and the flexor carpi ulnaris and extensor carpi ulnaris are elevated from the bone as needed (VII-13).

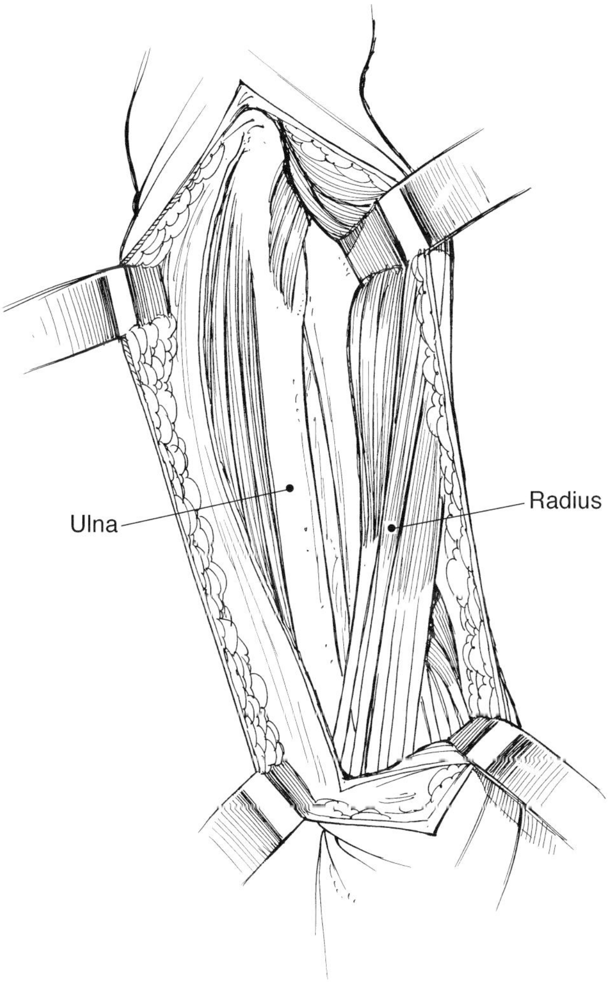


**FIGURE VII–11**

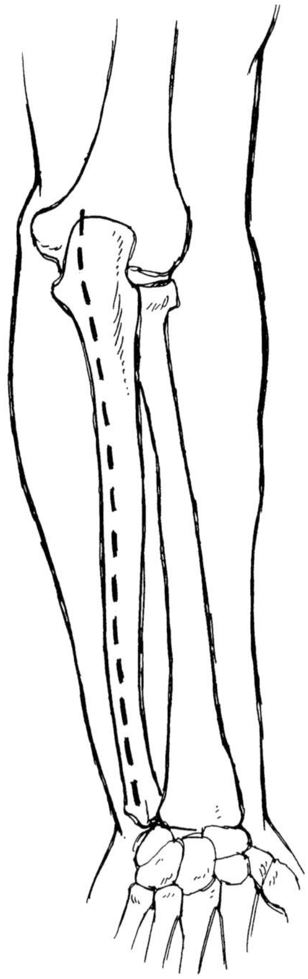

**FIGURE VII–12**

# Compartment Resection in the Forearm

The entire extensor compartment of the forearm may be resected for malignant tumors if necessary. This soft tissue resection can be combined with removal of a segment of the radius or ulna. An incision is made from the lateral supracondylar ridge of the humerus to the middorsal wrist in a gentle S curve (VII-24). The fascia is incised longitudinally with the skin. The radial nerve is identified in the proximal margin and transected. The extensor tendons are identified at the wrist, tagged, and transected (VII-25). The entire muscle mass can then be elevated from the radius, ulna, and interosseous membrane. The posterior interosseous artery and perforating branches of the anterior interosseous artery are ligated as they are encountered. If the tumor involves a segment of bone, the segment is isolated proximally and distally through the anterior compartment and excised with the muscles. The extensor function can be restored by flexor-to-extensor tendon transfers. The segmental defect in the radius or ulna can be restored with an autologous fibula transfer or by creation of a one bone forearm with a radioulnar synostosis.

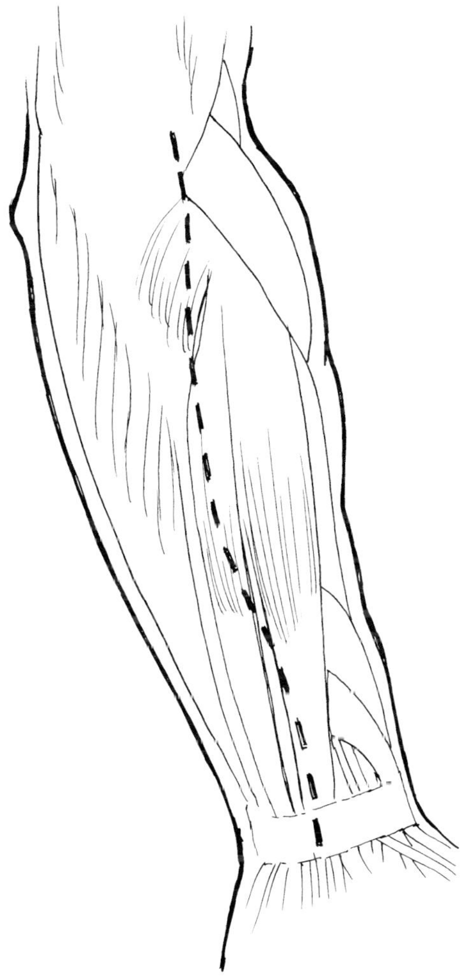

**FIGURE VII–24**

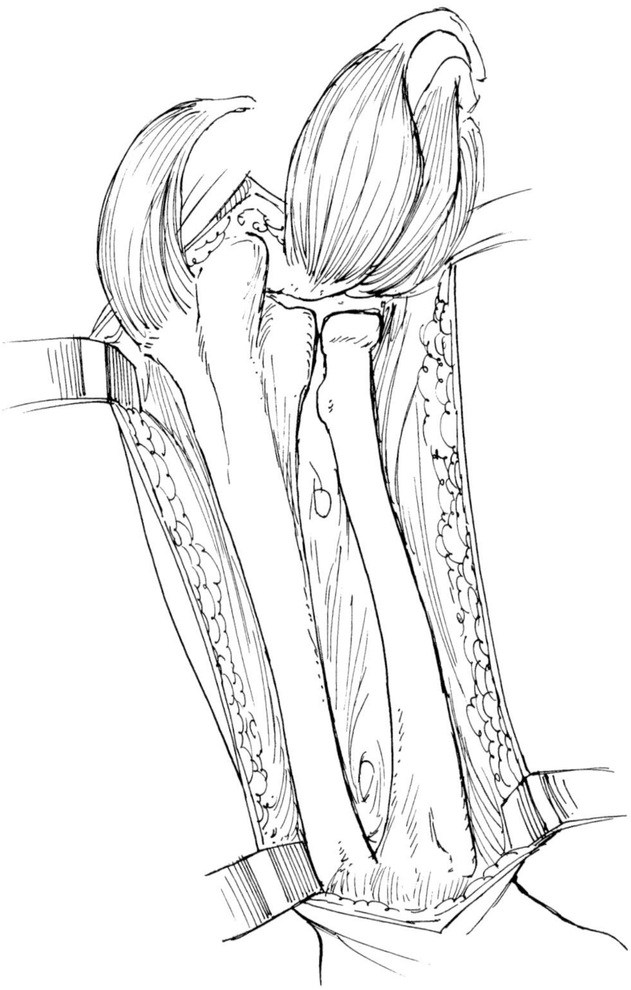

**FIGURE VII–25**

Excision of the anterior compartment is not practical since it would require removal of the major vascular trunks to the hand as well as the median and ulnar nerves. Excision of one axial segment (radial or ulnar) still preserves a reasonably functional hand. In these dissections, the skin flap should be carried deep to the fascia to preserve the collateral vascular supply. Incisions directly over bony prominences or hardware should be avoided.

# References


1. Boyd HB. Surgical exposure of the ulna and proximal third of the radius through one incision. Surg Gynecol Obstet 1940;71:86.
2. Henry AK. Extensile Exposures, 2nd ed. Baltimore: Williams & Wilkins, 1970:100–106.

# VIII

# SURGICAL APPROACHES TO THE WRIST AND HAND

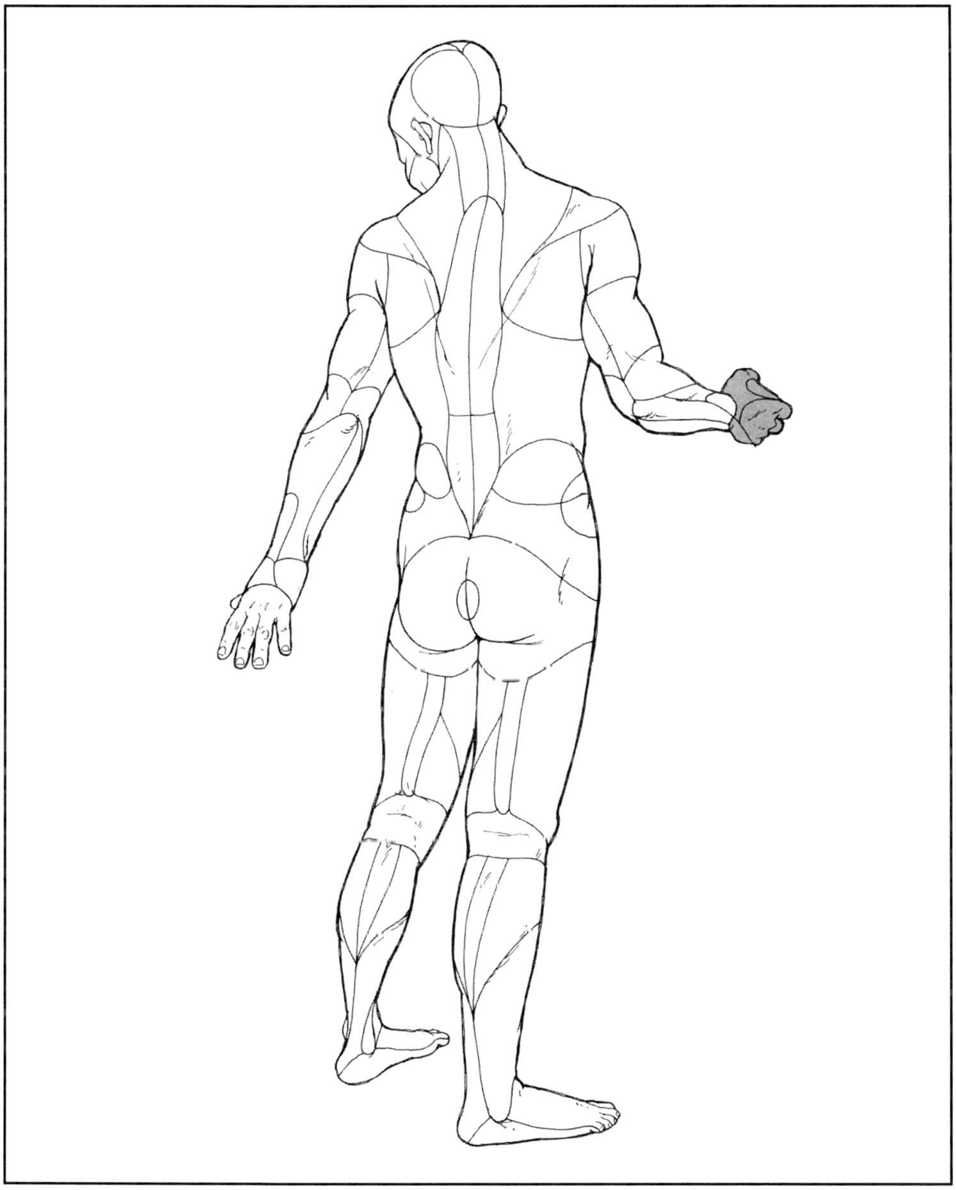

## General Principles and Complications

Skin incisions in the hand and wrist must provide not only adequate exposure of the deep structures with preservation of the blood and nerve supply but also cosmetically acceptable scars without producing joint contractures (1). In the hand and fingers, exuberant scarring not only produces an unsightly scar, but it can create contractures that restrict joint motion. The dorsal skin of the hand is thin and mobile while the volar skin is thick and firmly adherent to the deep fascia. The arterial supply to the skin of the hand is from perforating branches of the superficial and deep palmar arches. The skin of the fingers is supplied by longitudinally arranged digital vessels. There is a plexus of large subcutaneous veins on the dorsum of the hand that should be preserved to provide adequate venous drainage. The critical innervation of the skin on the dorsum of the hand is from the dorsal branch of the ulnar nerve and the superficial branch of the radial nerve (VIII-1). On the palmar surface, the palmar cutaneous branches of the median and ulnar nerves are critical (VIII-2). Incisions that cross the major sensory nerves can result in entrapment of the nerve, creating a painful neuroma. In general, to minimize scarring, incisions on the dorsal surface of the wrist and hand should be transverse while incisions on the volar surface should be made within the palmar creases. If an incision must be extended across a crease, it should be placed at an oblique angle to the crease to minimize the risk of contracture. On the fingers, the dorsal surface can be exposed by S-shaped incisions with the central line in the joint crease and the proximal and distal limbs in the midlateral line. The volar aspects of the fingers and the metacarpals can be approached by longitudinally oriented midlateral incisions or by a zig-zag volar (Bruner) incision (2).

## Surgical Anatomy

### *Dorsal Wrist*

The dorsal wrist is covered by the extensor retinaculum which spans from the anterolateral border of the radius to the pisiform and triquetrum. It receives fibrous septae projecting from the carpal bones to its deep surface to divide the extensor tendons into six compartments. The compartments are numbered from lateral to medial and contain the following (VIII-3):

1. Abductor pollicis longus and extensor pollicis brevis.
2. Extensor carpi radialis longus and extensor carpi radial brevis. These tendons run lateral to Lister's tubercle and make the floor of the anatomic snuff box.
3. Extensor pollicis longus which passes medial to Lister's tubercle.
4. Extensor indices and extensor digitorum communis.
5. Extensor digiti minimi.
6. Extensor carpi ulnaris.

### *Dorsal Hand and Fingers*

The long extensor tendons crossing the dorsum of the hand are interconnected by the juncturae tendinea just proximal to the metacarpophalangeal joints (VIII-4A). The extensor tendons blend with the dorsal capsule of the metacarpophalangeal joints. At that level, they became wider and divide into three "slips" which project onto the dorsum of the proximal phalanx. The central slip inserts into the base of the middle phalanx. The two marginal slips receive the insertions of the interossei and lumbricals to form the broad extensor hood. The two marginal slips project onto the base of the distal phalanx. The intrinsic tendons join to each other over the middle phalanx by the transversely oriented "triangular ligament" (VIII-4B).

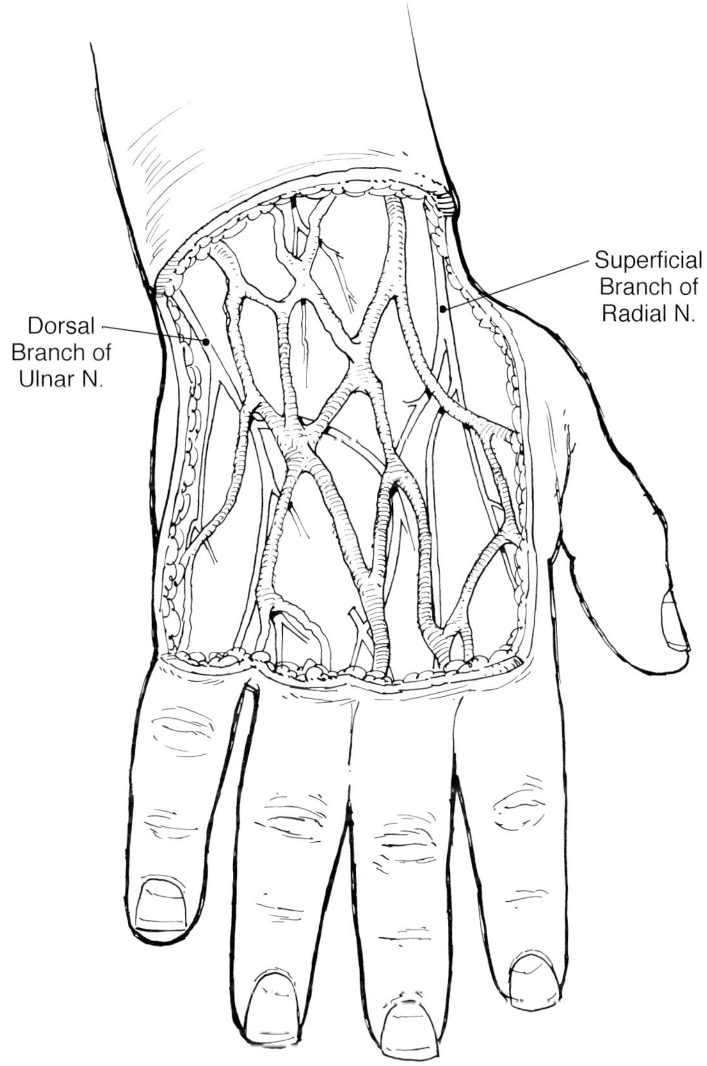


**FIGURE VIII–1**

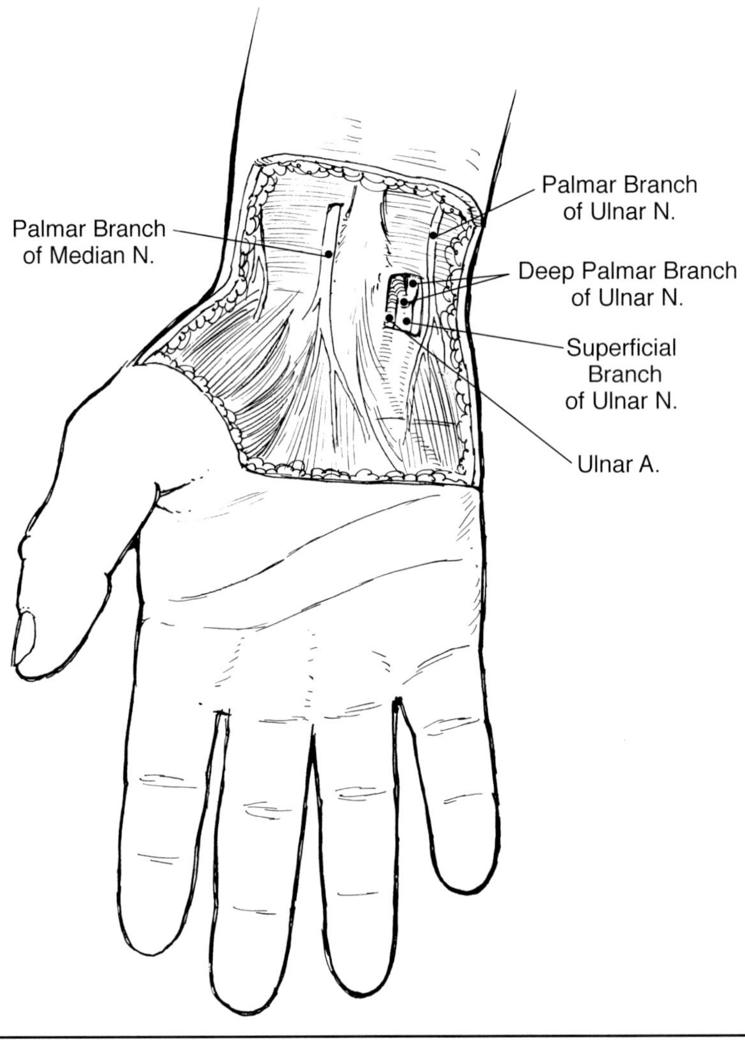


**FIGURE VIII–2**

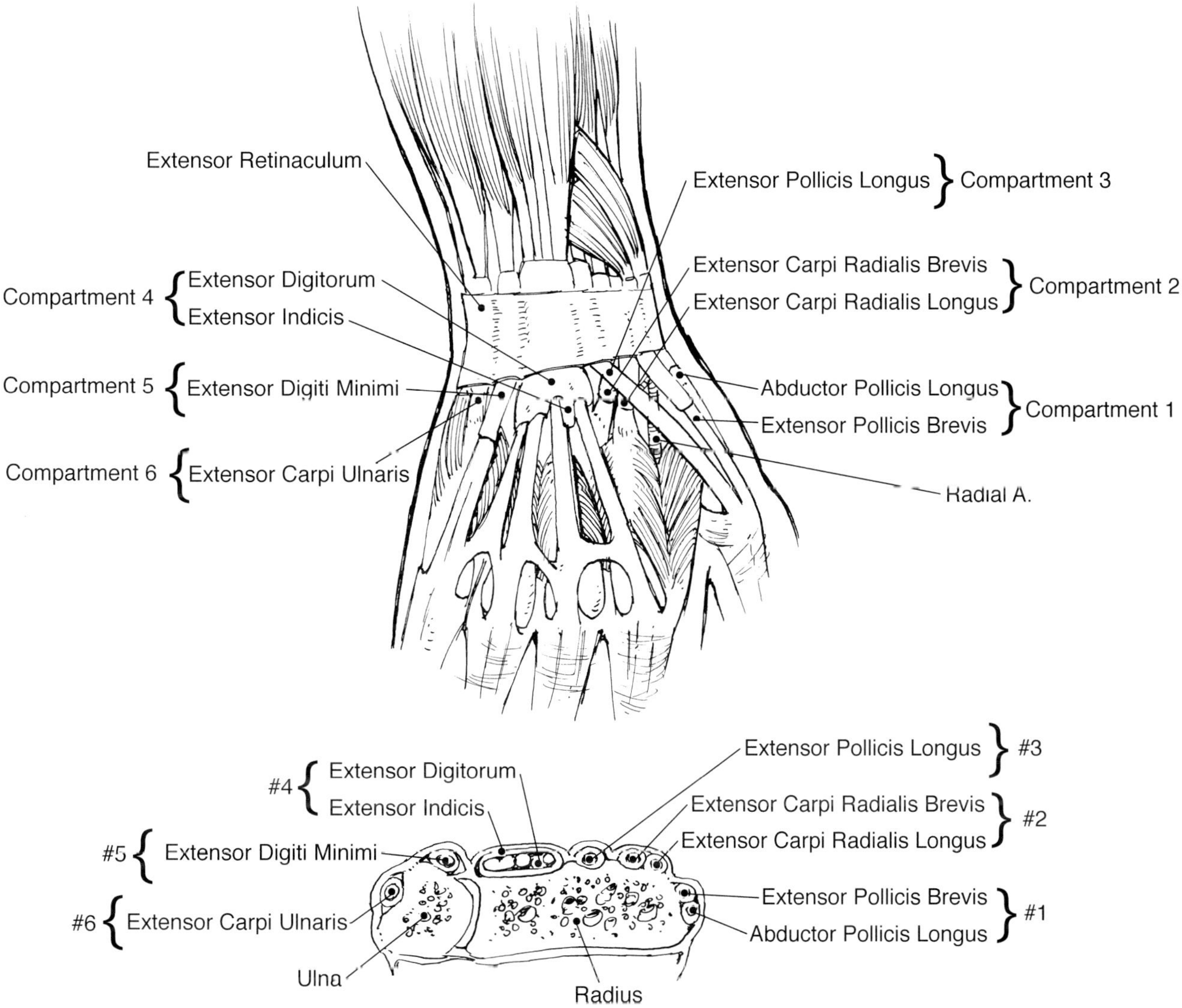


**FIGURE VIII-3**

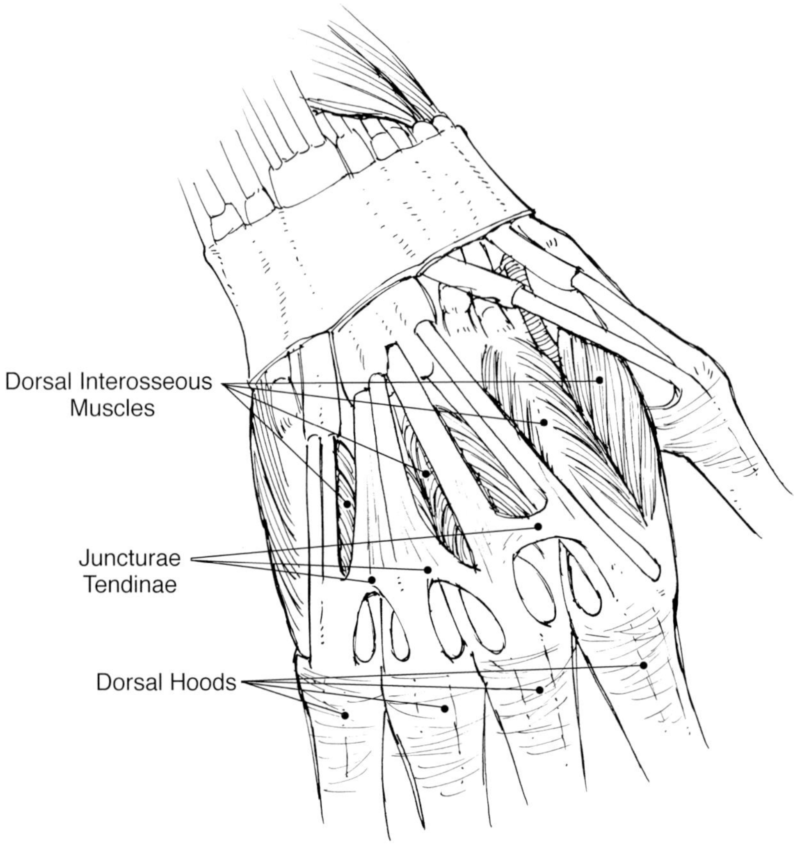


**FIGURE VIII-4A**

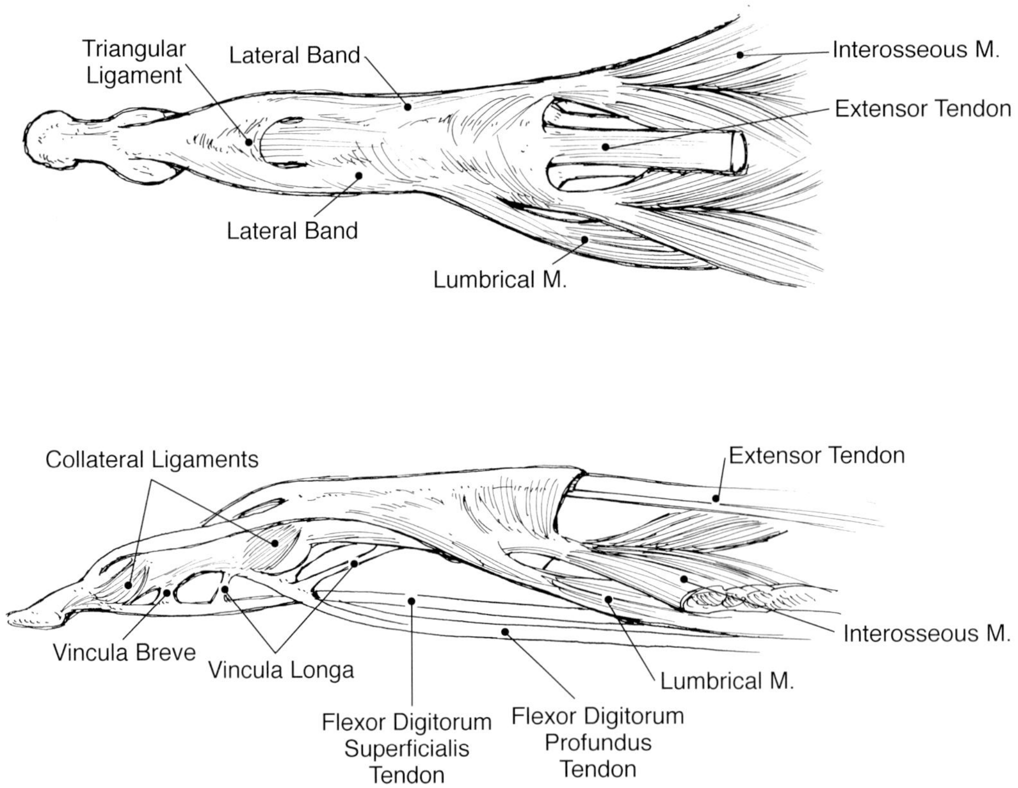


**FIGURE VIII-4B**

*Anterior Wrist*

The carpal tunnel is a fibro-osseous canal made up of the pisiform, hook of the hamate, ridge of the trapezius, and scaphoid tubercle. Its volar "roof" is the flexor retinaculum which attaches to these four bony landmarks (VIII-5). Four structures pass superficial to the flexor retinaculum: the tendon of the palmaris longus, the palmar cutaneous branch of the median nerve; and the ulnar nerve and artery (VIII-6). Just proximal to the wrist, the ulnar nerve and artery pass ventrally from

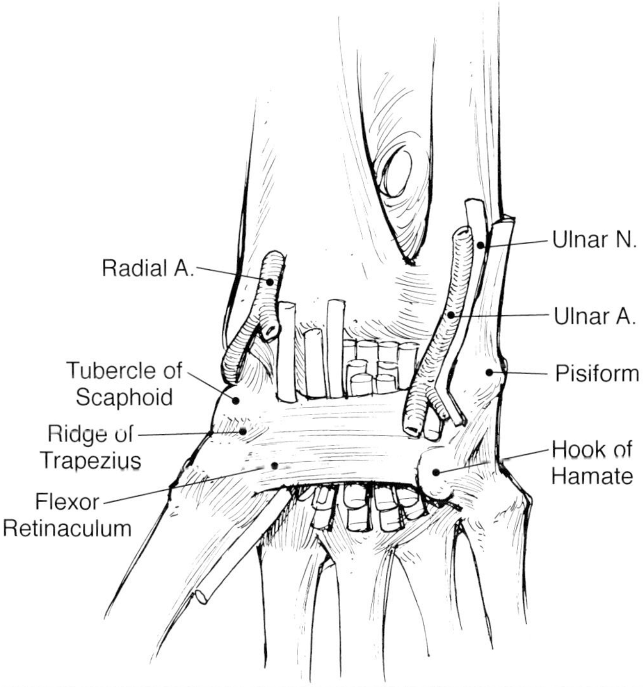


**FIGURE VIII-5**

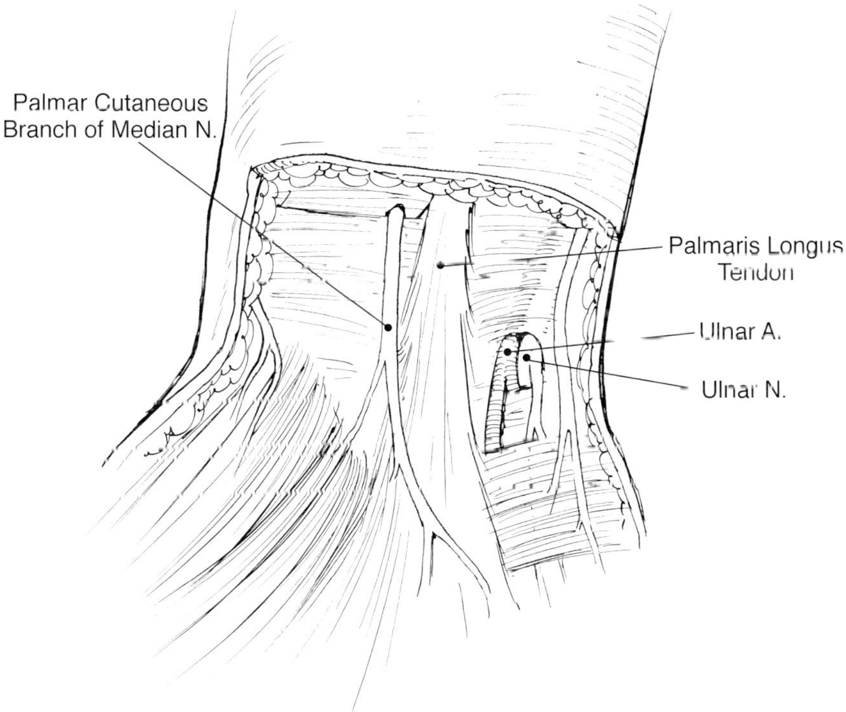


**FIGURE VIII-6**

under the flexor carpi ulnaris tendon to pass superficial to the flexor retinaculum and enter the canal of Guyon. This canal consists of the pisiform medially, the hamate laterally, the flexor retinaculum dorsally, and the transverse carpal ligament anteriorly (VIII-7). The median nerve and long flexor tendons pass through the carpal tunnel, deep to the flexor retinaculum. The median nerve lies superficial to the flexor digitorum superficialis tendons at the wrist, between the tendons of the palmaris longus and flexor carpi radialis.

### *The Palm*

The palm is divided into three compartments: thenar, central, and hypothenar. The palmar aponeurosis covers the anterior surface of the central compartment. It is a fibrous sheath continuous with the tendon of the palmaris longus (VIII-8). The palmar aponeurosis has deep fibrous connections to the first and fifth metacarpals which divide the palm into the three compartments. The nerves and vessels lie immediately deep to the palmar aponeurosis. The central compartment contains the long flexor tendons to the fingers, the adductor pollicis muscle, the digital nerves, and the superficial and deep palmar arches and their branches. The deep palmar space is a potential space between the long flexor tendons and the interossei and adductor pollicis muscles (VIII-9). The deep palmar space is divided sagittally by the oblique septum which projects from the third metacarpal to the flexor tendons of the middle fingers. This septum subdivides the deep palmar space into a medial (midpalmar) space and a lateral (thenar) space (VIII-10). The medial space contains the lumbricals to the middle, ring, and little fingers. Its deep boundary is composed of the interossei and metacarpals of the third and fourth spaces.

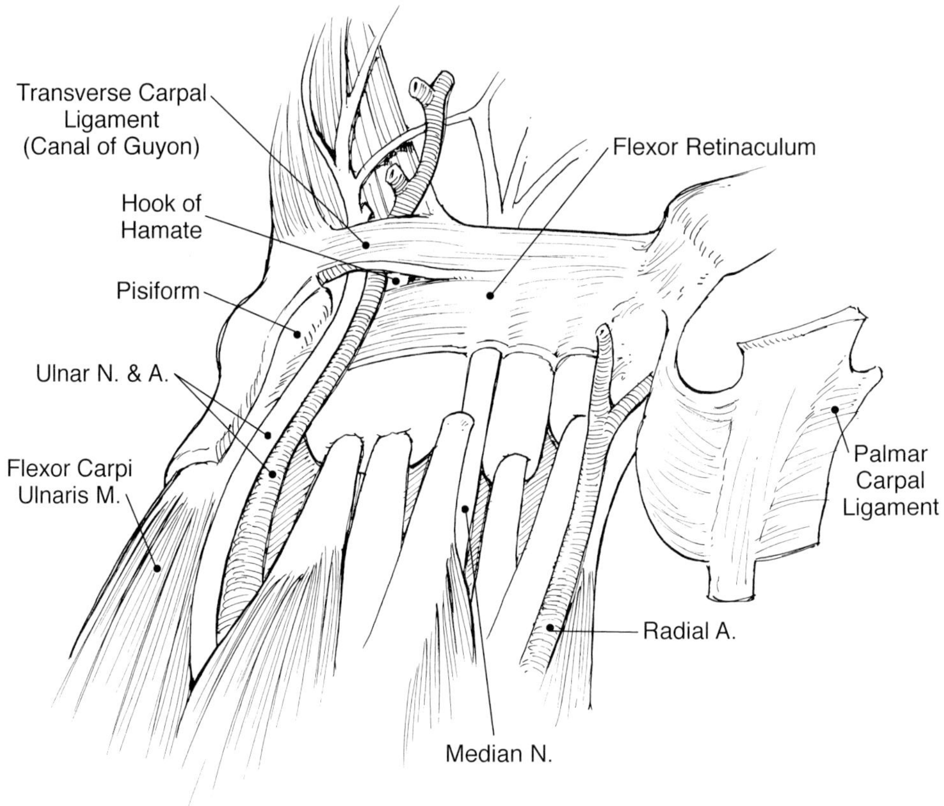


**FIGURE VIII–7**

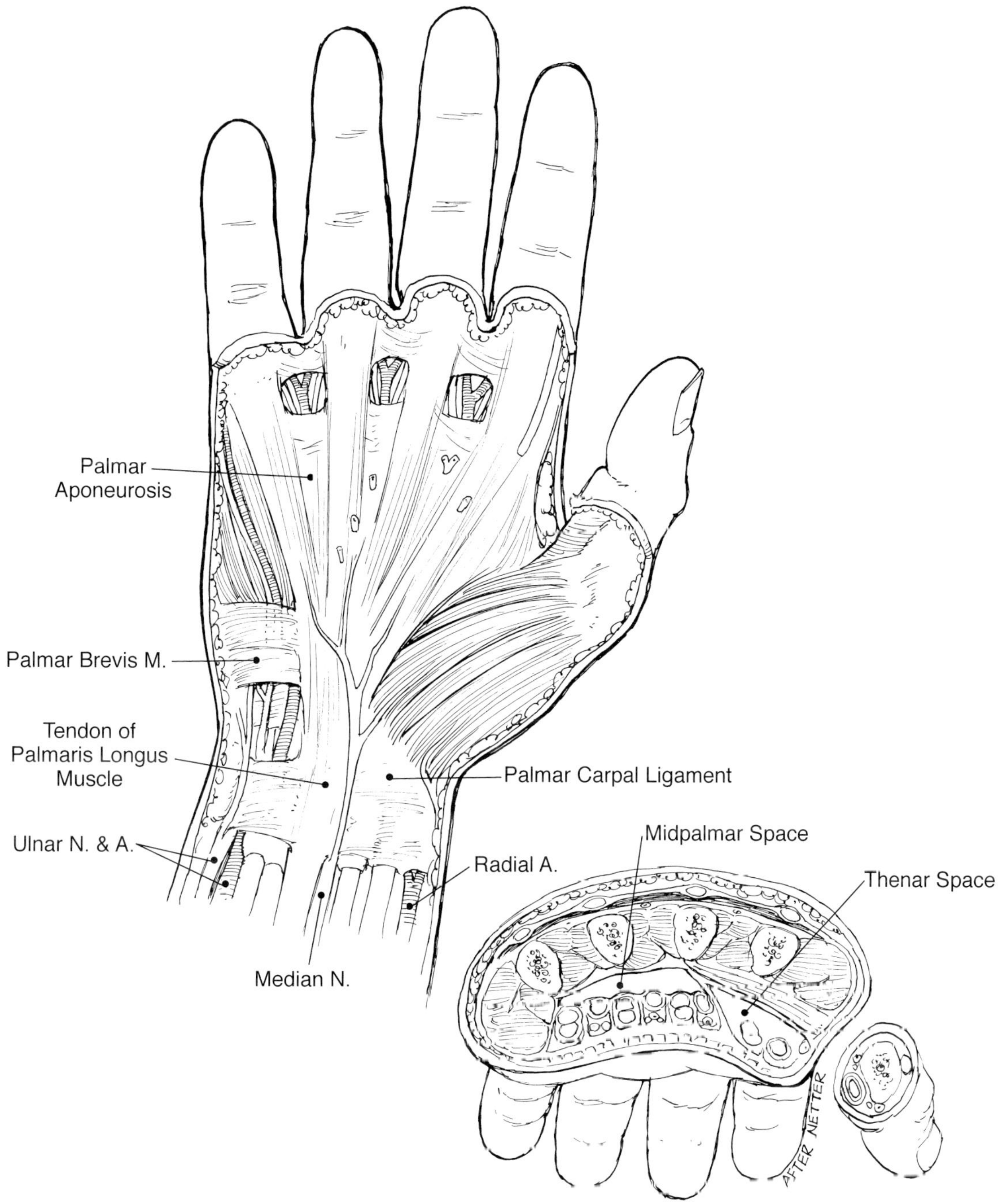


**FIGURE VIII–8**

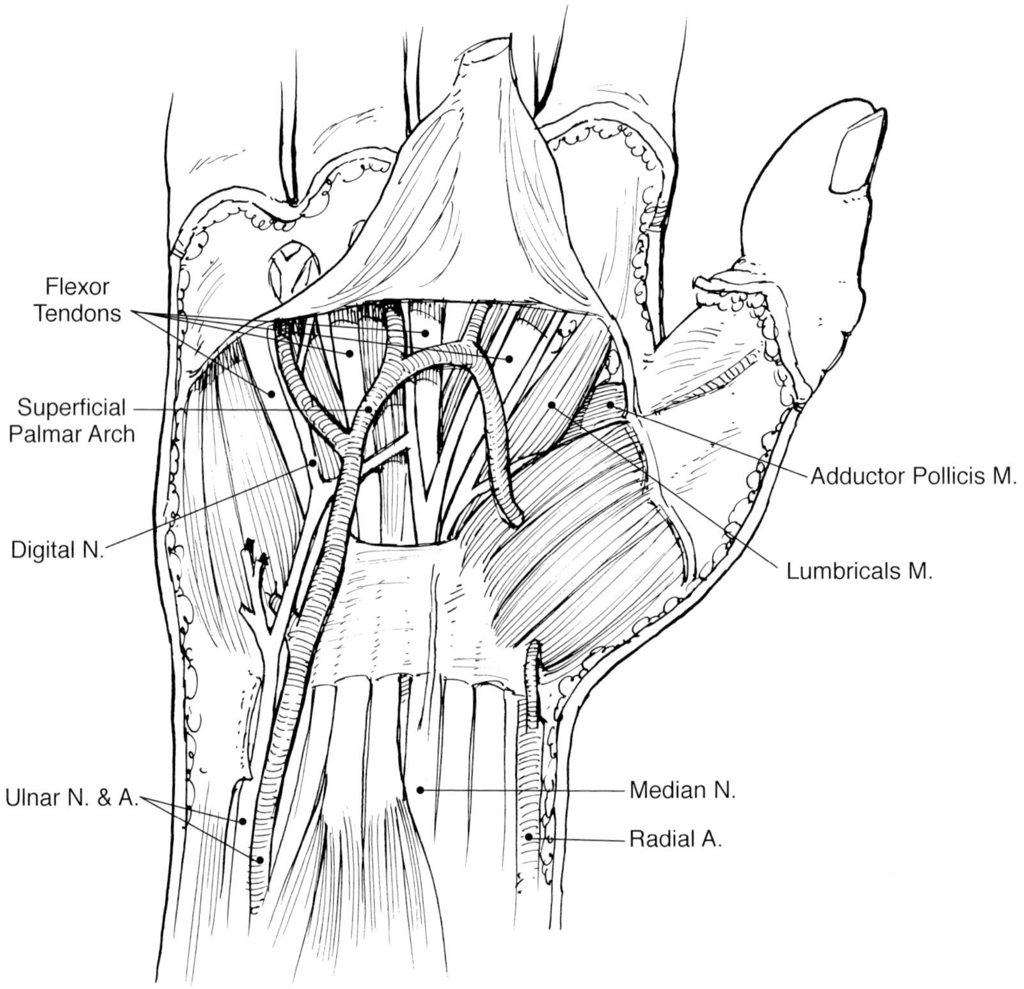


**FIGURE VIII–9**

The lateral space contains the first lumbrical which runs to the index finger flexor tendon. The deep surface of this space is the adductor pollicis (VIII-11).

The thenar eminence consists of the abductor pollicis brevis, flexor pollicis brevis, and opponens pollicis. All three are innervated by the median nerve except for the deep head of the flexor pollicis brevis which receives its nerve supply from the ulnar nerve.

The hypothenar eminence consists of the abductor digiti minimi, flexor digiti mini, and opponens digiti minimi. These muscles are innervated by the motor branch of the ulnar nerve.

The superficial palmar arch is formed largely, if not entirely, by the ulnar artery. It connects to the superficial palmar branch of the radial artery. Four palmar digital arteries arise from the arcade, pass superficial to the nerves of the palm and distribute to the ulnar four fingers. It does not provide branches to the thumb or the radial side of the index finger. The long flexor tendons pass deep to the superficial palmar arch and digital nerves. The lumbrical muscles arise from the flexor profundus tendons and pass around the radial side of the metacarpophalangeal joint to insert on the extensor tendon expansions over the proximal phalanx. The deep palmar arch lies deep to the long flexor tendons. It consists of the terminal branch of the radial artery (which enters the palm between the heads of the adductor pol-

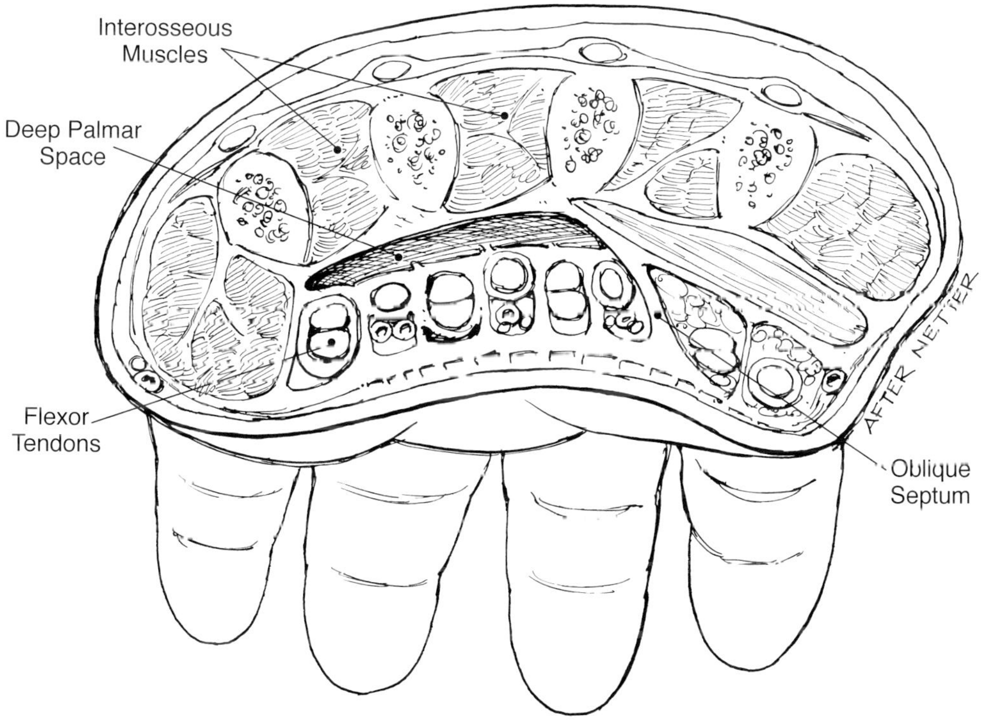


**FIGURE VIII-10**

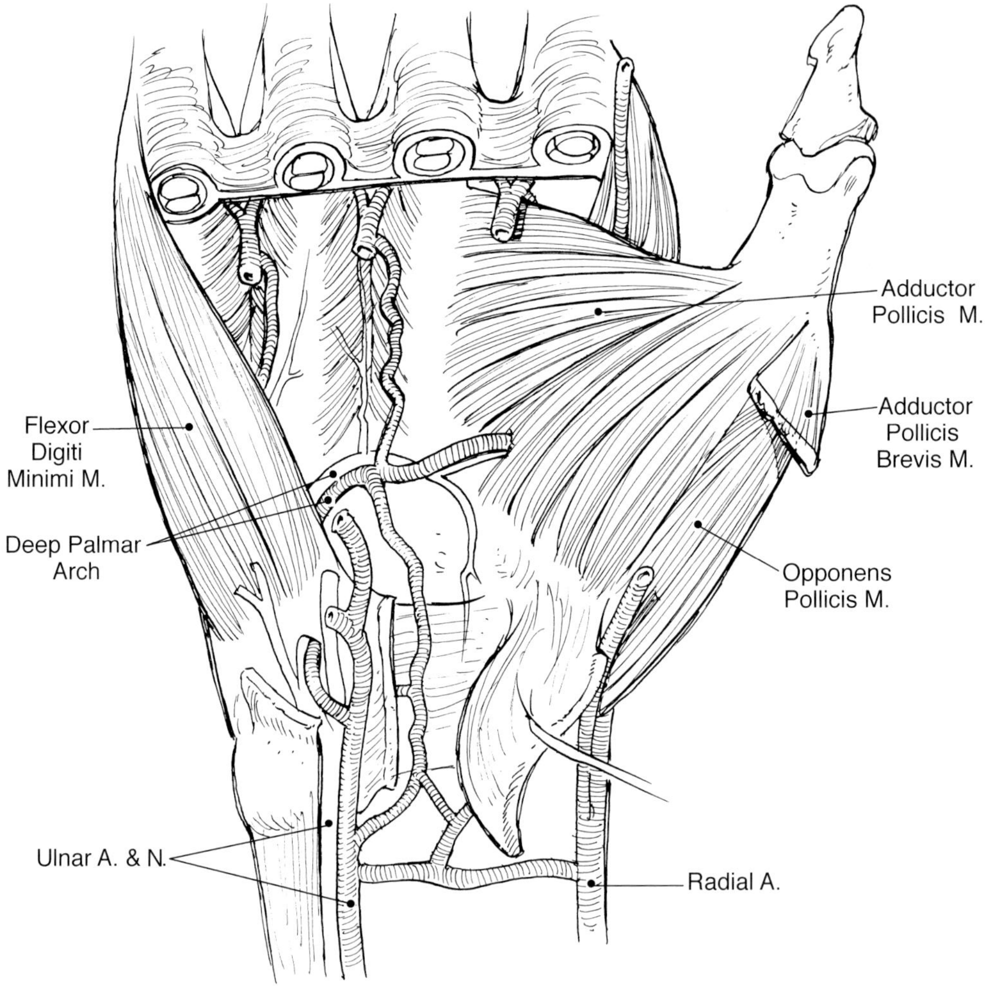


**FIGURE VIII-11**

licis) and the deep branch of the ulnar artery. The deep branch of the ulnar nerve runs with the ulnar artery to supply the interossei. The interossei are divided into dorsal and palmar groups. The dorsal interossei abduct the fingers away from the middle finger, the palmar interossei adduct the fingers toward it.

The radial artery passes deep to the first compartment extensor tendons to lie on the surface of the scaphoid in the anatomical snuff box. It then passes between the two heads of the first dorsal interosseus muscle. At this point, it gives off the radialis indices and princeps pollicis arteries to the index finger and thumb (VIII-12). The main trunk then continues between the heads of the adductor pollicis to enter the palm and form the deep palmar arch.

The ulnar nerve exits Guyon's canal and divides into superficial and deep branches. The superficial branch distributes with the superficial palmar arch. The deep branch passes between the bellies of origin of the opponens digiti minimi to distribute to the interossei in the same plane as the deep palmar arch. There are three web spaces between the four fingers. They extend from the edge of the skin to the metacarpophalangeal joints. They contain the superficial and deep transverse ligaments, the digital nerves and vessels, and the tendons of the interossei and lumbricals. The superficial transverse ligament (natatory ligament) lies immediately deep to the palmar skin to support the margins of the webs. It runs superficial to the digital nerves and vessels and attaches to the palmar aponeurosis. The deep transverse metacarpal ligament interconnects the volar plates of the metacarpophalangeal joints. It runs 3 cm proximal to the superficial transverse metacarpal ligament. The tendons of the interossei pass dorsal to the deep transverse metacarpal ligament, while the digital nerves and vessels and lumbricals pass volar to it. The transverse metacarpal ligaments do not exist in the first web space. The first web space is filled with the first dorsal interosseous muscle and the transverse head of the adductor pollicis.

The finger flexor tendons are arranged in five zones from proximal to distal as described by the classification of Milford (3). Zone 5 is in the anterior compartment of the forearm proximal to the flexor retinaculum (VIII-13). Here the tendons are surrounded by a synovial sheath and not enclosed in a tight canal. Tendon repairs are usually successful in this zone. Zone 4 is the space in the carpal

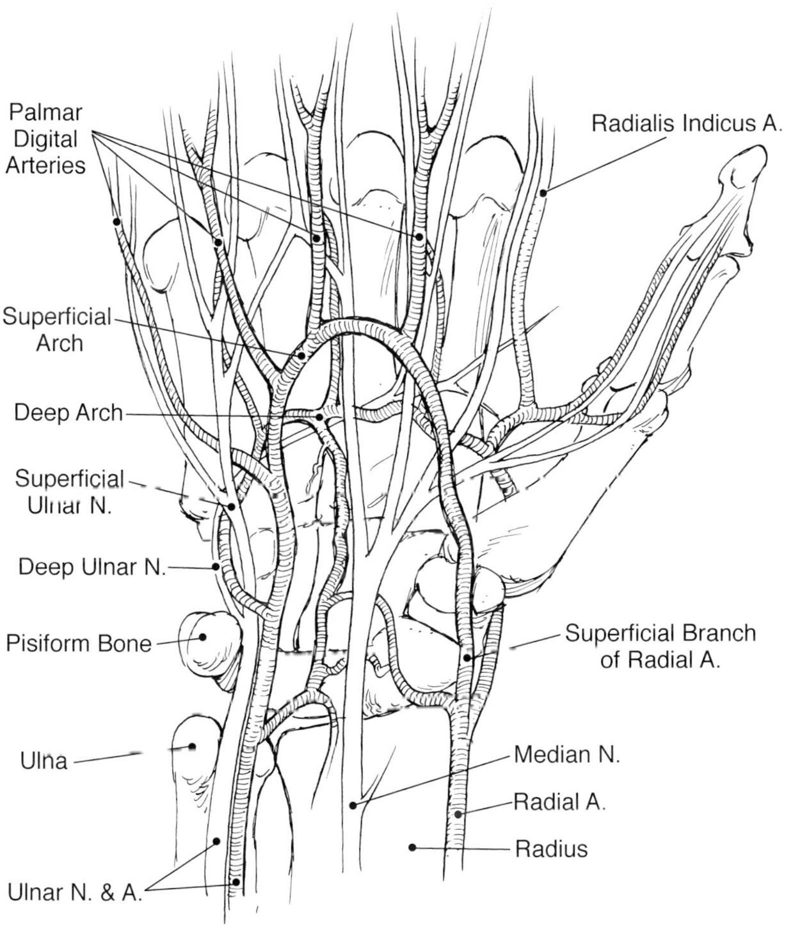


**FIGURE VIII–12**

tunnel. Here the tendons are in a common synovial sheath. Tendon repairs are usually successful in this zone but are more likely to form adhesions. Zone 3 is the midpalm in the area of the origin of the lumbricals. When lacerated along with the flexor tendons, the lumbricals are not usually repaired because doing so results in scarring that can lead to fixed flexion deficits of the metacarpophalangeal joint and loss of flexion of the interphalangeal joints (an "intrinsic plus" hand). Zone 2 extends from the distal palmar crease to the middle of the middle phalanx. The long flexor tendons run in a common fibro-osseous sheath in each digit. The sheath is made up of seven pulleys, divided into annular (A1 through A4) and cruciate (C1 through C3) types. The cruciate pulleys are interposed in sequence between the annular pulleys and are not critical for flexor tendon function. The A1 pulley is volar to the metacarpophalangeal joint. The A2 pulley is at the level of the proximal end of the proximal phalanx. It must be preserved or, if cut, it must be repaired to prevent bowstringing of the flexor tendons. The A3 pulley overlies the proximal interphalangeal joint. The A4 pulley is located at the middle of the middle phalanx and is also necessary for function of the flexor tendons (VIII-14). The sublimis tendon splits at the level of the proximal phalanx (in the A2 pulley) and passes around the profundus tendon to insert on the base of the middle phalanx. Therefore, laceration of the flexor tendons in Zone 2 is most likely to result in tendon adhesions during healing. Zone 1 is distal to the insertion of the super-

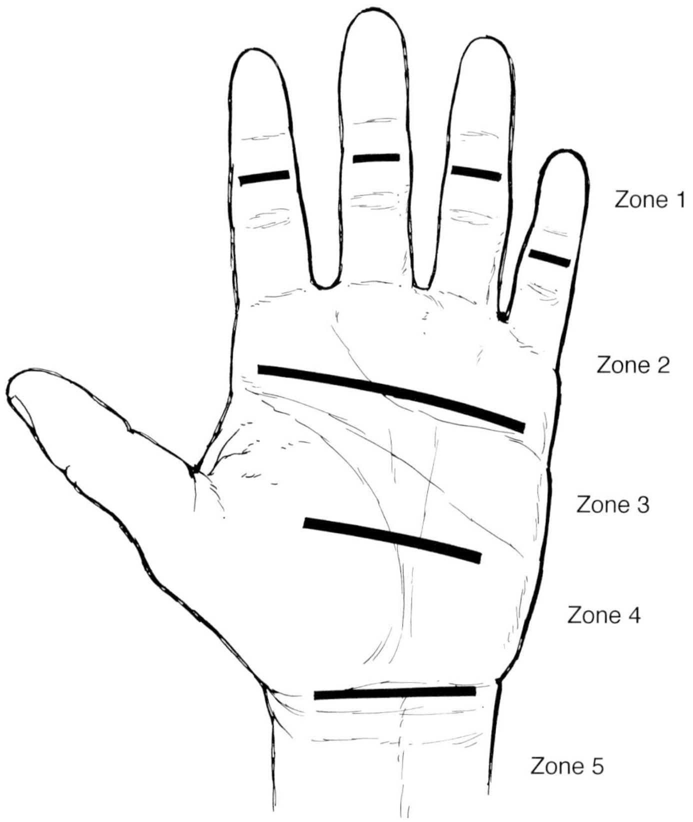


**FIGURE VIII–13**

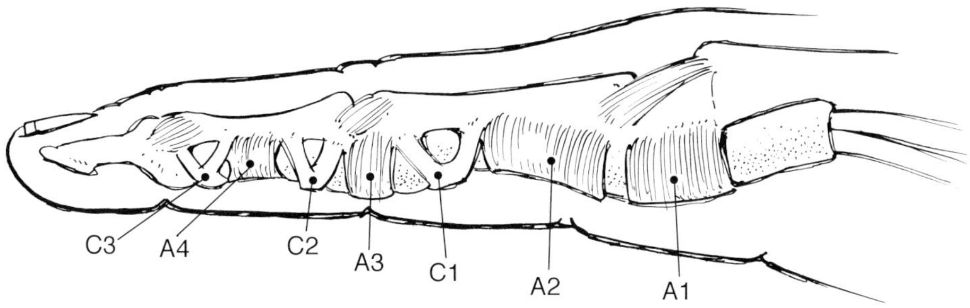


**FIGURE VIII-14**

ficialis tendon and contains only the profundus tendon. Each flexor tendon receives a blood supply from a long and short vinculum on its dorsal surface.

# Dorsal Approach to the Wrist

***Applications***

There are a multitude of reasons for surgery on the dorsum of the wrist including tendon lacerations, ruptures or transfers, reconstruction of the wrist for bone or ligament injuries, open reduction and internal fixation of fractures or dislocations, wrist fusion or synovectomy, or excision of tumors.

***Technique***

The patient is placed supine with the forearm pronated on an arm board. The incision is made transversely through a dorsal wrist crease and can be extended through a proximal zig-zag if necessary (VIII-15). This exposes the extensor retinaculum and extensor tendons and the proximal half of the dorsal hand. The dorsal veins should be preserved as much as possible. The flaps are raised deep to the fascia proximally and directly over the extensor tendons in the hand. The extensor retinaculum is preserved (VIII-16). For broad exposure of the wrist, the extensor retinaculum can be incised longitudinally over the second compartment (extensor carpi radialis longus and brevis) (VIII-17). The ulnar side of the retinaculum is then elevated and reflected ulnarward, transecting the fascial projections from the wrist to unroof the remaining four compartments (VIII-18). The wrist is then opened by elevating the tendons of the fourth compartment (extensor digitorum communis and extensor indices proprius) and incising the dorsal wrist capsule longitudinally (VIII-19). The exposure is extended by subperiosteal elevation of the wrist capsule from the distal radius and carpus. Alternatively, the retinaculum can be opened directly over the fourth compartment, the tendons can be elevated, and the joint capsule can be incised and elevated.

***Dangers***

The major concerns are injury to the superficial radial nerve and the dorsal cutaneous branch of the ulnar nerve, which can produce a painful neuroma. Disruption of the dorsal veins can lead to persistent edema and poor healing of the wound.

***Limitations***

This approach should provide wide access to the dorsum of the wrist and proximal hand. It can be extended into the forearm as a dorsal approach to the radius if necessary.

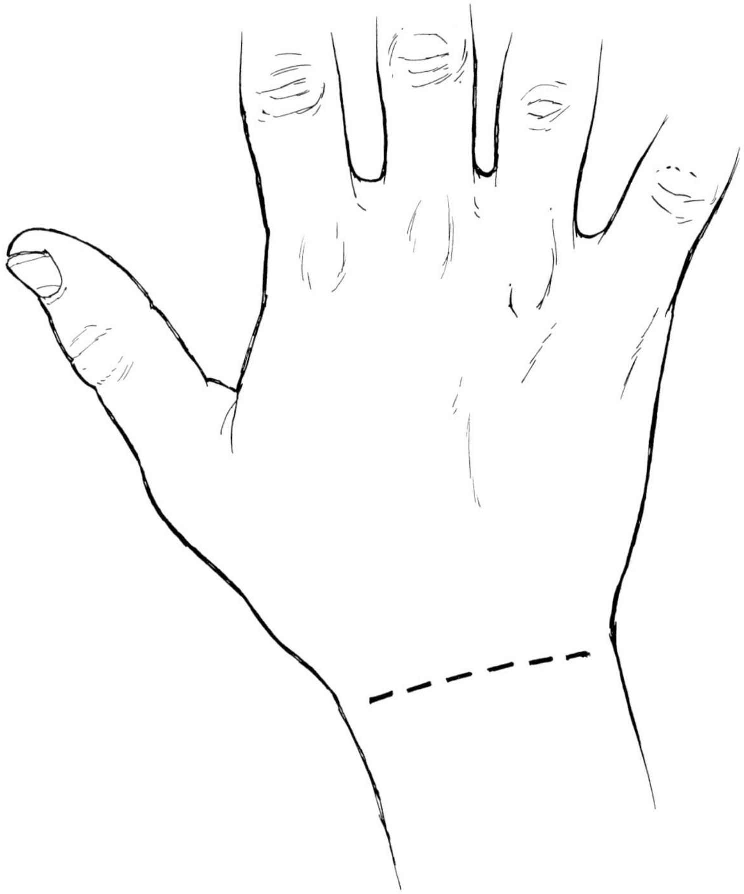

**FIGURE VIII–15**

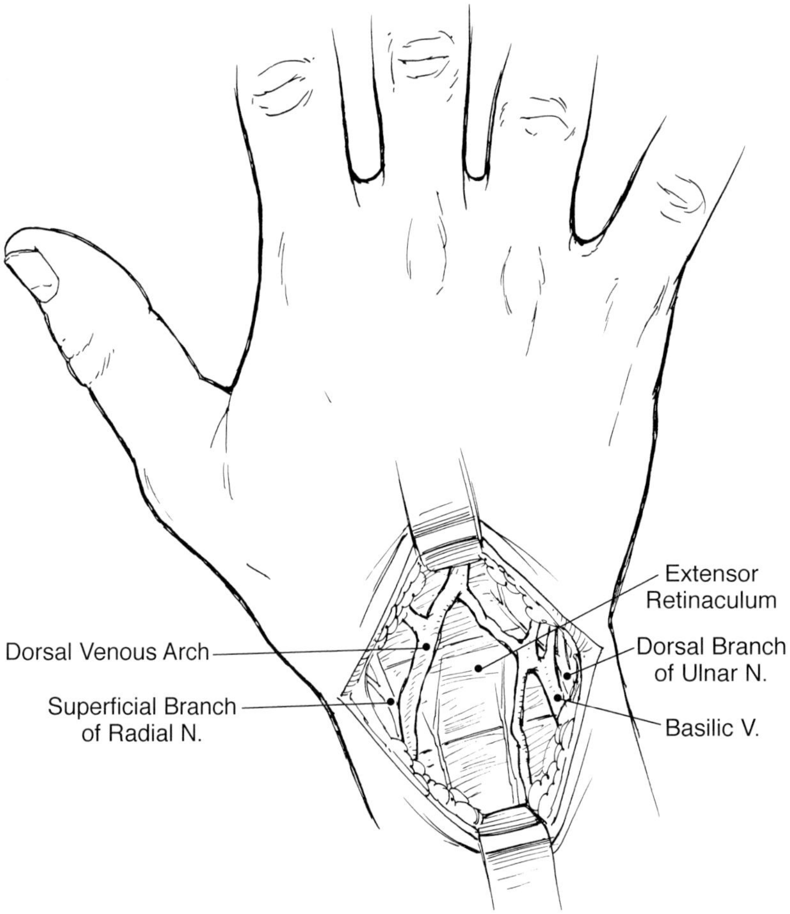


**FIGURE VIII–16**

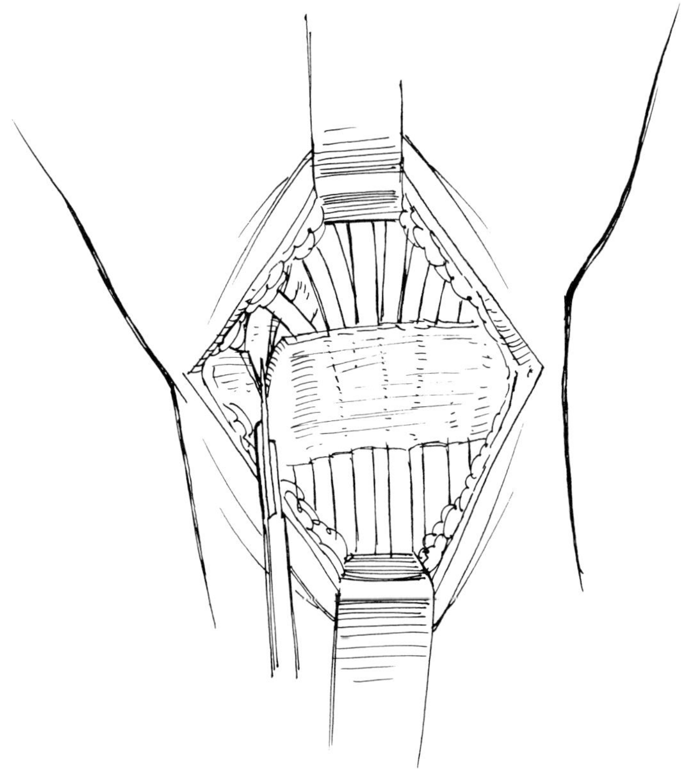

**FIGURE VIII–17**

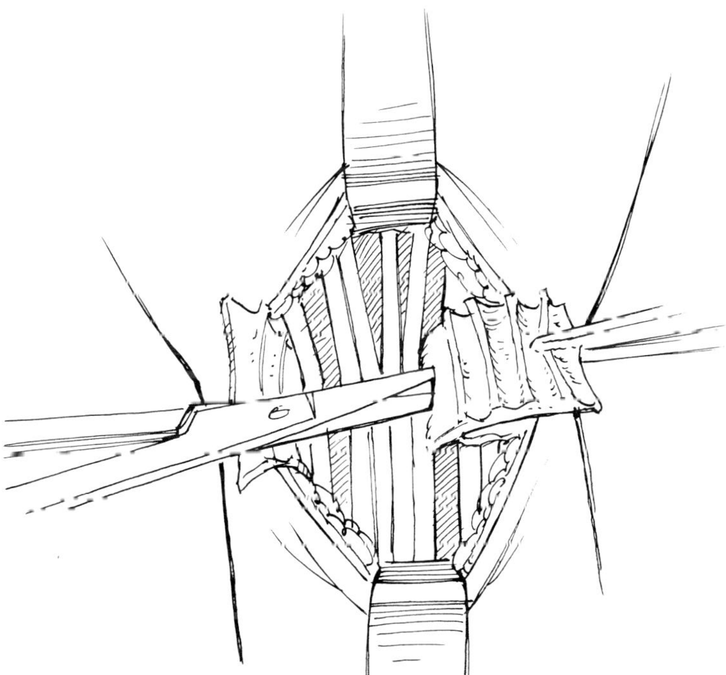

**FIGURE VIII–18**

# Volar Approach to the Wrist

***Applications***

This approach is used for decompression of the median nerve, flexor tendon synovectomy, repairs of lacerations of tendons or nerves, repair of ligament injuries associated with wrist dislocations and open reduction internal fixation of volar distal radius fractures.

***Technique***

The patient is supine with the arm supinated on an arm board. The incision begins proximal to the flexion crease of the wrist on the ulnar side of the palmaris longus tendon. It is carried down to the flexion crease and then carried in the flexion crease to the thenar crease. It is then carried in the thenar crease as far as is necessary (VIII-20). The subcutaneous fat and superficial palmar fascia are opened in line with the incision. The skin flaps are retracted to expose the palmaris longus tendon and flexor retinaculum (VIII-21). The retinaculum is incised on the ulnar side of the palmaris longus tendon longitudinally to expose the median nerve and flexor tendons (VIII-22). A blunt retractor can be placed in the carpal tunnel and the retinaculum and palmar aponeurosis are opened onto the retractor to protect the median nerve (VIII-23). The flexor tendons may be elevated from the floor of

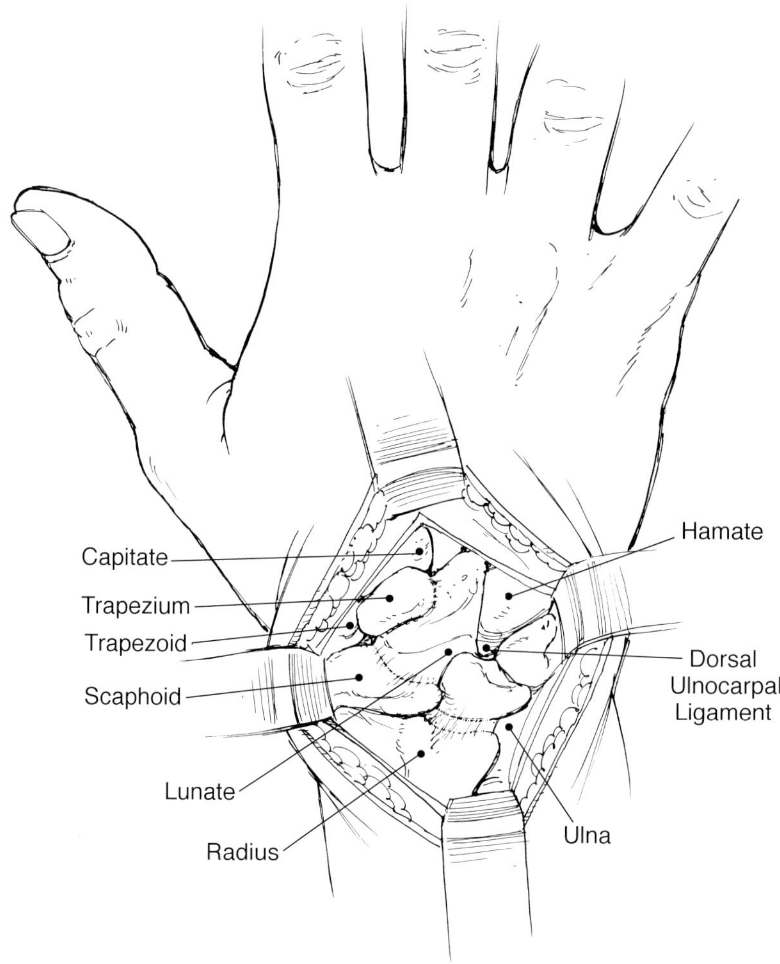


**FIGURE VIII–19**

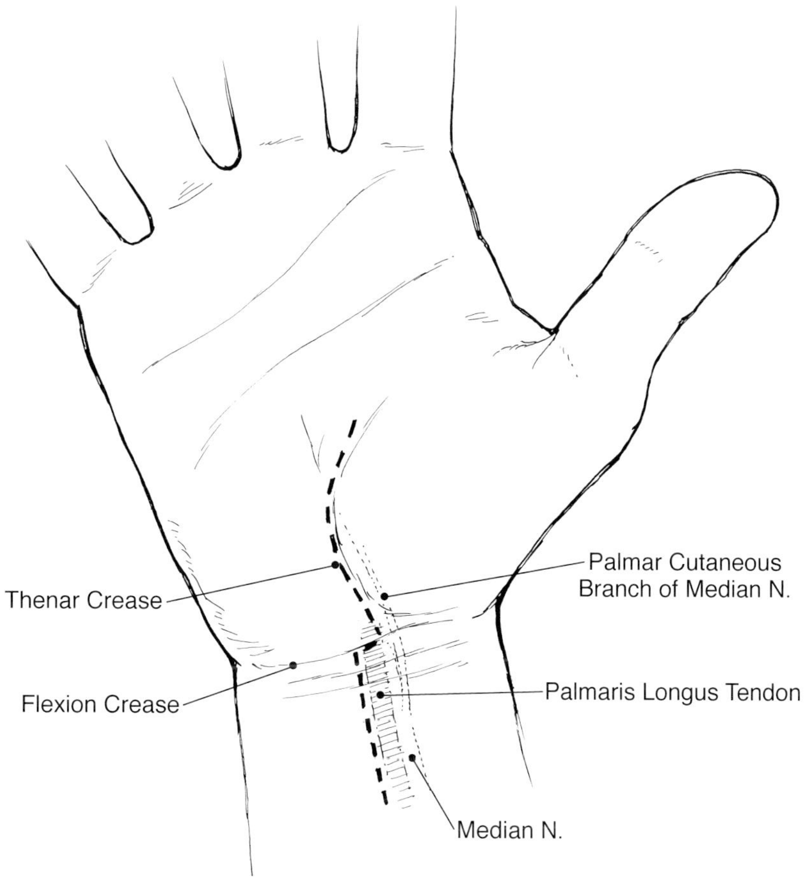


**FIGURE VIII–20**

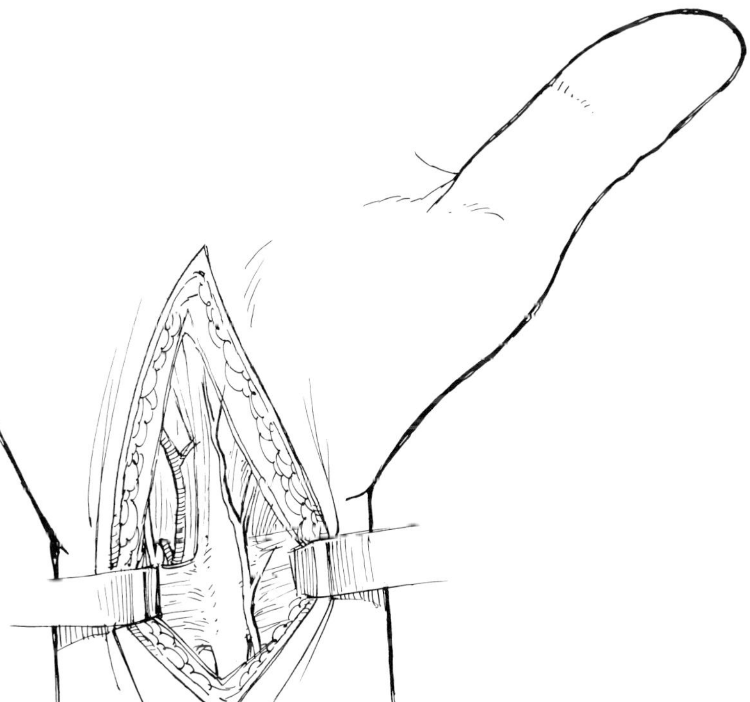

**FIGURE VIII–21**

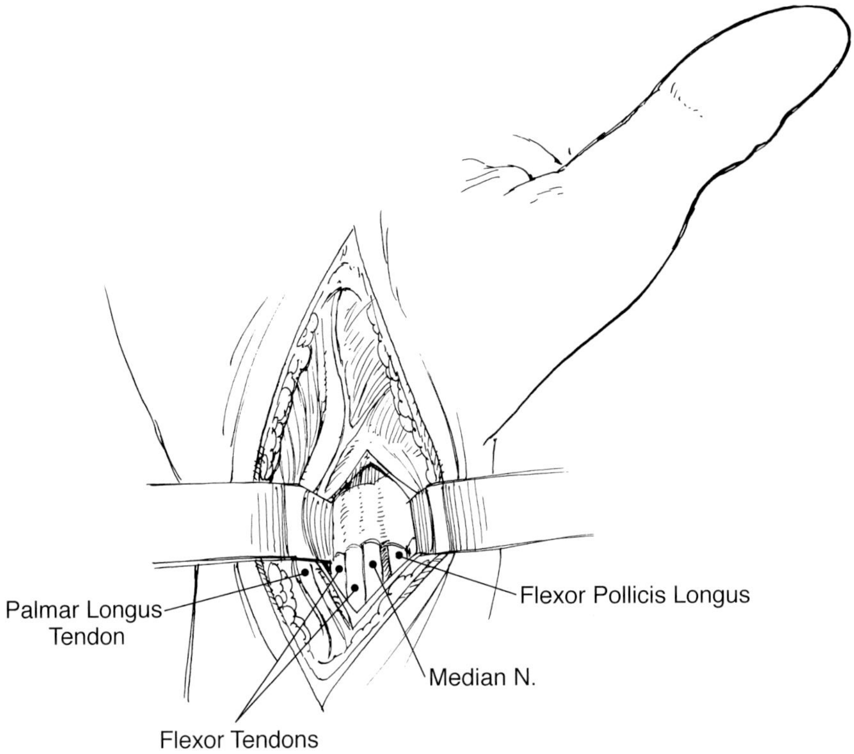


**FIGURE VIII–22**

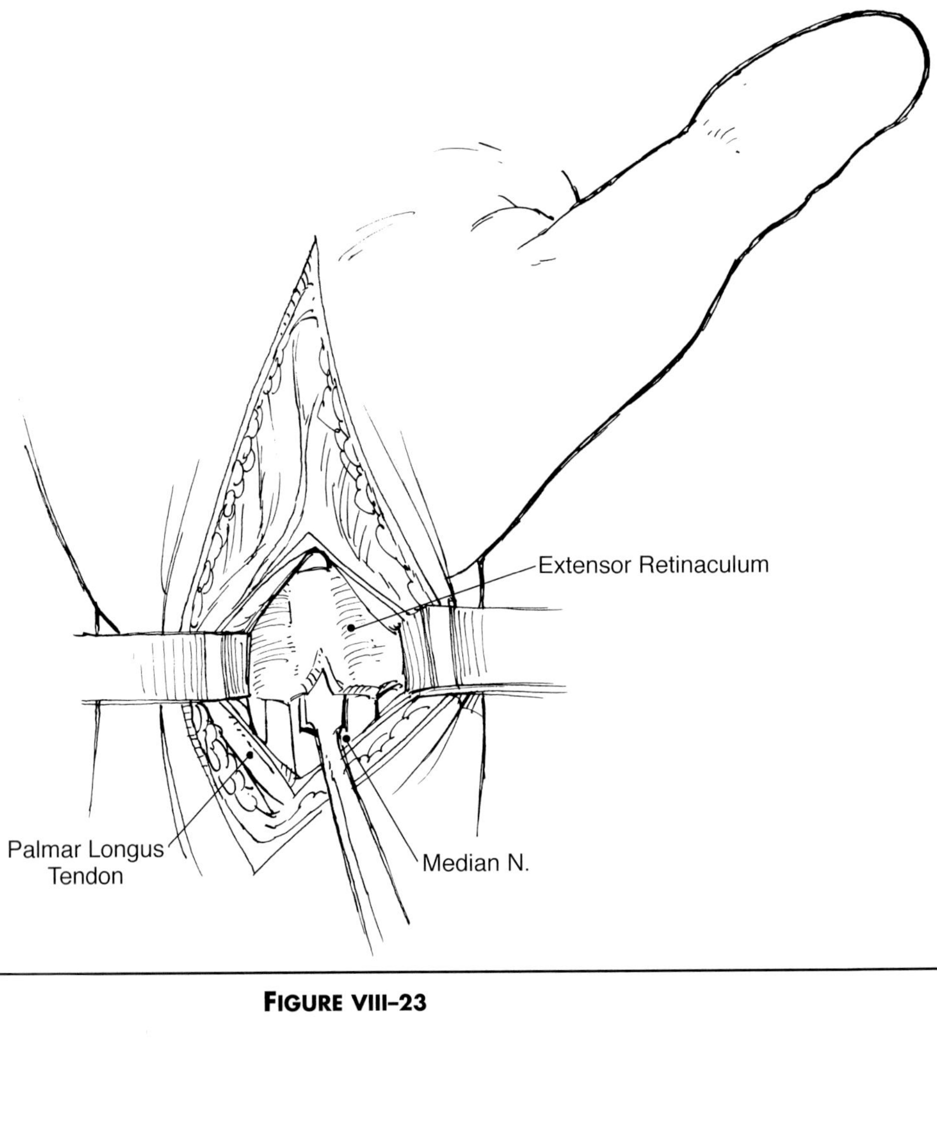


**FIGURE VIII–23**

the carpal tunnel ulnar to the median nerve to prevent traction on the motor branch of the median nerve. The motor branch is found entering the thenar eminence just distal to the carpal tunnel on the anterolateral side of the nerve. Elevation of the flexor tendons exposes the volar surface of the radius and wrist joint (VIII-24).

***Dangers***

The palmar cutaneous branch of the median nerve runs along the ulnar side of the flexor carpi radialis tendon to pass superficial to the flexor retinaculum and can be damaged by straying into the radial side of the carpal tunnel in the subcutaneous tissue. The motor branch of the median nerve is variable in location and vulnerable to injury in the proximal palm. The superficial palmar arch crosses the distal end of this approach, just deep to the palmar aponeurosis.

***Limitations***

This approach can be extended into the volar forearm as a zig-zag incision as needed and continued in a zig-zag across the palm and into the fingers or thumb, if necessary.

# Dorsal Approach to the Hand

***Applications***

This approach is used for repair of extensor tendons or for tendon transfers, open reduction and internal fixation of metacarpal fractures, metacarpophalangeal joint reconstruction or replacement, and debridement of infections.

***Technique***

The best cosmetic result is obtained with transverse incisions (1). The proximal half of the hand can be reached by a transverse incision through the extensor crease of the wrist. The distal half may be reached by a transverse incision directly over the area of the planned procedure. The entire distal half of the dorsum of the hand may be reached by scalloped incisions which run distally over the apices of

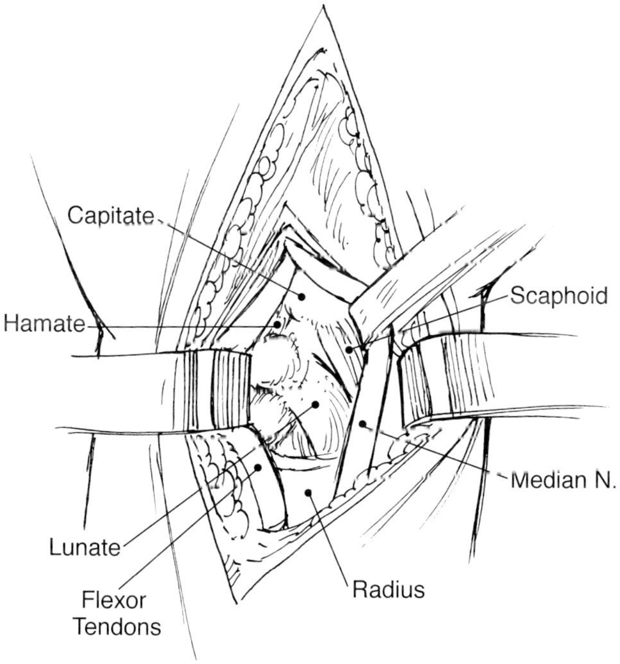


**FIGURE VIII–24**

the flexed metacarpophalangeal joints and curve proximally into the intermetacarpal spaces (VIII-25). The incision is through the skin onto the extensor tendons. It is imperative to preserve the dorsal veins as much as possible to prevent persistent edema and facilitate wound healing. Longitudinal incisions will heal, but with a significantly larger scar. For ray amputations or resection of malignant tumors of the dorsum of the hand or wrist, a longitudinal or zig-zag incision may be necessary to minimize adjacent tissue contamination. Incisional biopsy tracts for possibly malignant tumors should always be placed longitudinally to allow a minimal amount of soft tissue resection at the time of definitive tumor removal. The skin is elevated superficial to the extensor tendon for exposure as far proximally as necessary. Direct exposure of a metacarpal is made by lifting the extensor tendon and incising the periosteum on the dorsum of the metacarpal, then elevating the interosseous muscles subperiosteally.

***Dangers***

The concerns of this approach are excessive disruption of the dorsal skin veins which can lead to chronic edema of the hand and fingers and compromise wound healing. A transverse incision placed more proximally on the dorsal hand may injure branches of the superficial radial nerve or the dorsal branch of the ulnar nerve that may result in a painful neuroma.

***Limitations***

Extension of the transverse incisions can be obtained by lengthening the incision transversely or converting it to a zig-zag incision. Retracting skin flaps limits visibility and access to the dorsum of the hand to approximately half the length of the metacarpals.

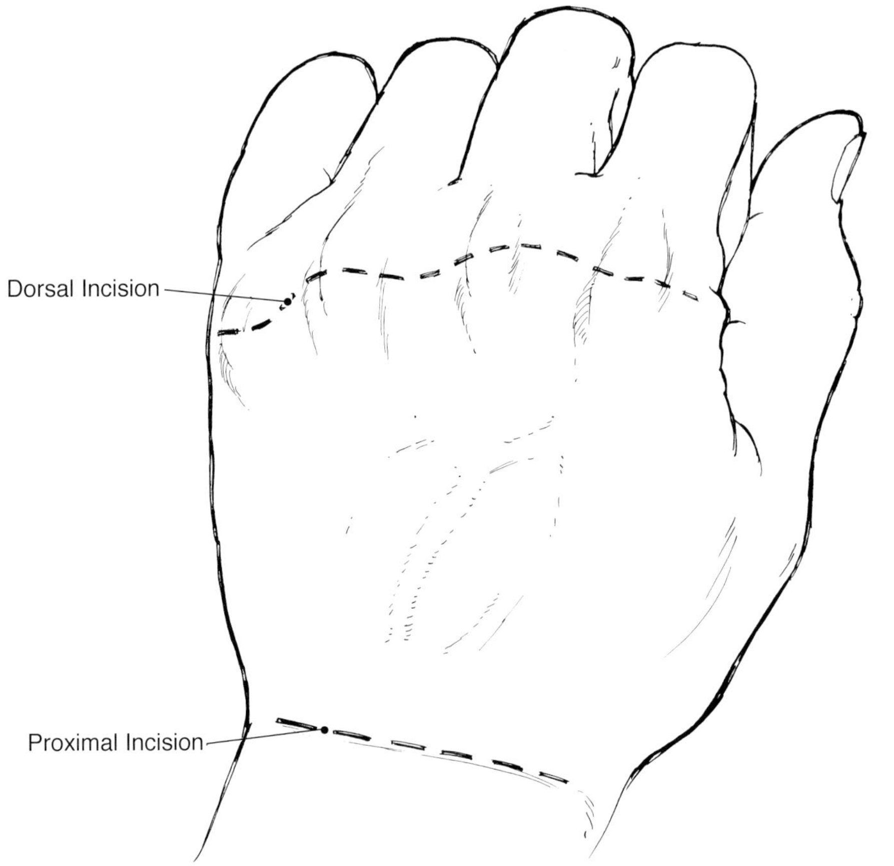


**FIGURE VIII–25**

# Surgical Approach to the Palm and Web Space

### *Applications*

Access to the palm is most often needed for repair of flexor tendon or digital nerve lacerations, resection of palmar fascia for Dupuytren's disease, and drainage of abscesses.

### *Technique*

Skin incisions are placed within the thenar crease to expose the thenar eminence, in the hypothenar crease to expose the hypothenar eminence, and in the proximal or distal transverse palmar crease to expose the midpalmar space (VIII-26). For more extensive exposures, these incisions may be converted into zig-zag incisions crossing the palmar creases at oblique angles, and they may be extended across the wrist or onto the fingers as necessary. The web space may be reached by any arcuate incision just proximal to the edge of the web and following it (VIII-27). The skin is incised and retracted with skin hooks to expose the subcutaneous fat. The fat and fascia are then incised longitudinally. The nerves and vessels are separated from the flexor tendon sheaths by longitudinal spreading of the adventitial tissue. The dissection can be carried deeply by opening the interval between the radial edge of the flexor sheath and the neurovascular bundle, spreading longitudinally (VIII-28). The flexor sheath is opened longitudinally if necessary. The metacarpals can be exposed deep to the flexor tendon sheath, but there is rarely a need to

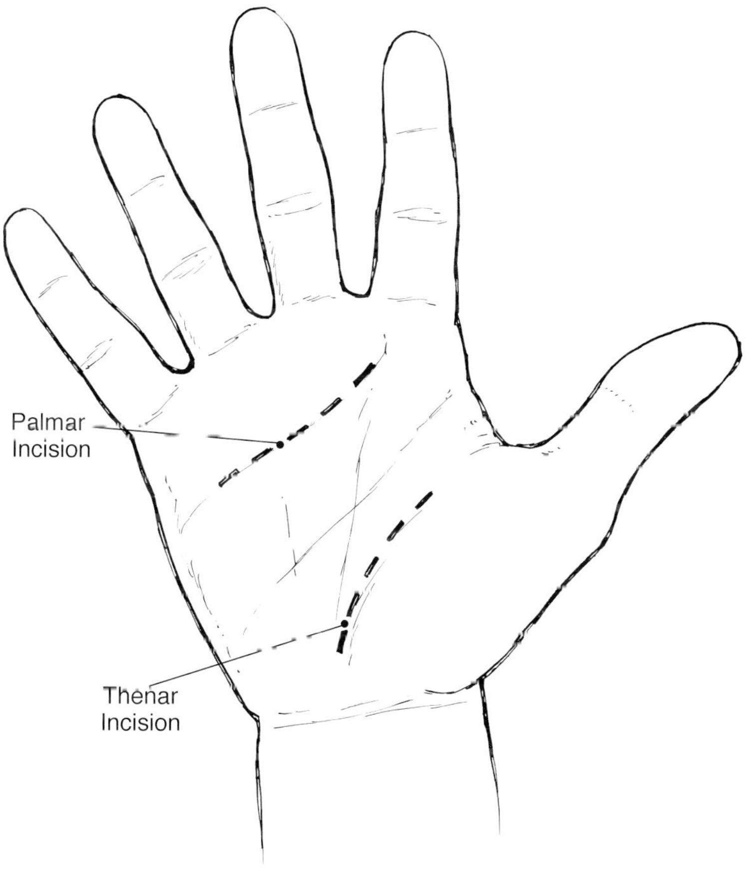


**FIGURE VIII–26**

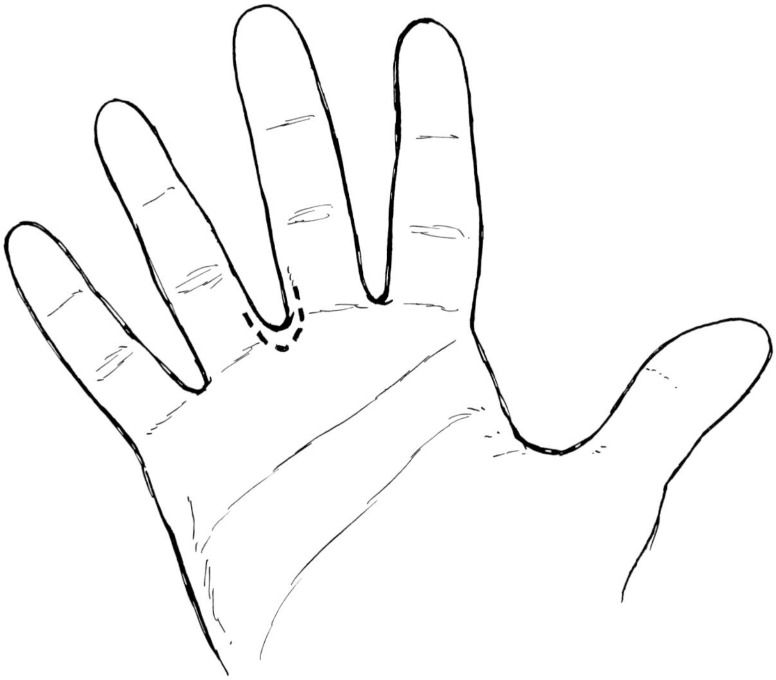

**FIGURE VIII–27**

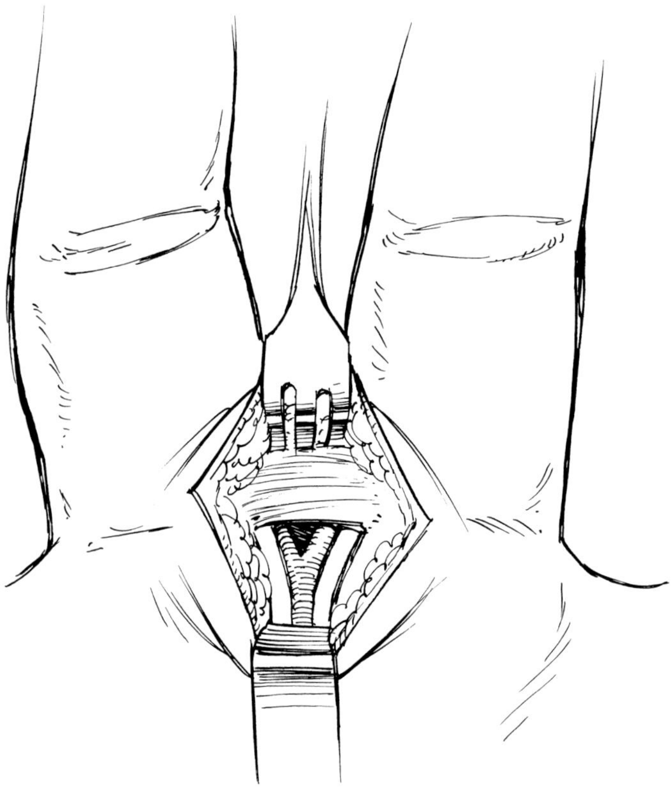

**FIGURE VIII–28**

expose the metacarpals from the volar surface since they are much more easily and safely reached by a dorsal approach. Extension of the dissection around the flexor tendon will likely lead to adhesions and permanent loss of finger motion.

***Dangers***

Broad subcutaneous skin flaps may result in necrosis of the skin. Digital nerves and vessels may be damaged by transverse dissection. Disruption of the flexor tendon sheath may produce adhesions leading to permanent loss of finger motion.

***Limitations***

The incision may be extended proximally onto the forearm and distally onto the fingers as needed. Multiple longitudinal incisions should be spaced as widely as possible to avoid vascular compromise of the skin flaps. The metacarpals are poorly exposed from this approach.

## Dorsal Approach to the Fingers

***Applications***

This exposure is often needed for removal of foreign bodies, repair of extensor tendon lacerations, or reconstruction of interphalangeal joints.

***Technique***

The proximal and distal interphalangeal joints and their adjacent phalanges may be approached by an S-shaped incision with the transverse limb overlying the joint crease. The proximal and distal limbs should be just dorsal to the midlateral line. The skin is incised to expose the extensor tendon and the flaps raised off of the surface of the tendon (VIII-29). The interphalangeal joints may be reached by a longitudinal split in the midline of the extensor tendon and joint capsule and further exposed by subperiosteal elevation of the capsule (VIII-30). The capsule and extensor tendons are then carefully repaired with interrupted sutures.

***Dangers***

Sharp angles on the skin flaps or skin dissection that is too superficial can result in skin necrosis. Extending the incision volar to the midlateral line can injure the digital neurovascular bundles.

***Limitations***

This exposure provides access to the interphalangeal joints, extensor tendons, and phalanges. It does not allow exposure to the flexor tendons and requires extensive subcutaneous dissection to adequately expose the digital nerves and vessels.

## Volar (Bruner) Approach to the Fingers

***Applications***

This approach gives wide exposure of the flexor tendon sheaths, flexor tendons, and digital nerves and vessels for repair or reconstruction (2).

***Technique***

The skin incision is made in a zig-zag pattern obliquely across the phalanges, connecting the midlateral line on alternating sides at the flexor creases (VIII-31). Full thickness skin flaps are elevated from the apices of the angles. The digital nerves and vessels will be exposed along the edges of the incision. The flexor tendon sheath may be exposed as far longitudinally as necessary (VIII-32).

***Dangers***

The greatest concern is preservation of the digital nerves and vessels during the initial exposure. If the flexor tendon is incised, then the annular pulleys A2 and A4 must be reconstructed to prevent bowstringing of the tendons.

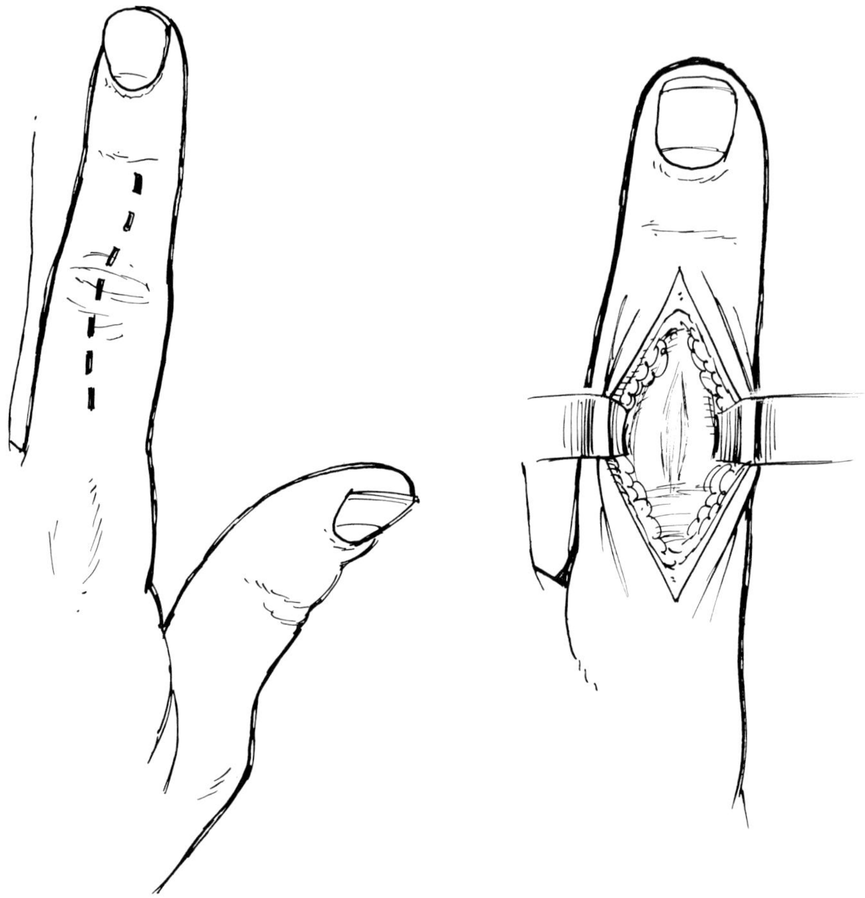

**FIGURES VIII-29 & 30**

*Limitations*

This dissection may be carried distally over the distal phalanx and proximally into the palm as needed. It does not provide exposure of the extensor mechanism.

## Midlateral Approach to the Fingers

*Applications*

This approach is useful for the thumb and fingers. It provides access to the phalanges, the flexor tendon sheath and tendon, and the neurovascular bundle on the side of the incision. It may be used for repair of injuries to any of these structures. This approach creates a long volar flap containing the digital nerve and vessels. It is usually performed on the radial side of the digit.

*Technique*

The finger is flexed and a line is drawn connecting the apices of the flexor creases. The incision is then made along this line or slightly dorsal to it (VIII-33). The volar flap is created by dissecting longitudinally toward the midline to expose the phalanx and flexor tendon sheath. The digital nerves and vessels will be found along the edge of the volar flap. The approach can be carried across the flexor sheath by dissecting on its surface.

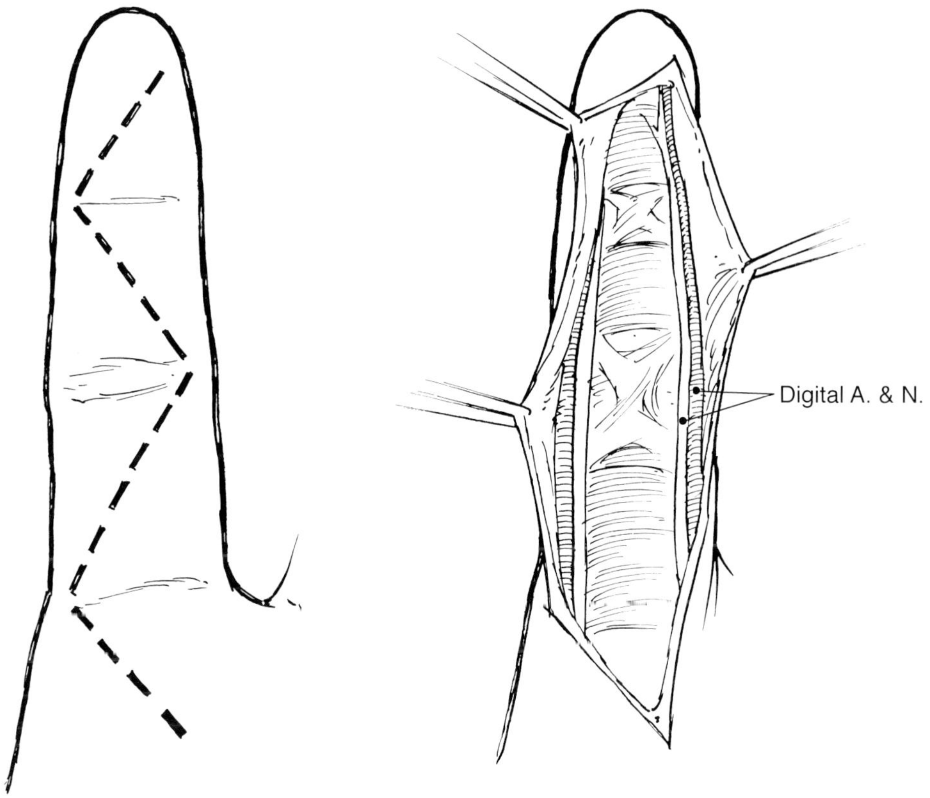


**FIGURES VIII–31 & 32**

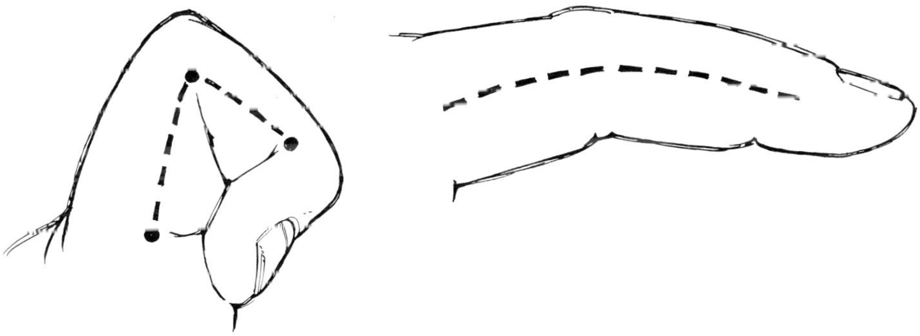

**FIGURES VIII–33**

***Dangers***

The major hazard is injury to the digital nerve or vessels. The skin over the proximal interphalangeal joint is thin and care must be taken to not dissect into the joint.

***Limitations***

This approach can be extended onto the palm by a zig-zag incision, but to do this requires crossing the neurovascular bundle and increases the risk of injury to it.

# References

1. Adamson JE, Fleury AF. Incision in the hand and wrist. In: Green DP, ed. Operative Hand Surgery. New York: Churchill Livingstone, 1982:1263–1281.
2. Bruner JM. The flexor tendons in the hand. J Bone Joint Surg 53:84, 1973.
3. Milford L. The hand. In: Edmonson AS, Crenshaw AH, ed. Campbell's Operative Orthopaedics, St. Louis: C.V. Mosby, 1980.

# IX

# SURGICAL APPROACHES TO THE PELVIS

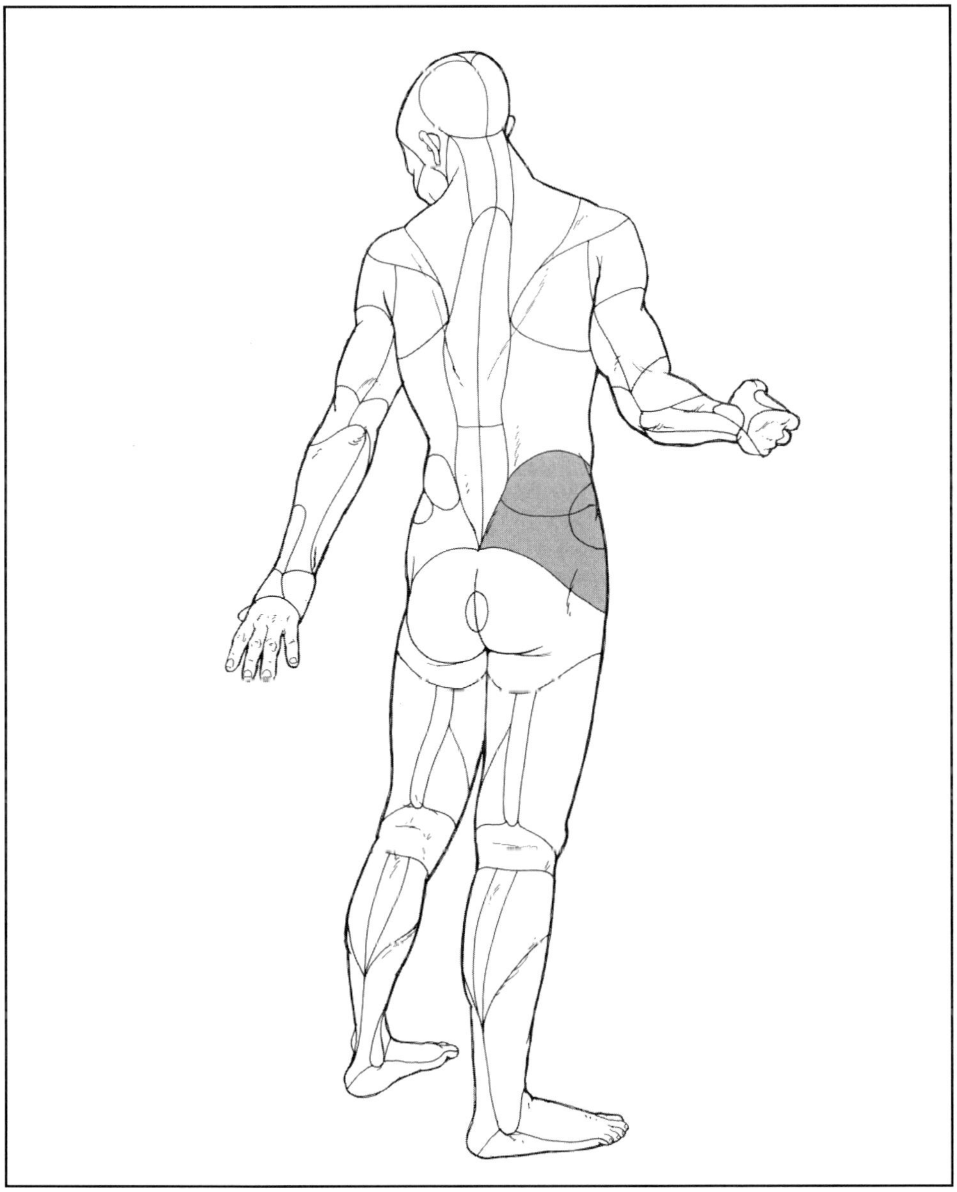

# General Principles and Complications

Many orthopaedic problems in the pelvis, such as complex pelvic ring and acetabular fractures, periacetabular or sacral tumors, or infections have historically been treated non-operatively with mediocre results (1). As our knowledge and experience in surgical anatomy have improved, enthusiasm for surgical management of these problems has increased. Nevertheless, orthopaedic surgery in and about the pelvis has been fraught with some of the most severe complications seen in orthopaedics, including loss of limb and life.

When considering open reduction of pelvic ring and periacetabular fractures, the surgeon must first be aware that patients with this injury usually have numerous other injuries. These most frequently include closed head and spine injury, blunt chest and abdominal trauma, urologic or rectal injury, and extremity injuries. In addition, patients with pelvic fractures can be expected to have massive blood loss from disruption of the pelvic veins, along with additive blood loss from the concomitant injuries. For example, the average acute blood loss in a patient with an open Malgaigne fracture is 18 units (2), which must be replaced promptly during the initial resuscitation.

Therefore, precedence must be given to stabilizing the patient's pulmonary, hemodynamic, and multiple organ involvement, as well as preventing infection prior to surgical management of the pelvic fracture. Conversely, there is a sense of urgency to stabilize the skeleton to allow mobilization of the patient. Mobilization is necessary to minimize the severity of secondary problems such as pneumonia, skin breakdown, and late infections. Experience has already shown that uncontrolled blood loss from immediate open reduction of the pelvis will increase patient mortality (3). Therefore, at the present time, it is recommended that in most cases the ideal time to undertake internal fixation of pelvic fractures is 5 to 10 days after the injury.

A second consideration in planning surgery for fractures of the pelvis is to assess the severity of soft tissue damage. Not only is major pelvic vein disruption at the time of injury to be expected, but there may also be major arterial injury, especially of branches of the internal iliac system that are relatively fixed against the bone. These vessels provide the major collateral blood supply to the muscles and skin about the pelvis. In addition, there can be massive crush injury to the soft tissues which will compromise their viability. A poorly planned surgical approach through devitalized skin and muscle can produce major problems with wound dehiscence, infection, and rhabdomyolysis. Thus, the surgeon must thoroughly evaluate the vascular supply to the pelvis, plan the surgical procedure to minimize the extent of dissection, and plan the dissections through viable tissue with a reliable blood supply (4).

Third, in dealing with pelvic fractures, there is an increased incidence of common complications which occur in surgery about the hip and pelvis. In particular, these patients are at significant risk of developing deep venous thrombosis in the thigh and pelvis, where the thrombi are more likely to produce symptomatic or fatal pulmonary emboli. The surgeon must plan a regimen of prophylaxis to minimize this risk. This may include a combination of mechanical antiembolic devices (compressive stockings and sequential compression devices) and pharmacologic agents (heparin, aspirin, and warfarin). No single method has been proven superior; therefore, the surgeon must select a method that he believes provides adequate prophylaxis with minimal complications.

Fourth, the surgical approach must be designed to allow adequate exposure of the bony pelvis for the procedure, to minimize the amount of muscle damage, and to prevent injury to the nerves and vessels inside and outside the pelvis. Disruption of the origin of the hip muscles from the pelvis produces significant weakness, resulting in a permanent limp. Therefore, the surgical approach should be designed to minimize dissection through, or detachment of, the hip muscles, especially the abductors. Furthermore, disruption of the origin of these muscles will often lead to heterotopic bone formation that may severely compromise hip motion. If the muscles are damaged at the time of injury or during the dissection, the surgeon should consider prophylactic treatment, such as low dose radiation, to prevent heterotopic bone formation.

# Surgical Anatomy

The bony pelvis is a complex ring of three bones interconnected by three joints. The sacroiliac joints are supported by massive broad ligaments to withstand the vertical load of the trunk on the pelvis (IX-1A). Therefore, the most powerful and most important ligaments in the pelvic ring are those of the posterior sacroiliac ligament complex (IX-1B and IX-1C). They are augmented by the sacrospinous and sacrotuberous ligaments, which help to resist rotation. The retinaculum of the pubic symphysis and the anterior sacroiliac ligaments are weaker and secondary in importance. The spine is supported on the sacrum by the lumbosacral disc, the ver-

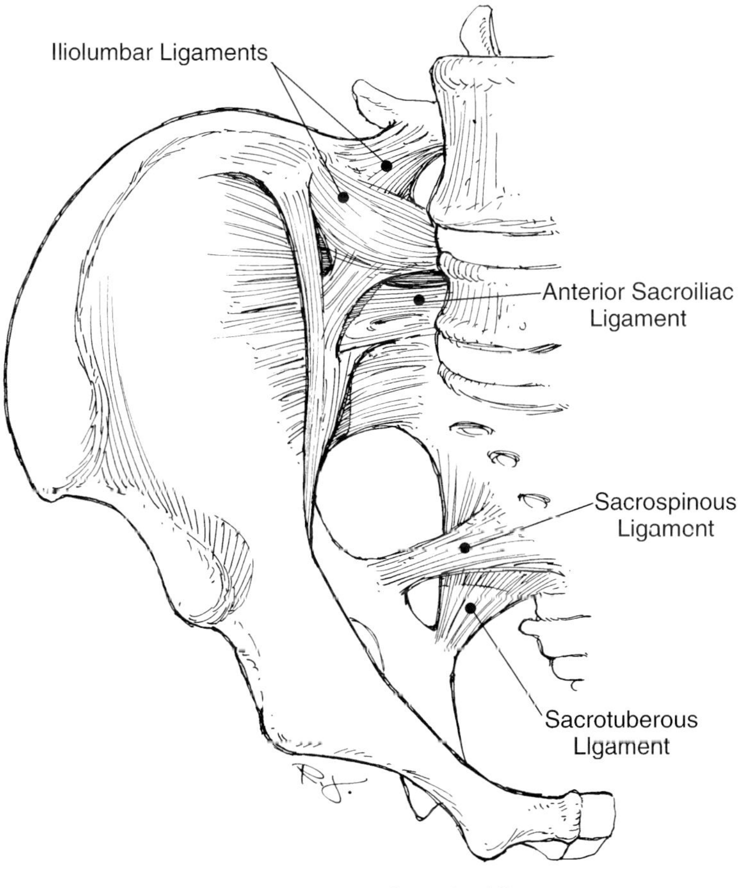


**FIGURE IX-1A**

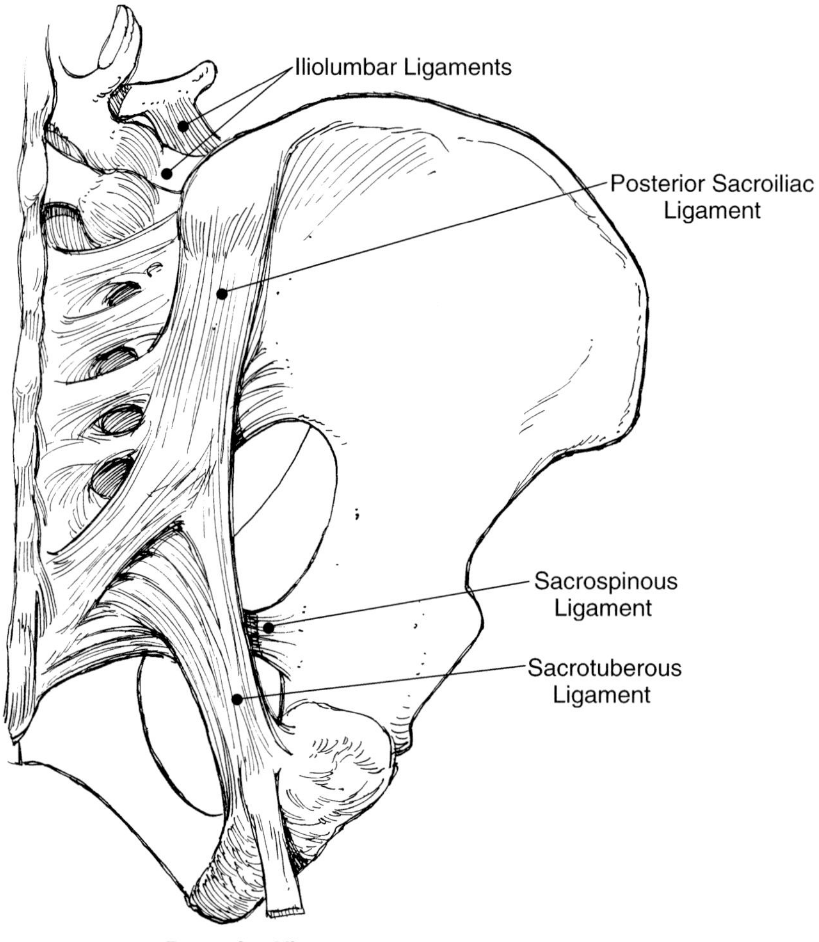
Iliolumbar Ligaments
Posterior Sacroiliac Ligament
Sacrospinous Ligament
Sacrotuberous Ligament
Posterior View

**FIGURE IX-1B**

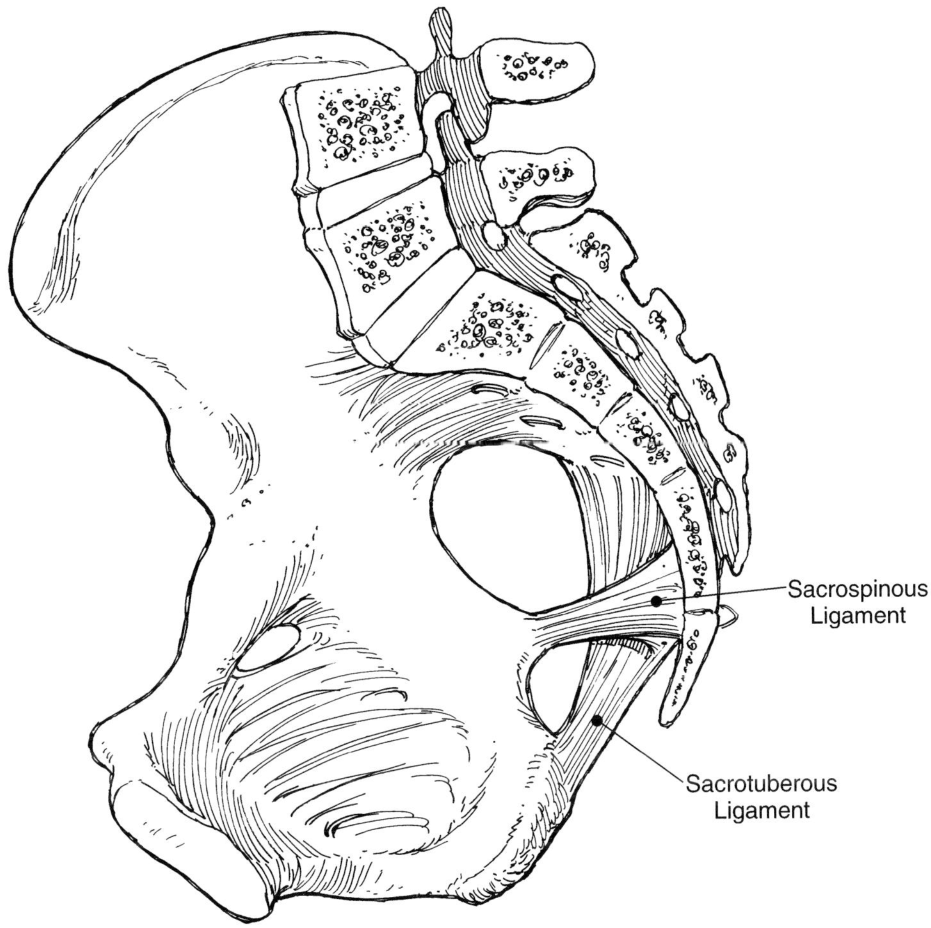


**FIGURE IX-1C**

tebral facets, and the iliolumbar ligaments (IX-2). The latter produce a tenacious suspension between the transverse processes of the fifth lumbar vertebrae and the iliac wing.

From the mechanical standpoint, the innominate bone is described as an inverted Y encircling the acetabulum (IX-3). The two caudal arms are divided into the anterior "iliopubic" column and the posterior "ilioischial" column. The iliopubic column includes the anterior portion of the iliac crest and extends to the pubic symphysis. It includes the anterior half of the iliac wing, the anterior half of the acetabulum, the pecten of the pubis, and the superior pubic ramus and symphysis. Externally, on the bone of the anterior column are the insertion of the external abdominal oblique muscles and the origin of the gluteus medius and minimus, rectus femoris, pectineus, adductor longus and brevis, tensor fascia lata, and sartorius (IX-4A, IX-4B, IX-4C, and IX-4D). Internally, in the false pelvis, the bony surface is covered by the iliacus muscle, and anteriorly, the superior pubic ramus is covered by the psoas major. The inner table of the superior pubic ramus is covered by the insertion of the arcus tendineus and the origin of the levator ani that bridge over the origin of the obturator internus (IX-5A).

The posterior column has the origin of the hamstring muscles and of the superior gemellus on its external surface. Internally, originating from the posterior col-

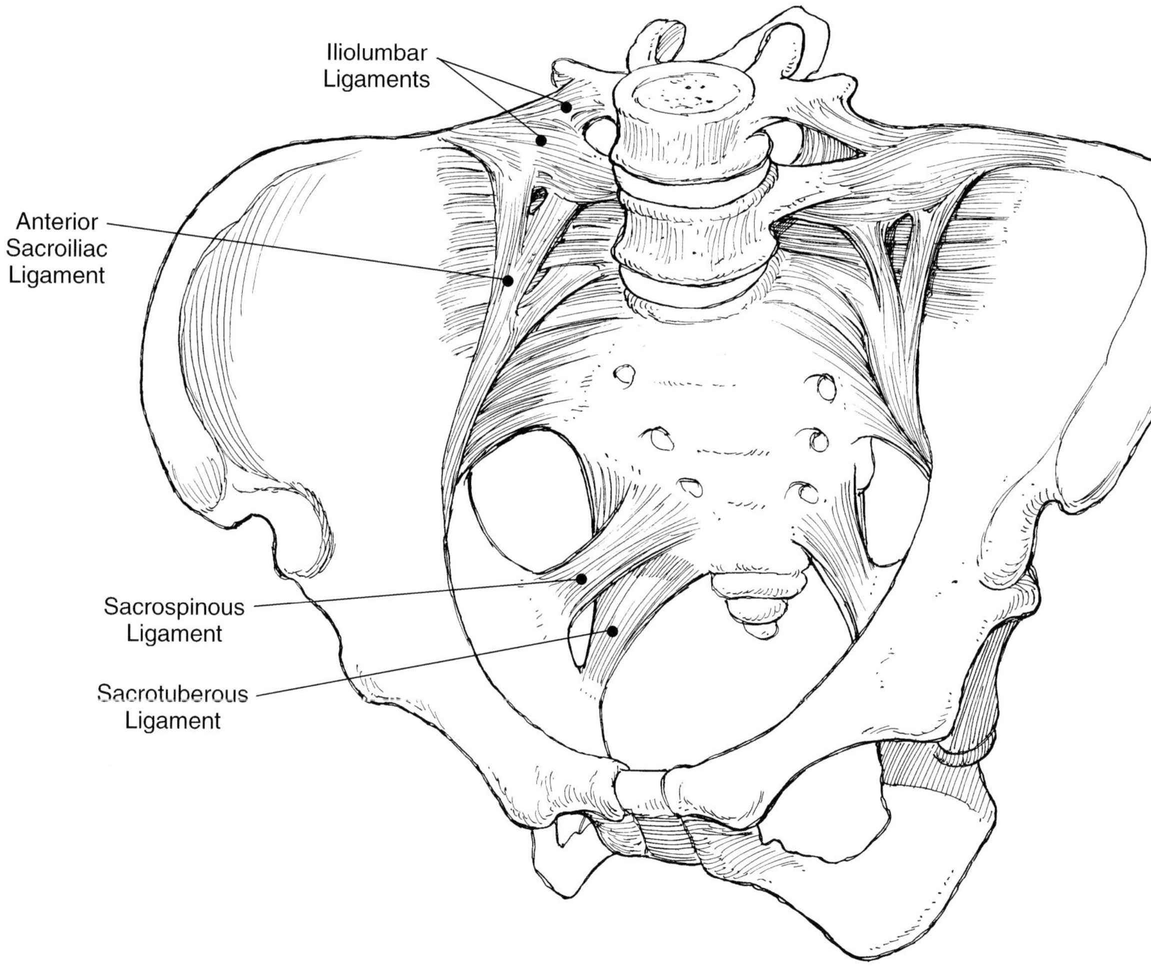


**FIGURE IX-2**

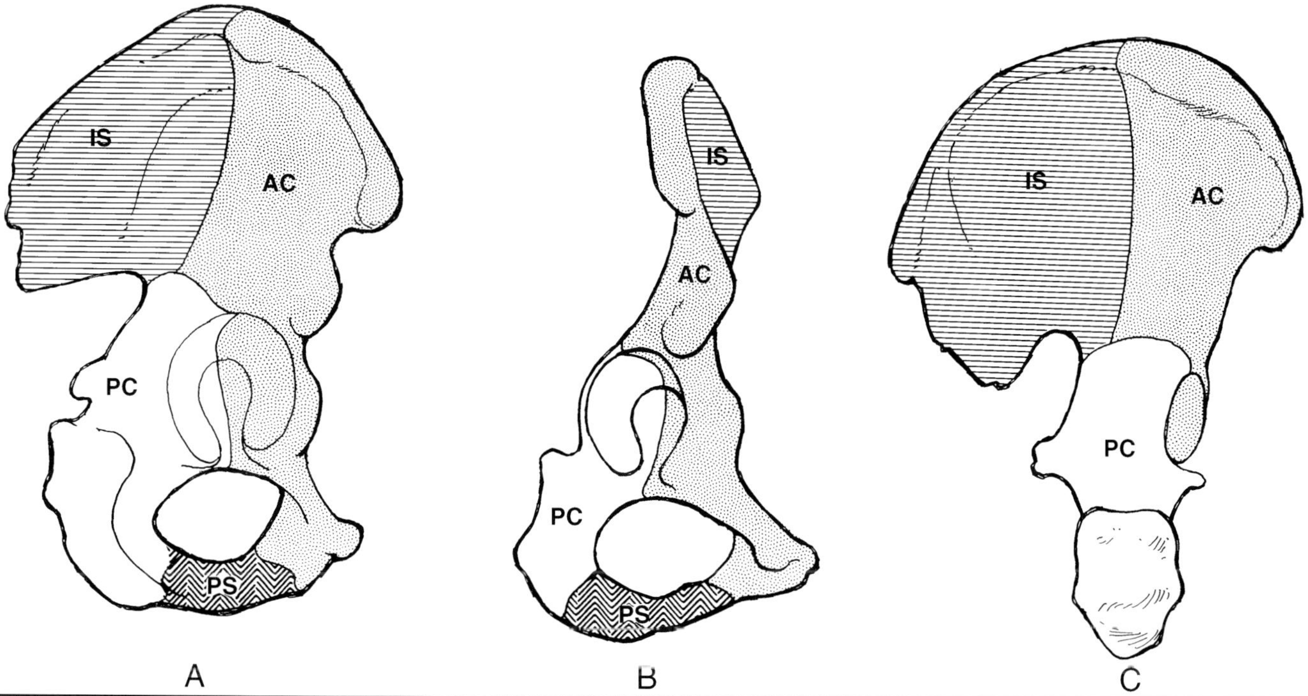


**FIGURE IX-3**

umn, are the coccygeus and the inferior gemellus. The posterior column extends caudally to approximately the posterior margin of the urogenital diaphragm (IX-4D). The major boundary to the inside of the anterior and posterior columns is the pelvic diaphragm, which consists of the levator ani and the coccygeus muscles and their investing fascia. These provide a soft tissue boundary separating the contents of the pelvis from the perineum and create an anatomic barrier to exposure of the internal surface of the superior pubic ramus, the medial wall of the acetabulum, and the ischium below the sciatic notch. The margin of the arcuate tendon (the origin of the levator ani) lies at about the level of the dome of the acetabulum (IX-5A, IX-5B, and IX-5C). The arterial and venous branches of the internal iliac arteries and veins and the branches of the lumbosacral plexus perforate the peroneal musculature deep to the pelvic diaphragm, making dissection in this area precarious. These vessels are deep in the basin of the pelvis and are fixed to the pelvic walls (IX-6). Inadvertent disruption of these vessels can lead to massive uncontrolled bleeding. For major pelvic resections, such as internal hemipelvectomy, this massive blood loss can be minimized by early ligation of the internal iliac artery and vein or preoperative selective arterial embolization. The vascular tree must be carefully dissected and preserved during intrapelvic approaches to the true pelvis, especially for exposure of displaced fracture fragments. When there has been significant displacement of the fracture fragments, an arteriogram of the internal iliac system to assess the remaining arterial supply to the pelvic musculature is an important element of preoperative planning (4). Arteriography may also be used therapeutically to embolize any actively bleeding arterial branches.

Attention must also be given to the pelvic visceral contents: the urogenital system and rectum (IX-7A and IX-7B). The urinary bladder, prostate, and ureters lie in the retroperitoneal space and must be recognized and retracted during intrapelvic dissection, especially in exposure of the anterior column through the retropubic space. The rectum is in direct contact with the anterior sacral wall and

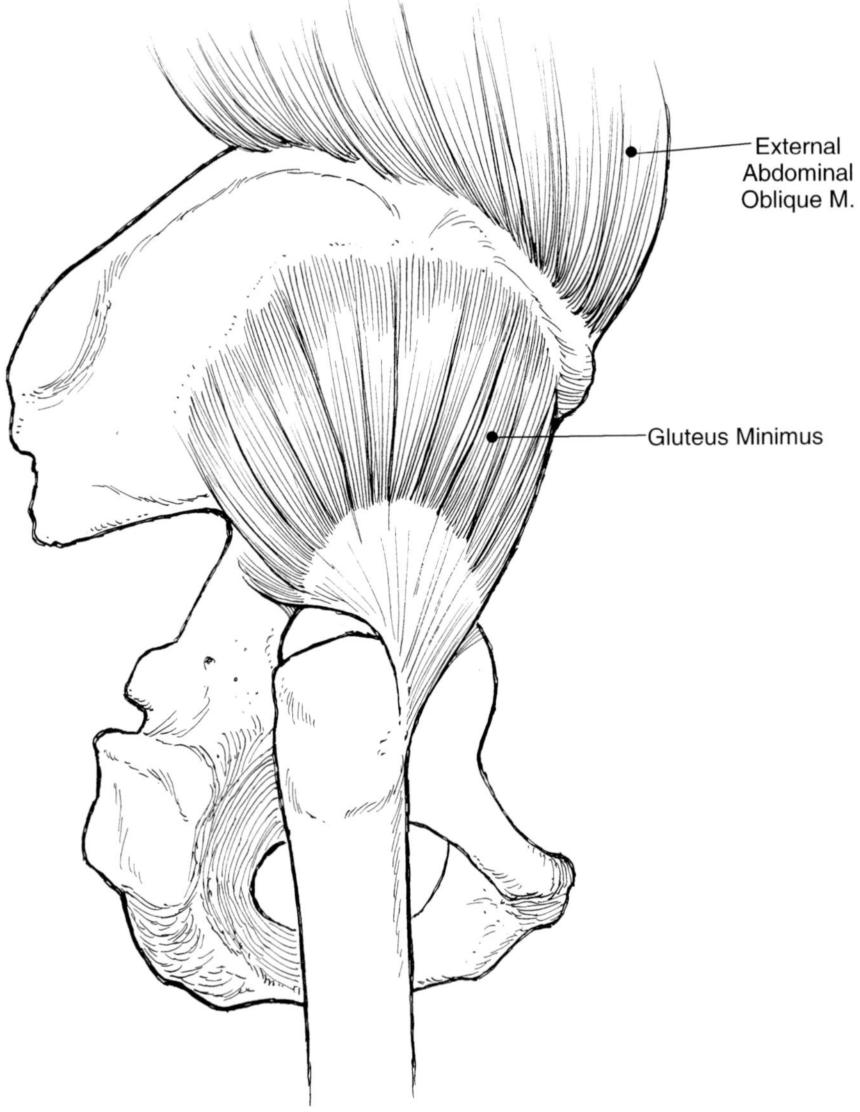


**FIGURE IX-4A**

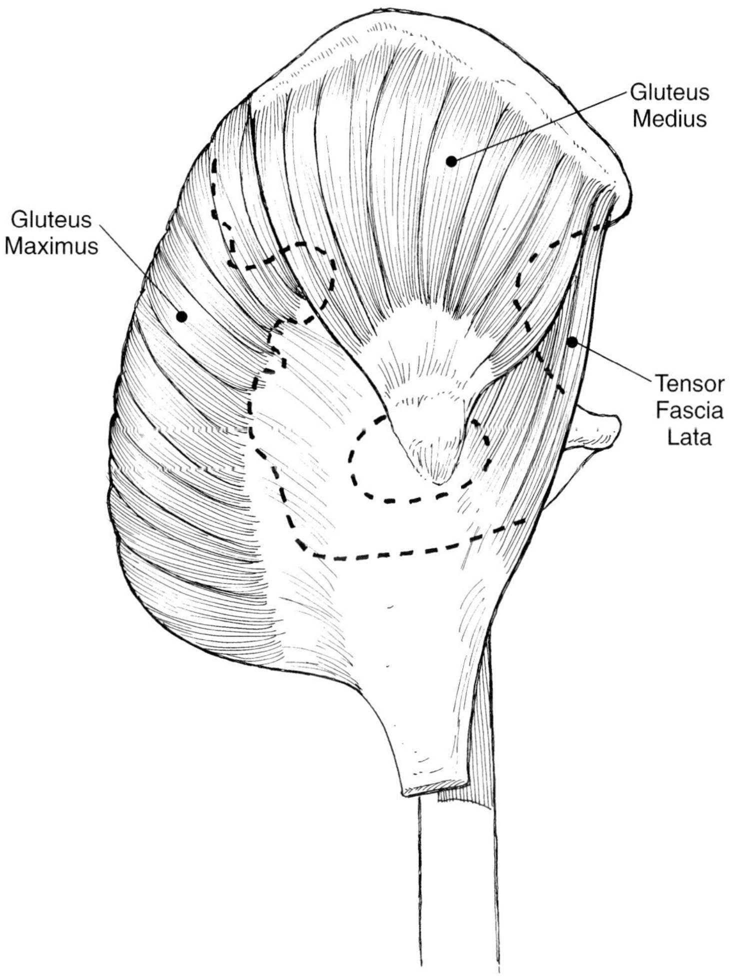


**FIGURE IX-4B**

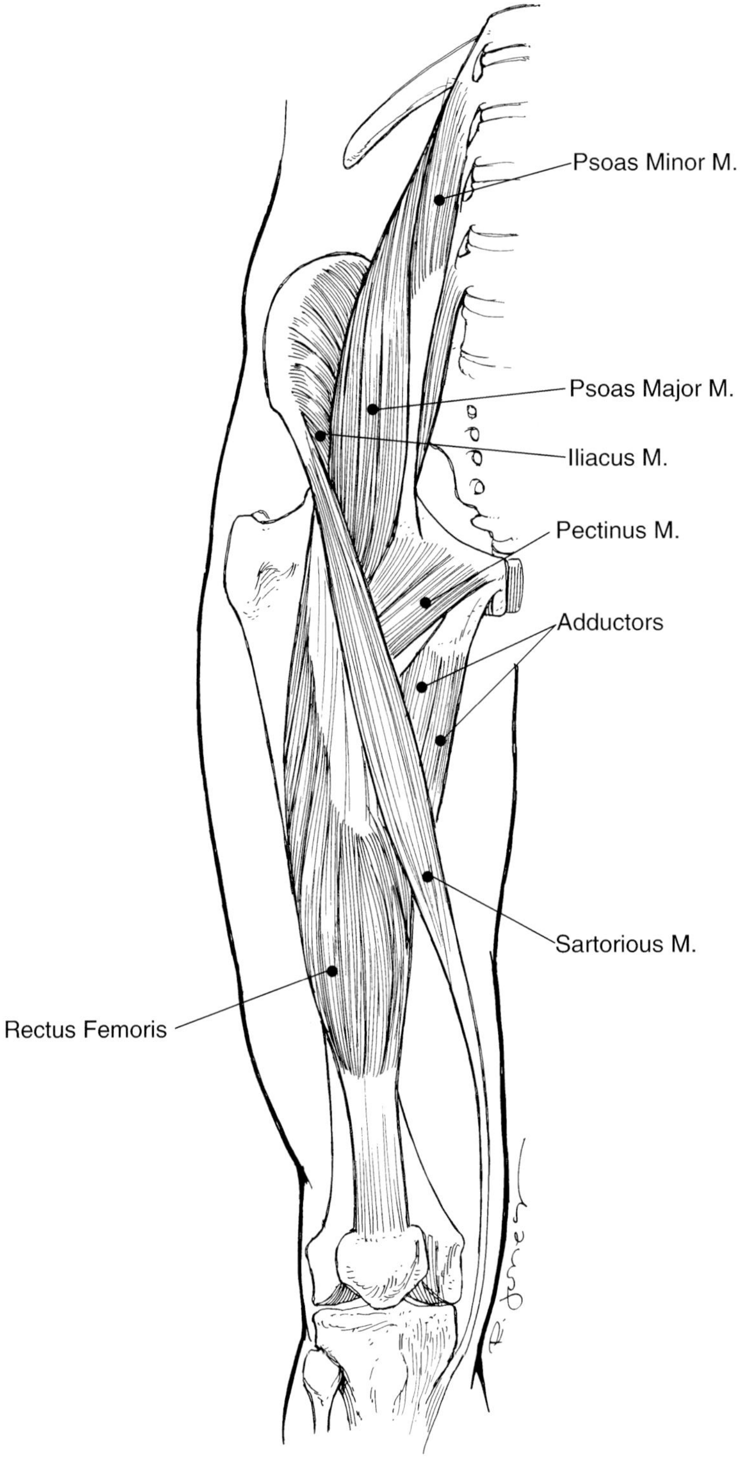
Psoas Minor M.
Psoas Major M.
Iliacus M.
Pectinus M.
Adductors
Sartorious M.
Rectus Femoris

**FIGURE IX-4C**

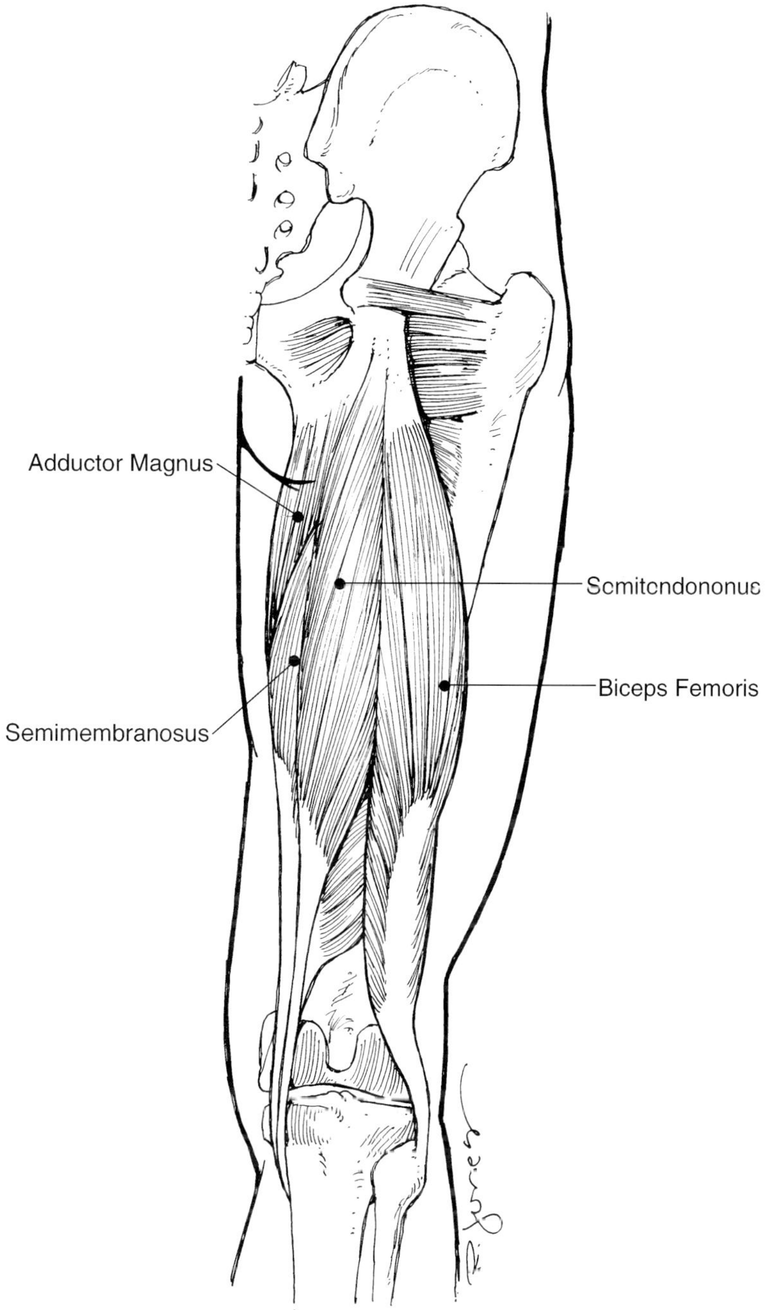
Adductor Magnus
Semitendononus
Biceps Femoris
Semimembranosus

FIGURE IX-4D

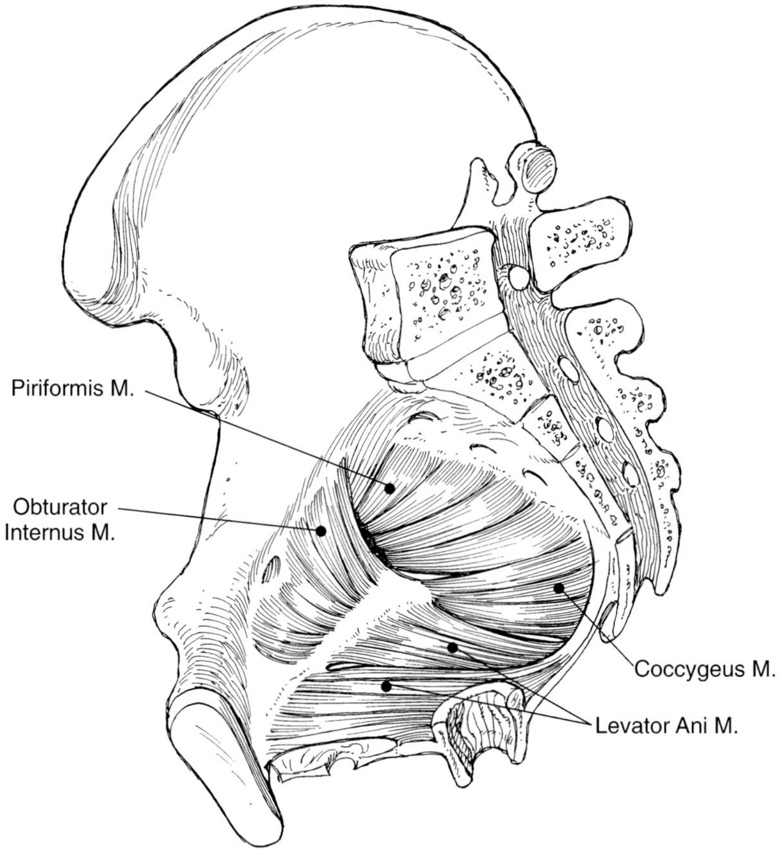


**Pelvic Diaphragm**
**(Medial View)**

**FIGURE IX-5A**

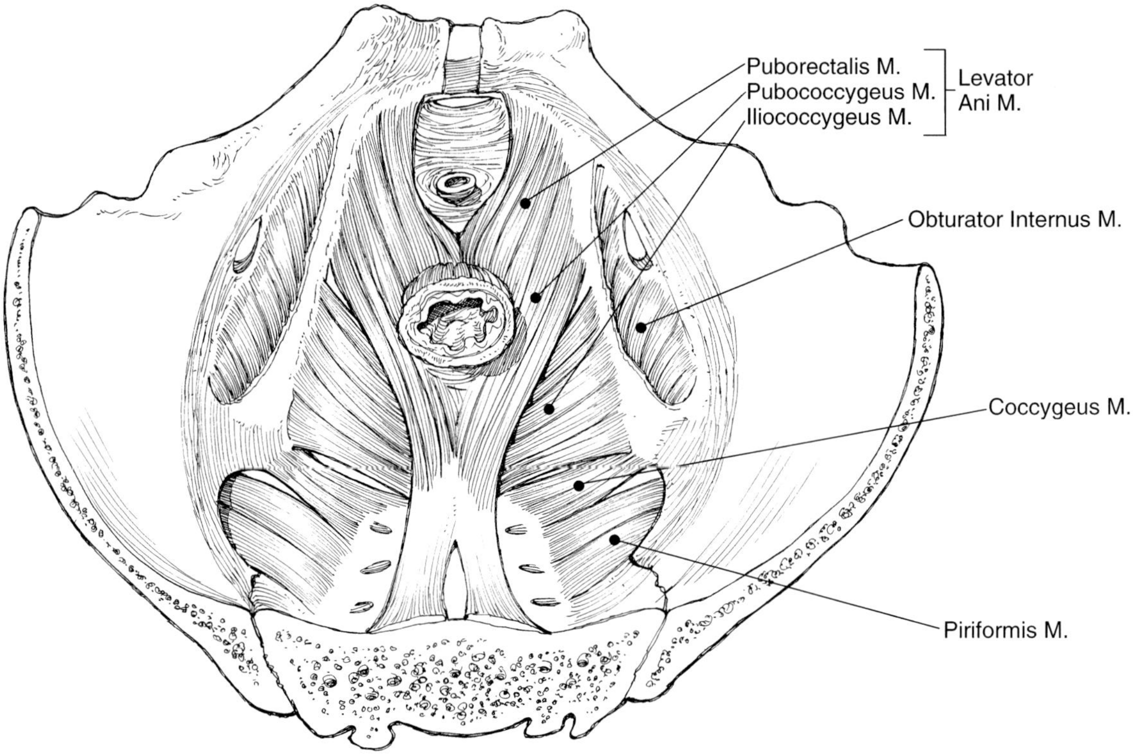


**FIGURE IX-5B**

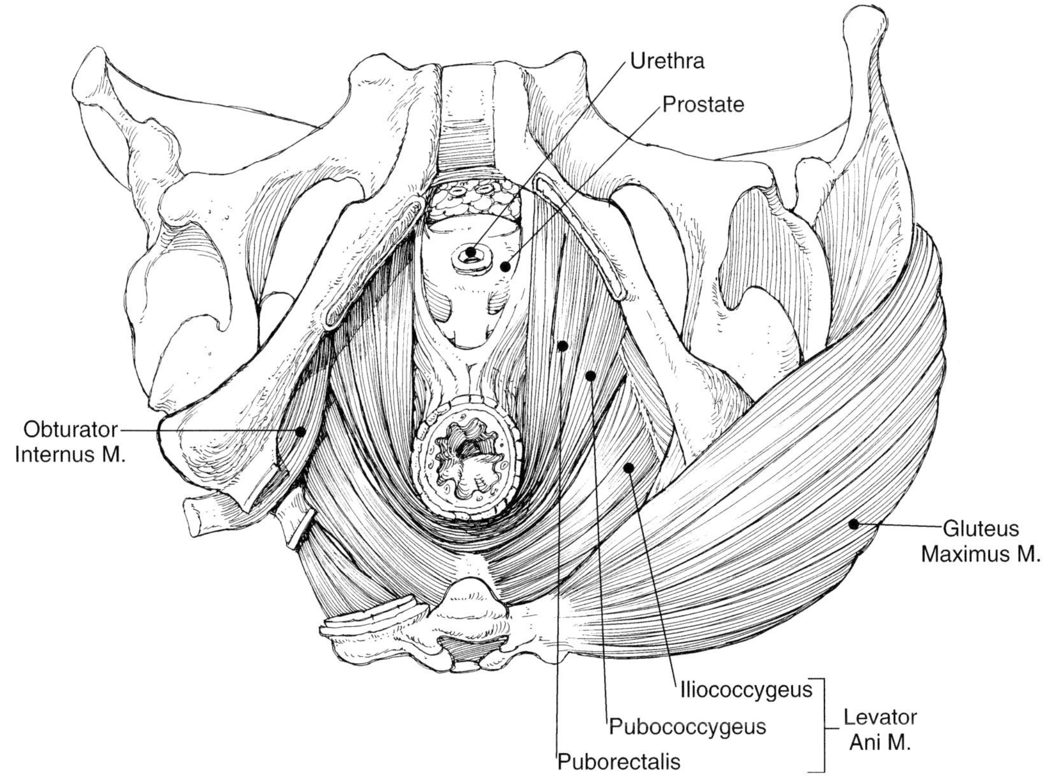


**FIGURE IX-5C**

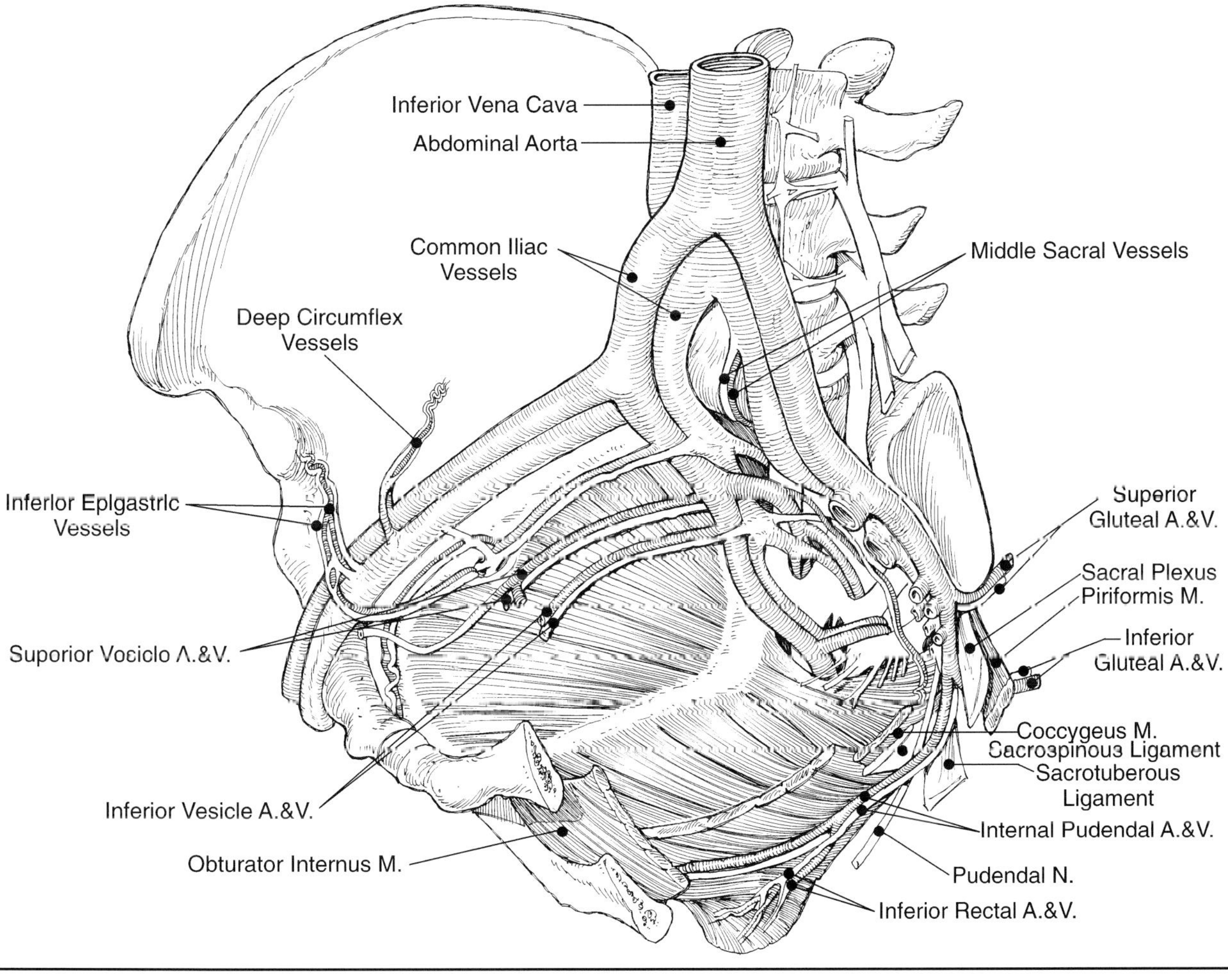


**FIGURE IX-6**

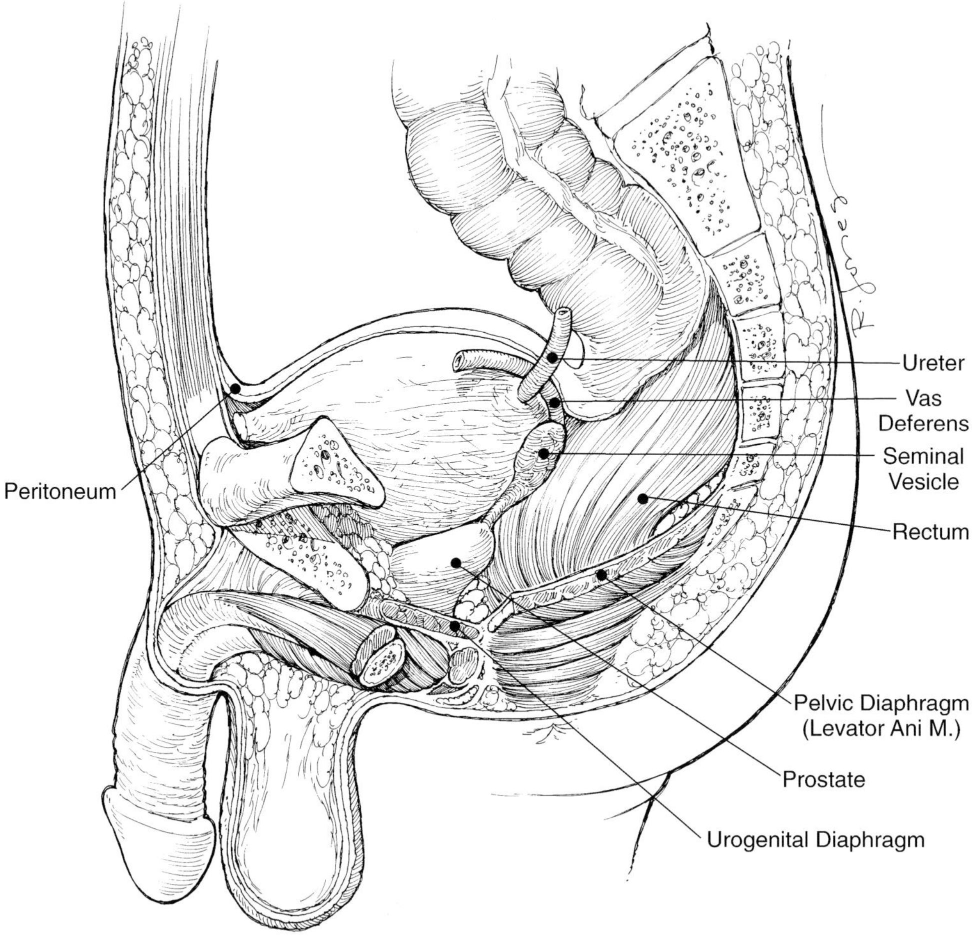


**FIGURE IX-7A**

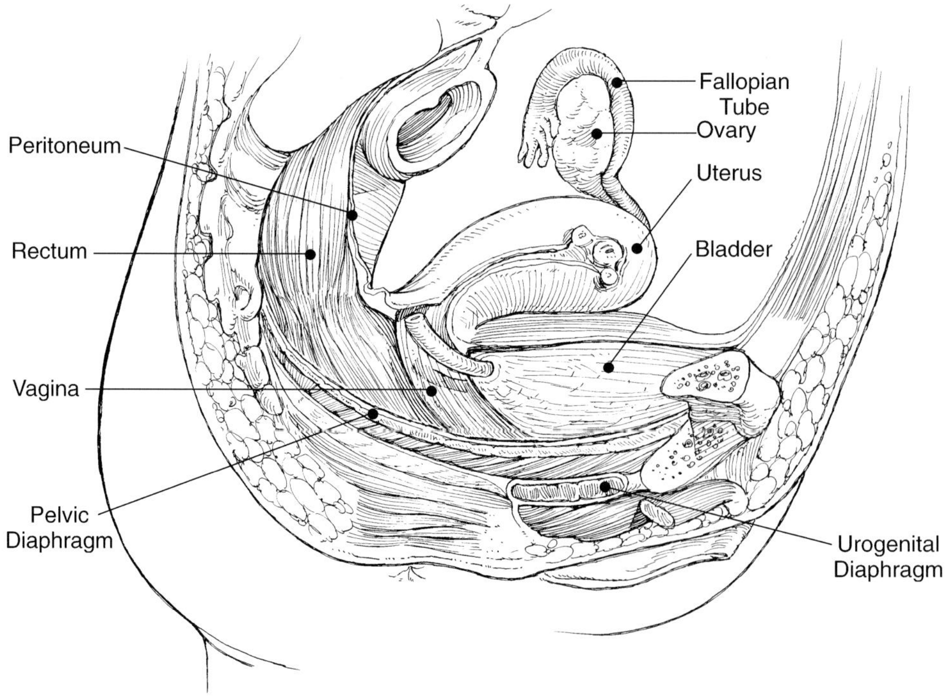


**FIGURE IX-7B**

must be mobilized during dissection of the sacrum (IX-8A). For excision of large tumors of the pelvis, preoperative assessment of the position of the visceral structures is necessary to prevent inadvertent damage or inadequate surgical resection. Therefore, the surgeon may need to consider contrast enhanced computed tomography (CT) scan, intravenous pyelogram, or barium enema to evaluate precisely the location of these structures, especially when the pelvic anatomy has been distorted. For surgical dissection into or through the sacrum, the surgeon must be aware of the position of the sacral nerve roots and dura (IX-8B). One must also be aware of the rich venous anastomoses through the sacrum connecting the epidural (Batson's) venous plexus with the internal iliac veins.

# Extensile Ilioinguinal Approach

*Applications*

This approach is one of the most utilitarian routes to the pelvis. It provides wide exposure to the inner surface of the false pelvis as far as the inner table of the dome of the acetabulum, the sciatic notch, and the pubis. It can be used for open reduction and internal fixation of many acetabular fractures involving the anterior column and weight-bearing dome of the acetabulum, for internal fixation of sacroil-

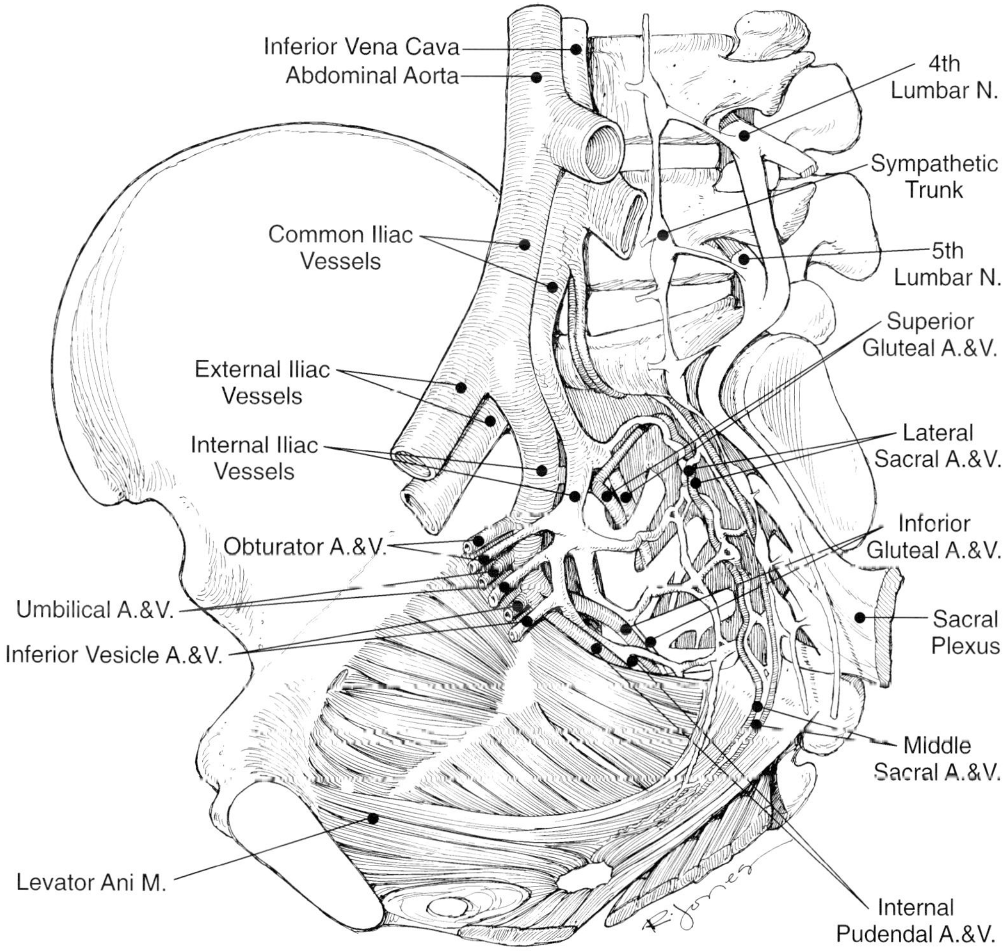


**FIGURE IX-8A**

iac joint disruptions, and for resection of periacetabular tumors. It can be used in conjunction with another incision, such as the Kocher-Langenbeck approach, to stabilize both column acetabular fractures or with a transtrochanteric approach for failed total hip arthroplasty with massive protrusion. The major advantage of this approach is that it allows wide access to the bone without disruption of the hip abductors, extensors, flexors, or adductors. It provides direct access to the iliac wing and anterior column for placement of reconstruction plates for structural grafts or to stabilize fractures.

## *Technique*

This approach has been classically described as a dissection through the abdominal wall, cephalad to the inguinal ligament (5). It requires mobilization of the contents of the inguinal canal and rectus sheath and subsequent repairs of these structures; however, it can be modified by approaching the pelvis *below* the inguinal ligament, mobilizing the contents of the femoral triangle as a unit, and performing subperiosteal elevation of the abdominal wall tendinous insertions so that there is, therefore, minimal disruption of the anatomy of the abdominal wall.

The patient is placed in the lateral decubitus position at 45° from the supine position, supported with a bolster under the trunk with the entire hindquarter draped free.

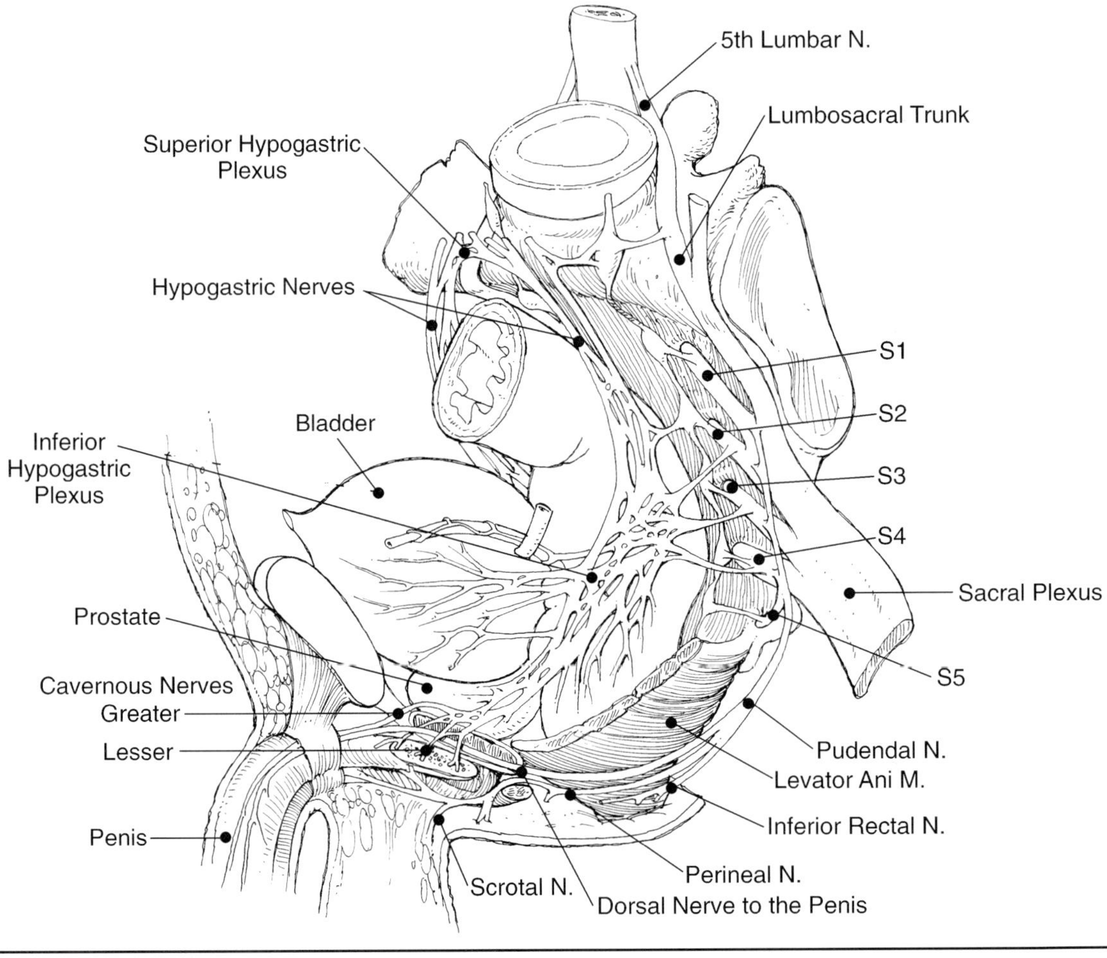


**FIGURE IX-8B**

For complete exposure of the iliac wing or the anterior sacroiliac joint, the incision may be started as far posteriorly as the posterior superior iliac spine. The incision is carried parallel to the iliac crest, approximately 1 cm above it, then in an arc to the level of the anterior superior iliac spine (ASIS), and then transversely 1 cm below the inguinal ligament, to just above the pubic symphysis in the midline (IX-9). The periosteum of the iliac crest is incised sharply in its midline, and the incision is carried from the sacroiliac joint to the ASIS (IX-10). The lateral femoral cutaneous nerve is then identified and mobilized proximally and distally by incision of the overlying fascia. The fascia lata is incised over the femoral triangle, exposing the iliopsoas belly and sartorius (IX-11). By staying below the inguinal ligament, dissection of the spermatic cord can be avoided as the dissection is carried medially toward the pubic tubercle. The contents of the femoral sheath can be preserved without dissection. The inguinal ligament is then detached subperiosteally from the ASIS. Next, the abdominal wall muscles are elevated subperiosteally from the iliac crest, and the iliacus muscle mobilized with them (IX-12). A 1-inch Penrose drain can then be passed around the iliopsoas muscle and the femoral sheath contents (IX-13). Mobility of the psoas muscle over the pelvic brim is facilitated by maintaining the hip in approximately 45° of flexion. The pelvis is then exposed through two "windows" medial and lateral to the psoas muscle. Medially, further dissection along the superior pubic ramus, as far as the pubic symphysis, can be accomplished by subperiosteal elevation of the rectus sheath. Care must be taken to identify any accessory or aberrant obturator artery arising from the exter-

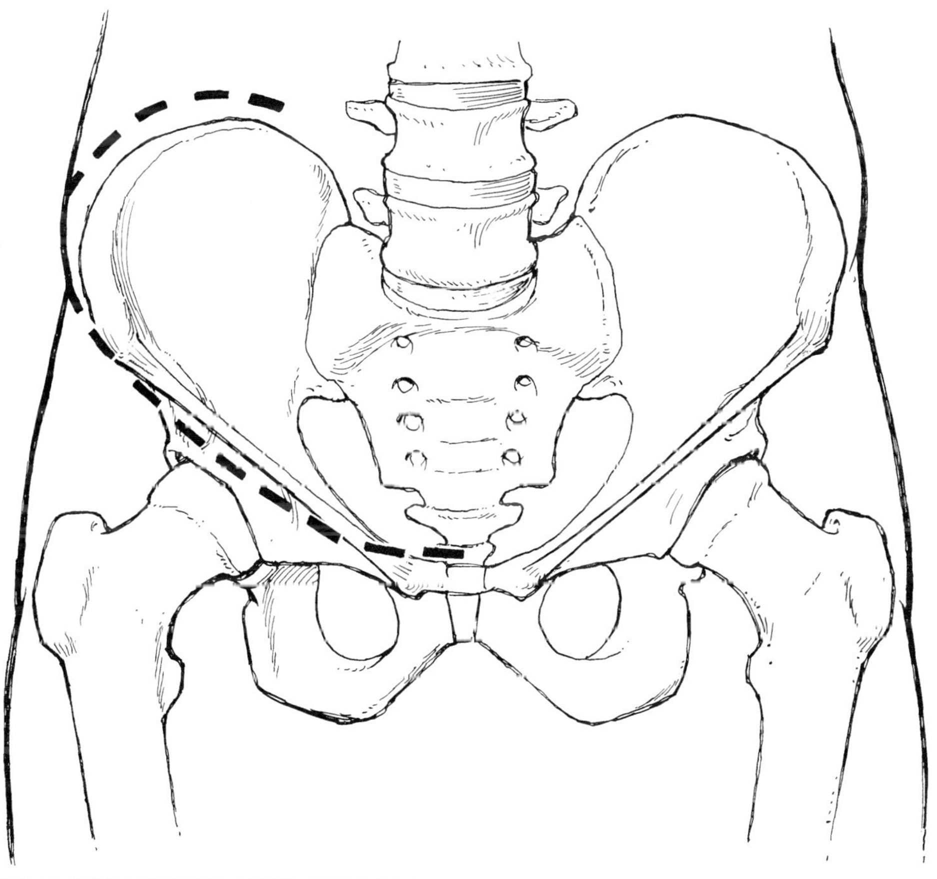

**FIGURE IX-9**

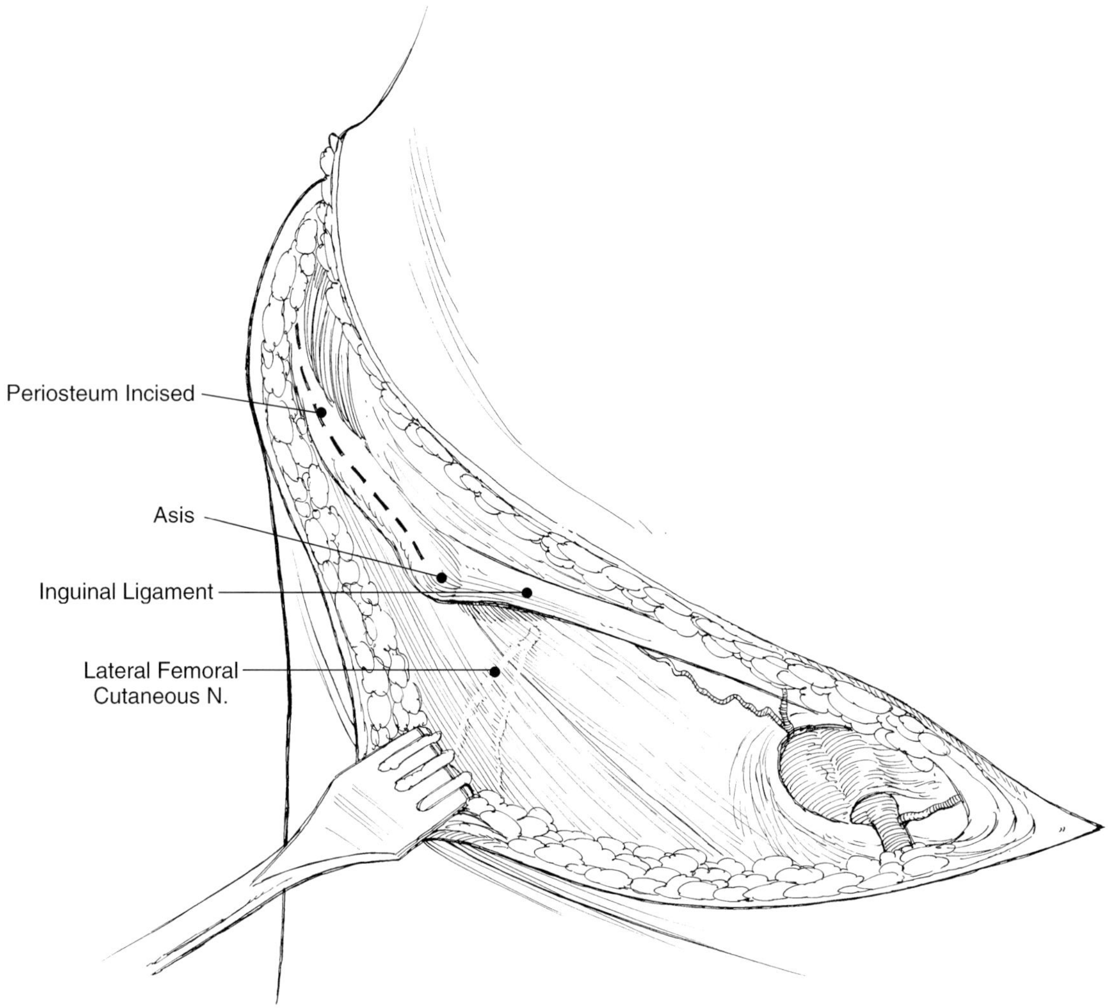
Periosteum Incised
Asis
Inguinal Ligament
Lateral Femoral
Cutaneous N.

**FIGURE IX-10**

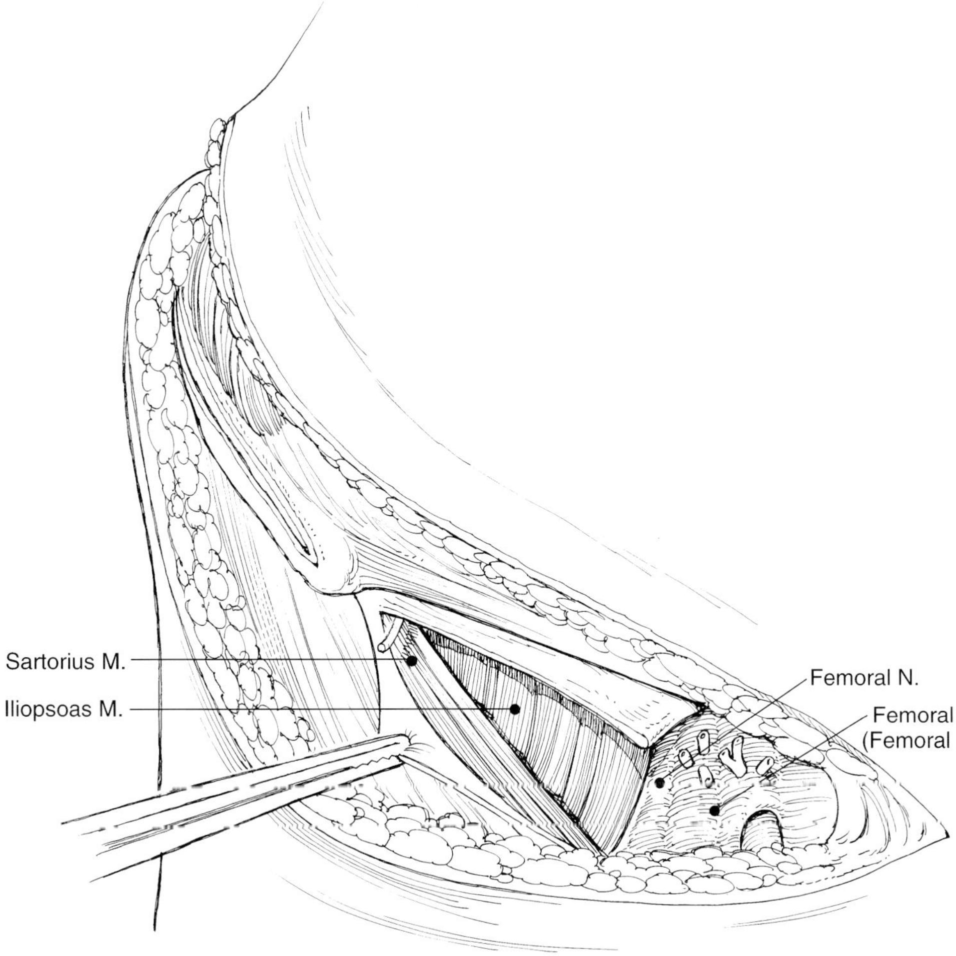


**FIGURE IX-11**

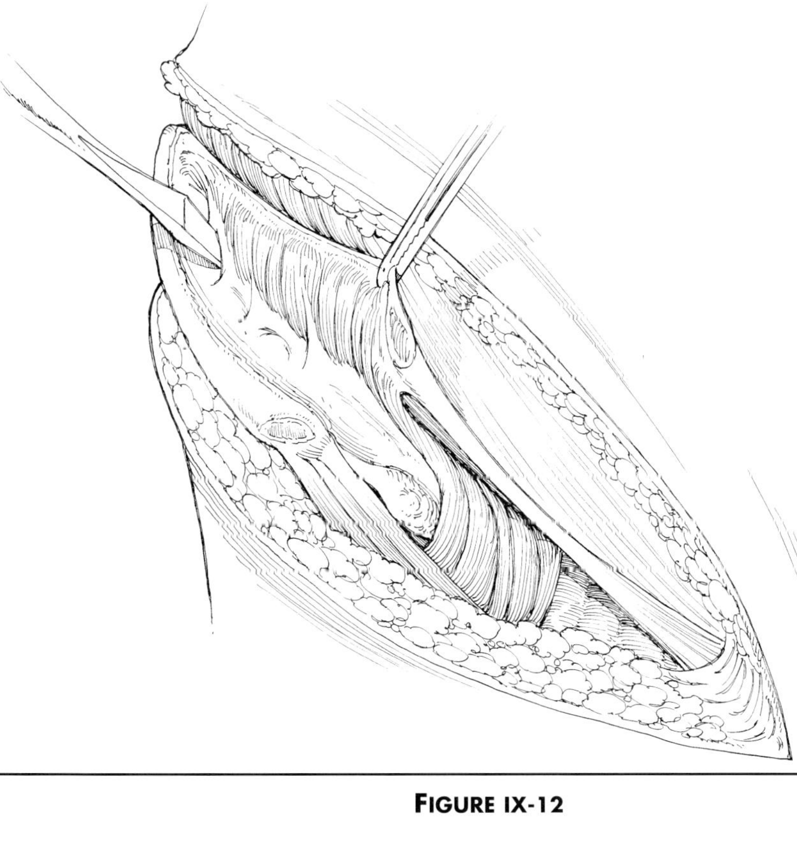

**FIGURE IX-12**

nal iliac or inferior epigastric artery at the level of the inguinal ligament (IX-13). If found, it must be ligated and transected to prevent uncontrolled bleeding. The inner table of the superior pubic ramus can be exposed by subperiosteal elevation of the tendinous insertion of the levator ani. This dissection is into the retropubic space, so the surgeon should carefully protect the urinary bladder and the prostate gland in males (IX-14). The obturator nerve, artery, and vein must be identified and protected as they pass through the obturator membrane. Dissection can be extended to the inferior margin of the pubic symphysis or across the midline to the contralateral superior pubic ramus if necessary. For unusual cases such as bilateral sacroiliac joint disruptions with a pubic symphysis diastasis, bilateral dissections can be performed.

### *Dangers*

The major hazard to this approach is inadvertent injury to the internal iliac arterial and venous branches. The internal iliac trunks may be ligated unilaterally without significant sequelae in most patients. For patients who have sustained unstable pelvic ring fractures or lateral compression-type acetabular fractures, however, the surgeon should take care to preserve blood supply to the gluteal muscles and their overlying skin. Thus, if the patient has sustained a significant crush injury to the anterior pelvis, the superficial iliac circumflex or profunda femoris arteries may be injured, leaving the superior gluteal artery as the remaining vascular supply to the soft tissue of the lateral pelvis. The superior gluteal artery lies in the posterior corner of this approach adjacent to the sciatic nerve. When the dissection must be carried to or through the sciatic notch, the artery should be identified and protected

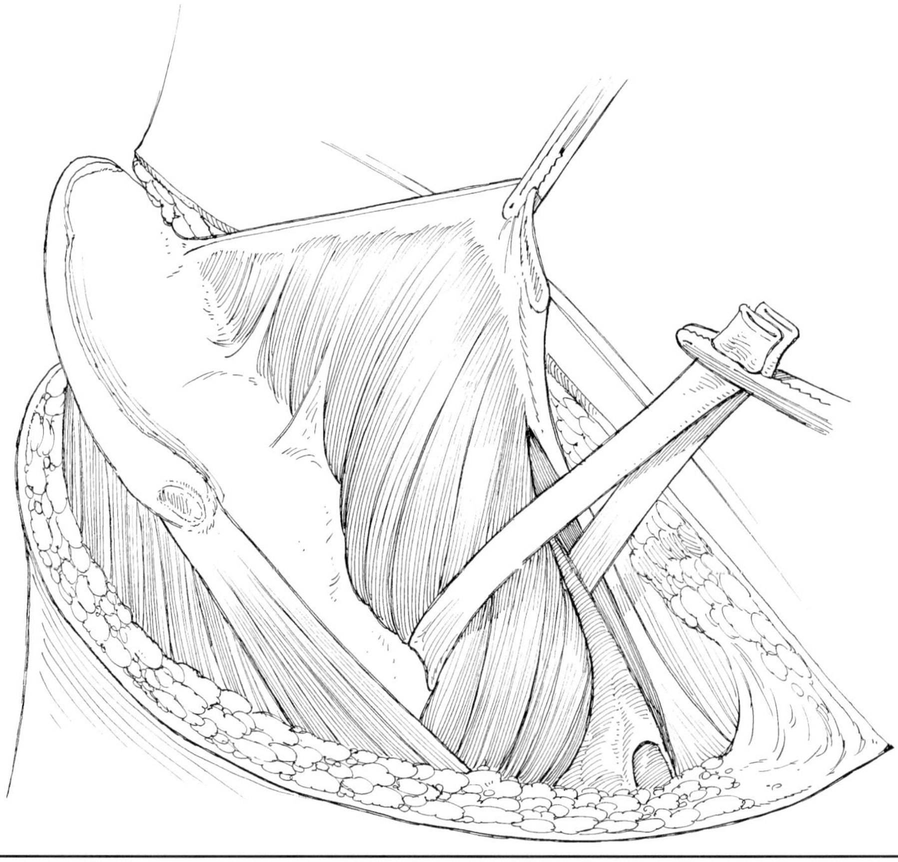

**FIGURE IX-13**

along with the sciatic nerve. The obturator neurovascular bundle and any aberrant obturator artery must be identified and preserved.

### *Limitations*

The principal limitation is the caudal boundary of the dissection defined by the pelvic diaphragm. Attempts to dissect deep to this structure may result in injury to nerves or vessels, such as the pudendals, in the true pelvis which cannot be visualized through this approach. The inferior half of the acetabulum cannot be safely exposed from the inner pelvis. Similarly, the posterior column beginning approximately 2 cm distal to the apex of the greater sciatic notch can be more safely

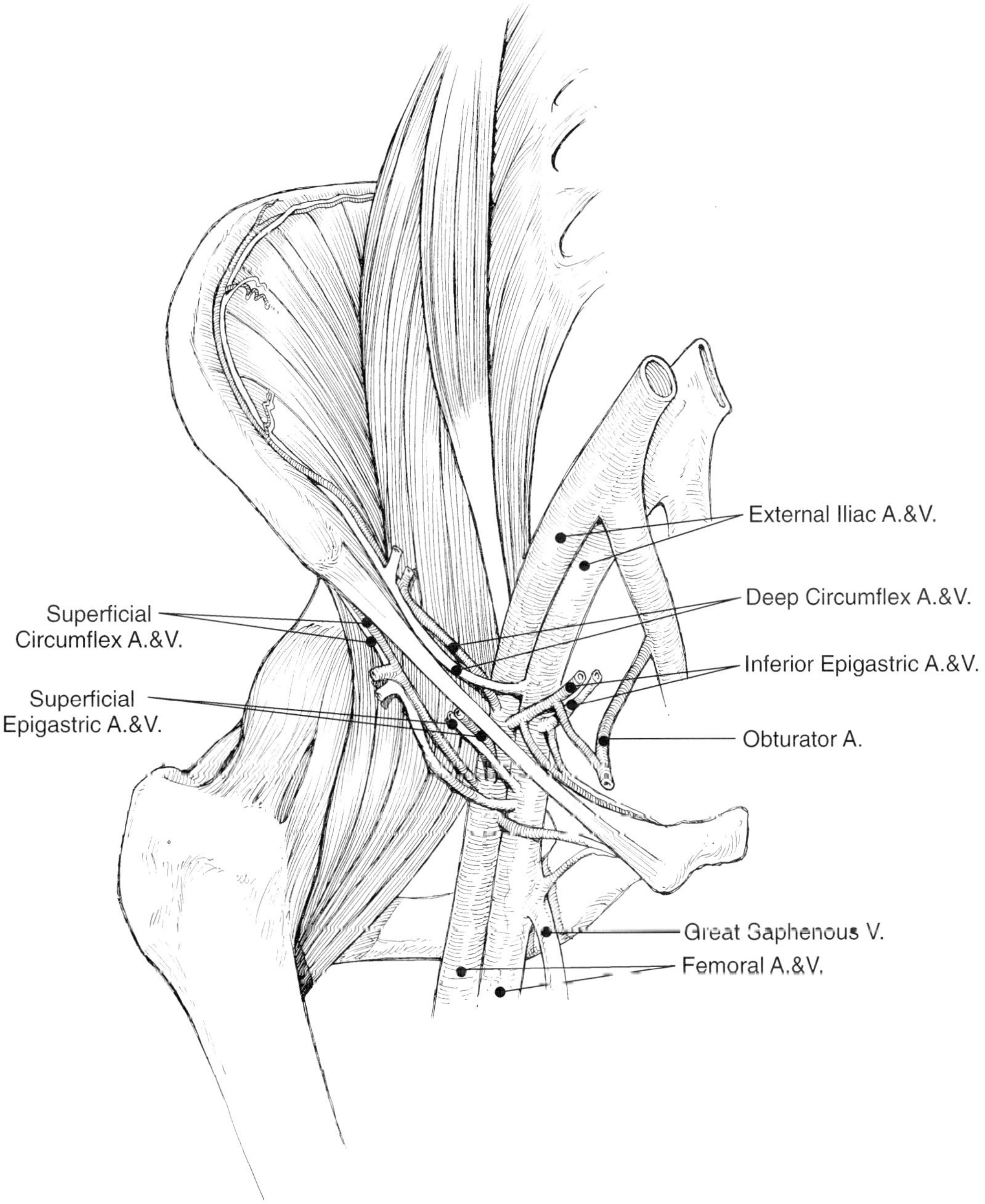


**FIGURE IX-14**

reached by an extrapelvic exposure. The hip joint cannot be completely visualized by this approach. Any limited visualization of the femoral head and acetabular articular surface can be achieved through a medial wall fracture line, if one is present.

## Extensile Iliofemoral Approach

***Applications***

The "extended iliofemoral approach" described by Letournel and Judet (5) provides complete exposure to the internal and external surfaces of the pelvis, acetabulum, and hip joint. It is rarely needed for fixation of pelvic fractures, and this approach has received some criticism because of the significant rate of postoperative infections that occurs with its use. Its usefulness is, therefore, limited to resection of tumors of the ilium, hip, and acetabulum.

***Technique***

The patient is placed in the lateral position with the hindquarter draped free to allow manipulation of the hip. The incision is an inverted J beginning at the posterior superior iliac spine, following the arc of the iliac crest to the ASIS, continuing down the anterior thigh to the level of the base of the greater trochanter. Some surgeons then arc the incision posteriorly, or it can be extended distally for further retraction of the posterior flap.

An alternative incision that provides easier access to both the anterior or posterior pelvis is a T-shaped one. The proximal skin incision is the same as that described for the ilioinguinal approach. It is then intersected by a vertical incision placed at approximately the posterior margin of the tensor fascia lata. The vertical incision is curved to intersect the transverse incision at 90°. The vertical incision can then be carried over the greater trochanter distally, as far as necessary (IX-15). When the latter skin incision is used, fasciocutaneous flaps are created anteriorly and posteriorly. They must be raised deep to the gluteal fascia to preserve the vascularity of the skin. In severe lateral impaction fractures or fractures associated with significant displacement, the vascularity of these flaps should be assessed by preoperative arteriogram.

The inner table of the ilium can be exposed by the technique described for the extensile ilioinguinal approach. The outer portion of the ilium and hip joint can be exposed from anterior to posterior by subperiosteal elevation of the tensor fascia lata and gluteus medius. This part should only be necessary if the iliac wing is to be resected. For exposure of the hip joint and posterior column, the fasciocutaneous flaps can be created anteriorly and posteriorly until the entire body of the gluteus medius is visualized. If the hip joint is to be entered or excised, the abductor muscle can be rotated cephalad by osteotomy of the greater trochanter (IX-16), providing complete exposure of the superior surface of the hip joint. The anterior capsule can be exposed by elevation of the reflected head of the rectus femoris (IX-17). The posterior capsule and posterior column can then be exposed by detachment of the obturator internus and piriformis from their insertions on the greater trochanter (IX-18). These tendons should be marked with sutures prior to detachment, and a stump of tendon should be left on the greater trochanter for repair. A blunt tipped retractor can be placed deep to the bellies of these muscles and into the sciatic notch to retract the posterior flap, including the sciatic nerve which is protected by these muscles (IX-19). The outer surface of the posterior column is then visualized. It can be further exposed to the level of the ischial tuberosity by elevation of the origins of the hamstrings (IX-20). For resection of the caudal half of the pelvis, the ischial spine should be visualized. The internal pudendal artery and vein and pudendal nerve should be identified wrapping around the sacrospinous ligament (IX-21). The sacrotuberous ligament can be transected close to its insertion on the ischial tuberosity to gain wide exposure of this region. Doing so allows retraction of the gluteus maximus that is draped over this region.

The hip joint can be entered by a T-shaped capsular incision creating anterior and posterior flaps as needed.

If the entire hemipelvis is to be resected, the anterior column is further exposed by detachment of the origin of the direct head of the rectus femoris (IX-22). The superior pubic ramus can be further exposed by detachment of the psoas tendon insertion on the femur through an osteotomy of the lesser trochanter. This allows the iliopsoas belly to be retracted superiorly, exposing the superior pubic ramus medially to the pubic symphysis (IX-23). Further dissection of the inferior pubic ramus is discussed in the extensile ischiopubic approach.

***Dangers***

The critical neurovascular structures exposed during this dissection include the sciatic nerve and superior gluteal artery, internal pudendal artery and vein, pudendal nerve, and femoral neurovascular bundle (IX-24). The surgeon must be cognizant of the importance of preserving the superior gluteal artery and superficial iliac circumflex vessels to maintain viability of the large soft tissue flaps created by this dissection. Complete exposure of the external surface of the iliac wing by

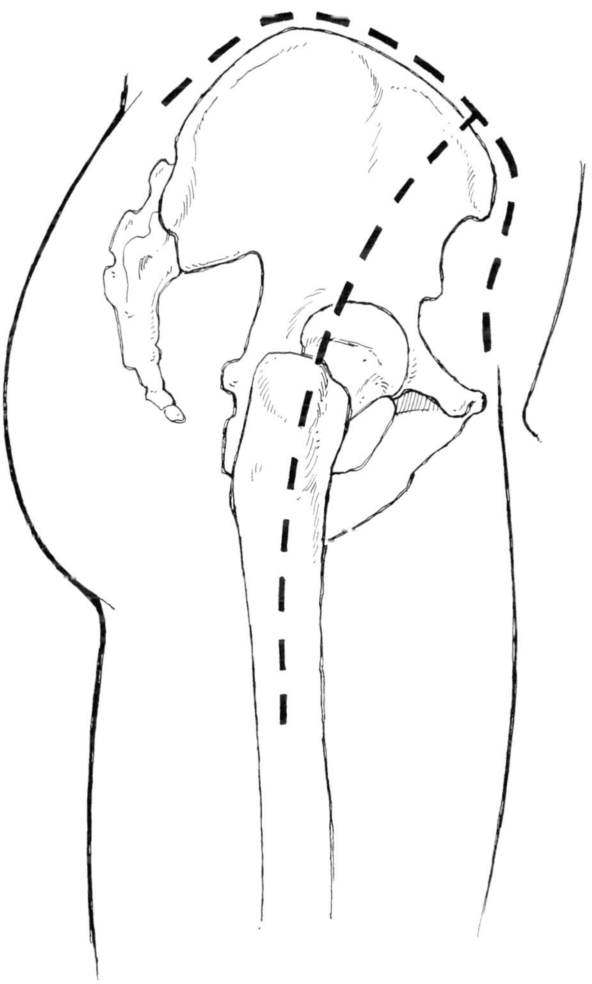

**FIGURE IX-15**

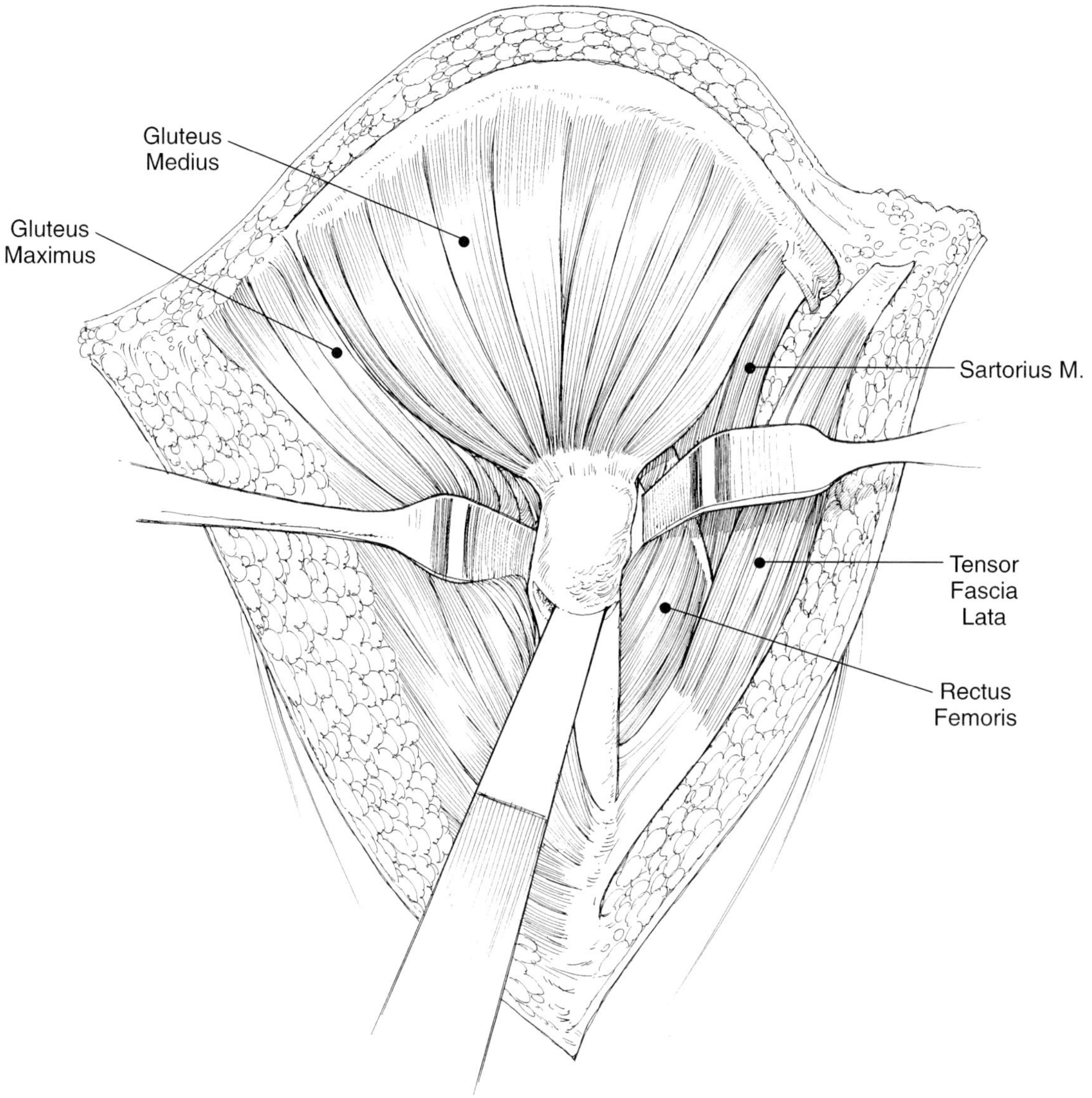
Gluteus Medius
Gluteus Maximus
Sartorius M.
Tensor Fascia Lata
Rectus Femoris

**FIGURE IX-16**

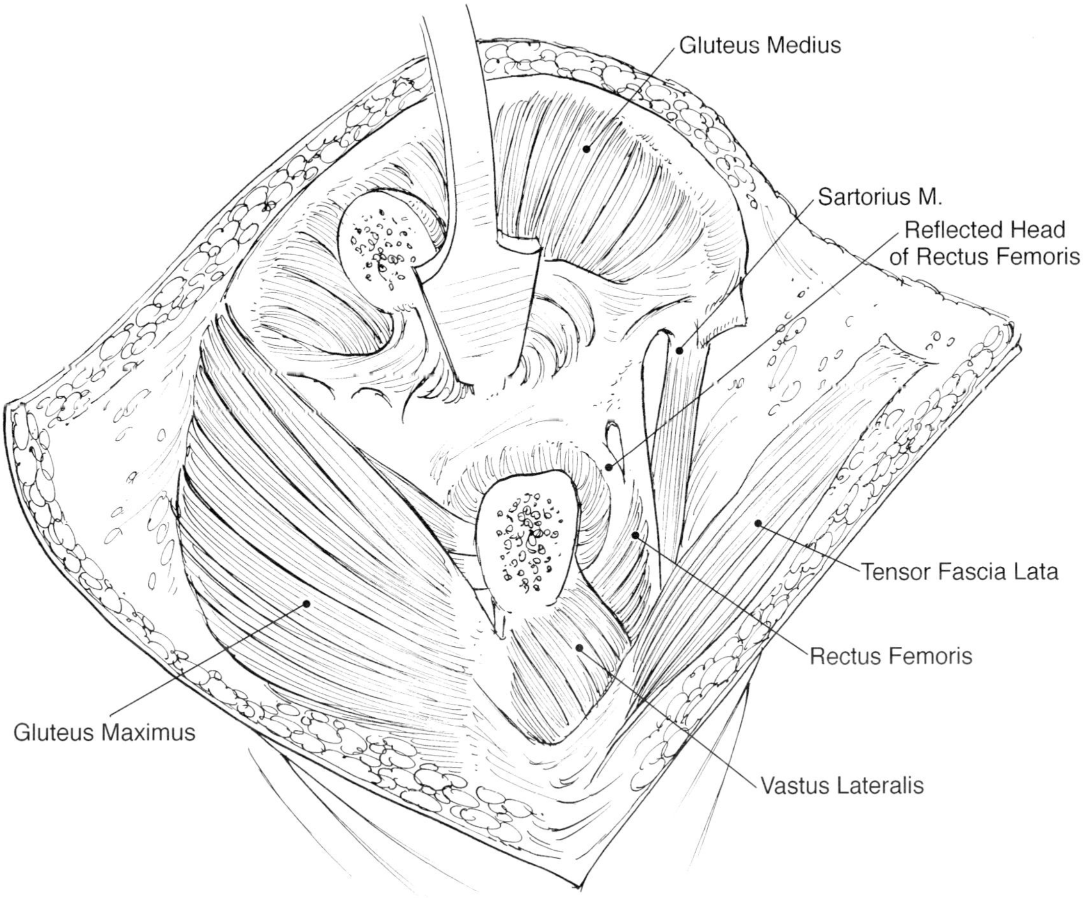
Gluteus Medius
Sartorius M.
Reflected Head of Rectus Femoris
Tensor Fascia Lata
Rectus Femoris
Gluteus Maximus
Vastus Lateralis

**FIGURE IX-17**

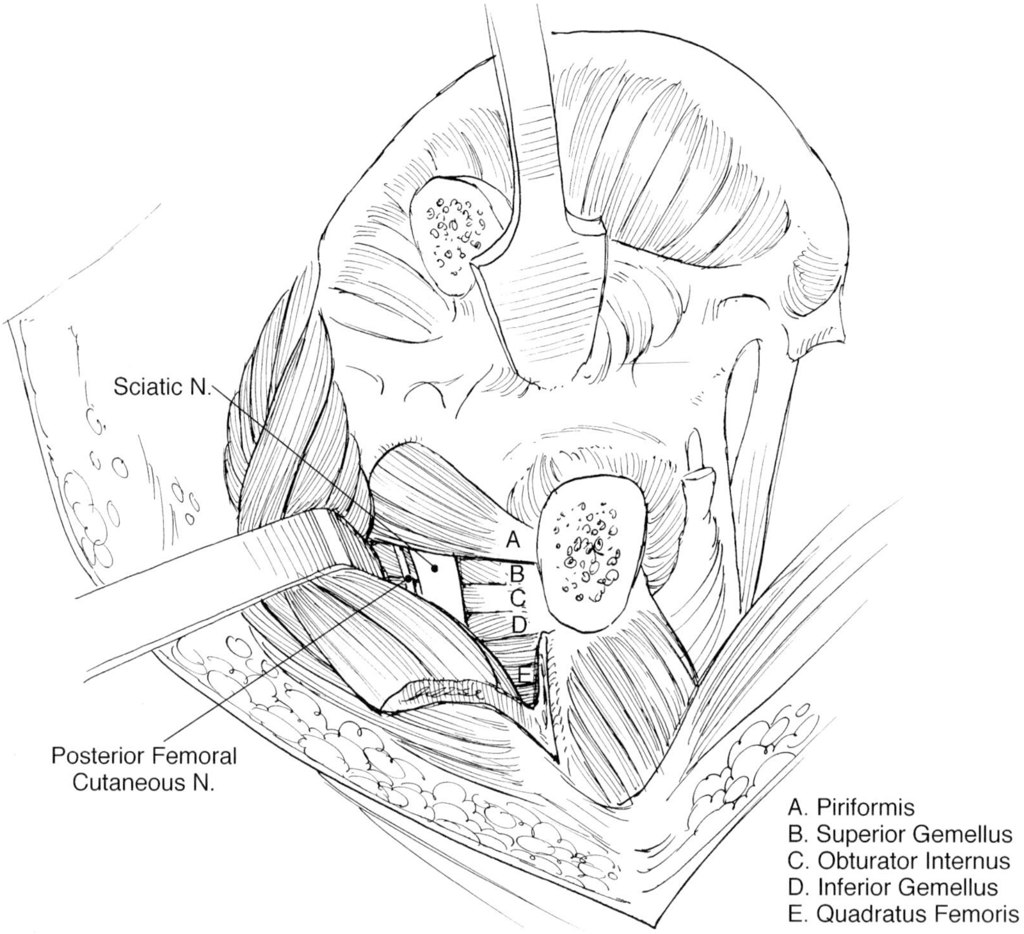
Sciatic N.
A
B
C
D
E
Posterior Femoral Cutaneous N.
A. Piriformis
B. Superior Gemellus
C. Obturator Internus
D. Inferior Gemellus
E. Quadratus Femoris

**FIGURE IX-18**

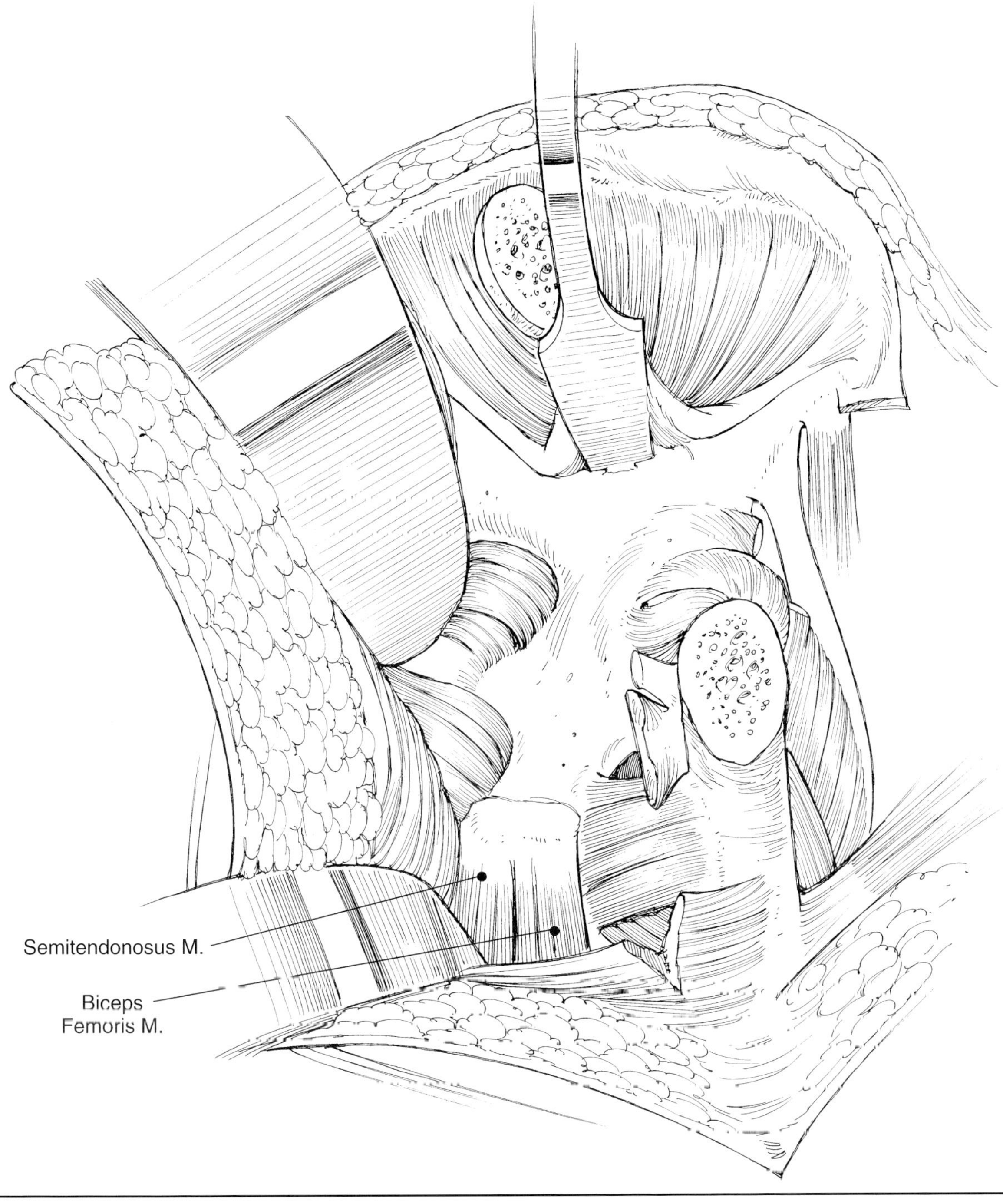


**FIGURE IX-19**

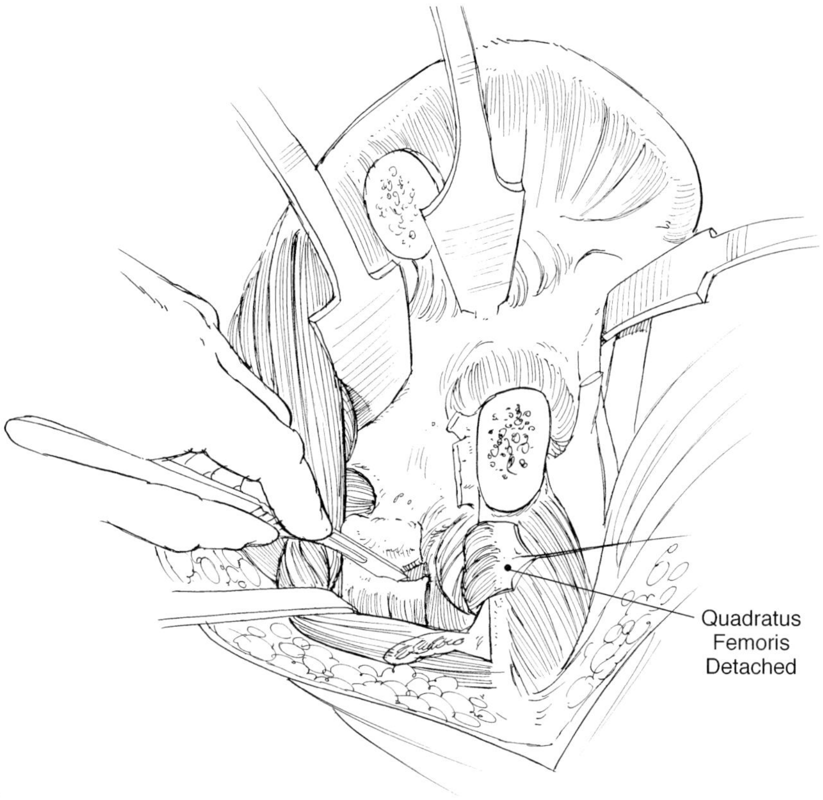


**FIGURE IX-20**

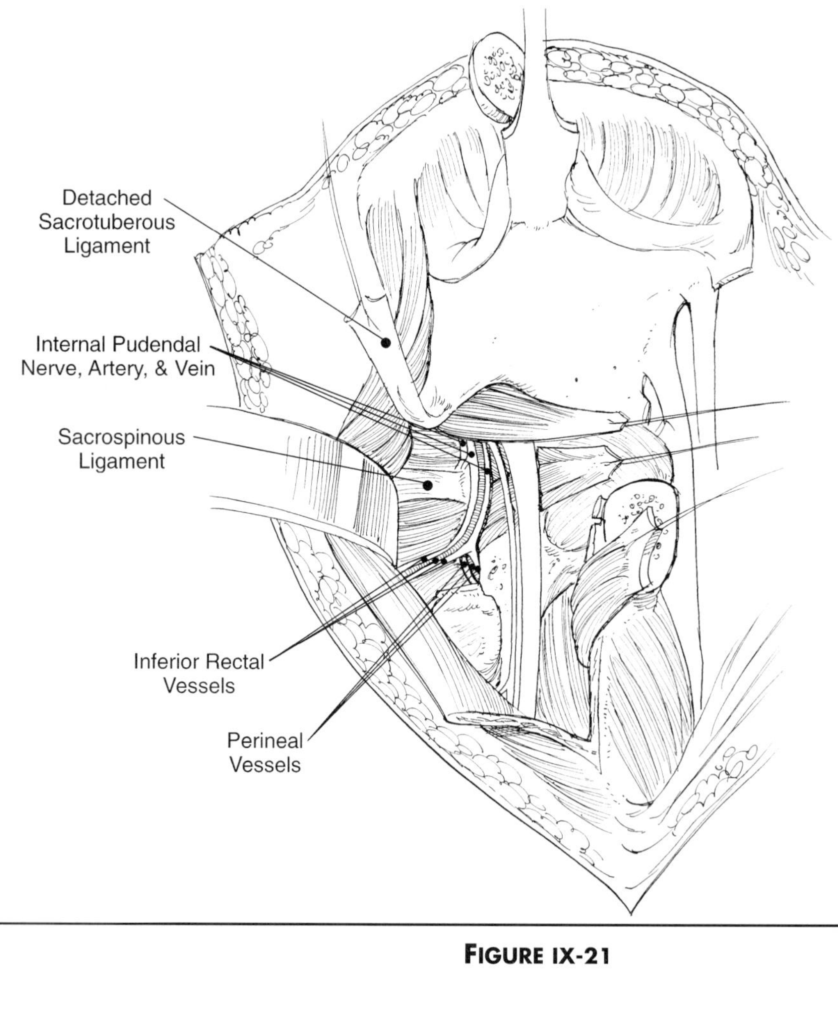


**FIGURE IX-21**

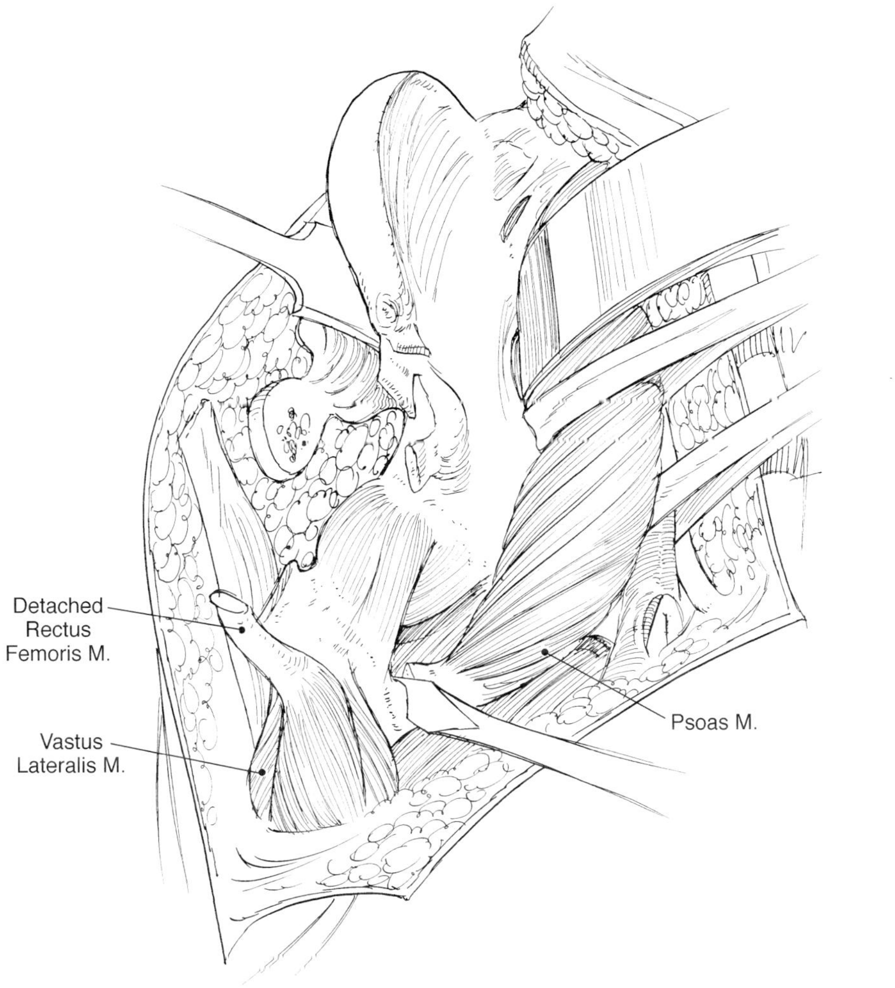


**FIGURE IX-22**

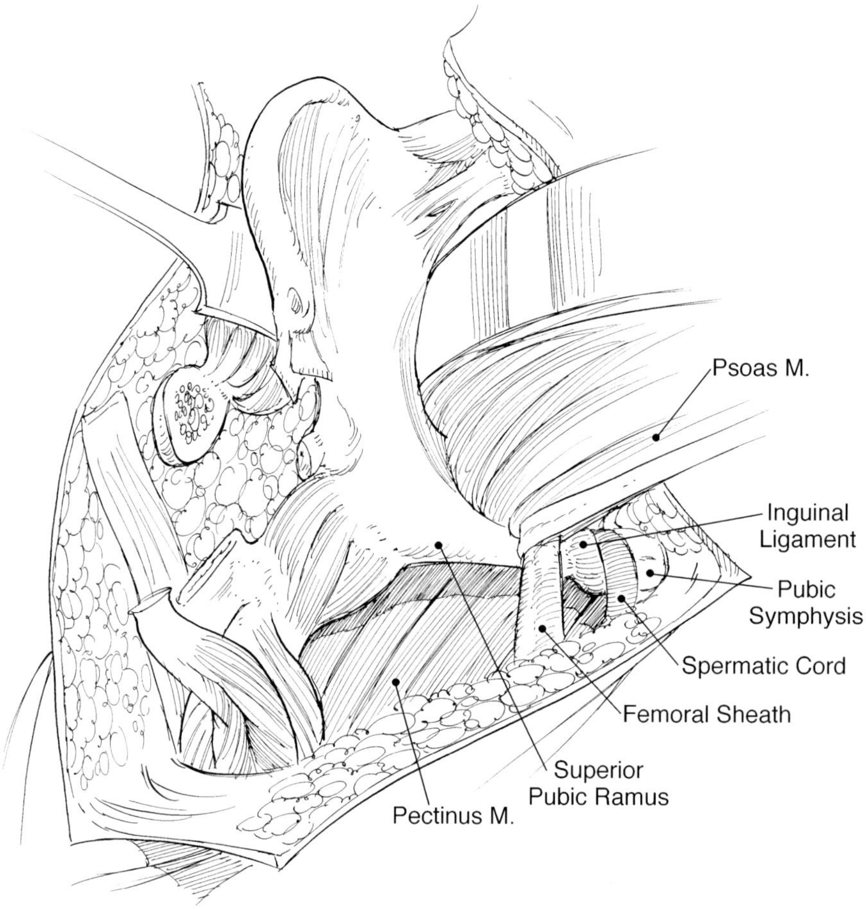
Psoas M.
Inguinal Ligament
Pubic Symphysis
Spermatic Cord
Femoral Sheath
Superior Pubic Ramus
Pectinus M.

**FIGURE IX-23**

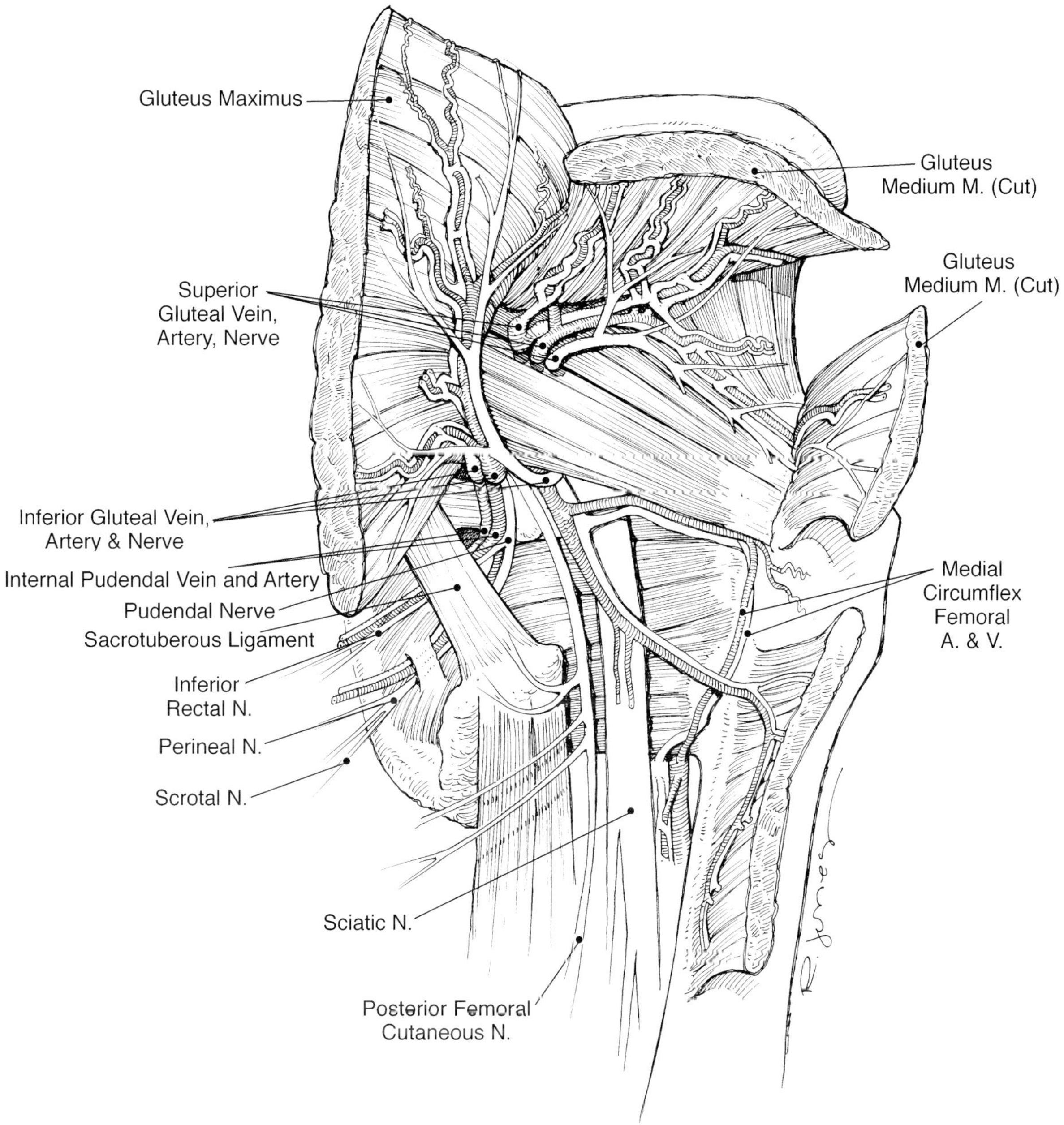
Gluteus Maximus
Gluteus Medium M. (Cut)
Gluteus Medium M. (Cut)
Superior Gluteal Vein, Artery, Nerve
Inferior Gluteal Vein, Artery & Nerve
Internal Pudendal Vein and Artery
Pudendal Nerve
Sacrotuberous Ligament
Inferior Rectal N.
Perineal N.
Scrotal N.
Medial Circumflex Femoral A. & V.
Sciatic N.
Posterior Femoral Cutaneous N.

**FIGURE IX-24**

detachment of the origins of the gluteus medius and minimus can lead to heterotopic bone formation. It is expected that patients who have undergone this exposure will have permanent abductor weakness and will have at least a mild abductor lurch. When the abductors are left in situ, the posterior exposure is limited by the superior gluteal artery and vein and the motor branch to the abductors. Disruption of the nerve or vessels can lead to necrosis of the hip abductor and a severe limp. Extensive detachment of the gluteus maximus from the iliotibial band and proximal femur can lead to weakness of hip extension, manifested by difficulty rising from the sitting position or climbing stairs. Extensive disruption of the iliopsoas muscle origin or insertion will weaken hip flexion. The patient will complain of "lack of control" of the hip in trying to lift the limb to walk up stairs. Extensive collateral blood flow in this region may produce dramatic bleeding in patients undergoing hemipelvic resections for tumor. In these patients, preoperative arteriography and embolization of the major branches feeding the tumor is recommended; however, the surgeon must review these findings with the radiologist to prevent complete disruption of both the anterior and posterior blood supply to the external soft tissues.

***Limitations***

The inverted J incision is more limited in exposure than the T incision because of the limited mobility of the abductor muscles. The entire hemipelvis can be resected through the T incision by elevation of the adductor muscles, pelvic diaphragm, and urogenital diaphragm as described in the extensile ischiopubic approach. The entire acetabulum and hip joint can be resected and reconstructed through this approach. The major limitation is preexisting vascular insufficiency in the lateral hip region from a direct muscle crush injury, arterial or venous disruption from displaced fractures, or prior radiation. Using the extensile approach in the presence of these complicating factors can lead to massive ischemic necrosis and infection, requiring hemipelvectomy for a cure.

## Extensile Posterior (Kocher-Langenbeck) Approach

***Applications***

This approach provides direct access to the posterior pelvis, from the apex of the greater sciatic notch to the ischial tuberosity. The acetabulum and posterior column are well visualized, allowing reduction of posterior column and acetabular rim fractures with the sciatic nerve exposed (5). This approach can be used in conjunction with an anterior approach for fixation of both column fractures.

***Technique***

The patient is placed in the lateral decubitus position and the lower extremity is draped free. The hip and knee can then be maintained in a flexed position to minimize traction on the sciatic nerve and allow manipulation of the limb. The incision begins approximately 6 cm distal to the posterior superior iliac spine and is carried in an arc to the anterior margin of the greater trochanter and then parallel to the femoral shaft for 15 to 20 cm (IX-25). The gluteal fascia is opened over the greater trochanter and the fascia lata divided vertically along the femoral shaft. The gluteal fascia and muscle fibers are then split with scissors or blunt dissection. The subgluteal bursa is explored to identify the superior gluteal artery and sciatic nerve as they exit the greater sciatic notch (IX-26). The piriformis and obturator internus tendons are identified, tagged, and detached from the greater trochanter through their tendinous insertions (IX-27). The muscles are then retracted posteriorly by the sutures so they can be draped over the sciatic nerve to protect it. The retraction provides wide exposure of the posterior column and posterior acetabular rim. If exposure to the ischial tuberosity is needed, the quadratus femoris mus-

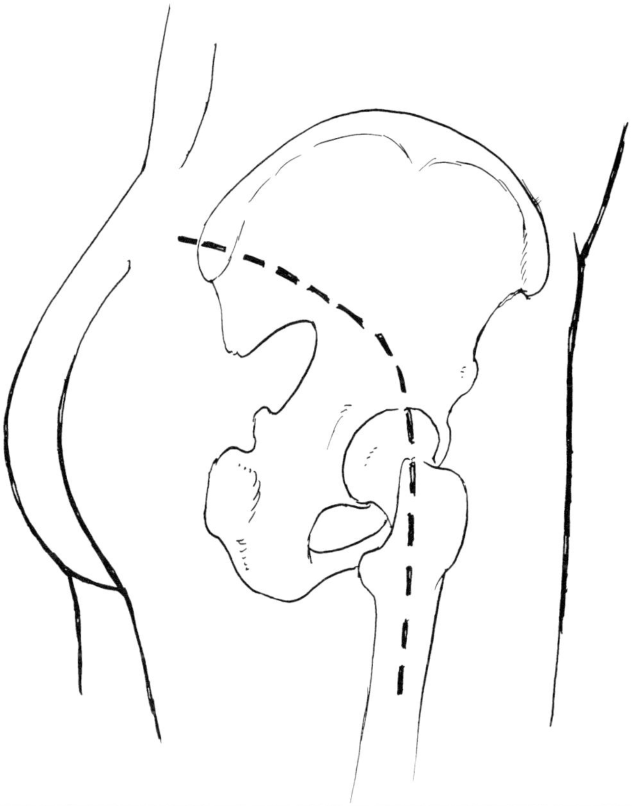

**FIGURE IX-25**

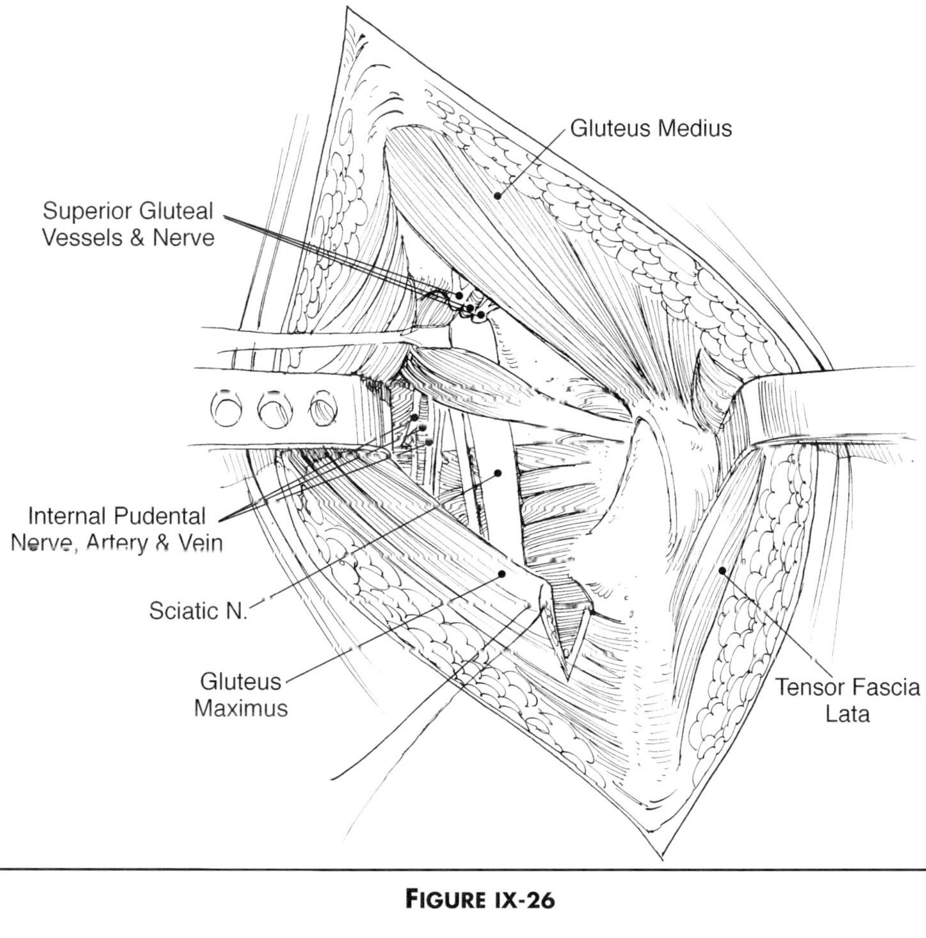


**FIGURE IX-26**

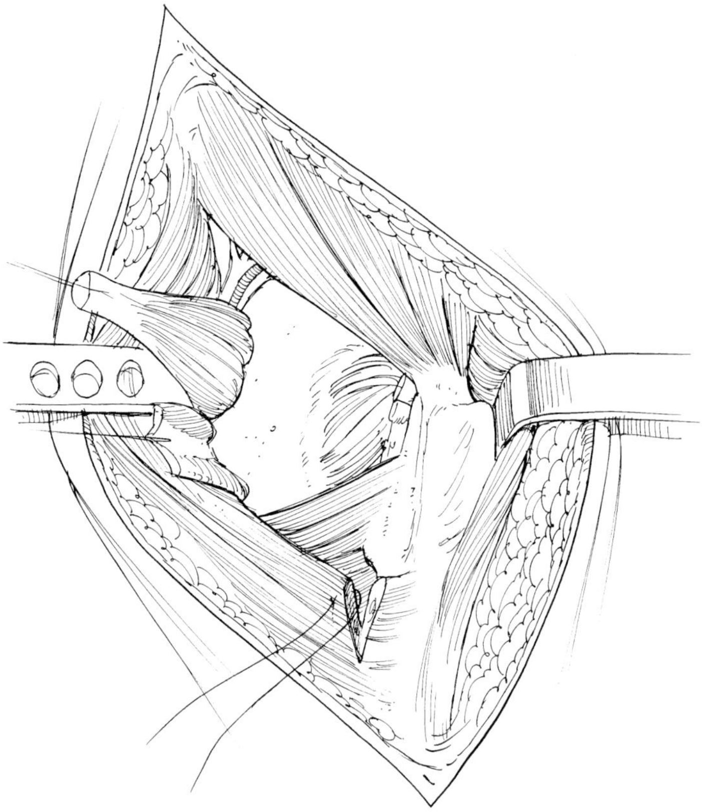

**FIGURE IX-27**

cle can be elevated from its origin on the ischium and reflected anteriorly to minimize risk of injury to its blood supply or to the posterior femoral circumflex artery (IX-28). The tendinous insertion of the gluteus maximus onto the linea aspera may be divided for 1 to 2 cm as necessary to visualize the ischium without excessive traction on the muscle or sciatic nerve.

***Dangers***

The major neurovascular structures susceptible to injury from this approach include the sciatic nerve, superior gluteal artery, pudendal nerve, and internal pudendal artery and vein as they pass over the ischial spine. The sciatic nerve may be found between bone fragments in displaced posterior column fractures.

***Limitations***

The gluteus maximus is innervated by the inferior gluteal nerve. If the muscle is split too far proximally, the superior portion of the muscle may be denervated. Denervation will lead to permanent weakness that the patient will notice when attempting to stand up from a sitting position or when climbing stairs. The superior gluteal nerve to the gluteus medius and minimus and tensor fascia lata may also be injured by excessive proximal dissection. There is very limited access to the medial wall of the acetabulum and true pelvis through this approach. By placing a finger through the greater sciatic foramen distal and lateral to the sciatic nerve, the medial edge of the ilium can be palpated almost to the anterior pelvic rim. A finger placed into the lesser sciatic foramen can displace the obturator internus muscle medially to gain circumferential access to the ischium and to the cotyloid notch portion of the acetabulum. This may be useful for defining boundaries for tumor resection or to aid in reduction of acetabular fractures.

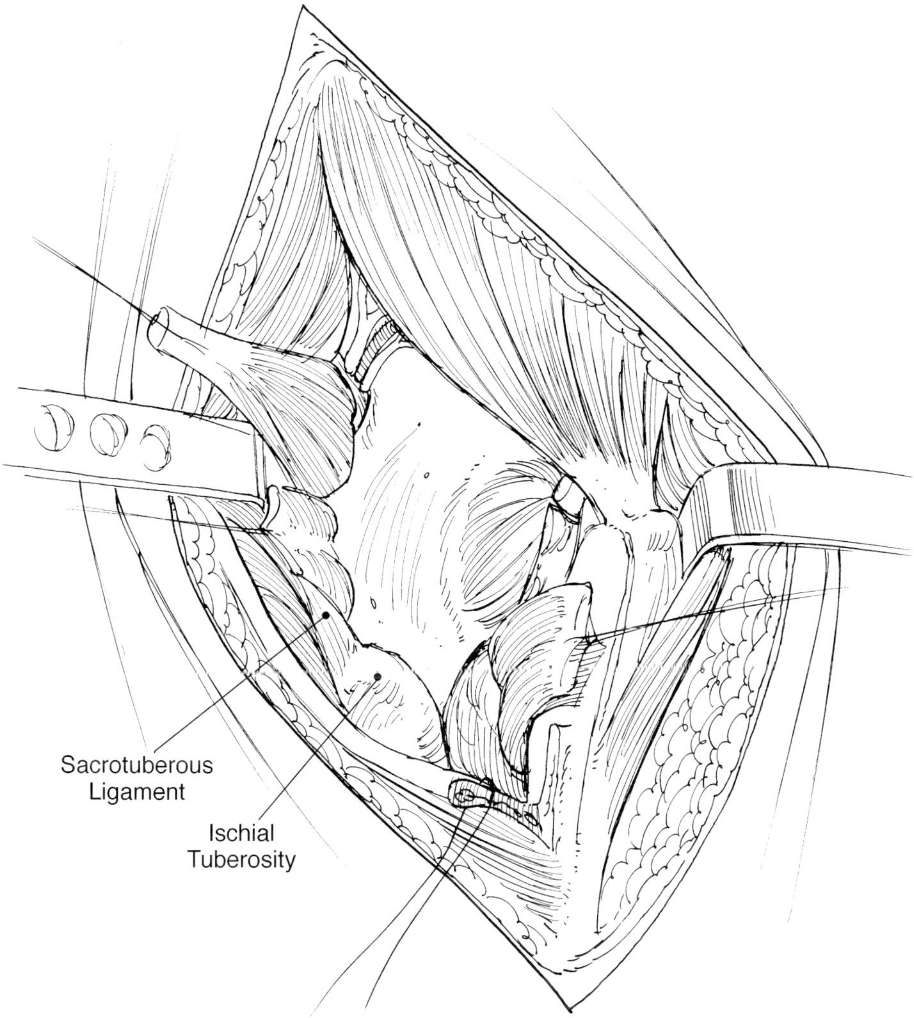


**FIGURE IX-28**

# Extensile Ischiopubic Approach

***Applications***

This approach is used for resection of the superior and inferior pubic rami, the pubic symphysis, and the ischium up to the posterior limit of the ischial tuberosity. This approach is not needed for fracture fixation. It is necessary for access to the bony true pelvis for treatment of infection or tumors of the bones or the soft tissue of the obturator region or proximal thigh (6). It can be combined with the extensile ilioinguinal or iliofemoral approach for a complete so called "internal hemipelvectomy" and reconstruction. The levator ani and obturator internus muscles provide anatomic barriers for tumor margins inside the pelvis, making wide resection of these bones possible.

***Technique***

The patient is placed supine with a bolster under the affected side. The limbs are placed in the lithotomy position. The dissection is much easier if the affected limb is left free and supported by an assistant so that it can be manipulated during the procedure. Most of the dissection is easiest when the limb is in a figure 4 position with the hip flexed, abducted, and externally rotated. The incision begins at the medial boundary of the femoral triangle, approximately 1 cm distal to the inguinal ligament (IX-29). This position can be approximated by palpating the femoral pulse and gracilis tendon and beginning the skin incision approximately halfway between them. The incision is then curved transversely across the medial thigh to the level of the ischial tuberosity, staying 1 cm lateral to the inguinal crease and perineum. The posterior limit of the incision may then be curved distally for 3 to 5 cm to allow better exposure of the ischium. The incision is carried through the fascia lata to enter the adductor compartment. The adductor tendons can then be followed to the inferior pubic ramus and outer table of the ischium.

The medial edge of the inferior pubic ramus and ischium are the lateral boundaries of the perineum. In the anterior half of the incision, the urogenital diaphragm tightly adheres to the periosteum of the inferior pubic ramus (IX-30). The diaphragm extends from the lateral edge of the symphysis posteriorly to the anterior edge of the ischial tuberosity. Posterior to this is the large potential space of the ischiorectal fossa. This space extends deep to the urogenital diaphragm (between it and the levator ani) and anteriorly to the pubic symphysis. Therefore, it is possible to open this space, lateral to the rectum, and bluntly mobilize the fat in the ischiorectal fossa to visualize the bone.

The internal pudendal artery and vein and pudendal nerve should be located along the edge of the ischiorectal fossa posterior to the urogenital diaphragm (IX-31). They can then be traced into the pudendal (Alcock's) canal. They run anteriorly within the narrow fascial canal adjacent to the bone, encased in the dense fascia of the urogenital diaphragm (IX-32). The fascia can be incised longitudinally to mobilize these vessels and allow them to be retracted medially. The deep fascia of the urogenital diaphragm can then be incised longitudinally to detach it from the bone (IX-33). As the anterior edge of the urogenital diaphragm is reached, care must be taken to identify the deep dorsal artery and vein of the penis or clitoris. These vessels must be retracted and protected while the pubic symphysis is

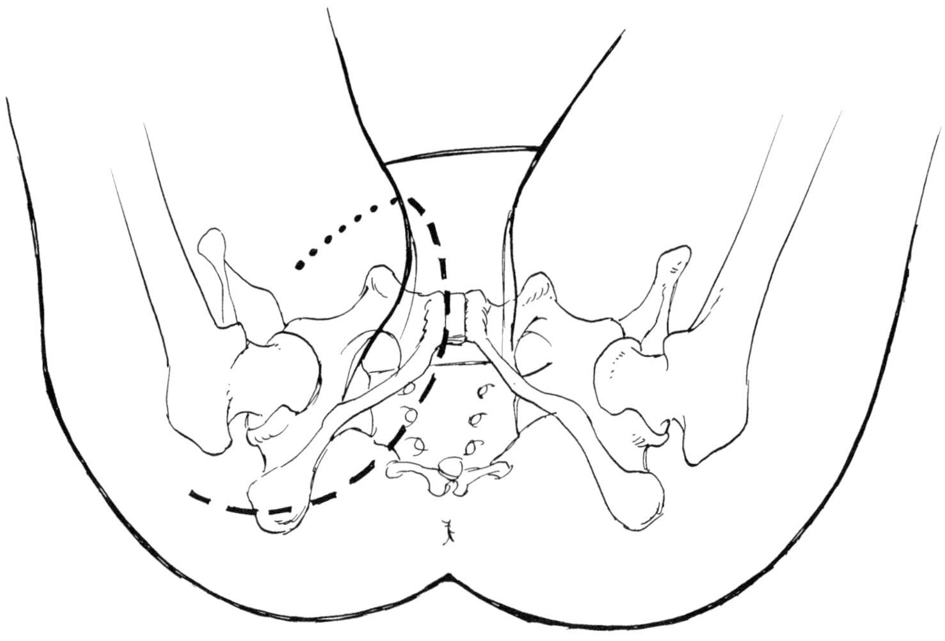

**FIGURE IX-29**

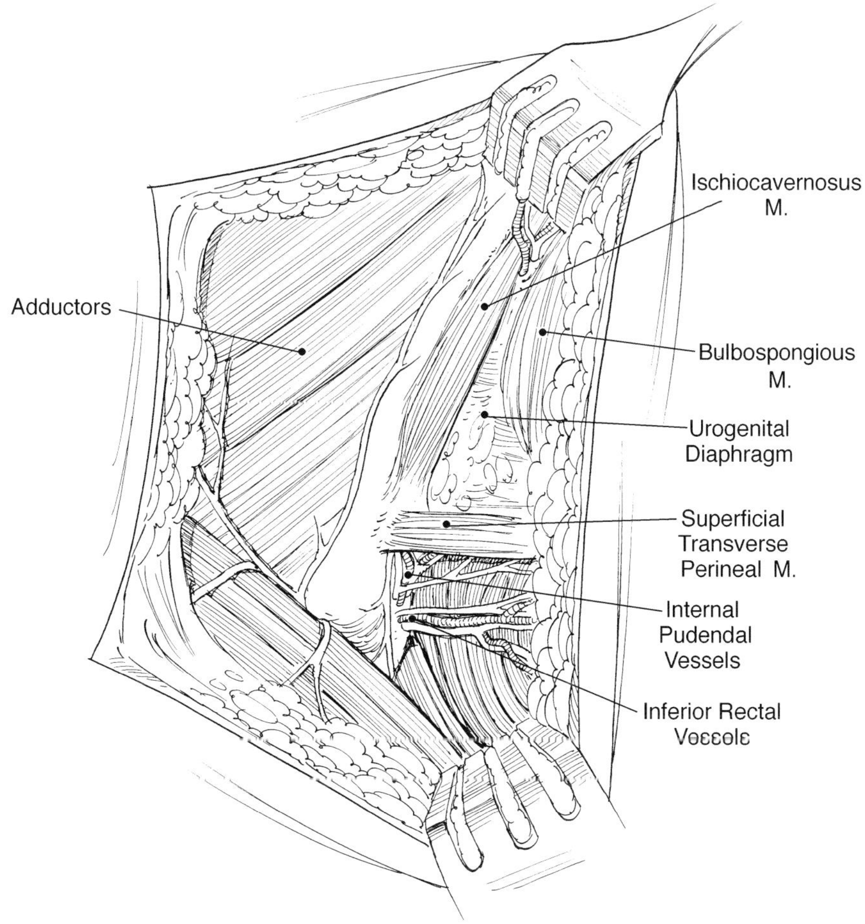


**FIGURE IX-30**

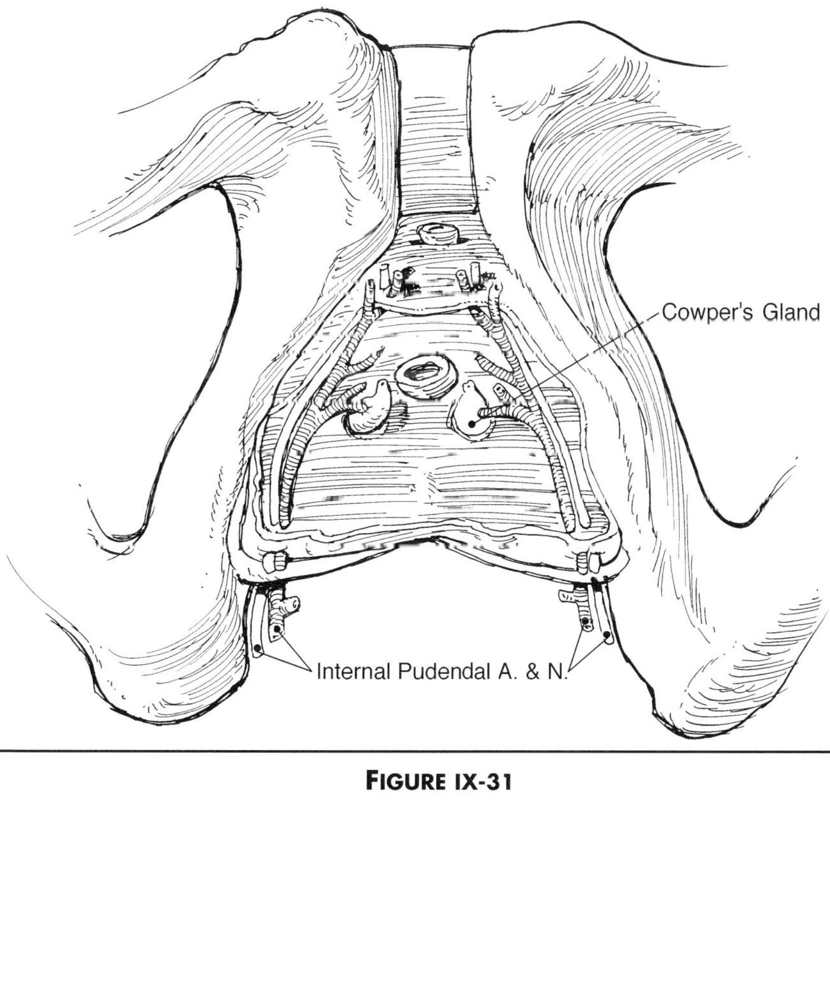


**FIGURE IX-31**

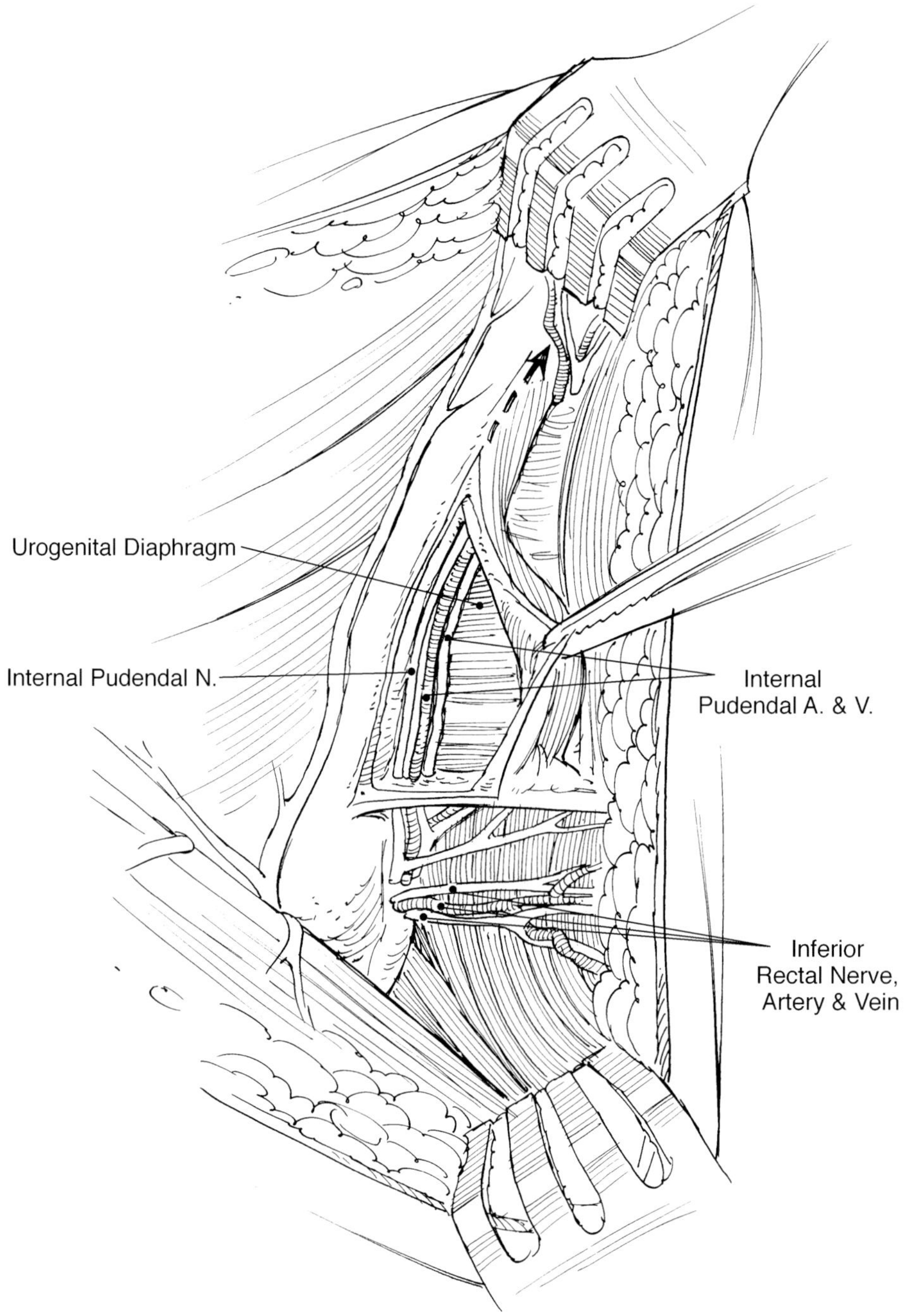
Urogenital Diaphragm
Internal Pudendal N.
Internal Pudendal A. & V.
Inferior Rectal Nerve, Artery & Vein

**FIGURE IX-32**

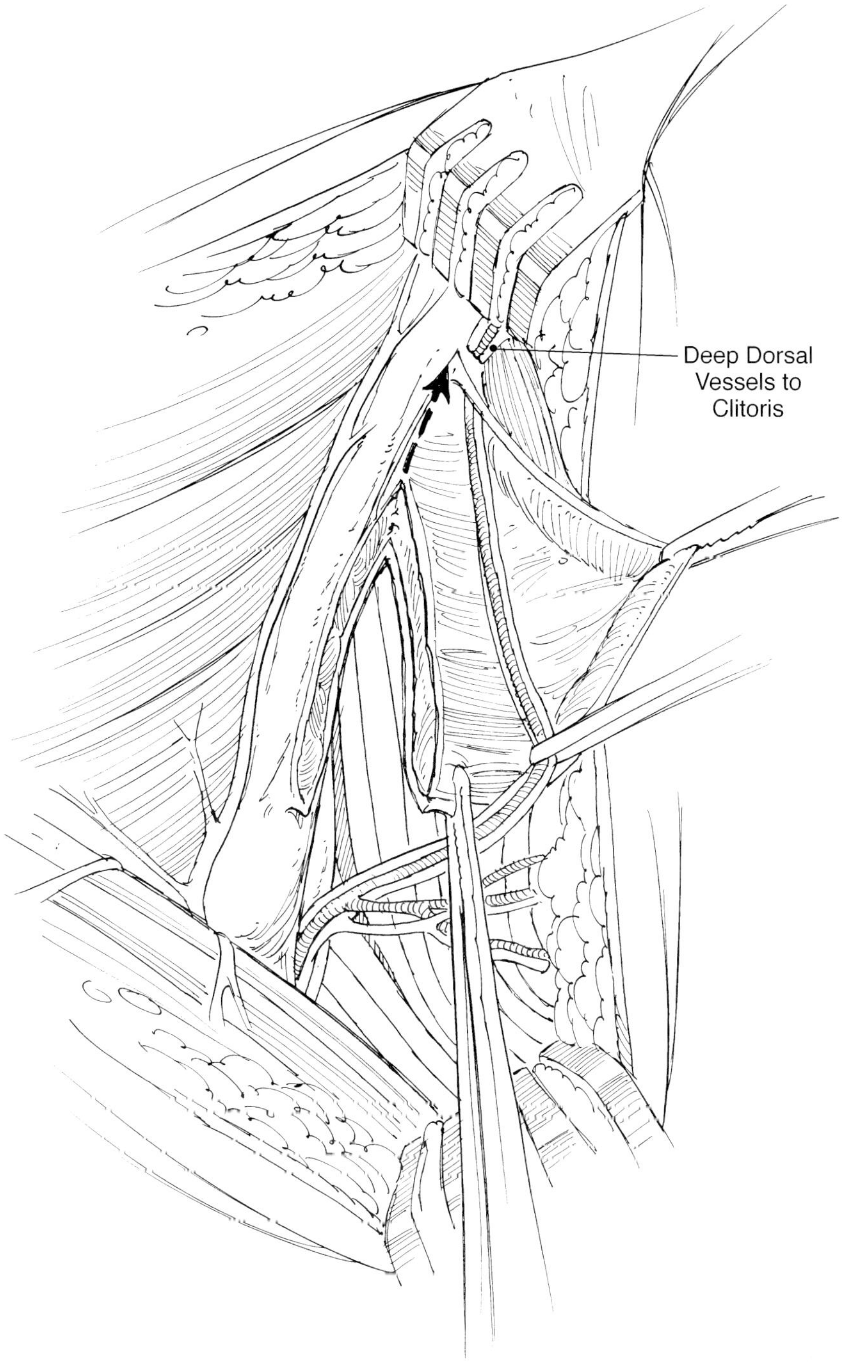


**FIGURE IX-33**

disarticulated. The crus of the penis or clitoris originates from the caudal surface of the urogenital diaphragm and need not be disturbed. In males, the prostate gland lies immediately on the deep surface of the urogenital diaphragm and can be visualized and protected after the fascia is detached from the pubic ramus. The extensive venous plexus around the prostate should not be disturbed. The inguinal ligament can be detached from the pubic tubercle to expose the superior pubic ramus (IX-34). The exposure along the superior pubic ramus can then be performed as described in the extensile ilioinguinal approach.

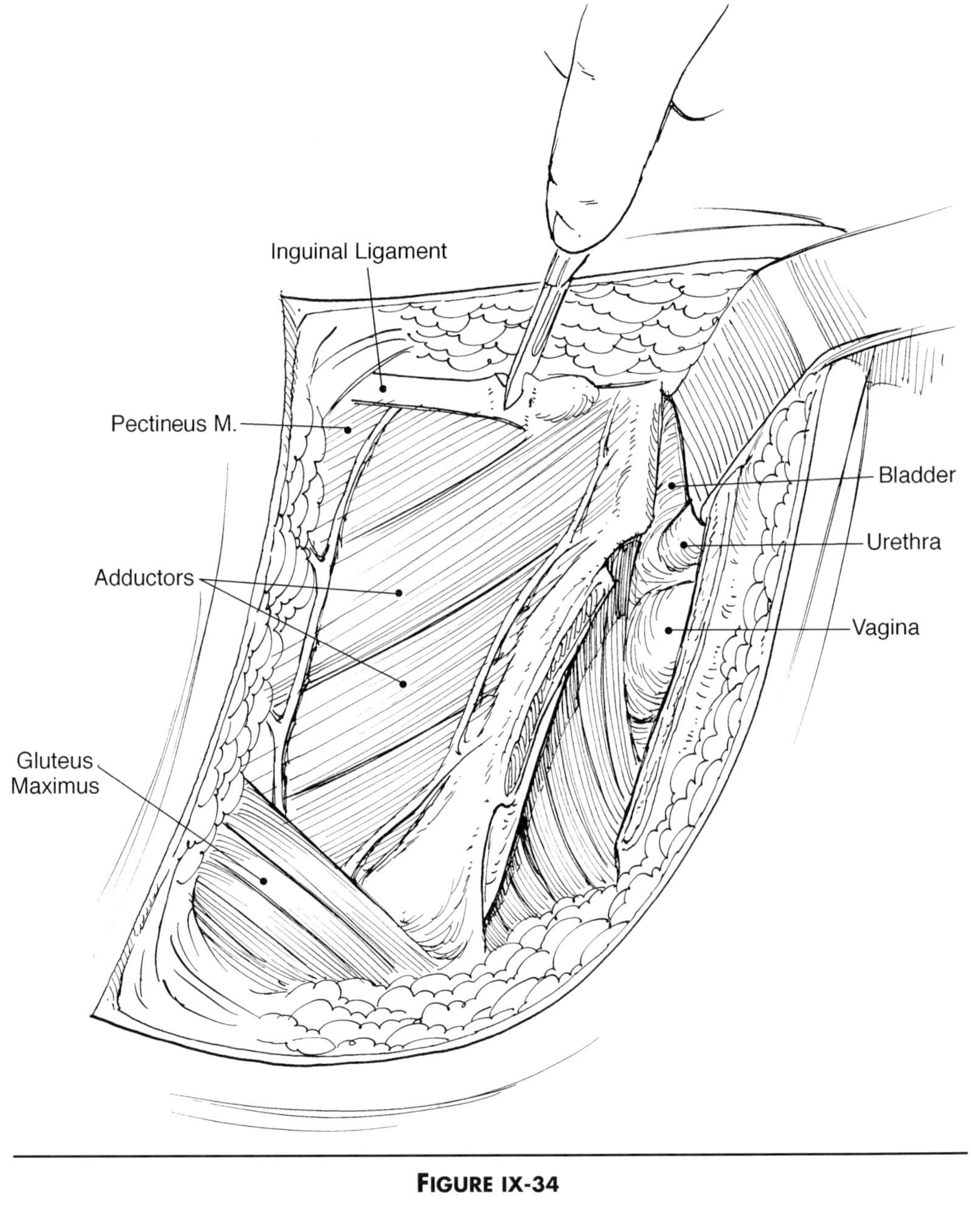


**FIGURE IX-34**

Posteriorly, the medial edge of the gluteus maximus must be retracted or divided to allow visualization of the ischial tuberosity. The sciatic nerve will be found along the lateral edge of this dissection (IX-35).

The extent of the deep dissection necessary for this procedure depends on the surgical margin needed. For simple excision of the bone, for osteomyelitis or benign tumors, the adductor muscle origins, obturator externus, urogenital diaphragm, and obturator internus may be detached subperiosteally by incising the periosteum along the visible perineal bone margin (IX-36). Resection of the ischium requires detachment of the sacrotuberous and sacrospinous ligaments from the ischium. Detaching the sacrotuberous ligament allows retraction of the gluteus maximus that originates on its external surface. The internal pudendal artery and vein and pudendal nerve should be traced over the ischial spine and protected before transecting the sacrospinous ligament.

For malignant tumors requiring wide resection, the muscles of the adductor compartment may be partially or completely excised. The iliopsoas and hamstrings will compensate for the resected adductors, even if they are completely excised with the obturator neurovascular bundle. The patient can expect to ambulate without a limp after this resection. For this dissection, the adductors can be transected as far distally as necessary. The divisions of the obturator nerve, artery, and vein should be identified anterior and posterior to the adductor brevis and transected

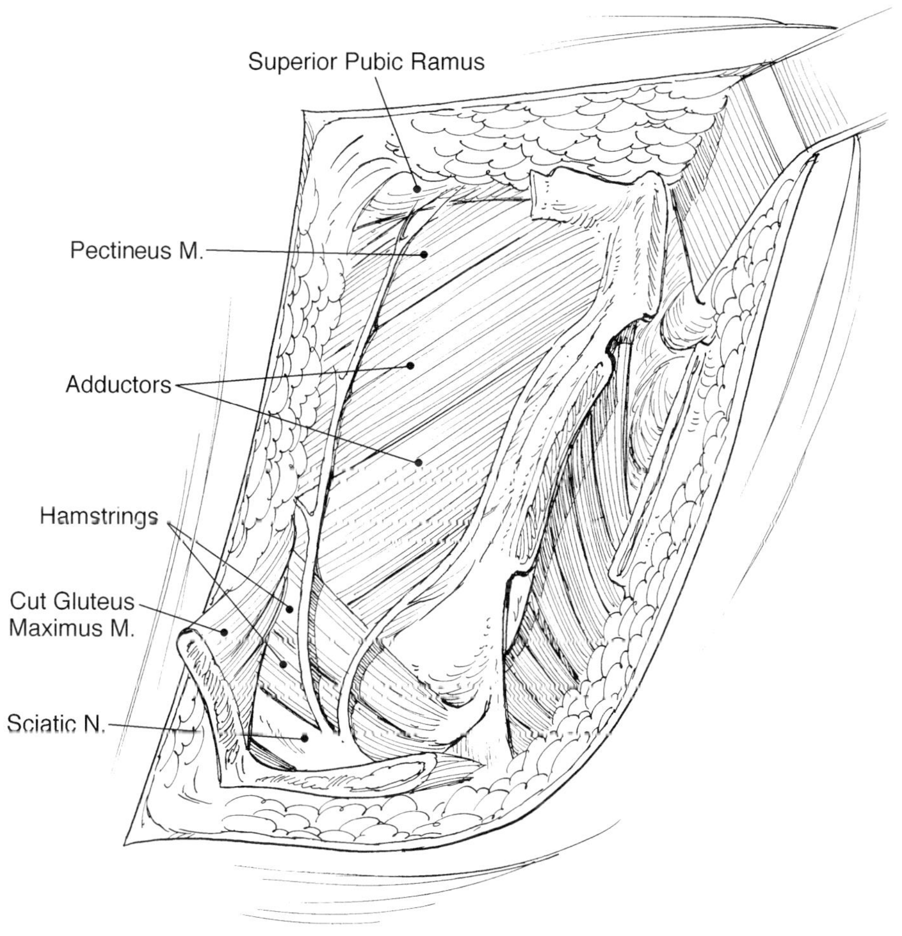


**FIGURE IX-35**

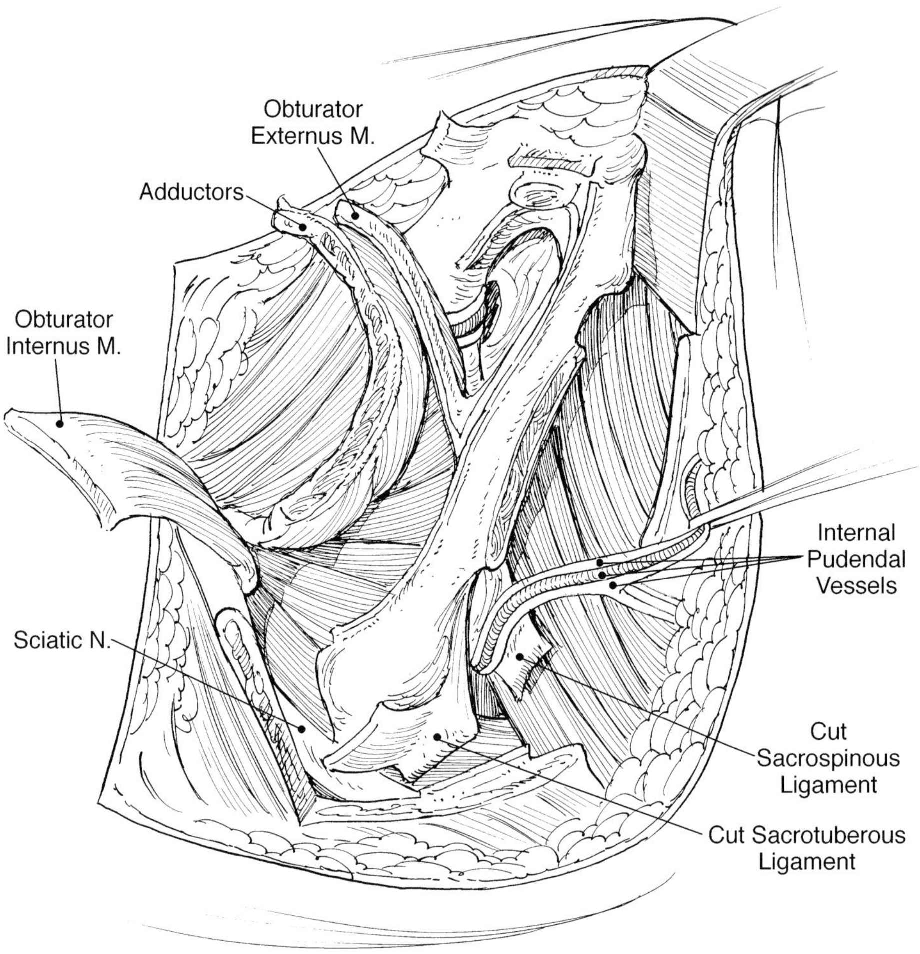


**FIGURE IX-36**

individually (IX-37). The psoas tendon can then be visualized and preserved. The quadratus femoris and obturator externus can be detached from either the ischium or the femur (IX-38). The dissection can then be carried medial to the ischium by mobilizing the pudendal neurovascular bundle and urogenital diaphragm. The obturator internus origin will be encountered on the deep ischial surface. If necessary, the entire muscle origin can be excised. In this case, the obturator vessels should be identified inside the pelvis and transected before they enter the obturator foramen. If the obturator muscles can be preserved, they can be elevated from the surface of the ischium and pubis and retracted (IX-39), the bone transected and removed, and the obturator nerve and vessels preserved.

A large cavitary wound is created which should be closed in layers. Care must be taken to close the fascia deep to the inguinal ligament to prevent a visceral herniation.

***Dangers***

With proper exposure and control of the vessels encountered during this dissection, bleeding should be minimal. Injury to the pudendal nerve may result in perineal numbness. Men must be informed of the possibility of impotence. The urethra, prostate, urinary bladder, and rectum are all immediately adjacent to the area of dissection and must be protected. The sciatic nerve is usually found laterally in this approach and does not limit the dissection.

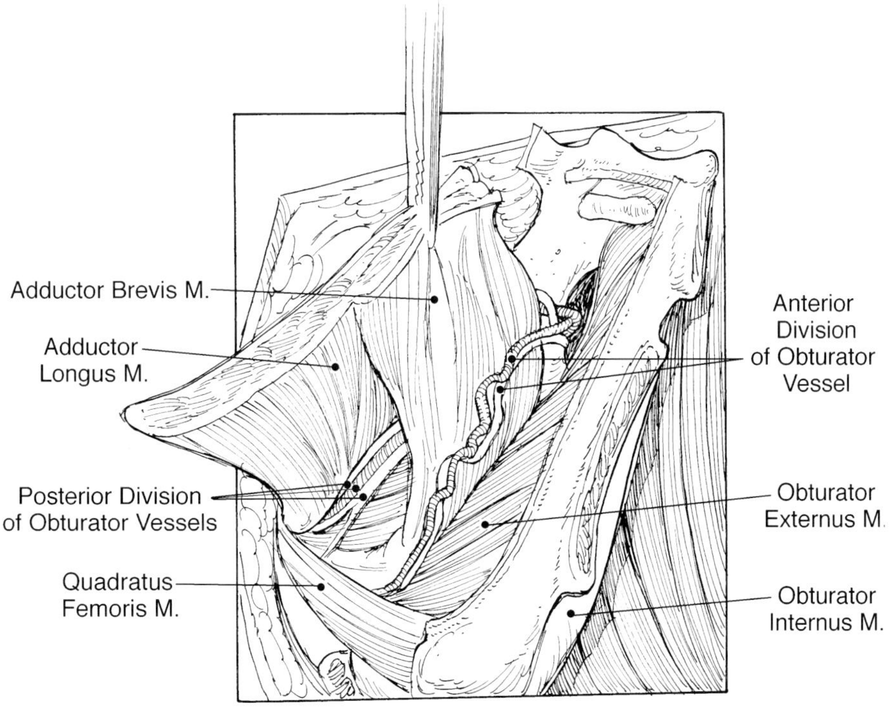


**FIGURE IX-37**

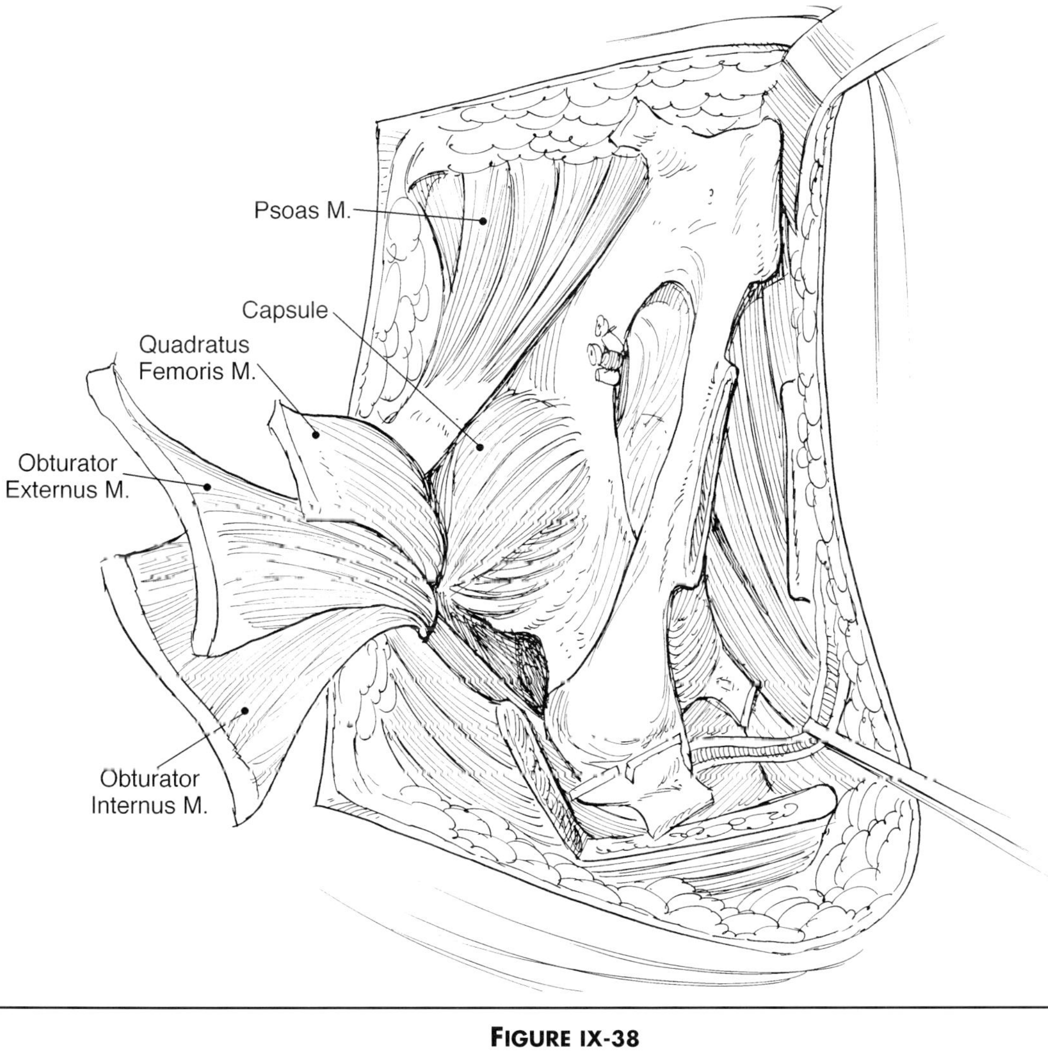


**FIGURE IX-38**

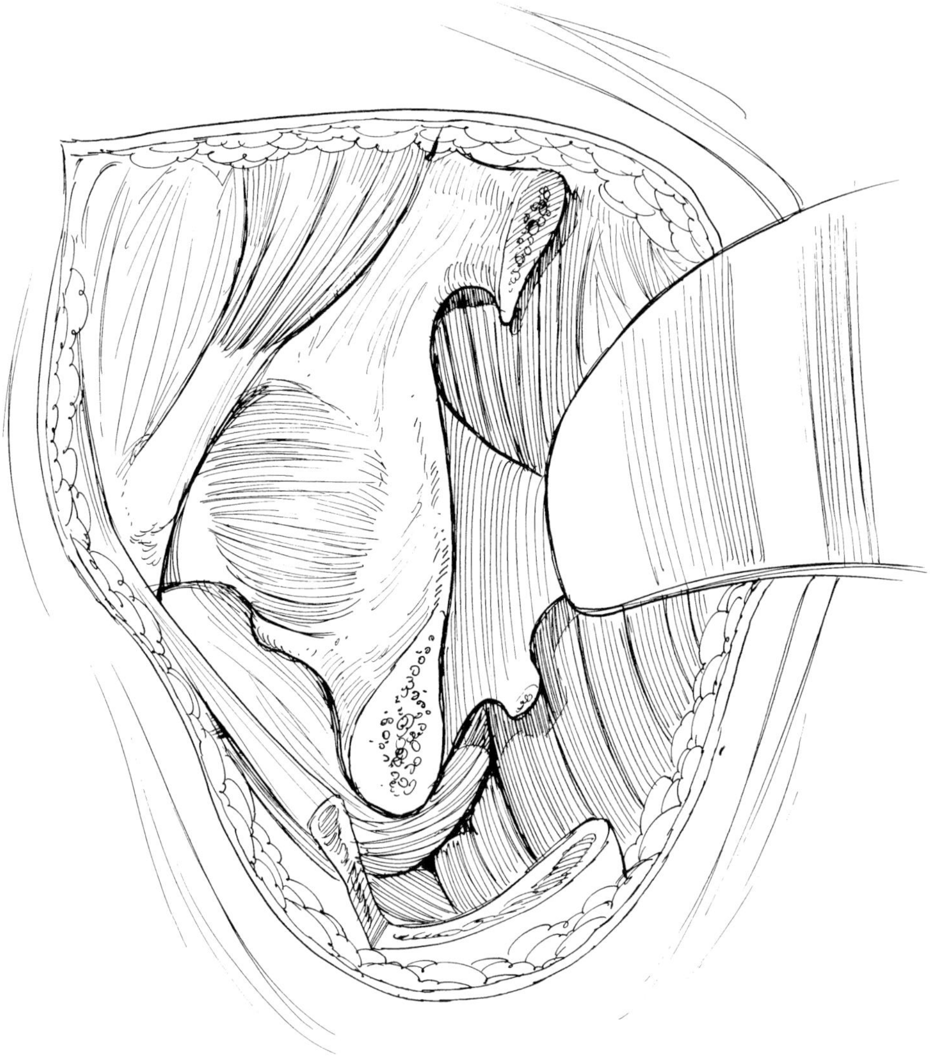

FIGURE IX-39

*Limitations*

This approach can be used for exposure of the true pelvis for as extensive a dissection as is needed. When combined with the extensile iliofemoral approach, the entire hemipelvis and hip joint can be resected, as is most commonly done for large chondrosarcomas of the juxtaacetabular region. The posterior boundary of this approach is the posterior edge of the ischial tuberosity. Further approach to the posterior column requires a posterior approach.

## Posterior Sacral Approach

*Applications*

This dissection is used for open reduction and internal fixation of comminuted pelvic fractures involving the sacral ala and for partial or total sacrectomy. For malignant tumors of the sacrum or posterior pelvis, it may be combined with an anterior approach to mobilize the viscera from the anterior sacral surface. Total sacrectomy should only be undertaken for an attempted curative resection of a tumor such as a chordoma or chondrosarcoma (7). The morbidity of this operation does not justify its use for palliation. A diverting colostomy and/or a ureteroileal conduit may be performed as a staged procedure prior to sacral resection or as a single procedure at the same time. Preoperative arteriography and embolization of all of the major vessels entering the tumor region can significantly decrease the blood loss. A compiete bowel prep is necessary. Placement of ureteral stints can minimize the risk of inadvertent ureteral damage. The patient must undergo extensive preoperative counseling and psychiatric assistance is recommended for support throughout the perioperative period because the patient can be expected to become depressed during the prolonged recovery from this procedure.

### *Technique*

Extensive preoperative planning is necessary for successful completion of this procedure, as noted above.

The sacrum can be exposed posteriorly by a vertical midline incision, transverse incision, or T incision. If a T incision is used, the transverse limb of the T should be at the level of the iliac crests. The vertical incision should be at the midline for exposure of the entire sacrum, or it may be at the level of the posterior iliac crest for lateral hemisacral exposure (IX-40). A fasciocutaneous flap can be elevated over the paravertebral muscles. For exposure of the dorsal sacrum, the paravertebral muscles can be elevated from the bone, beginning at the caudal end (IX-41). The dural sac and cauda equina can be exposed by a dorsal sacral laminectomy (IX-42). The sacrum may be resected by disarticulation of the sacroiliac joints or by excision of the posterior iliac wing. For sagittal hemisacrectomy, the nerve roots on the resected side may be ligated and transected within the spinal canal to allow exposure of the sacral body. For total sacrectomy, the dura may be ligated and transected at the lumbosacral junction. The posterior iliac crest is exposed by elevation

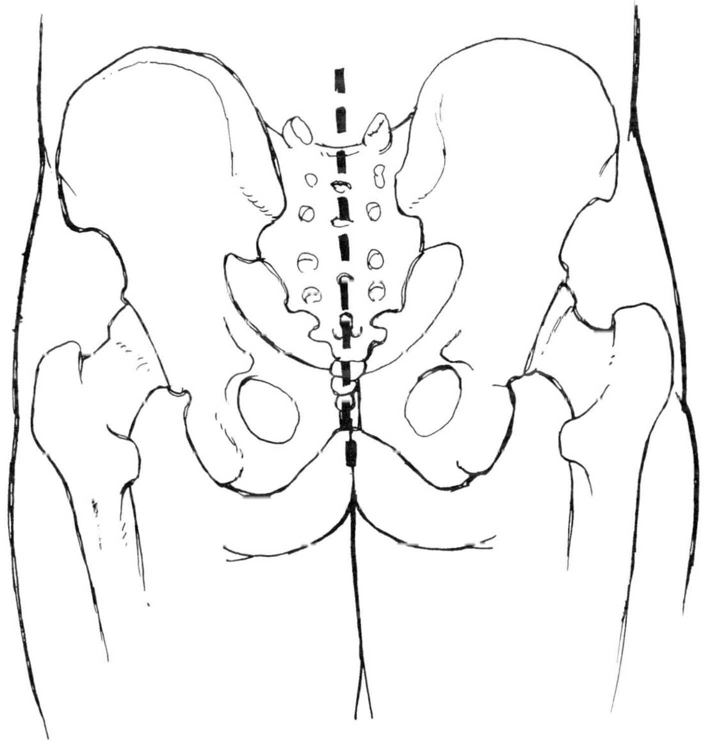

**FIGURE IX-40**

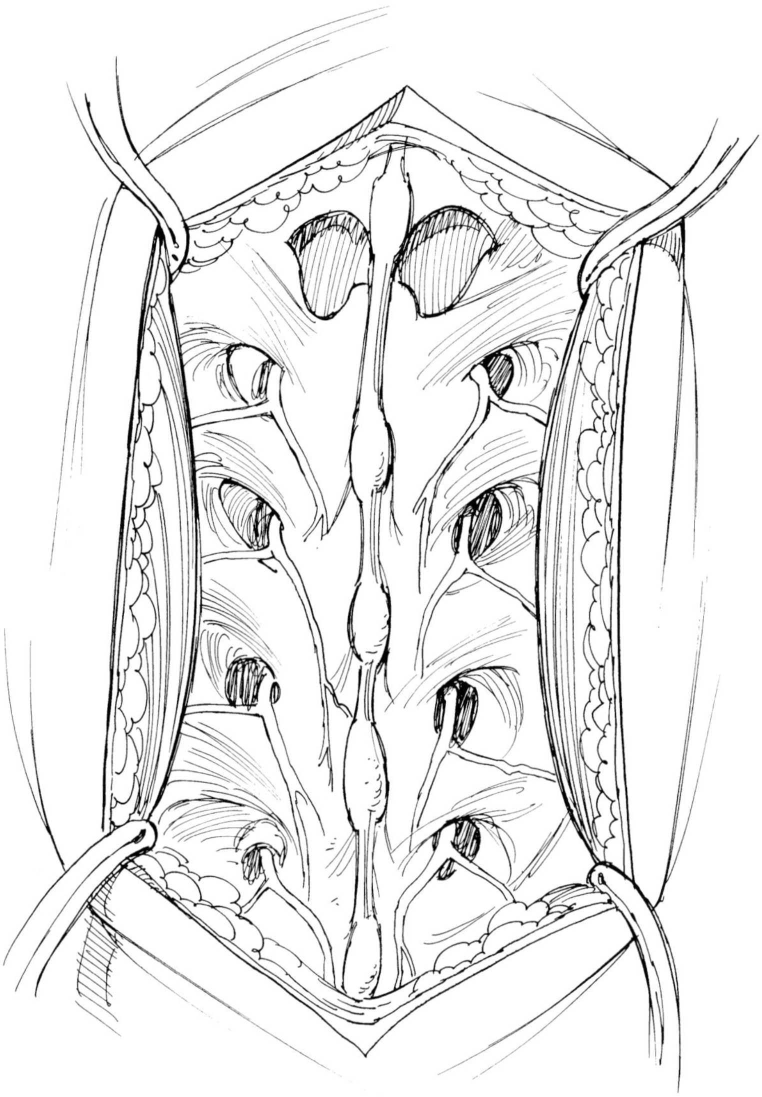

**FIGURE IX-41**

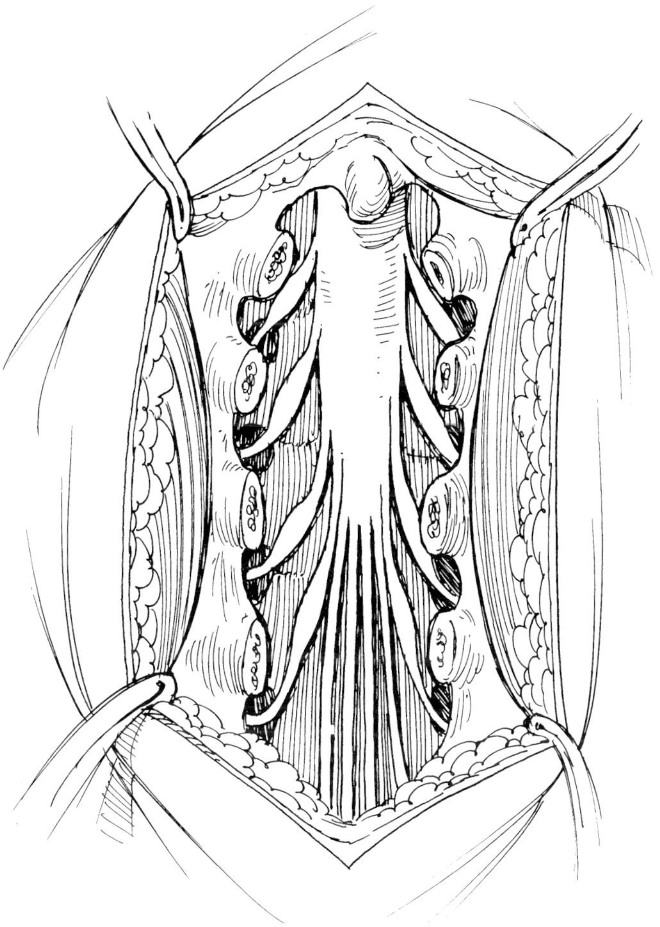

FIGURE IX-42

of the gluteus maximus and abdominal wall muscles. This elevation exposes the sciatic notch and the piriformis muscle, superior gluteal artery and vein, and sciatic nerve as they exit the notch (IX-43). The superior gluteal vessels may be ligated or mobilized and preserved. The sacrotuberous ligaments and sacrospinous ligaments should be divided. The coccygeus muscle can be detached from the tip of the coccyx (IX-44).

Anterior exposure of the sacrum and mobilization of all structures to be resected with the sacrum is performed prior to the posterior dissection. For anterior exposure, the sacrum can be approached by either a transabdominal or a unilateral or bilateral retroperitoneal approach. The middle sacral artery, ascending lumbar arteries, and other branches of the internal iliac system must be mobilized and ligated to allow retraction of the common iliac vessels. The psoas muscles and quadratus lumborum must be transected. The femoral nerve, lateral femoral cutaneous nerves, and lumbosacral trunk should be preserved if possible. For total sacrectomy, the lumbosacral disc can be excised. For partial sacrectomy, the sacrum is divided with an osteotome. For radical sacrectomy, the iliac wings are transected and the iliolumbar ligaments divided to allow removal of the sacrum. For resection of large tumors or radical dissections of recurrent rectal carcinoma, the aorta may be cross clamped at the time of sacral excision to decrease blood loss.

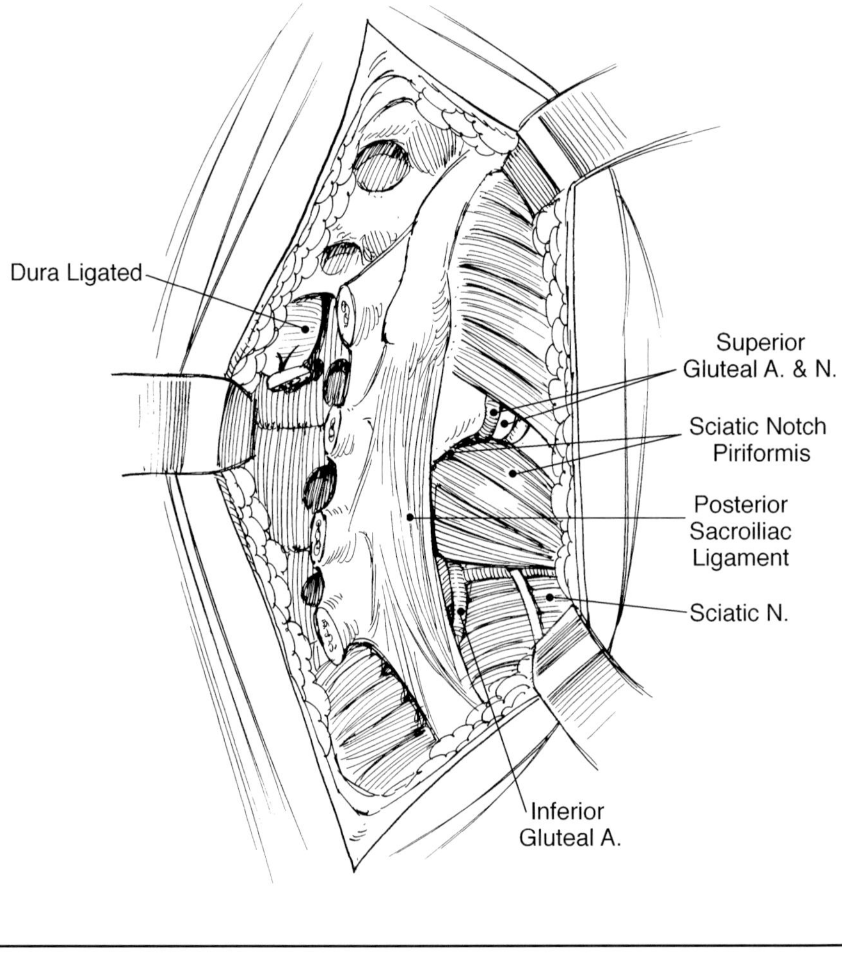


**FIGURE IX-43**

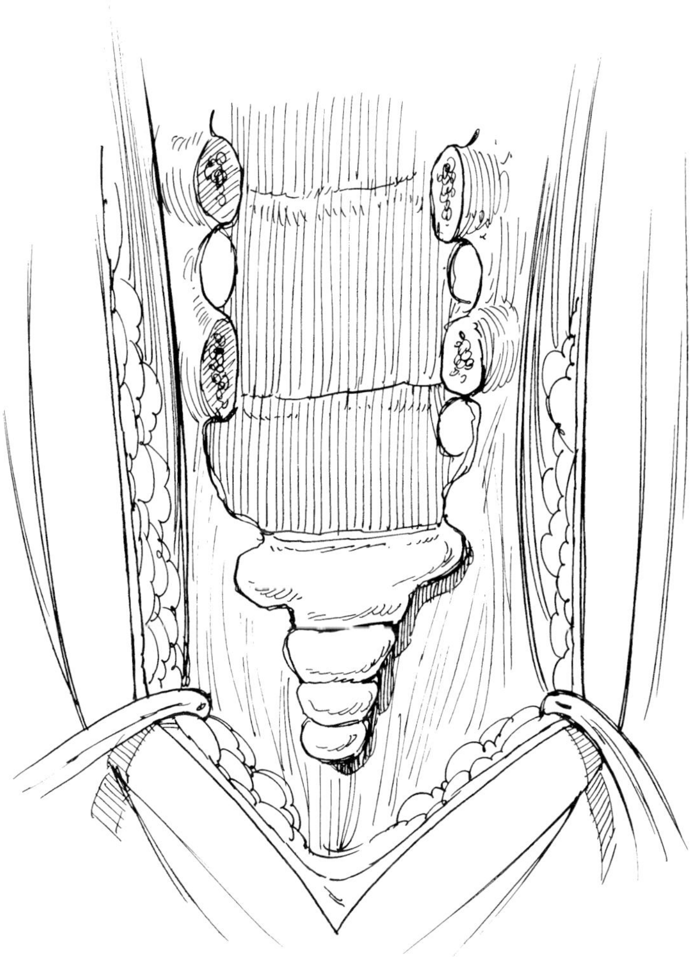

**FIGURE IX-44**

In most cases, the anterior dissection is completed, the wound is packed with sponges, and the anterior wound is closed. The patient is then repositioned prone for the posterior dissection.

The large cavity created by sacrectomy should be filled with either a gluteal rotation flap, vascularized free muscle, or composite flaps. The spine can be stabilized by instrumentation of the lower lumbar spine to the iliac wings. This step can be facilitated by closing the defect by compressing the iliac wings, for example, with Harrington bolts. The large cavitary wound will accumulate fluid easily and should be drained with chest tubes at low suction until the drainage subsides. Some authors have advocated cementing an antibiotic impregnated spacer in the cavity at the time of initial resection. Four to 6 weeks later, the spacer is removed and the spine is stabilized to the iliac crest with instrumentation.

***Dangers***

Significant bleeding can be expected with sacral resection. Control of the major divisions of the internal iliac vessels will help to minimize the blood loss. Bleeding from the venous plexus within the sacral vertebrae and the anastomosis with the epidural venous plexus can be difficult to control when the sacral vertebrae are transected. Wide exposure of the area prior to transection of the bone and immediate use of clotting agents and bone wax can help to decrease the blood loss.

The rectum, ureters, lumbosacral trunk, and sacral nerve roots should be protected and preserved.

***Limitations***

The entire sacrum including the sacroiliac joints can be resected. It can be removed en bloc with the adjacent rectum and entire pelvic contents if necessary. The patient must be willing to accept the morbidity of loss of bowel and bladder control, colostomy, ureteral diversion, sexual dysfunction, motor and sensory loss in the lower extremities, and wound infection along with numerous other complications. Recovery from this procedure can be expected to last several months.

# References

1. Semba RT, Yasukawa K, El Guatillo RB. Critical analysis of results of 53 malgaigne fractures of the pelvis. J Trauma 23:535–537, 1983.
2. Perry JF, Jr. Pelvic open fractures. Clin Orthop 151:41–45, 1980.
3. Noam NH, Brown WM, Burdge RE, Kominski DL. Major pelvic fractures. Arch Surg 118:610–616, 1983.
4. Reinert CM, Boss MJ, Poka A, et al. A modified extensile exposure for the treatment of the complex or malunited acetabular fractures. J Bone Joint Surg 70A(3):329–337, 1988.
5. Letournel E, Judet R. General principles of surgical management. In: Elson RA, ed. Fractures of the Acetabulum. New York: Springer-Verlag, 1981:233–240.
6. Steel HH. Partial or complete resection of the hemipelvis. An alternative to hindquarter amputation for periacetabular chondrosarcoma of the pelvis. J Bone Joint Surg 60:719–730, 1978.
7. Shikoto J, Yamamuro T, Katouro Y, Mikaua Y, Iida H, Maetani S. Total sacrectomy and reconstruction for primary tumors. J Bone Joint Surg 70(1):122–125, 1988.

X

# SURGICAL APPROACHES TO THE HIP

*Jay D. Mabrey and Lorence W. Trick*

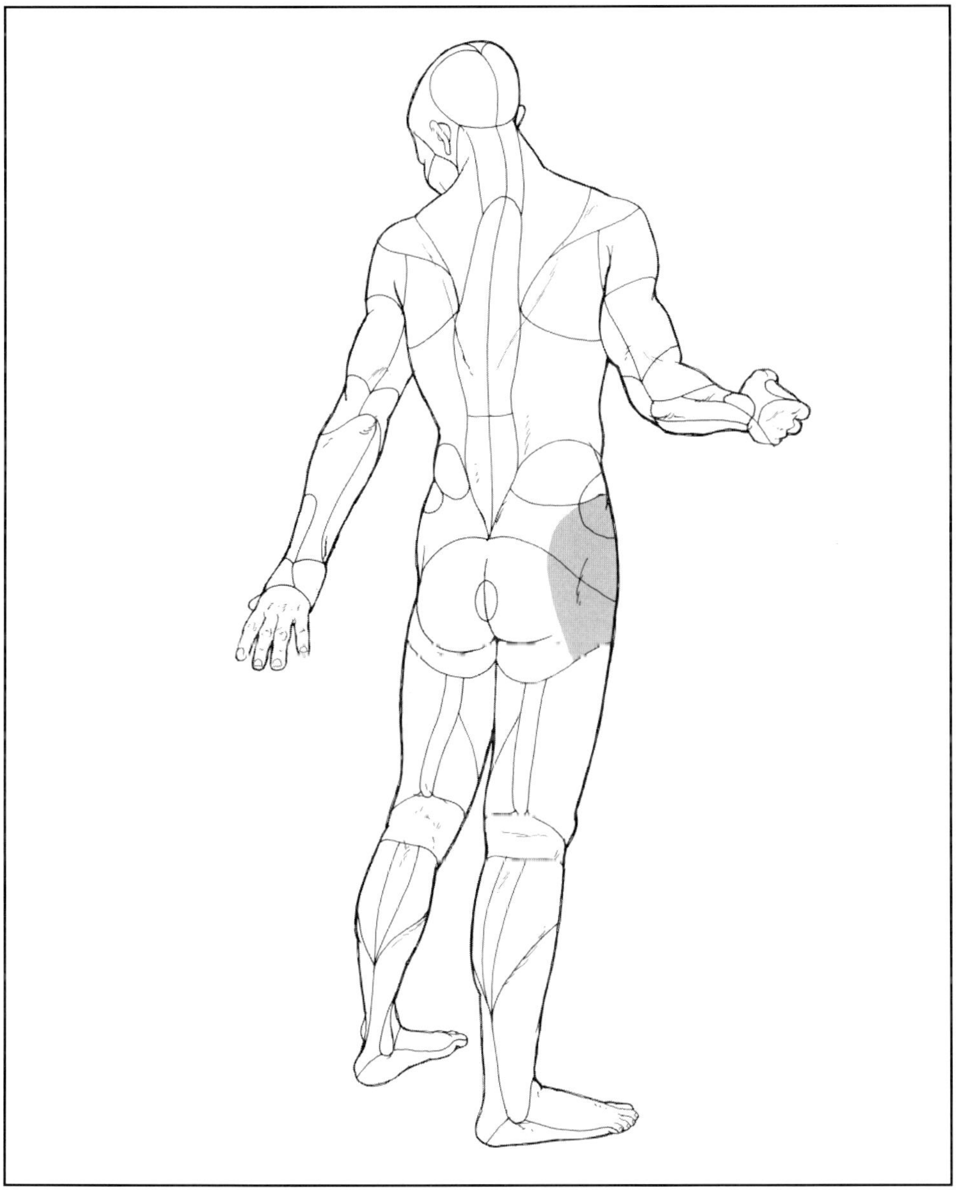

# General Principles and Complications

The advances made in recent years in total joint arthroplasty, musculoskeletal tumor surgery, and the treatment of complex fractures around the acetabulum have brought with them a plethora of surgical approaches to the hip, each carefully planned to provide a specific advantage for a given clinical situation.

Exposure of the hip takes the surgeon through one of the larger muscle masses of the body, the preservation of which is critical to maintain efficient ambulation. The skin incision should be positioned to allow access to the joint for visualization and instrumentation, without excessive soft tissue retraction. Draping should assure free mobility of the lower limb during the procedure. Most of the critical anatomic structures around the hip are not directly visualized during surgery. Therefore, the surgeon must have a thorough knowledge of the anatomic relationships about the hip and pelvis. Knowledge of the vascular anatomy is necessary to assure hemostasis and to avoid injury to major vascular trunks. Injury to the gluteal, femoral, and sciatic nerves is avoided with proper preoperative planning and careful retraction during the operation. The most serious complications associated with hip surgery are deep venous thrombosis and sciatic nerve palsy.

# Surgical Anatomy

For all operations on the hip joint, the anterior and posterior superior iliac spines should be draped into the field. The relationship of these two landmarks to the greater trochanter allows the surgeon to perceive the relationship of the pelvis to the femur. The femoral head and neck normally project at a 135° angle to the femoral shaft in the coronal plane and are anteverted 15° in the axial plane. The acetabulum also faces caudally and anteriorly in relation to the ilium. A line projecting straight medially from the apex of the greater trochanter when the thigh is in a neutral position should intersect the dome of the femoral head (X-1).

The hip is surrounded by a large muscle mass encapsulated in the thick fascia lata. The tensor fascia lata is engulfed by the fascia while the gluteus medius and gluteus maximus lie deep to the fascia. The gluteus maximus inserts onto the posterior aspect of the iliotibial band (X-2). The gluteus medius, gluteus minimus, and tensor fascia lata are all innervated by the superior gluteal nerve. This nerve passes anteriorly from the sciatic notch, deep to the gluteus medius (X-3). Anteriorly, the hip joint is crossed by the iliopsoas, rectus femoris, sartorius, and pectineus muscles. The femoral nerve, artery, and vein lie immediately anterior to these muscles as they pass through the femoral triangle (X-4). The "short external rotators" (the superior and inferior gemelli, obturator internus, and quadratus femoris) cover the posterior hip capsule and lesser trochanter, separating the sciatic nerve from the joint (X-5).

The adductor muscle group bridges the hip medially, with the obturator nerve and vessels passing through them.

The blood supply to the femoral head is a primary concern in any approach to the hip joint in which the femoral head is preserved. The arterial supply, in order of importance, is: (1) the medial femoral circumflex, (2) lateral femoral circumflex, (3) obturator, (4) superior gluteal, (5) ascending branch of the first profundus femoris perforator, and (6) inferior gluteal (X-6A and X-6B). Viability of the femoral head is most likely to be assured if the medial and lateral femoral circumflex vessels are preserved. The medial femoral circumflex artery arises from the profunda femoris and passes distally and medially about the insertion of the iliopsoas. It then passes inferior to the obturator externus and ascends superolaterally along the posterior surface of the femoral neck (X-6A). Its branches ascend deep to the synovium of the posterior neck to enter nutrient foramina along the outer rim of the articular surface of the femoral head. This creates a vascular ring around the medial, posterior, and superior two-thirds of the femoral neck. The lateral femoral circumflex artery supplies the bulk of the quadriceps muscles. It passes horizontally around the anterior femur at the level of the lesser trochanter. Its branches supply the greater trochanter and perforate the anterior, superior edge of the greater trochanter to supply the anterior neck (X-6B).

## Anterior Approach to the Hip (Smith-Petersen)

*Applications*

The anterior approach to the hip utilizes the interval between the sartorius and the tensor fascia lata. Surgical applications include open reduction of congenital dis-

*(continued on page 244)*

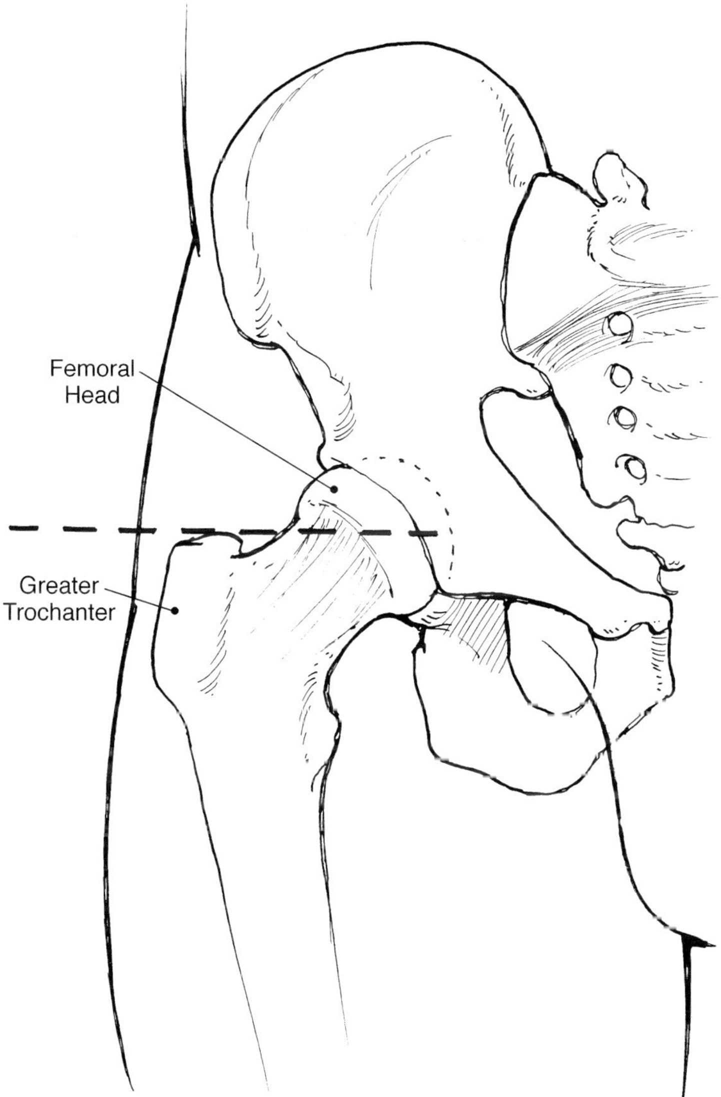


**FIGURE X-1**

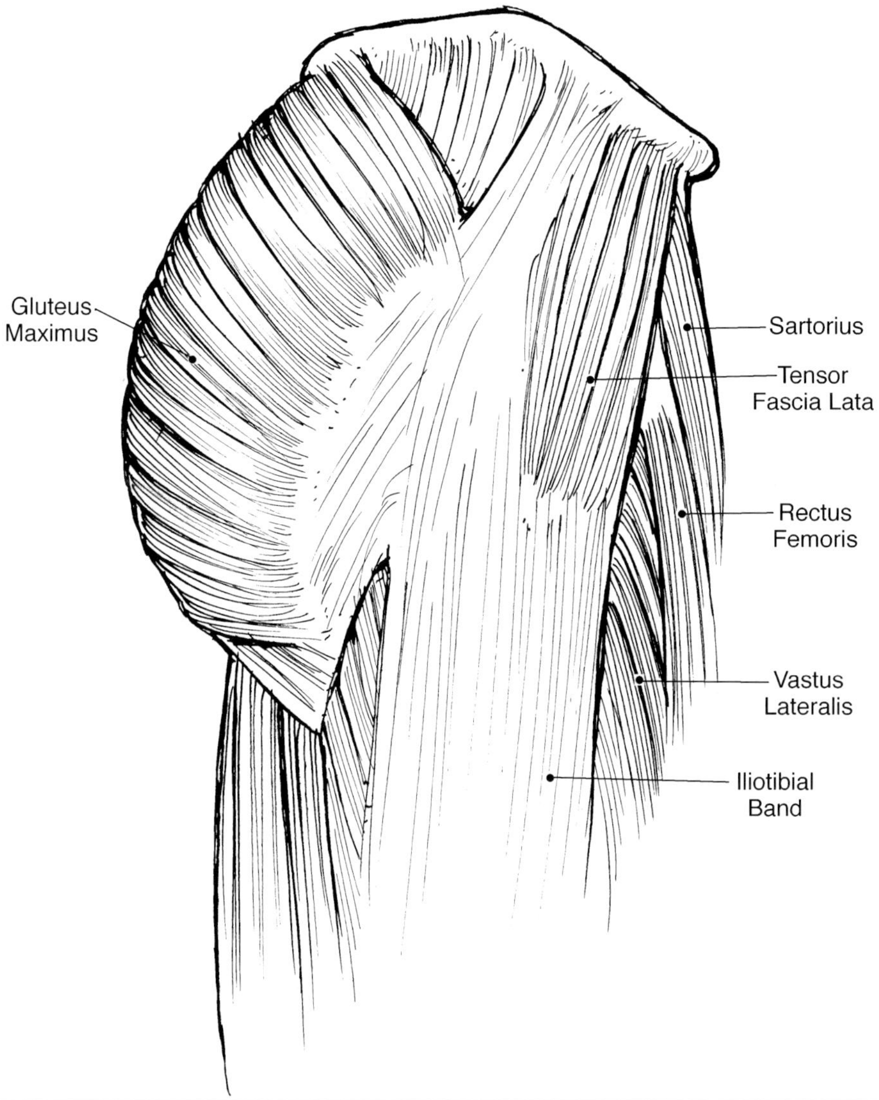
Gluteus Maximus
Sartorius
Tensor Fascia Lata
Rectus Femoris
Vastus Lateralis
Iliotibial Band

**FIGURE X-2**

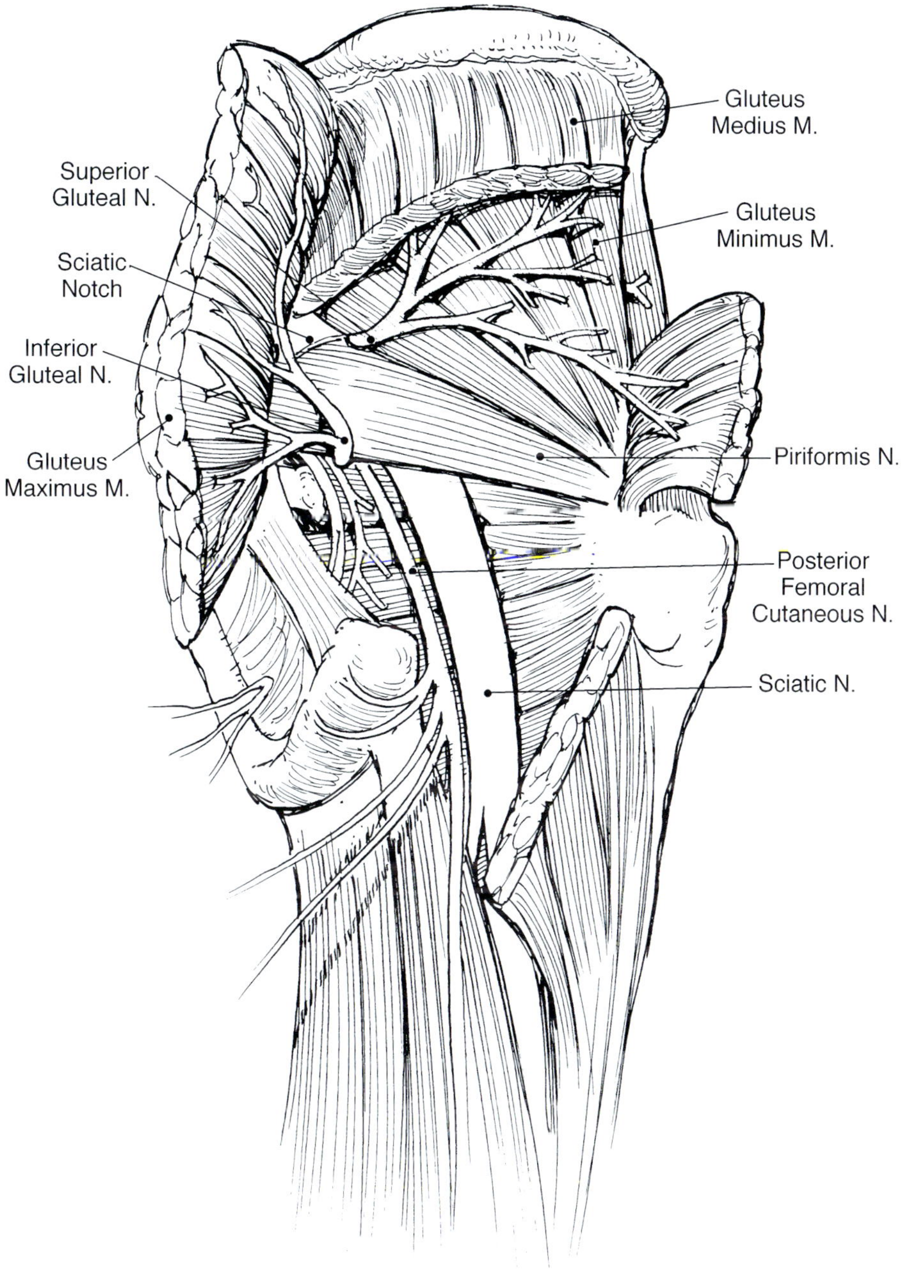
Gluteus
Medius M.
Superior
Gluteal N.
Gluteus
Minimus M.
Sciatic
Notch
Inferior
Gluteal N.
Gluteus
Maximus M.
Piriformis N.
Posterior
Femoral
Cutaneous N.
Sciatic N.

**FIGURE X-3**

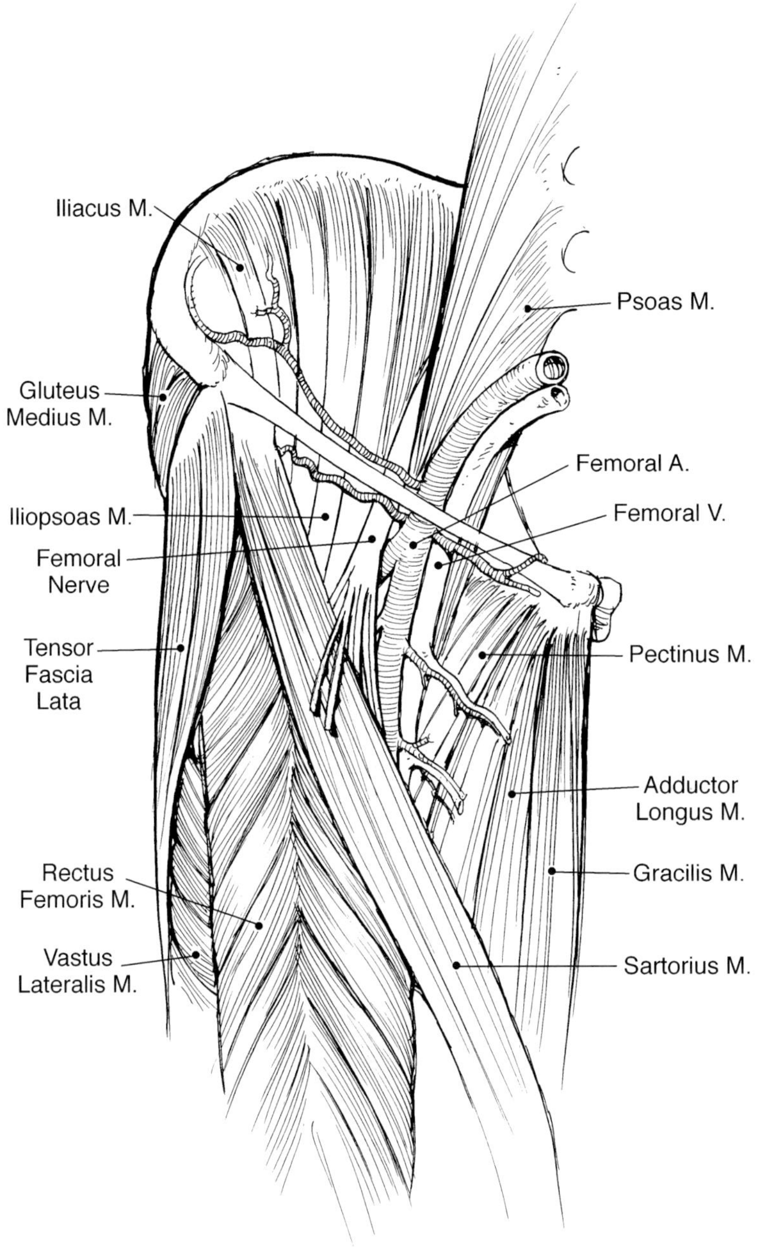
Iliacus M.
Psoas M.
Gluteus Medius M.
Femoral A.
Femoral V.
Iliopsoas M.
Femoral Nerve
Tensor Fascia Lata
Pectinus M.
Adductor Longus M.
Gracilis M.
Rectus Femoris M.
Vastus Lateralis M.
Sartorius M.

**FIGURE X-4**

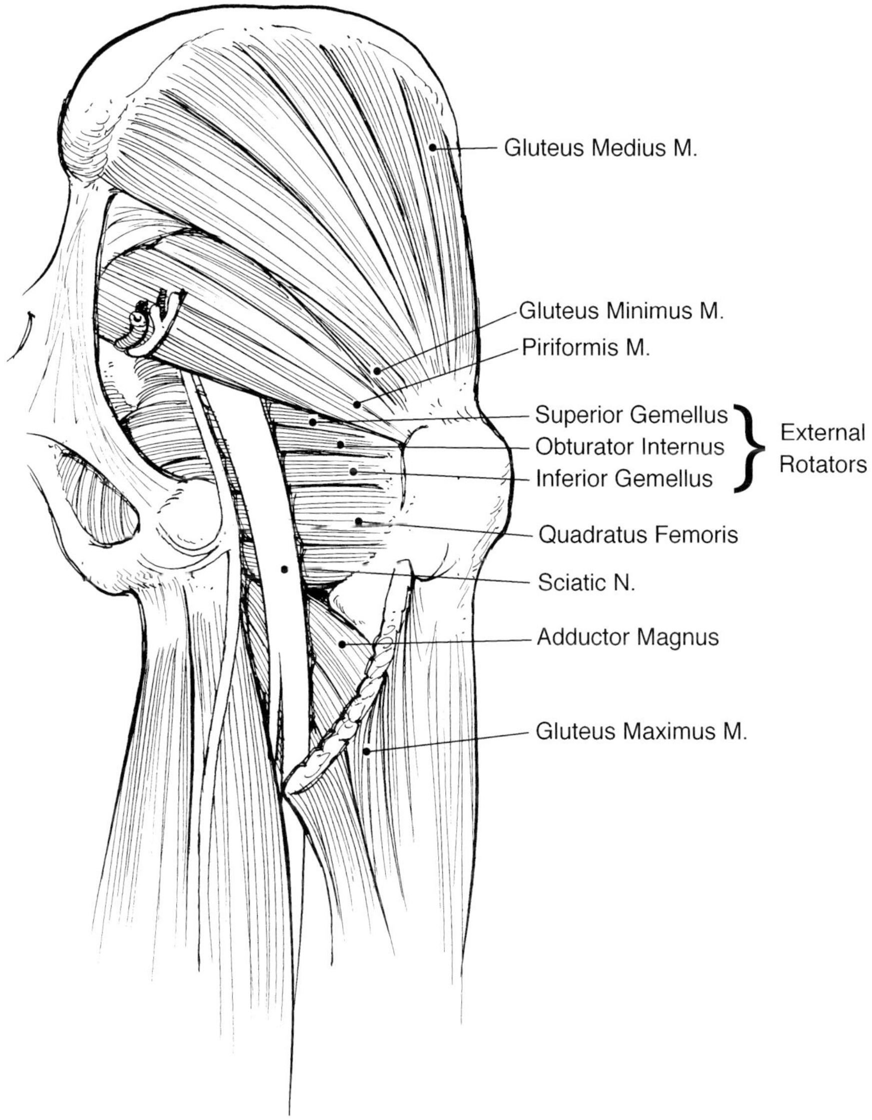
Gluteus Medius M.
Gluteus Minimus M.
Piriformis M.
Superior Gemellus
Obturator Internus
Inferior Gemellus
External Rotators
Quadratus Femoris
Sciatic N.
Adductor Magnus
Gluteus Maximus M.

**FIGURE X-5**

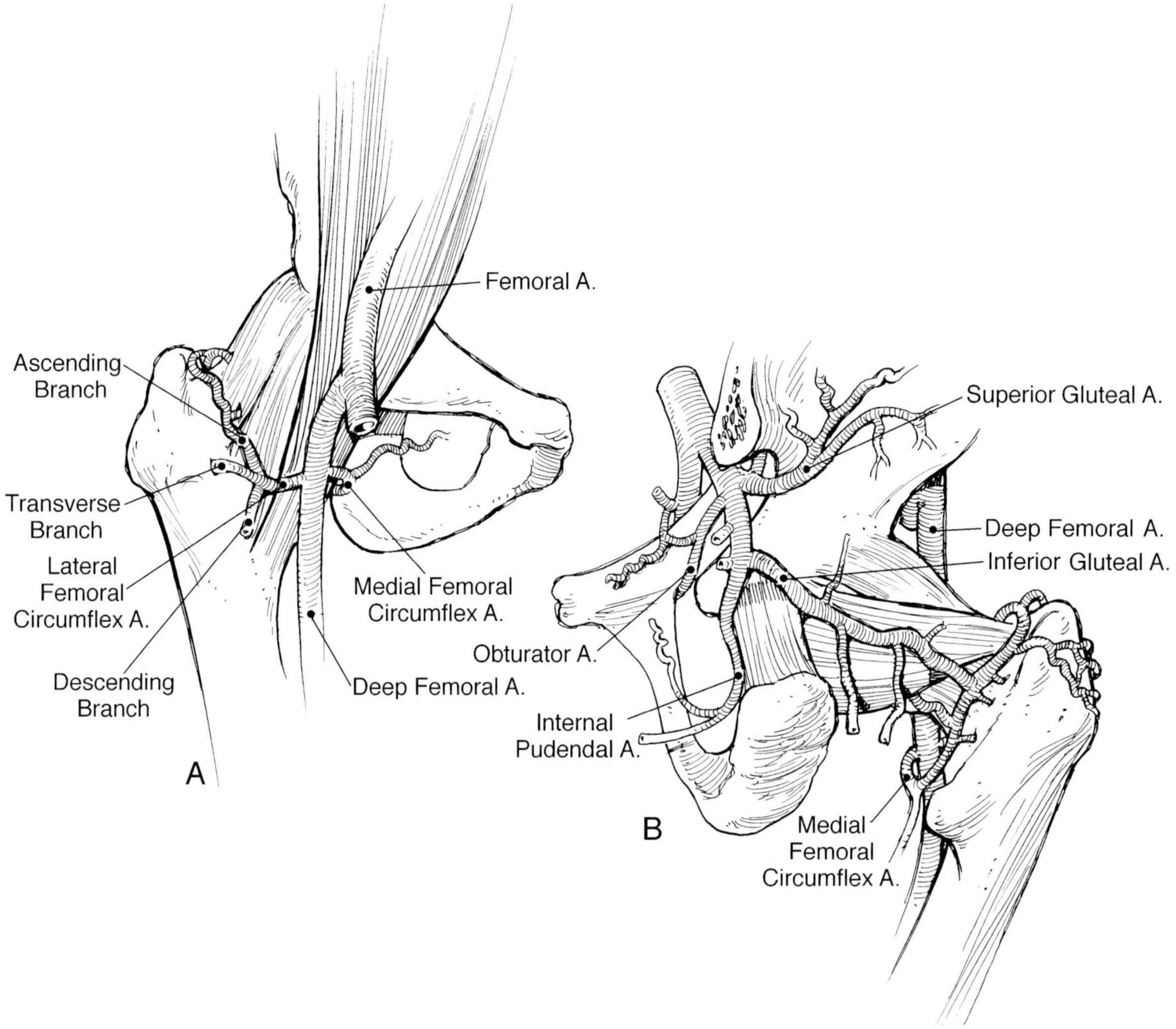


**FIGURE X-6A & B**

location, drainage of a septic joint, synovial biopsy, intraarticular hip fusion, hemiarthroplasty, and total hip arthroplasty (1). The femoral head must be dislocated anteriorly in this approach. A key advantage of this approach is that it avoids disruption of the abductor mechanism.

### *Technique*

The patient is placed supine on the operating table with a sandbag under the ipsilateral buttock to push the pelvis forward. This position can become uncomfortable for patients undergoing regional anesthesia. Alternatively, a well-molded beanbag placing the pelvis in the same forward tilted position provides more comfortable support.

Suggested incisions for the anterior approach are among the most varied about the hip. One of the more utilitarian incisions, originally described by Smith-Petersen, consists of a curvilinear incision following the anterior half of the iliac crest toward the anterior superior iliac spine (ASIS), then curving distally and longitudinally for another 10 cm toward the lateral edge of the patella (X-7). This inci-

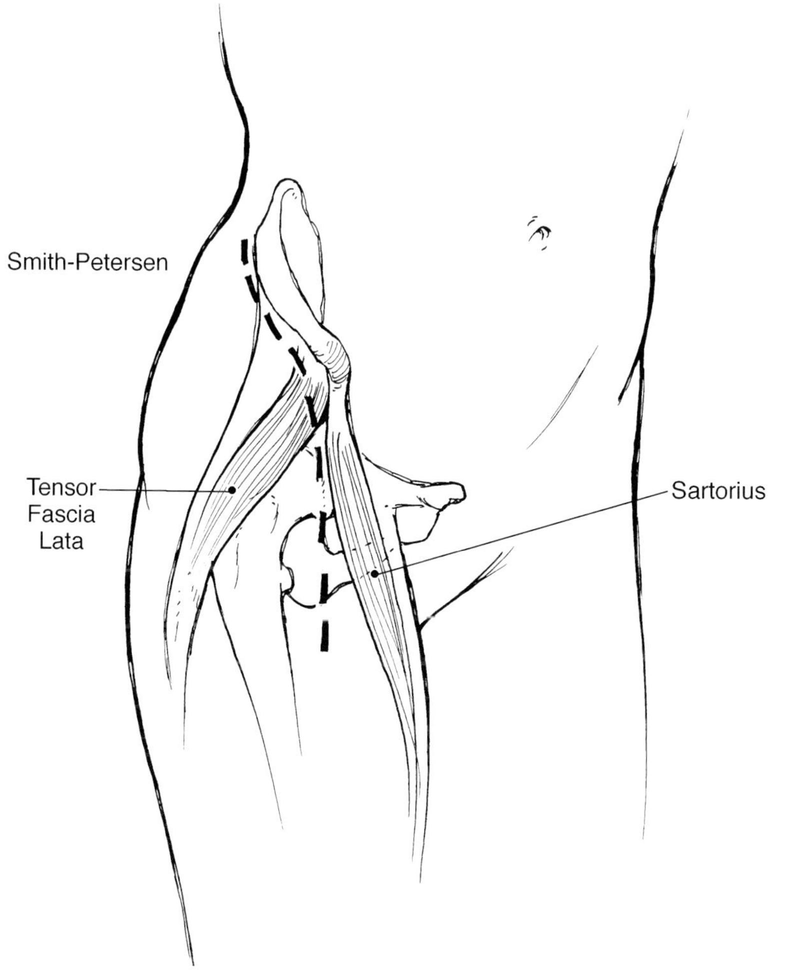


**FIGURE X-7**

sion offers an extensile approach to the anterior hip that can be extended both proximally and distally.

The hip is externally rotated to place tension on the sartorius to demonstrate the interval between the sartorius and the tensor fascia lata. This interval is best found 5 to 8 cm distal to the ASIS and along the line joining the ASIS and the lateral aspect of the patella. The lateral femoral cutaneous branch of the femoral nerve pierces the fascia at this level close to the intermuscular interval (X-8). The nerve is mobilized and retracted medially to avoid injury. Incising the deep fascia allows the sartorius to be retracted proximally and medially while the tensor is retracted laterally and distally (X-9). The origin of the tensor fascia lata along the iliac wing can be elevated subperiosteally to increase the exposure of the proximal femur.

The direct head of the rectus femoris arises from the ASIS and covers the anterior hip capsule. The reflected head originates from the superior rim of the acetabulum and anterior capsule. The space overlying the rectus femoris is largely filled with the belly of the iliopsoas (X-10). With the hip flexed and externally rotated, the psoas can be retracted to visualize the rectus femoris and hip. Access to the anterior rim of the acetabulum requires reflection of the rectus femoris from its origin (X-11). The ascending branch of the lateral femoral circumflex artery lies

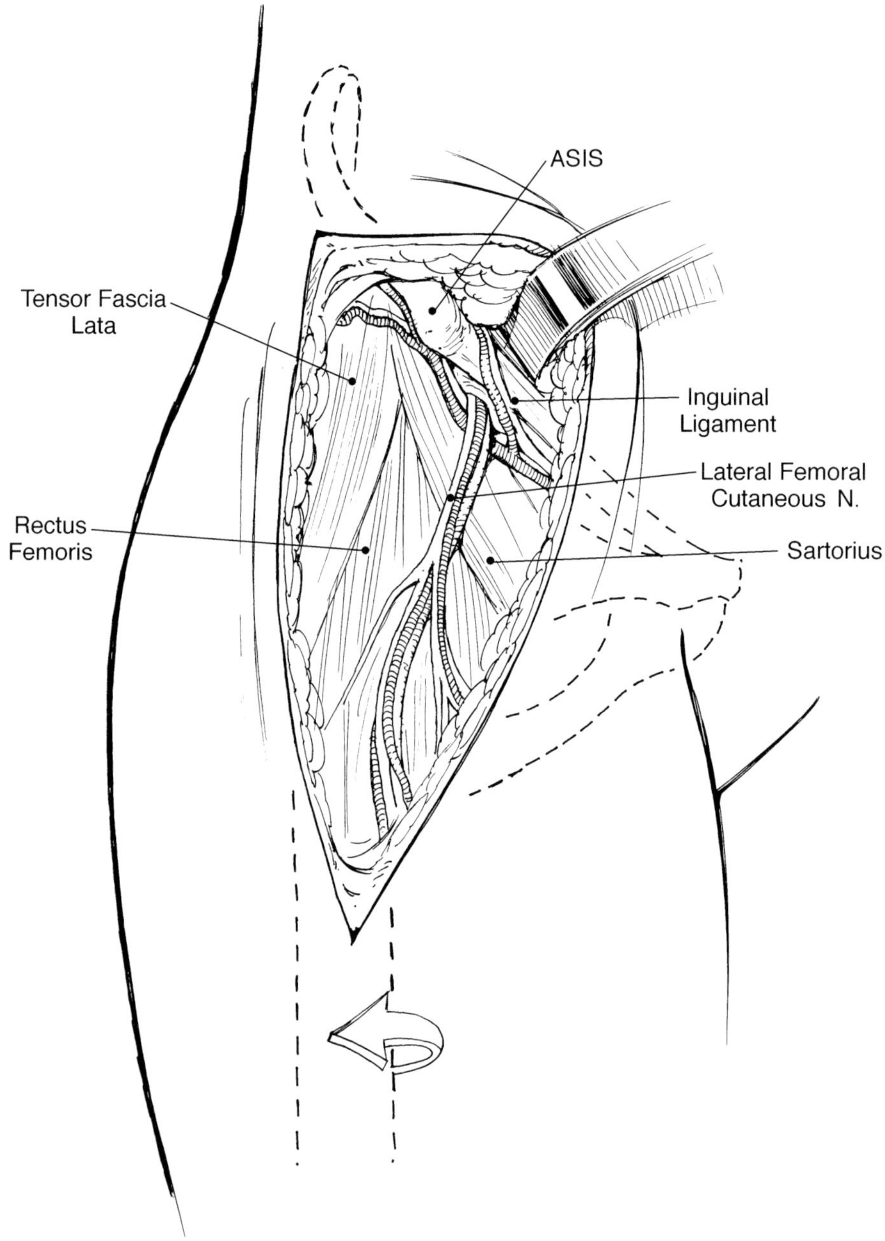
ASIS
Tensor Fascia Lata
Inguinal Ligament
Lateral Femoral Cutaneous N.
Rectus Femoris
Sartorius

**FIGURE X-8**

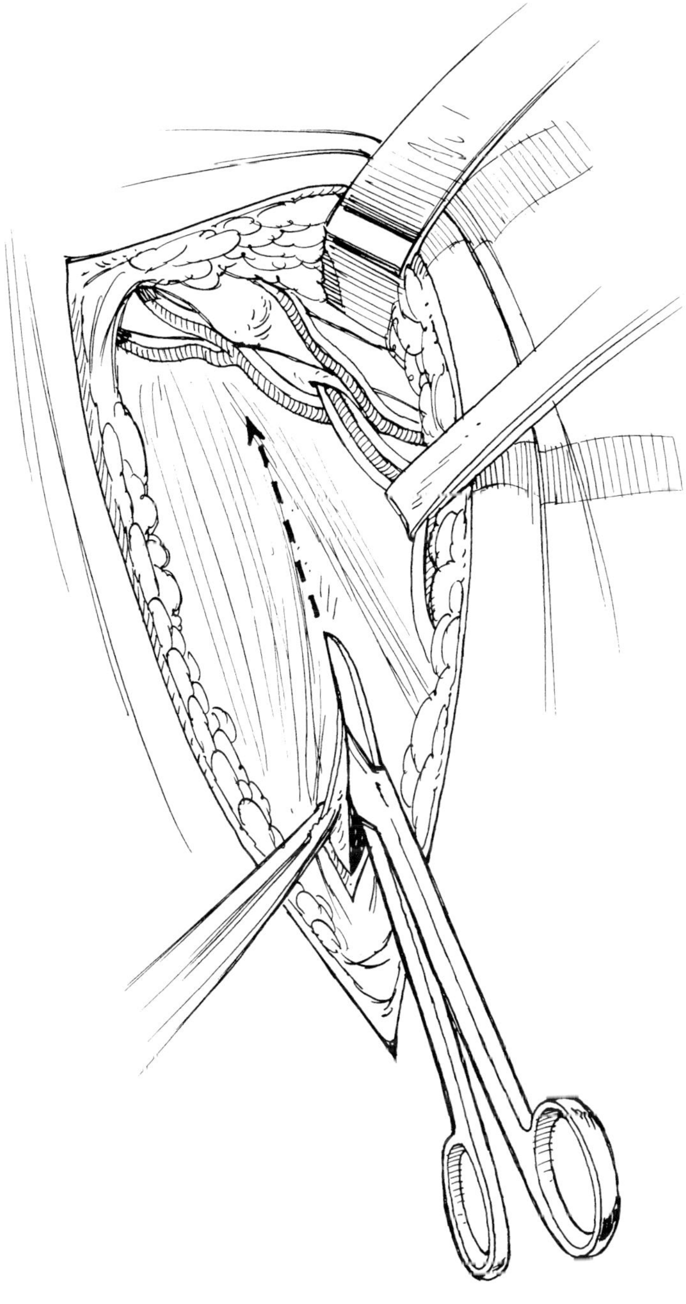

**FIGURE X-9**

anterior to the rectus, between the tensor and the sartorius at the level of the distal edge of the lesser trochanter. The gluteus medius is retracted laterally and the iliopsoas is retracted medially to visualize the anterior hip capsule (X-12).

A T-shaped incision can be made in the anterior capsule with the head of the T overlying the anterior rim of the acetabulum. Further external rotation of the hip dislocates the femoral head anteriorly (X-13).

***Dangers***

The lateral femoral cutaneous nerve can be injured in the initial dissection or by retraction. Mobilizing the tensor fascia lata from the ileum may avoid damage to the nerve. The femoral nerve overlies the hip joint but is medial to the rectus. The nerve should be safe unless one strays out of the plane of dissection. The femoral artery lies medial to the nerve; therefore, palpating the artery aids in orienting the surgeon to the proper plane of dissection.

***Limitations***

This approach provides a limited view of the anterior acetabulum and the femoral head and neck. Distal extension for access to the proximal femur requires ligation of the lateral femoral circumflex artery, which may compromise the blood supply to the proximal femur. Extension of this dissection superiorly by reflection of the hip abductors creates the risk of abductor weakness and limp and of heterotopic

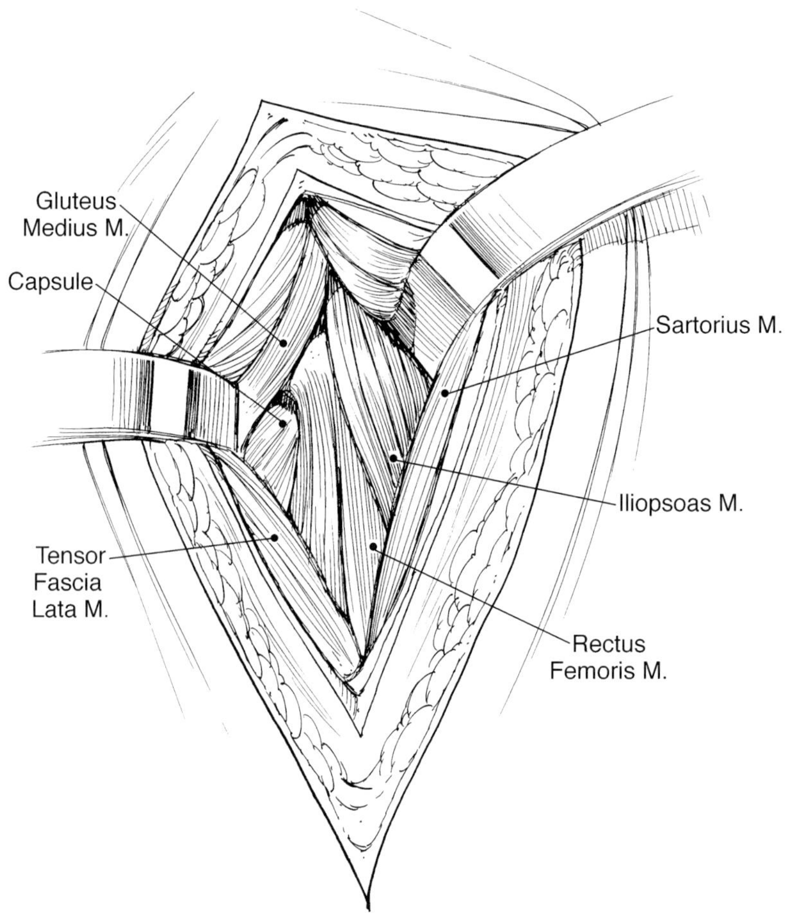


**FIGURE X-10**

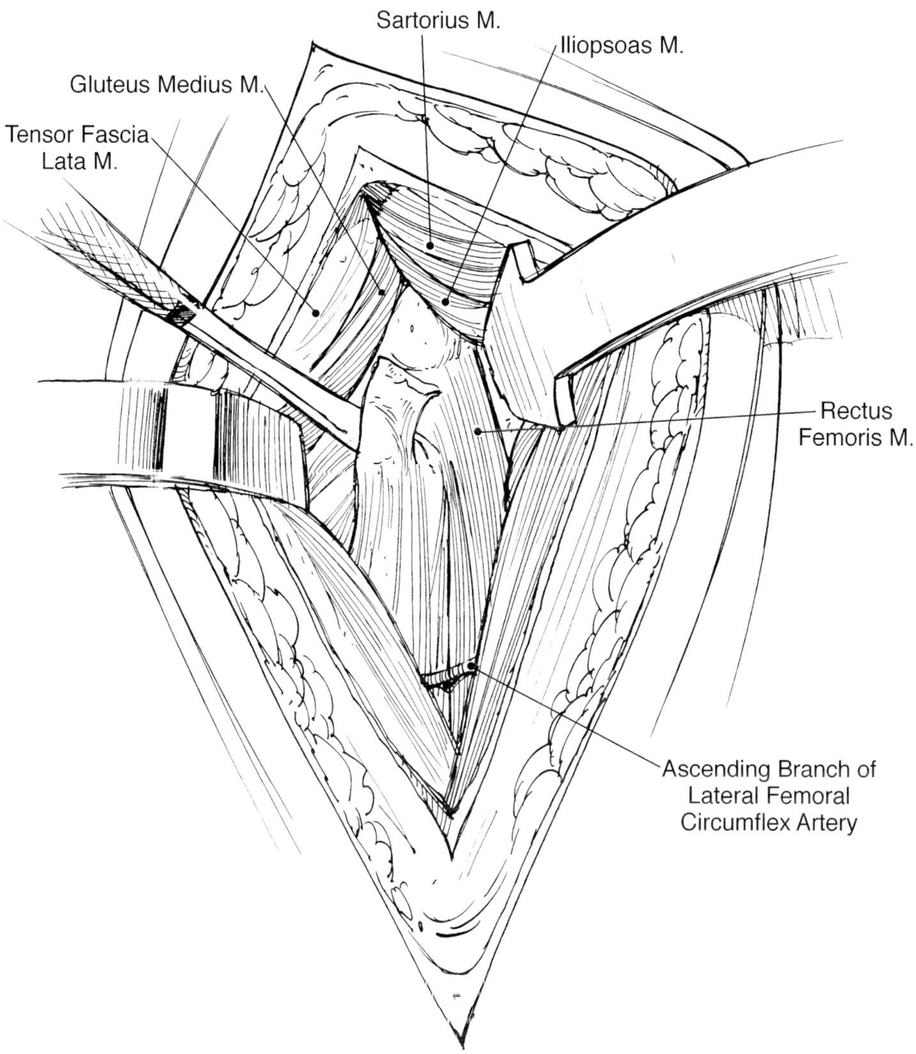
Sartorius M.
Iliopsoas M.
Gluteus Medius M.
Tensor Fascia Lata M.
Rectus Femoris M.
Ascending Branch of Lateral Femoral Circumflex Artery

**FIGURE X-11**

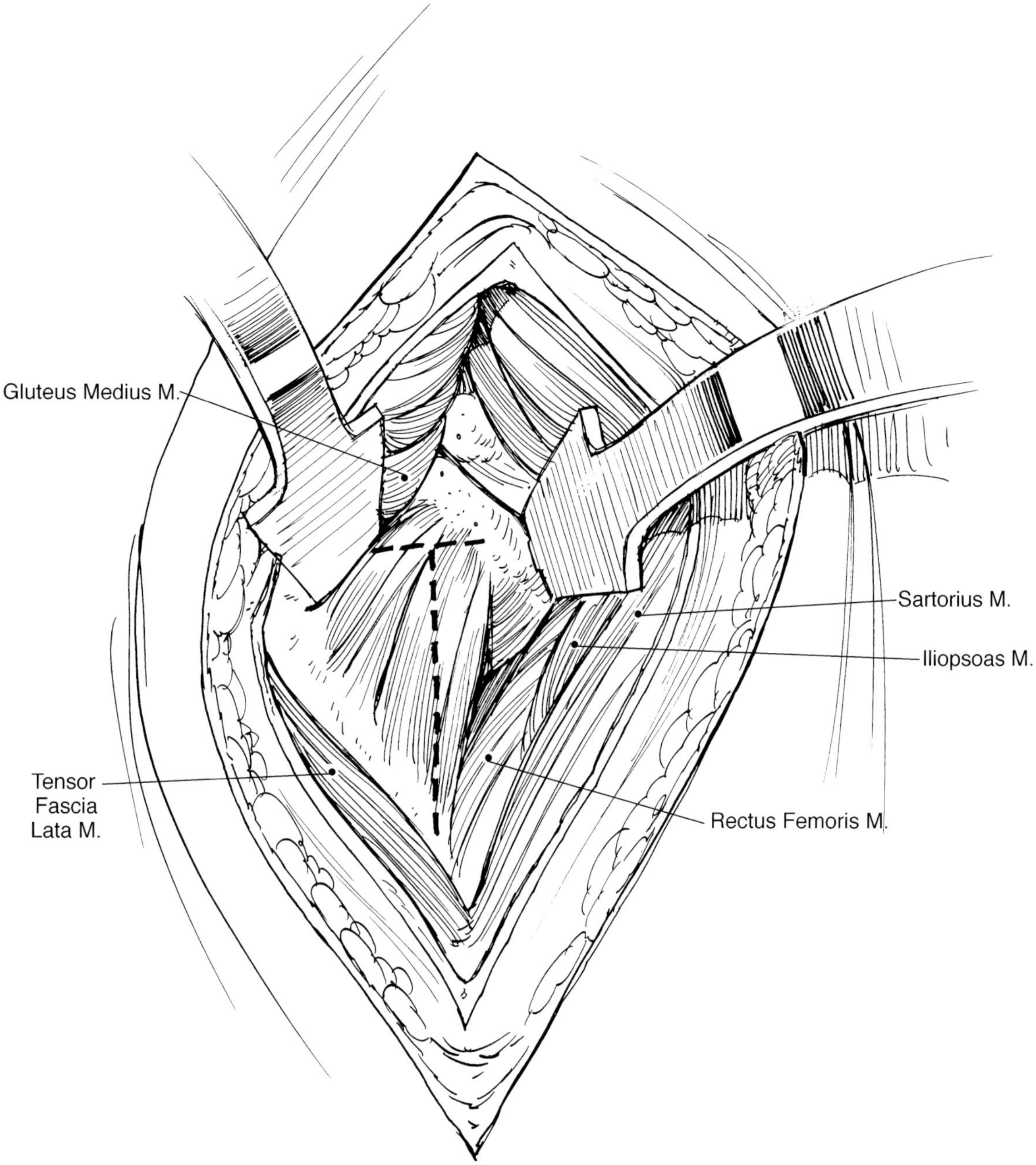
Gluteus Medius M.
Sartorius M.
Iliopsoas M.
Tensor Fascia Lata M.
Rectus Femoris M.

**FIGURE X-12**

ossification. The proximity of this dissection to the femoral neurovascular bundle makes it a poor choice for biopsy of a potentially malignant tumor of the hip joint.

## Anterolateral Approach to the Hip

***Applications***

The anterolateral approach is through the interval between the gluteus medius and the tensor fascia lata. This is not an internervous plane since both muscles are supplied by the superior gluteal nerve. It may be used for hip replacement, biopsy of the joint or femoral neck, and open reduction and internal fixation of fractures.

***Technique***

Either the supine or lateral decubitus position may be used for the anterolateral approach. For the supine technique, a sandbag is placed under the ischial tuberosity with the patient at the edge of the operating table so the affected buttock extends over the side. For the lateral decubitus position, the pelvis is rigidly supported and perpendicular to the table.

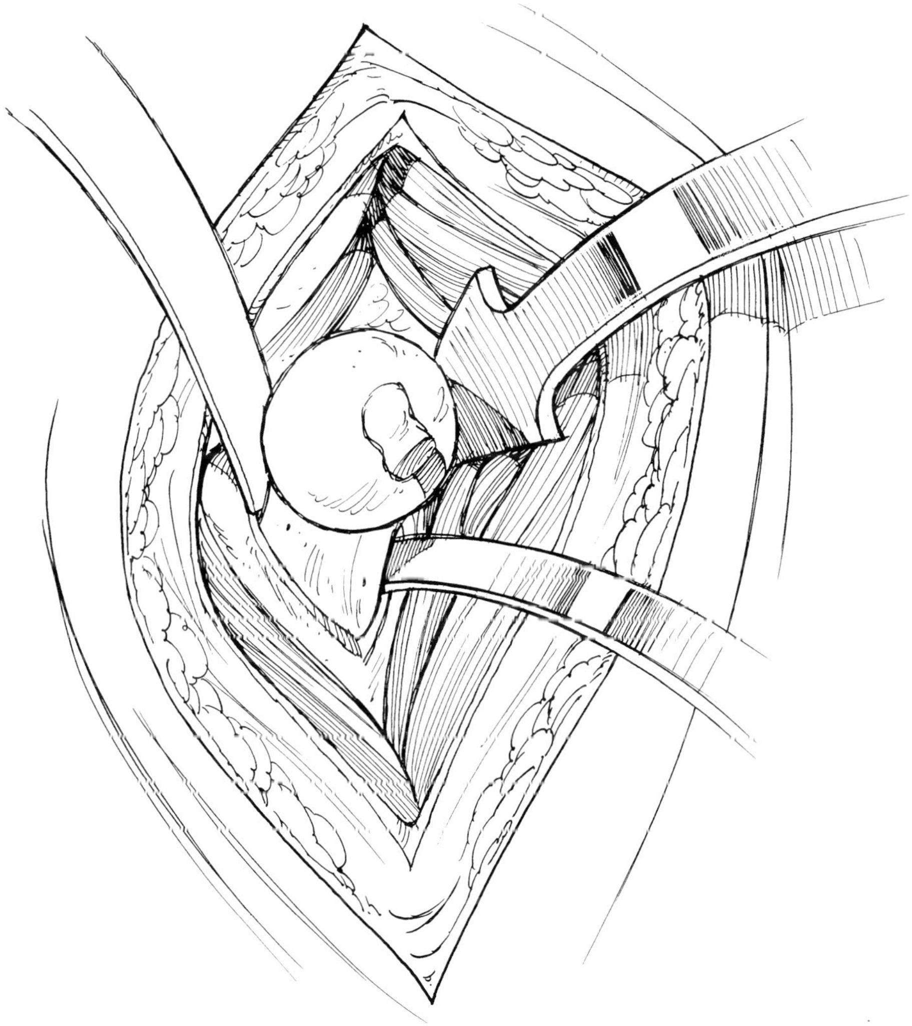

**FIGURE X-13**

The incision is centered directly over the midportion of the greater trochanter and directed distally along the line of the femoral shaft. Proximal to the greater trochanter, the incision is extended either in line with any previous incision or curved posteriorly. A posterior curve allows easier access to the medullary canal of the femur (X-14).

The iliotibial band is divided distally in line with the skin incision and proximally in the interval between the tensor fascia lata and the gluteus medius (X-15). Incising the fascia lata too far anteriorly will expose the muscle belly of the tensor fascia lata and make it difficult to develop a proper plane of dissection. This also makes exposure of the hip difficult because of the tension of the iliotibial band. The trochanteric bursa is excised to expose the greater trochanter and the insertion of the gluteus medius. The iliotibial band and the tensor fascia lata are retracted anteriorly and the gluteus maximus and the posterior iliotibial band are retracted posteriorly (X-16).

There are numerous modifications of the deep dissection for approach to the hip joint. The approach described by Watson-Jones (2) is anterior to the gluteus medius. The gluteus medius belly is retracted posteriorly. With the hip in a moderately flexed and externally rotated position, the anterior femoral neck and hip capsule can be palpated. The origin of the vastus lateralis and the fibers of the

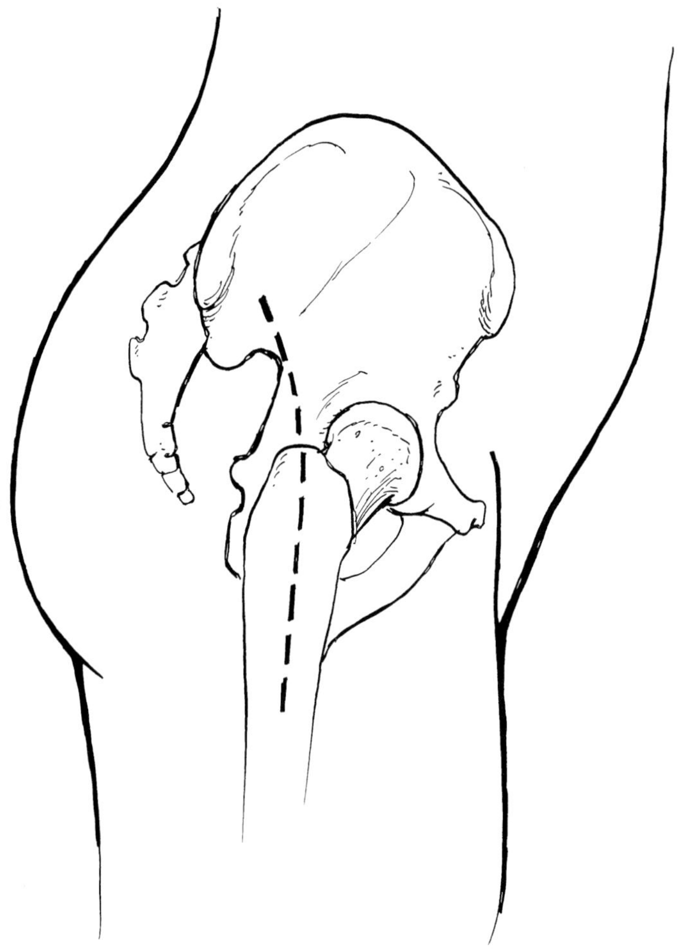

**FIGURE X-14**

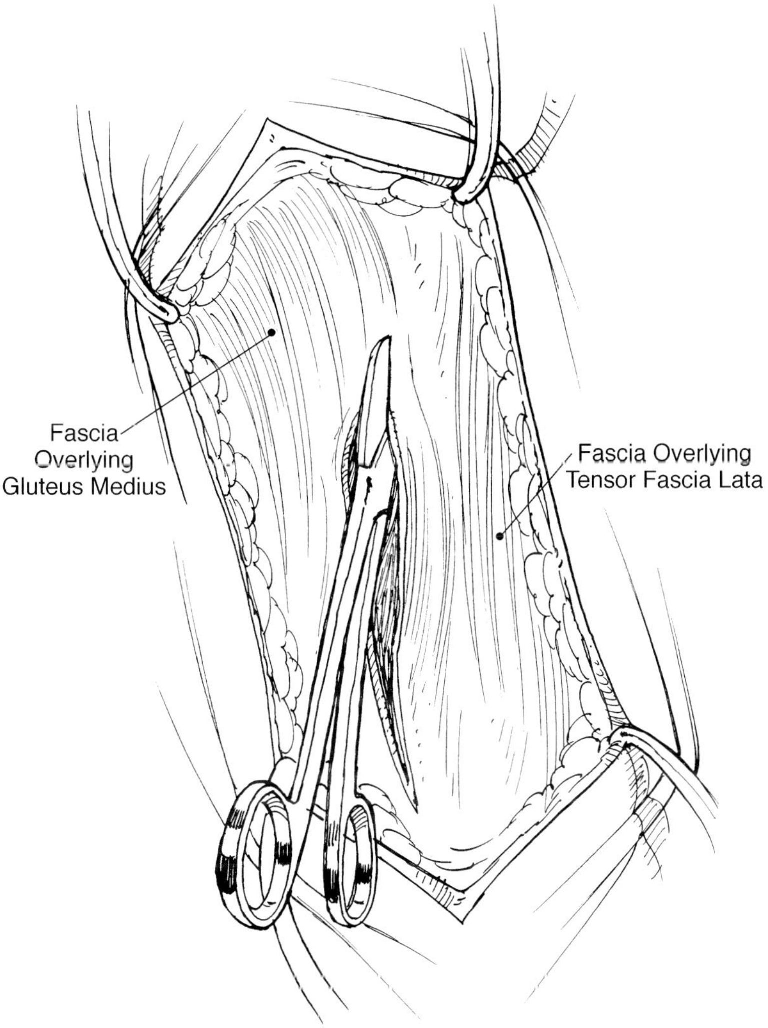
Fascia
Overlying
Gluteus Medius
Fascia Overlying
Tensor Fascia Lata

**FIGURE X-15**

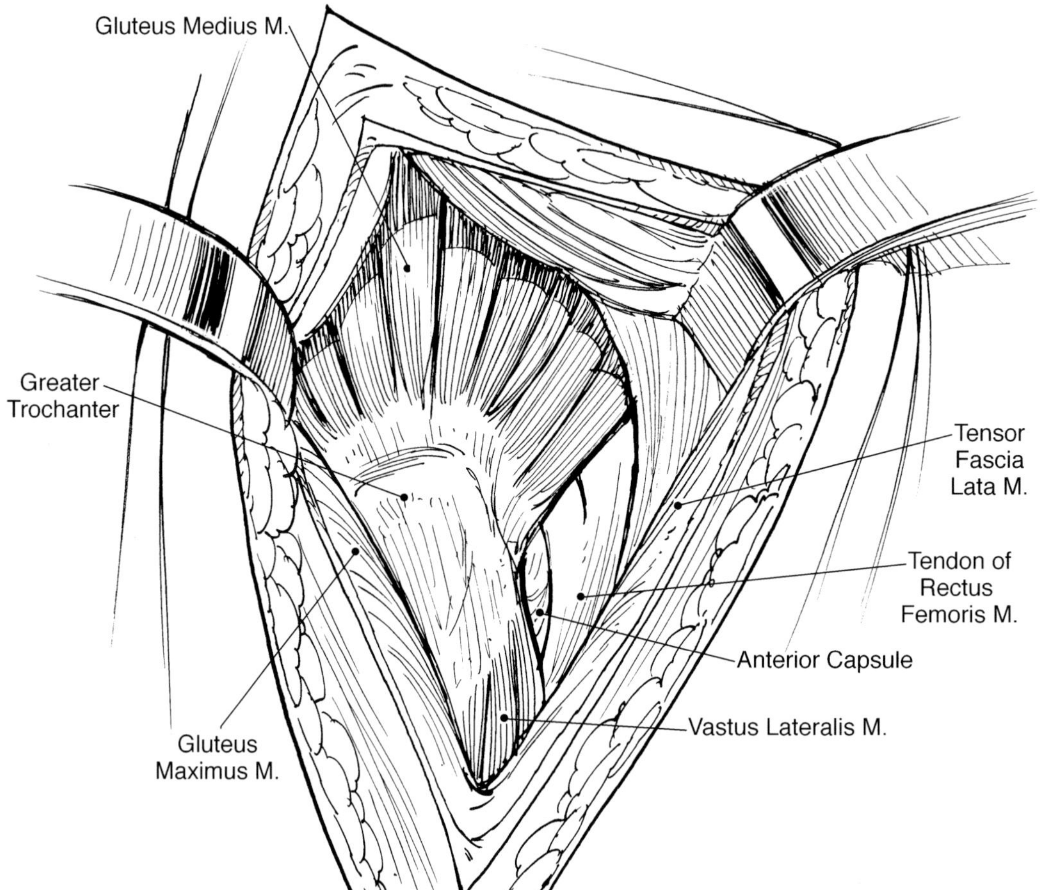
Gluteus Medius M.
Greater Trochanter
Tensor Fascia Lata M.
Tendon of Rectus Femoris M.
Anterior Capsule
Vastus Lateralis M.
Gluteus Maximus M.

**FIGURE X-16**

reflected head of the rectus femoris can be elevated from the anterior proximal femur and hip capsule. Doing so allows access to the femur neck, anterior hip joint, and intertrochanteric femur with minimal disruption of the blood supply to the femoral head (X-17). This approach is also well isolated from the major neurovascular bundles which makes it ideal for biopsy of tumors. It gives adequate exposure for removal of benign tumors of the femoral head, neck, or intertrochanteric region. This approach is limited by the inability to visualize the entire acetabulum if the hip is dislocated because of the broad expanse of the gluteus medius.

Hardinge (3) described a "direct lateral" approach with detachment of the anterior half of the gluteus medius from the greater trochanter by transection and proximal retraction of the tendon. To minimize the abductor weakness associated with transection of the abductor tendons, the anterior half of the gluteus medius, the tendon of the gluteus minimus, and the origin of the vastus lateralis can be reflected from the greater trochanter by subperiosteal dissection from posterior to anterior (4). This creates a longitudinally-oriented muscle flap which allows wide exposure of the hip joint (X-18A and X-18B). The repair is accomplished by placing the muscles back in their anatomic positions and suturing them to the bone through drill holes in the trochanter or to the remaining tendon and muscle. This concept has been further modified by reflection of the tendon of the anterior half

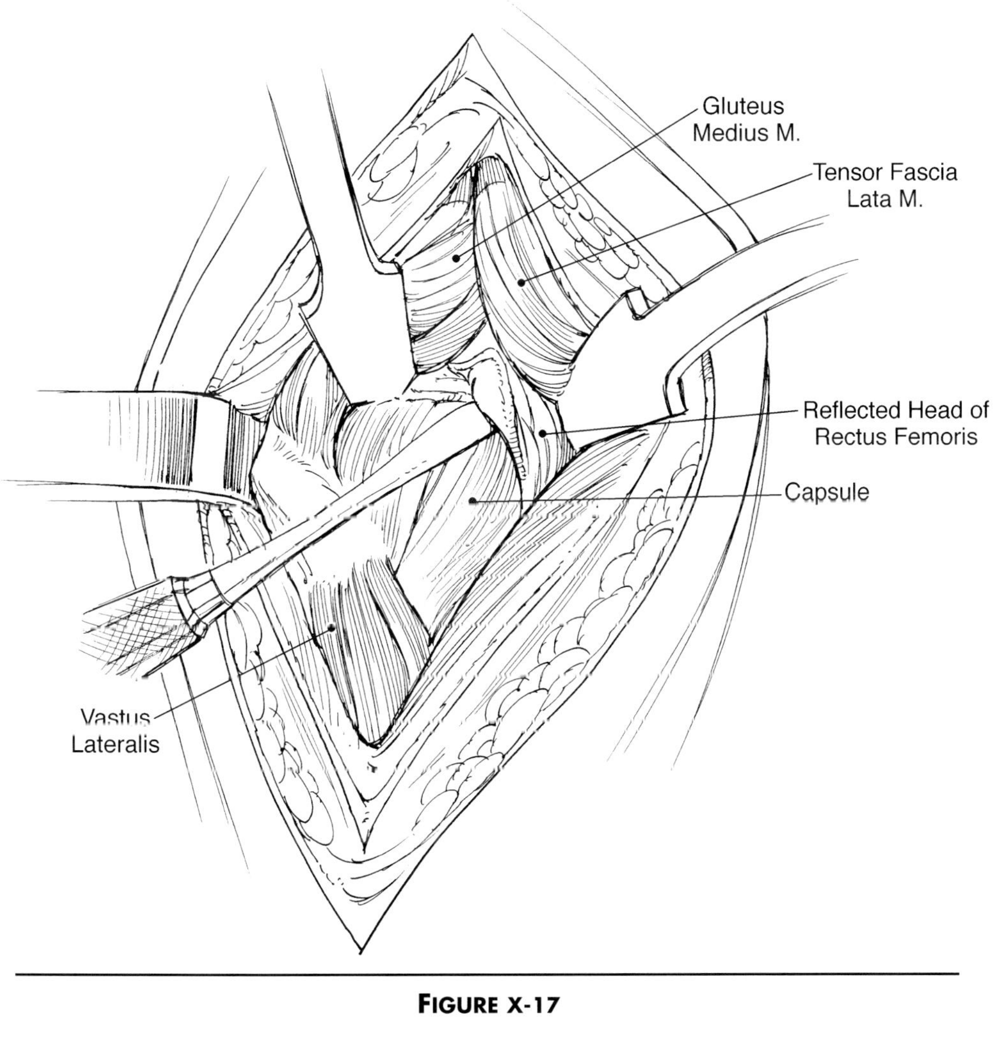


**FIGURE X-17**

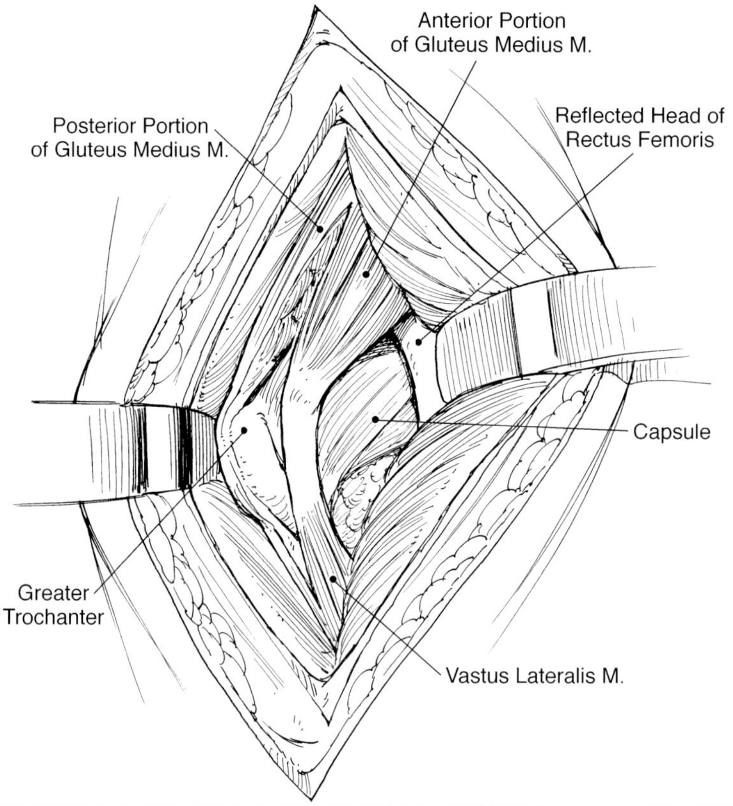


**FIGURE X-18A**

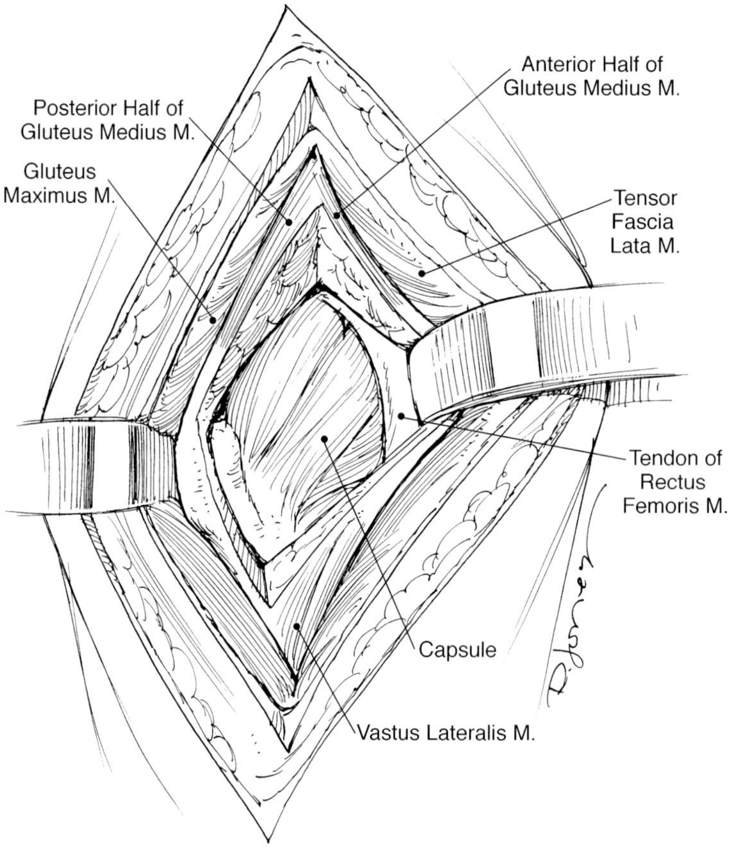


**FIGURE X-18B**

of the gluteus medius anteriorly and deepening the exposure with an osteotomy of the anterior rim of the greater trochanter (5). These modifications allow mobilization of the intact gluteus minimus which inserts on the bone block (X-19). The entire myo-osseous flap can then be retracted forward to expose the hip. This exposure can be extended distally by splitting the fibers of the vastus lateralis in line with the flap of the greater trochanter, allowing direct exposure of the proximal femur and hip. This flap can be reflected as far anteriorly and medially as the lesser trochanter, providing easy access to the acetabulum and proximal femur for proximal femur osteotomies or complex joint replacement. This flap is closed by anchoring the reflected bone block with attached tendons to the femur by nonabsorbable sutures passed through the bone.

***Dangers***

The major criticism of this approach is the potential for weakening of the hip abductors and creating a limp. Careful repair of the detached hip abductors is essential. Sciatic nerve palsy is a concern when the hip is dislocated anteriorly. Posterior retraction must avoid excessive traction on the nerve. When the limb is externally rotated and the hip is dislocated anteriorly, the entire extremity is being suspended by the posterior soft tissues. Therefore, the weight of the limb should be supported throughout the procedure to prevent prolonged traction on the nerve.

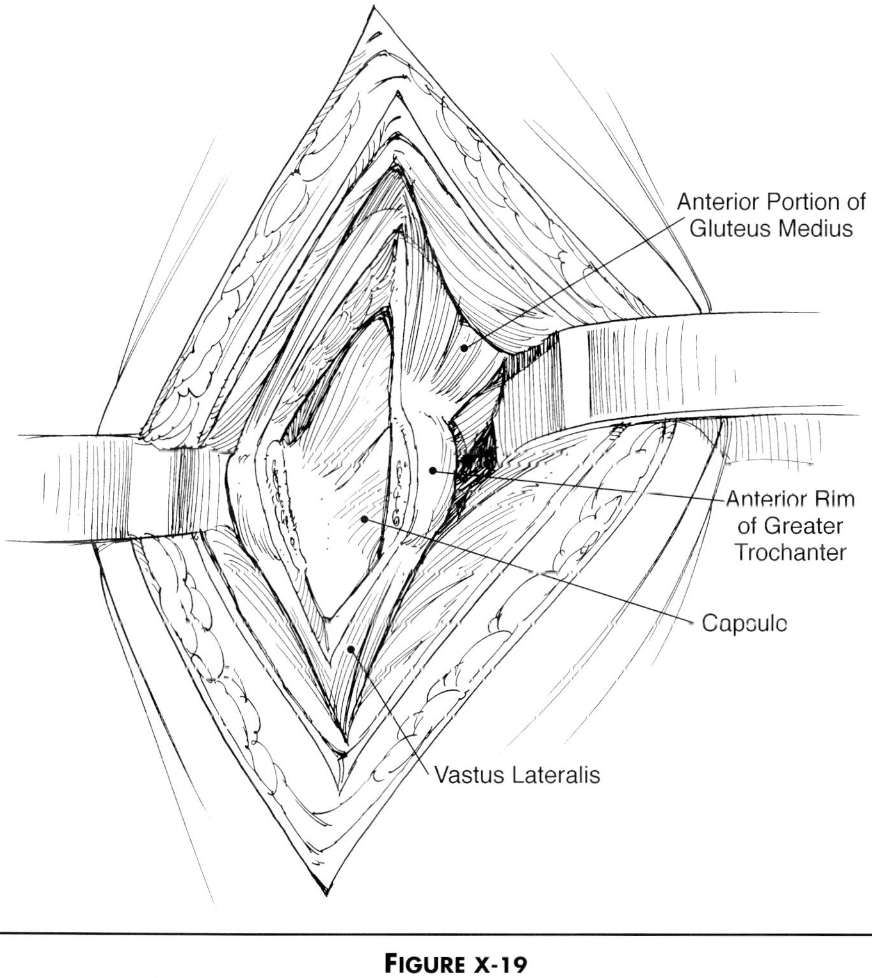


**FIGURE X-19**

*Limitations*

This approach can provide wide exposure to the acetabulum and proximal femur as necessary for revision total hip arthroplasty or proximal femoral replacement. It does not provide complete exposure of the posterior column of the pelvis or of the superior pubic ramus.

## Lateral (Transtrochanteric) Approach to the Hip

*Applications*

The lateral approach displaces the hip abductor mechanism by either transecting the tendons of the gluteus medius and minimus or by trochanteric osteotomy. The displacement provides direct access to the entire acetabulum and proximal femur. This exposure is ideal for open reduction and internal fixation of complex acetabular fractures that require dislocation of the femoral head to reconstruct the acetabulum. It is also useful for revision total hip arthroplasty, especially for complex acetabular reconstructions, and reconstruction of the acetabulum and proximal femur destroyed by tumor. This approach can be used in conjunction with the extensile ilioinguinal approach to the pelvis if access to the inner wall of the acetabulum is needed.

*Technique*

The patient is placed in the lateral decubitus position with the lower extremity draped free in the field. With the limb in the neutral position, the incision is centered over the greater trochanter and carried longitudinally from 8 cm distal to the trochanter to 8 cm proximal, curving the proximal portion posteriorly (X-20). The fascia lata is incised in line with the skin distally. The fibers of the gluteus maximus are split in line with the skin incision proximally. A retractor is then placed to spread the fascia for visualization of the greater trochanter and gluteus medius (X-21). The obturator internus and the gemelli are detached from their femoral insertion and retracted posteriorly. The upper half of the quadratus femoris is detached from the femur (X-22). A finger can then be placed anteriorly and posteriorly to palpate the medial edge of the greater trochanter. An incision is made through the vastus lateralis at the vastus ridge to expose the base of the greater trochanter. A 2-inch osteotome is used to detach the greater trochanter by cutting from distal to proximal, exiting at the base of the femoral neck (X-23). This allows the piriformis tendon to be retracted with the abductor mass. The greater trochanter with the attached tendons can then be retracted proximally to expose the superior rim of the acetabulum. Elevation of the fibers of the reflected head of the rectus femoris allows visualization of the entire anterior, superior, and posterior hip capsule (X-24). The capsule is incised along the superior surface from the acetabular rim to the top of the femoral neck. The femoral head is exposed and the capsule is reflected or excised as needed. The femoral head can then be lifted out of the acetabulum. If needed, the hip can be dislocated anteriorly or posteriorly. During closure, the greater trochanter is reattached using either lag screws or cerclage fixation.

There have been many modifications of this approach including the "trochanteric slide" (5) and the Stracathro approach (4), which provide more limited exposure but are designed to leave the muscle sleeve of the greater trochanter intact to decrease the risk of nonunion.

*Dangers*

For joint replacement, the detachment of the trochanter eliminates the tension of the abductor during the procedure. The surgeon must be careful to orient the prosthetic components in relation to the bony anatomy to prevent recurrent dislocation or excessive lengthening or shortening of the limb. Excessive lengthening is associated with an increased risk of sciatic nerve palsy. Nonunion of the greater trochanter has been reported to occur in approximately 7% of patients who have had joint replacement through this approach. Rigid fixation using screws, the Charnley wire technique (6), or cable clamp systems can minimize this risk.

*Limitations*

This approach can be extended proximally by elevating the origins of the gluteus medius and minimus from the iliac wing. This approach allows advancement of these muscles, if needed, for problems such as hip dysplasia. The gluteus maximus should not be split to the level of the posterior superior iliac spine as doing so will most likely damage the superior gluteal nerve, causing paralysis of the gluteus medius and minimus. The proximal femur can be exposed by circumferential elevation of the muscles, allowing complete excision of the proximal femur if needed.

## Posterior Approach to the Hip

*Applications*

The posterior approach is useful in a variety of situations including primary and revision total hip replacement or hemiarthroplasty, open reduction of posterior acetabular fractures and hip dislocations, and removal of loose bodies from the joint.

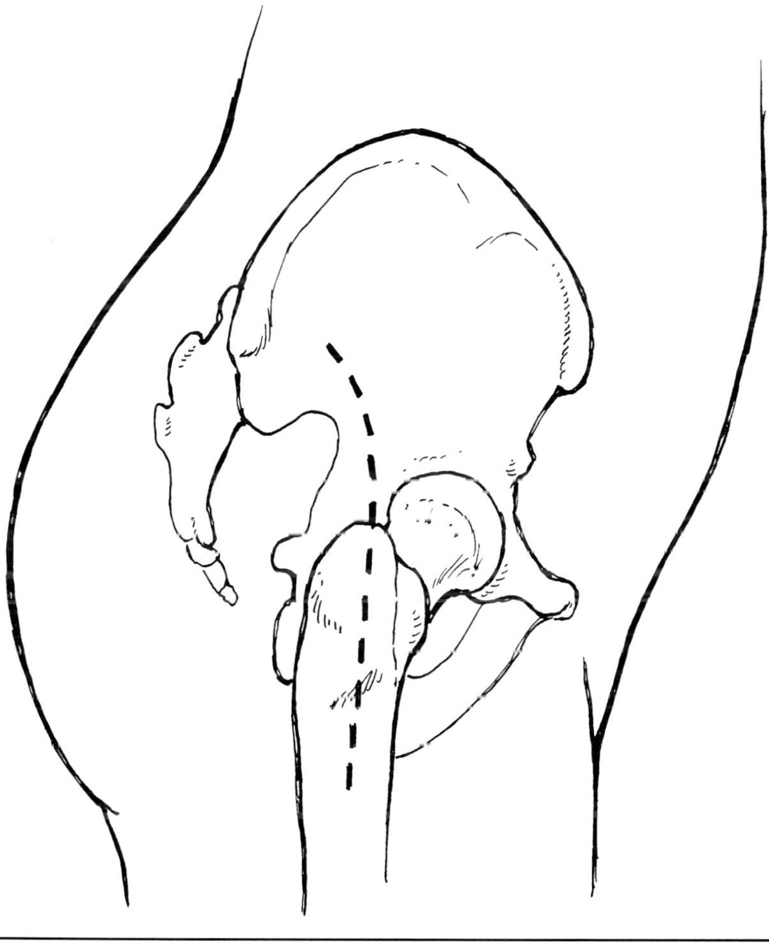

**FIGURE X-20**

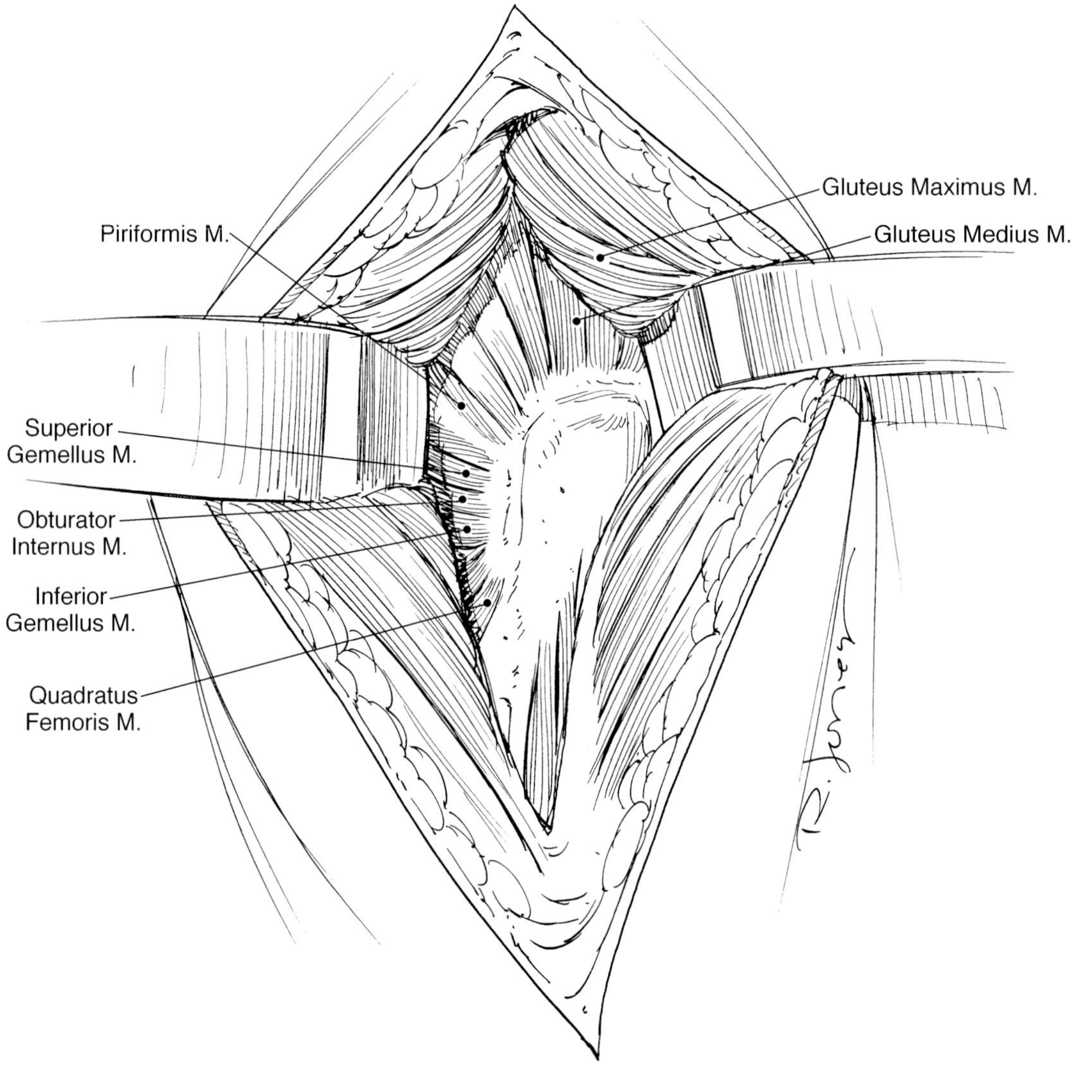
Gluteus Maximus M.
Gluteus Medius M.
Piriformis M.
Superior Gemellus M.
Obturator Internus M.
Inferior Gemellus M.
Quadratus Femoris M.

**FIGURE X-21**

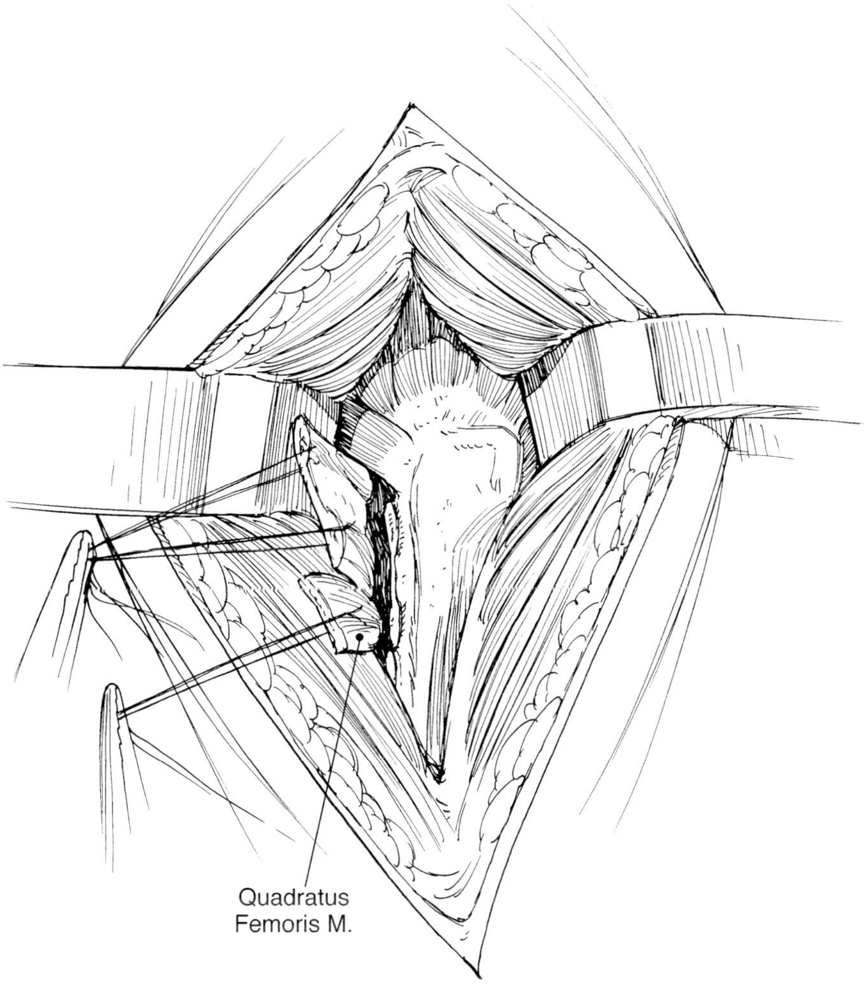


**FIGURE X-22**

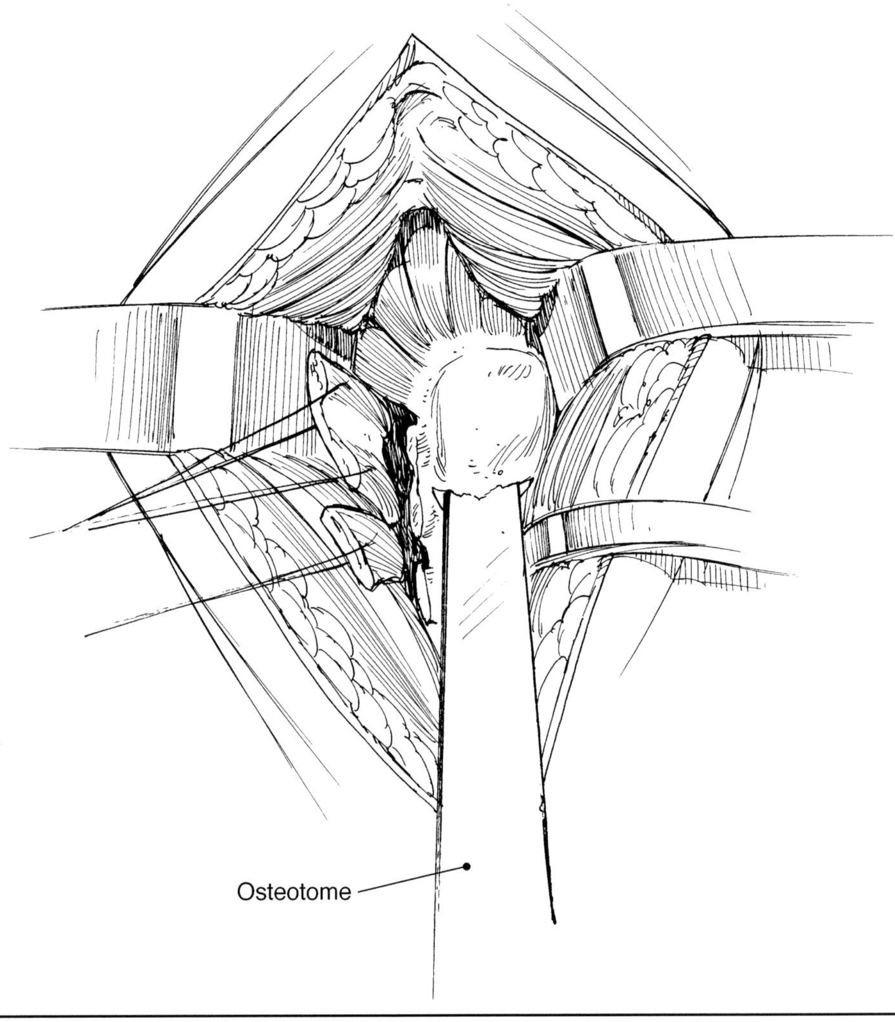


**FIGURE X-23**

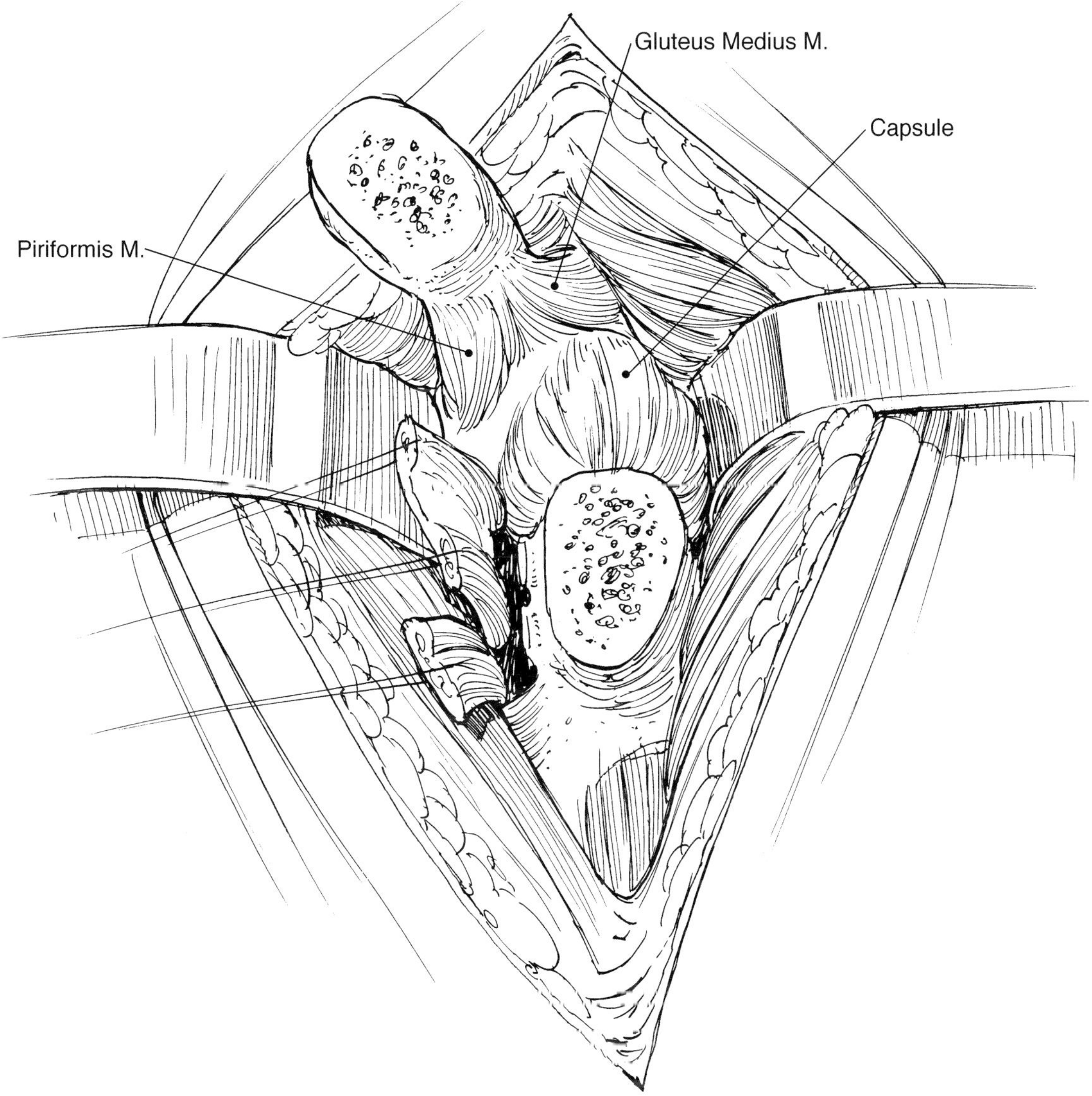


**FIGURE X-24**

### *Technique*

The patient is placed in the lateral decubitus position, supported either by a deflated bean bag or by pelvic supports attached to the table, or both. Problems with brachial plexopathy are avoided by placing an axillary roll one hand's breadth distal to the peak of the axilla and supporting the contralateral upper extremity with an airplane splint or securely stacked pillows. All bony prominences should be padded.

The incision is centered over the posterior half of the greater trochanter and extended distally along the shaft of the femur for 8 cm, curving posteriorly and proximally along the direction of the fibers of the gluteus maximus. Flexing the hip to 90° and marking a straight line along the femoral shaft, centered on the posterior half of the trochanter will also outline the incision (X-25).

The fascia lata is split in line with the skin incision distally. Palpating the greater trochanter and the proximal femur allows accurate placement of the blades of a pair of Mayo scissors to complete the split distally. Directing the incision posteriorly and proximally (the "dog leg" or "hockey stick") brings the line of dissection parallel with the fibers of the midportion of the gluteus maximus. The fibers of the

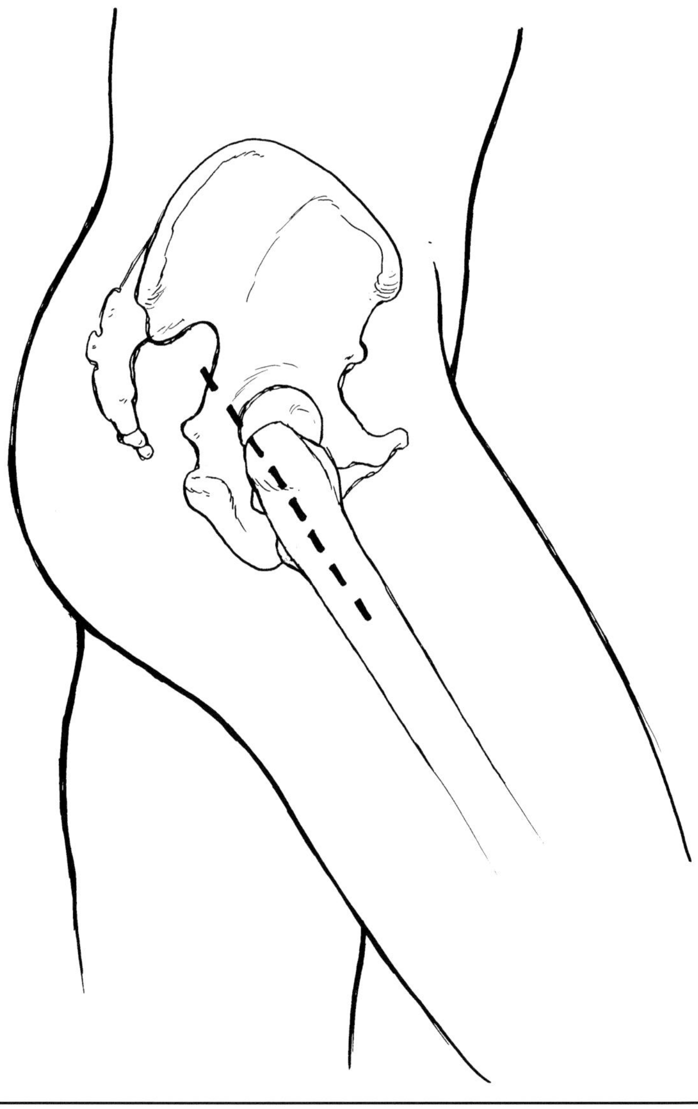

**FIGURE X-25**

gluteus maximus are split longitudinally with blunt dissection. Vessels are coagulated as they appear (X-26).

Internal rotation of the hip places the short external rotators on stretch. A blunt retractor placed between the capsule and the gluteus medius and minimus improves exposure of the short external rotators. They can either be divided en bloc or separately (X-27). Postoperative stability of the hip is enhanced if these muscles are reattached to the greater trochanter through drill holes. Tagging the tendons of these muscles, particularly the piriformis, at the time of initial dissection facilitates their identification and repair at the time of closure (X-28). Retraction of the short external rotators posteriorly helps to protect the sciatic nerve.

The posterior aspect of the hip capsule is incised with a T-incision along the length of the neck and along the rim of the acetabulum. In cases with a flexion contracture of the hip, it may be necessary to perform an extensive capsulectomy

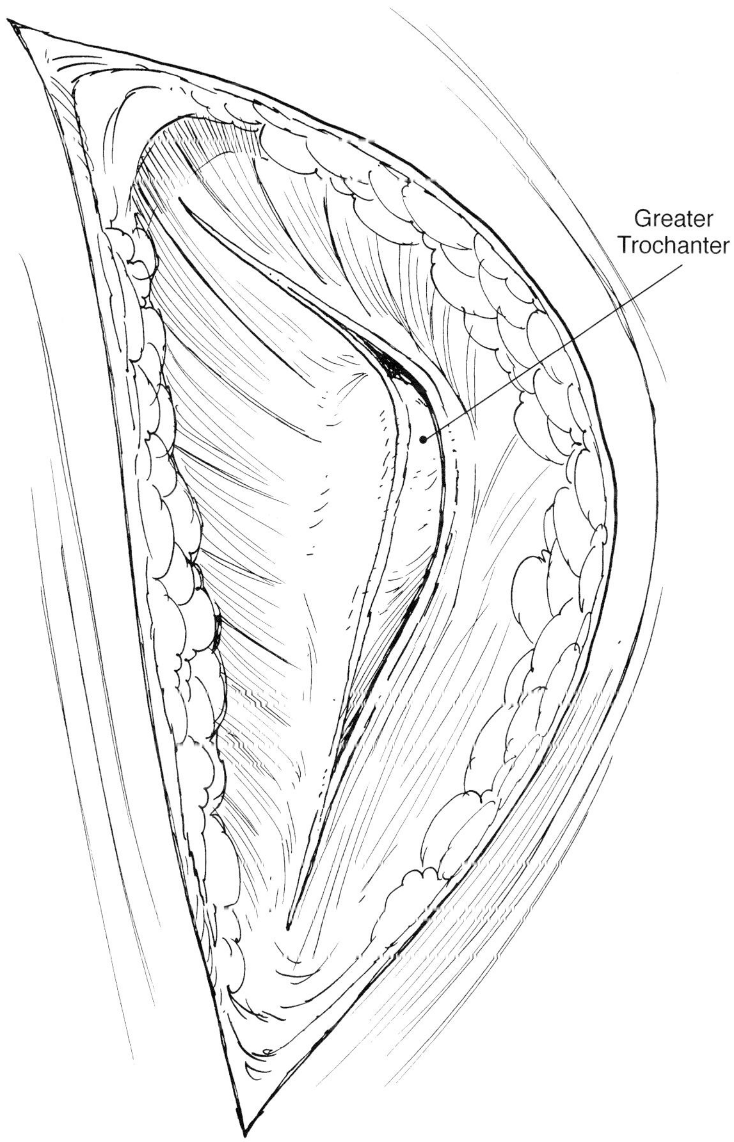


**FIGURE X-26**

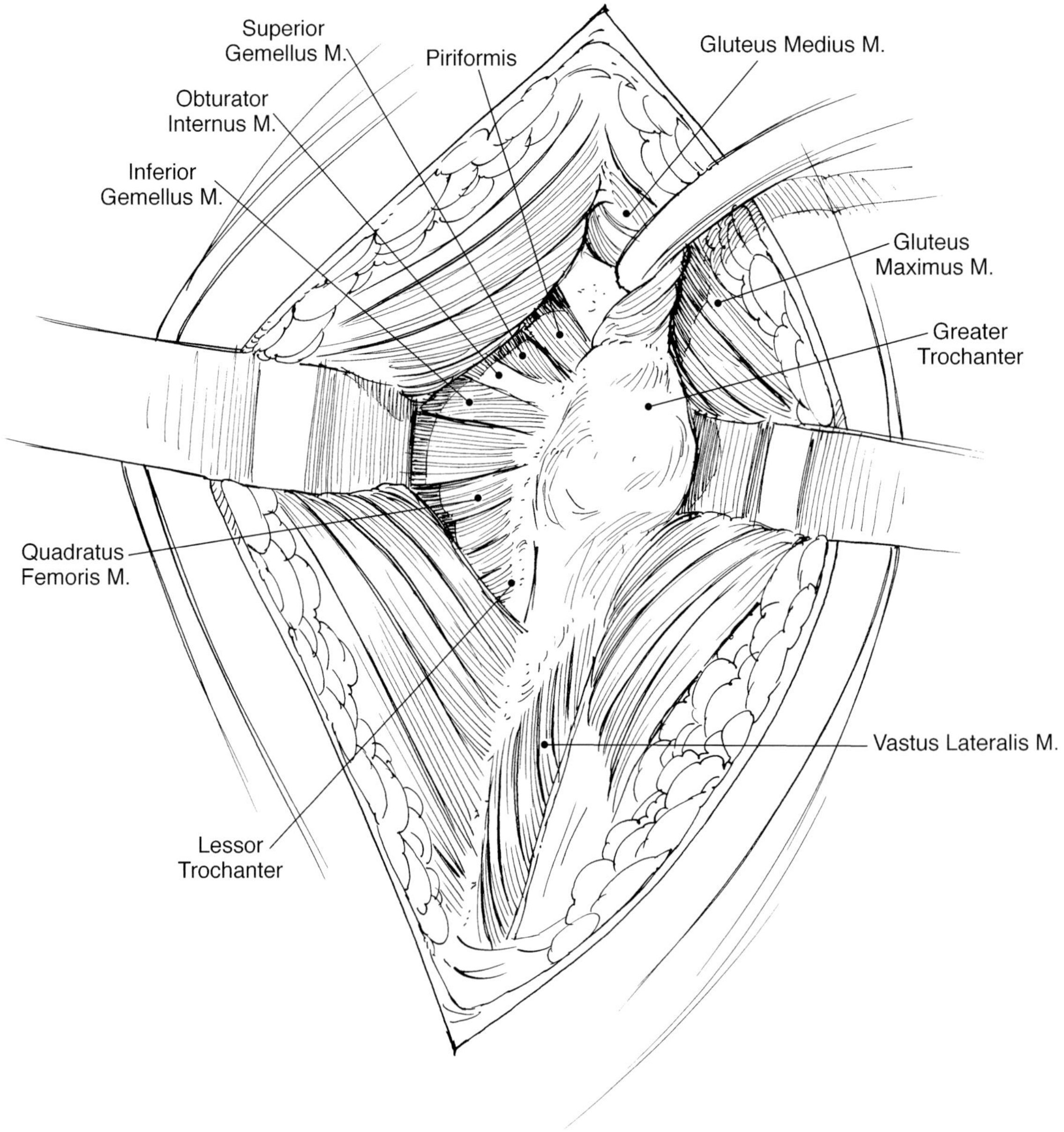
Superior
Gemellus M.
Piriformis
Gluteus Medius M.
Obturator
Internus M.
Inferior
Gemellus M.
Gluteus
Maximus M.
Greater
Trochanter
Quadratus
Femoris M.
Vastus Lateralis M.
Lessor
Trochanter

**FIGURE X-27**

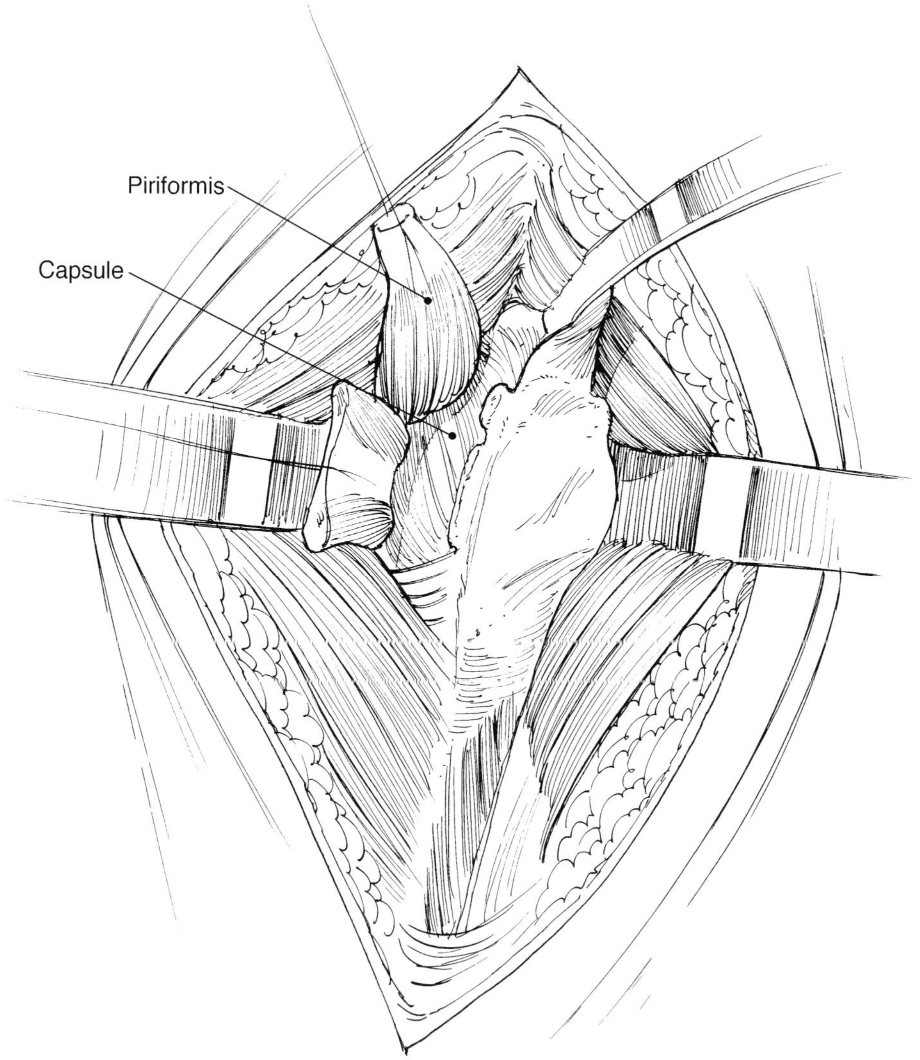


**FIGURE X-28**

in order to dislocate the femoral head safely. Extreme care should be exercised when dissecting anterior to the femoral neck from the posterior approach. In some cases, the posterior capsule can be salvaged and reattached to the posterior aspect of the greater trochanter along with the short external rotators.

Internal rotation and adduction of the hip brings the femoral head into view. Some patients, especially those with rheumatoid arthritis, may retain a tough ligamentum teres that must be sectioned prior to dislocating the femoral head (X-29).

*Dangers*

The sciatic nerve is located in the posterior aspect of the wound. Great care must be taken to prevent excessive traction on the nerve or inadvertent placement of a retractor against the nerve. Hip replacement through this approach has been reported to increase the risk of posterior dislocation of the prosthesis. Retractors placed along the anterior acetabulum should not be forced blindly into the soft tissue anteriorly since doing so can damage the femoral neurovascular bundle.

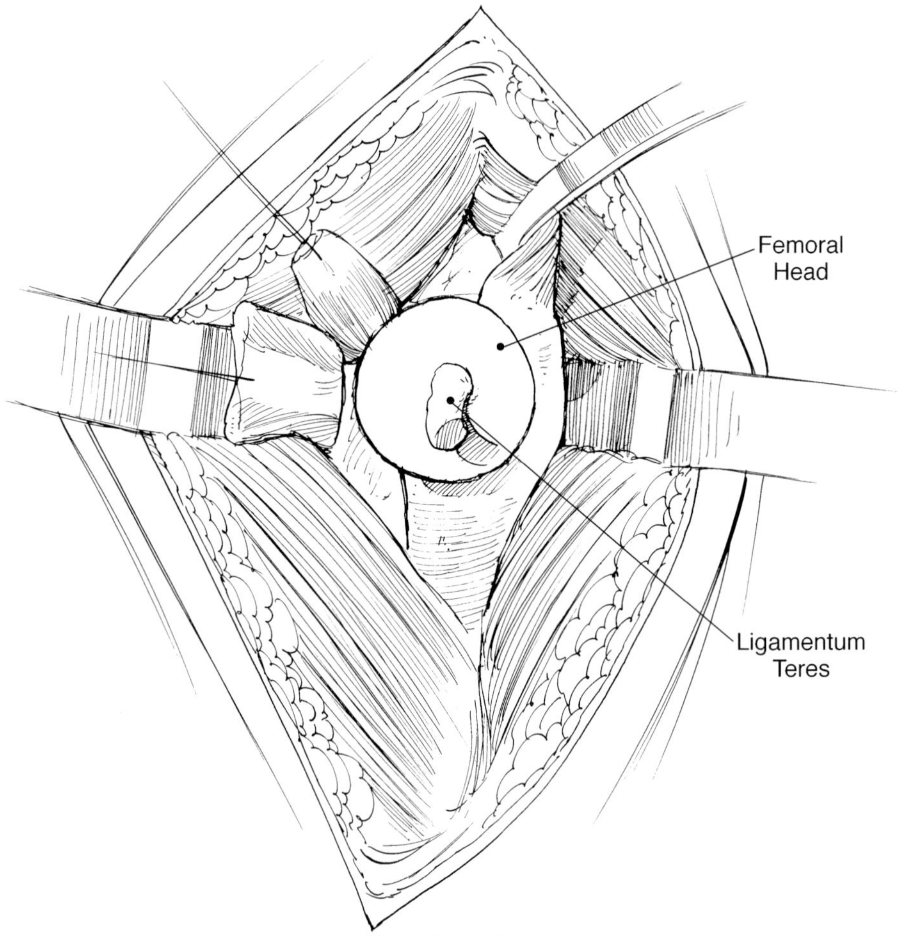


**FIGURE X-29**

***Limitations***

The fibers of the gluteus maximus should not be split as far proximally as the top of the sciatic notch because of the risk of transecting the superior gluteal nerve or artery. Access to the anterior pelvis is limited and retractors must be placed anterior to the hip capsule to allow complete visualization of the acetabulum.

## Medial (Ludloff) Approach to the Hip

***Applications***

First described by Ludloff in 1913 (7), the medial approach was designed for reduction of congenital dislocations of the hip. This approach may also be used for hip flexor and adductor muscle release for spasticity. Additionally, the medial approach provides exposure for biopsy of tumors of the inferior aspect of the femoral neck and the medial proximal femur.

***Technique***

The patient is placed in a supine position with the hip flexed, abducted, and externally rotated. The pubic tubercle and ischial tuberosity should be palpated for orientation. The tendons of the gracilis and adductor longus are palpable at their origins on the pelvis.

The skin incision is placed longitudinally, beginning 3 cm distal to the pubic tubercle and extending along the palpable tendon of the adductor longus (X-30). Dissection is carried out bluntly between the adductor longus anteriorly and the gracilis posteriorly (X-31).

Deep to the gracilis, the adductor brevis is identified. The adductor brevis is retracted anteriorly to open the interval between it and adductor magnus. The posterior division of the obturator nerve and vessels will be found adherent to the dorsal surface of the adductor brevis. The anterior division is found anterior to the adductor brevis (X-32). The lesser trochanter is palpable in the deep aspect of the dissection. The psoas tendon is detached from the lesser trochanter if the hip is to be opened (X-33). The inferior aspect of the hip capsule can be opened and the femoral neck can be exposed if necessary (X-34). If the adductor muscles are to be released, they should be transected close to their origins on the pelvis to minimize bleeding.

***Dangers***

The obturator vessels pass through the obturator foramen to enter this area. They are relatively fixed in that position. If torn, they may retract into the pelvis, making control of bleeding difficult. The medial femoral circumflex artery transverses the deep part of the dissection at the distal edge of the lesser trochanter. Injury to this vessel may compromise the blood supply to the femoral head.

***Limitations***

This is the most limited approach to the hip. It provides minimal exposure to the hip capsule and femoral neck. It is useful for open reduction of dysplastic hips if psoas recession and a medial capsulotomy are necessary to obtain reduction of the hip.

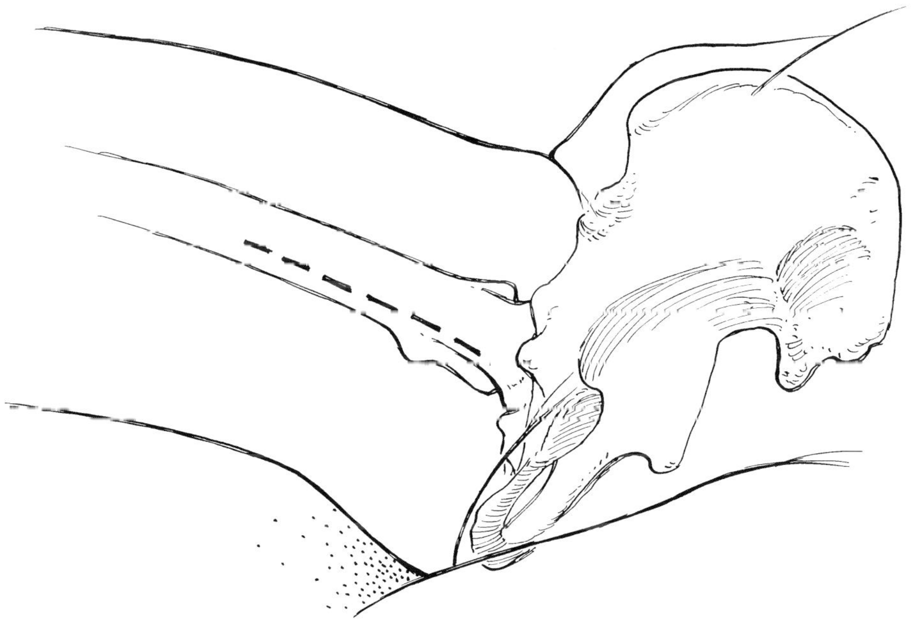

**FIGURE X-30**

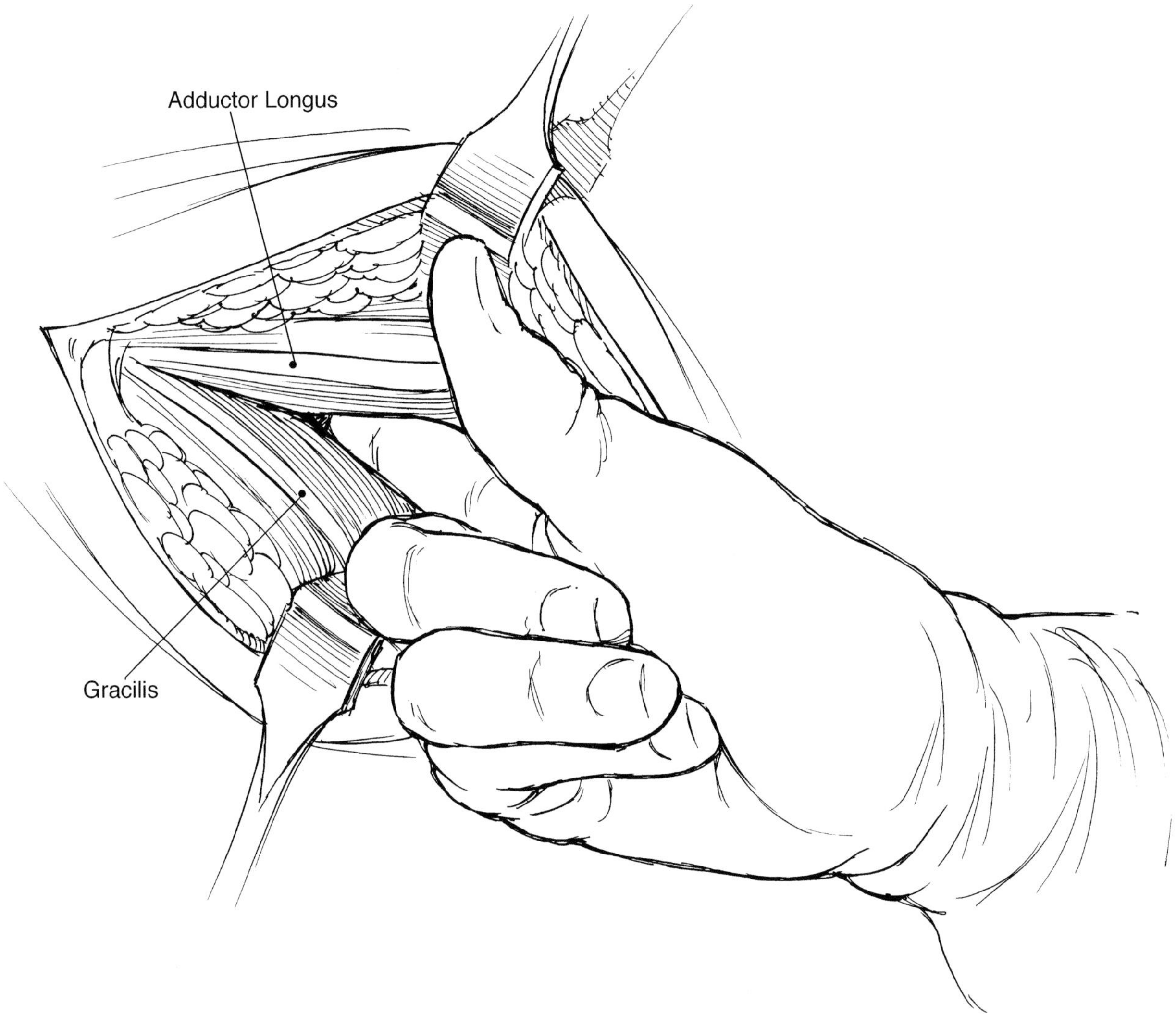


**FIGURE X-31**

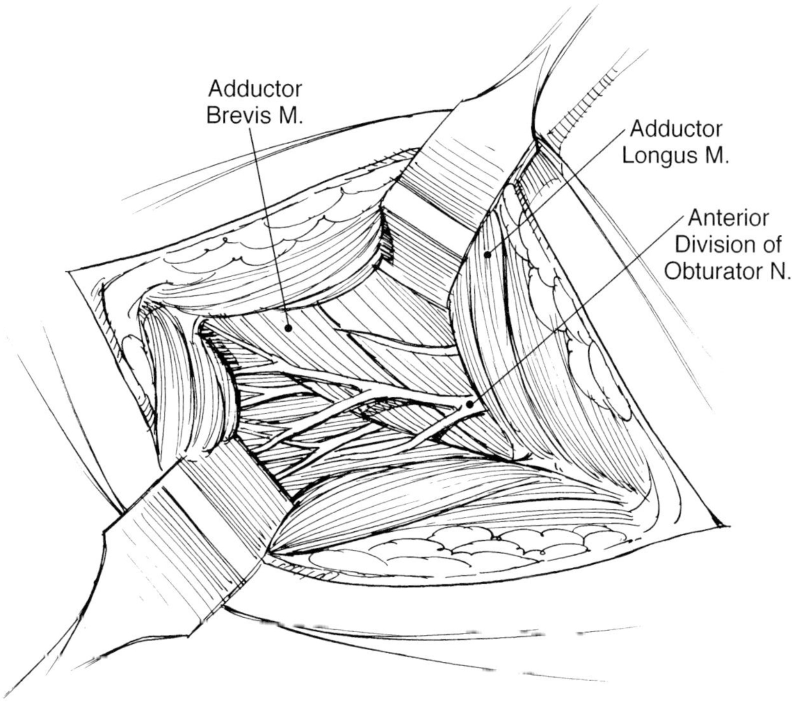


**FIGURE X-32**

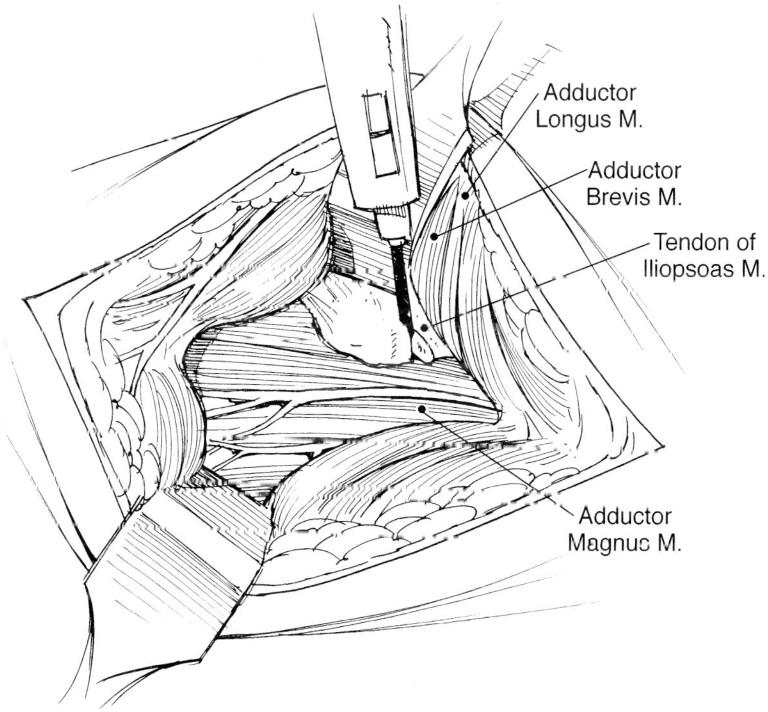


**FIGURE X-33**

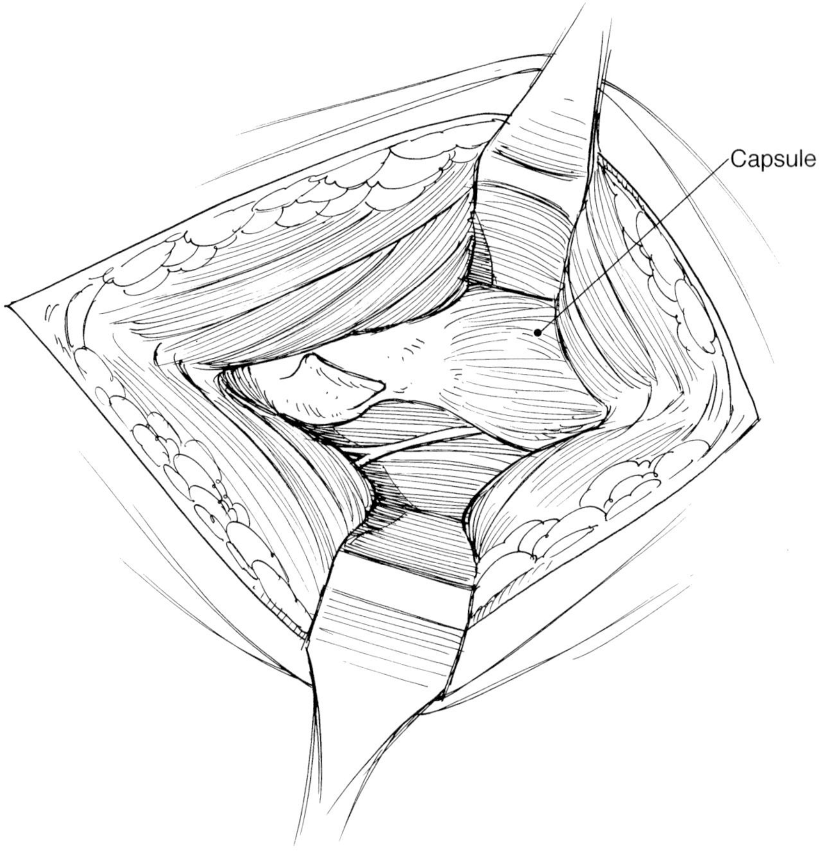


**FIGURE X-34**

# References


1. Smith-Petersen MN. Approach to and exposure of the hip joint for mold arthroplasty. J Bone Joint Surg 31:40, 1949.
2. Waston-Jones R. Fractures of the neck of the femur. Br J Surg 23:787–808, 1936.
3. Hardinge K. The direct lateral approach to the hip. J Bone Joint Surg 64B:17, 1982.
4. McLauchlan J. The Stracathro approach to the hip. J Bone Joint Surg 66B:30–31, 1984.
5. Glassman A, Engh C, Bobyn J. A technique of extensile exposure for total hip arthroplasty. J Arthroplasty 2(1):11–21, 1987.
6. Boardman K, Bocco F, Charnley J. An evaluation of a method of trochanteric fixation using three wires in the Charnly low friction arthroplasty. Clin Orthop 132:31, 1978.
7. Ludloff K. The open reduction of the congenital hip dislocation by an anterior incision. Ann J Orthop Surg 10:438, 1913.

# XI

# SURGICAL APPROACHES TO THE THIGH AND FEMUR

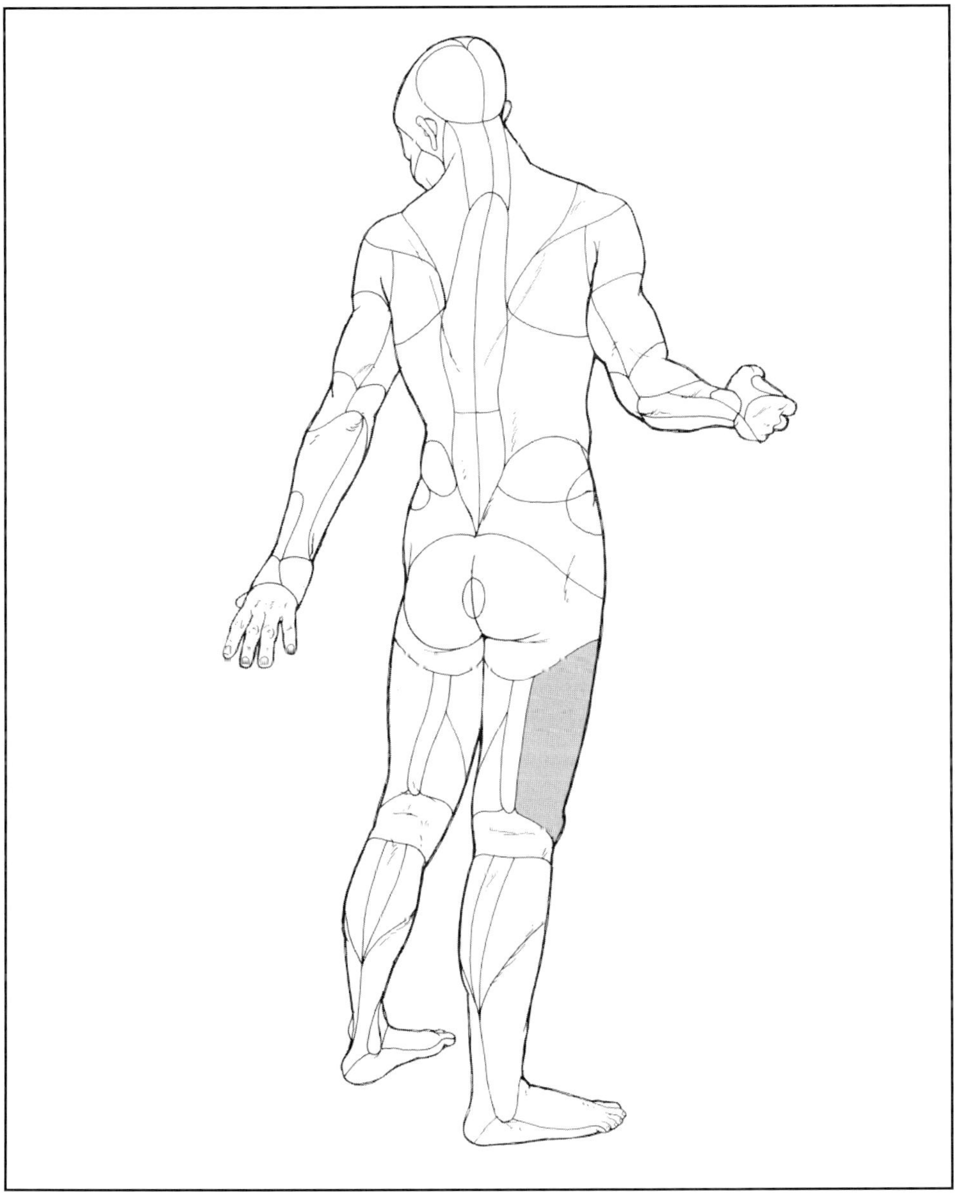

## General Principles and Complications

Operations on the thigh and femur are very common. Children require surgery for congenital or acquired deformities from problems such as fibrous dysplasia and for fractures involving the growth plates. Malignant tumors of the bone (osteosarcoma and Ewing's sarcoma) occur most frequently in adolescents and commonly arise in the distal femur. Young adults are frequently victims of comminuted fractures, especially from motor vehicle accidents. Benign tumors, such as giant cell tumors, are found most often in the distal femur in middle aged adults. In the fifth and sixth decades, the incidence of soft tissue sarcomas (such as liposarcoma and malignant fibrous histiocytoma) peaks. The majority of these tumors occur in the extensor and adductor compartments of the thigh. Metastatic carcinoma also frequently occurs in the proximal femur and femoral shaft. Elderly people are especially prone to osteoporosis-related proximal femur fractures. In addition, osteomyelitis of the femur can be a protracted, disabling problem for adults. This condition is most commonly encountered after open fractures or in intravenous drug abusers and diabetics.

Complications of surgery and fractures about the femur are similar to those discussed in surgical approaches to the pelvis. This is especially true for pulmonary emboli and infections. In addition, a significant volume of the femur is filled with fat (1). Severe pulmonary insufficiency, hypotension, and cardiovascular collapse can be caused by the fat emboli syndrome (2,3). The femur is surrounded by a large muscle envelope and, therefore, has an extensive blood supply; however, the subtrochanteric region is mostly thick, cortical bone that is relatively avascular and prone to nonunion. The long bones such as the femur have two blood supplies, from intramedullary and from periosteal vessels. Severely comminuted fractures may disrupt both blood supplies, making nonunion more likely. Reaming the medullary canal in preparation for internal fixation of a fracture will disrupt the intramedullary blood supply. Stripping of the periosteum from fracture fragments for surgical exposure disrupts the surface blood supply. Therefore, in selecting the type of fixation to use, the surgeon must consider the consequences of the surgical exposure. Periosteal stripping should always be kept to a minimum. The sciatic nerve and femoral artery traverse the thigh and are the most critical structures for preservation of the limb. The femoral artery can be replaced or bypassed if necessary; however, damage to or resection of the sciatic nerve can produce complete loss of sensation and motor function below the knee, as well as disabling problems with chronic pain or reflex sympathetic dystrophy. Angular deformity or limb length discrepancy from malunion or congenital deformity can produce disabling gait disturbances and may require elaborate leg lengthening and realignment procedures.

## Surgical Anatomy

The thigh contains three major muscle groups: medial, anterior, and posterior. The adductor (medial) group is supplied by the obturator nerve and vessels. The adductor magnus is the most posterior muscle of this group. The posterior ("hamstring") portion of the adductor magnus is innervated by the tibial component of the sciatic nerve. The extensor (anterior) compartment contains the quadriceps muscle and is supplied by the femoral nerve. The posterior compartment contains the biceps femoris laterally and the semimembranosus and semitendinosus medially, all of which are supplied by the sciatic nerve. There is no fibrous septum between the medial and posterior compartments.

The femoral artery enters the thigh under the inguinal ligament to traverse the femoral triangle. Its only major branch in the thigh is the profunda femoris artery. The femoral artery extends distally into the adductor (Hunter's) canal where it is covered by the sartorius on its anterior surface proximally and the vastus medialis distally (XI-1). It lies on the anterior surface of the adductor longus in the proximal thigh and on the adductor magnus distally. The artery exits the thigh into the popliteal fossa by passing through the adductor hiatus (a fibrous tunnel in the adductor magnus). The saphenous nerve (a continuation of the femoral nerve) runs with the artery in the femoral triangle, but exits the adductor canal through the vastus medialis to distribute to the skin along the medial side of the knee and leg. The femoral artery spirals around the femur, anteriorly to the proximal femur, medially to the mid-femur, and posteriorly to the distal femur. The femoral artery and vein also spiral around each other, with the vein lateral to the artery at the inguinal ligament and medial to the artery in the popliteal fossa. The femoral nerve lies lateral to the vein in the femoral triangle and distributes to all of the quadriceps, with the most distal motor branch extending into the vastus medialis.

The profunda femoris artery is the major blood supply to the thigh. It arises from the lateral side of the femoral artery, just below the inguinal ligament. It then

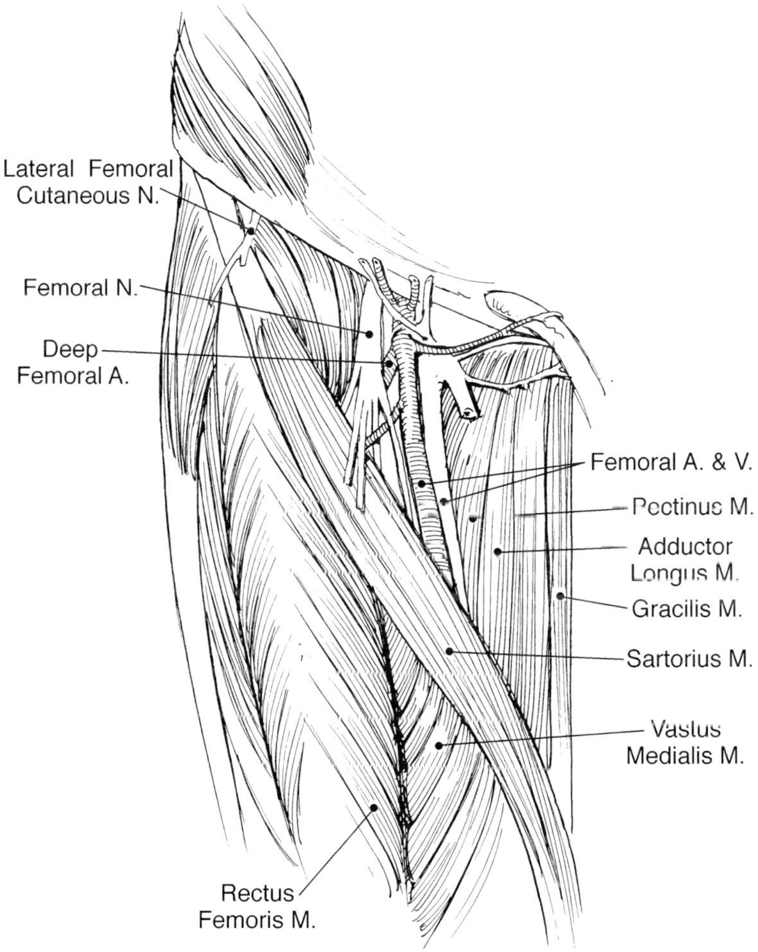


**FIGURE XI-1**

passes posterior to the adductor longus to run along its posterior surface. It terminates in multiple perforating branches which run medially and posteriorly around the femur, perforating the lateral intermuscular septum to distribute to the quadriceps muscle and to the skin of the anterior, lateral thigh (XI-2). The saphenous vein arises in the leg to pass along the posteromedial knee. It continues subcutaneously in the thigh to pierce the fascia lata at the fossa ovalis and terminates in the femoral vein (XI-3). The sciatic nerve runs down the middle of the posterior thigh between the medial and lateral hamstrings. It bifurcates at variable lengths along the thigh into its common peroneal and tibial portions. The common peroneal portion is lateral and runs laterally across the distal thigh to descend along the posteromedial edge of the long head of the biceps (XI-4). The tibial portion descends in the midline into the popliteal fossa.

## Lateral Approach to the Femur

***Applications***

This is the most commonly used and safest approach to the femur. It can be extended from the greater trochanter to the knee. It is used for open reduction and internal fixation of intertrochanteric, shaft or condylar fractures, bone grafting, debridement of osteomyelitis, and osteotomies.

***Technique***

The patient may be positioned supine or laterally, depending on the specific procedures and the surgeon's preference. An incision is made longitudinally along the lateral thigh, anterior to the iliotibial band. It may be extended along a line from

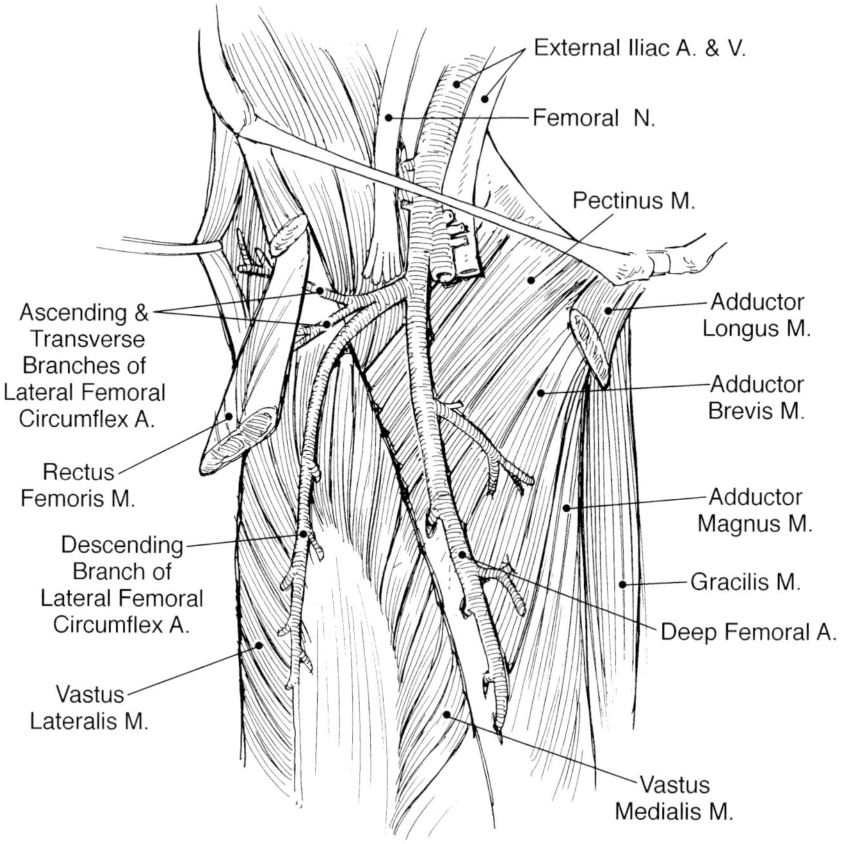


**FIGURE XI-2**

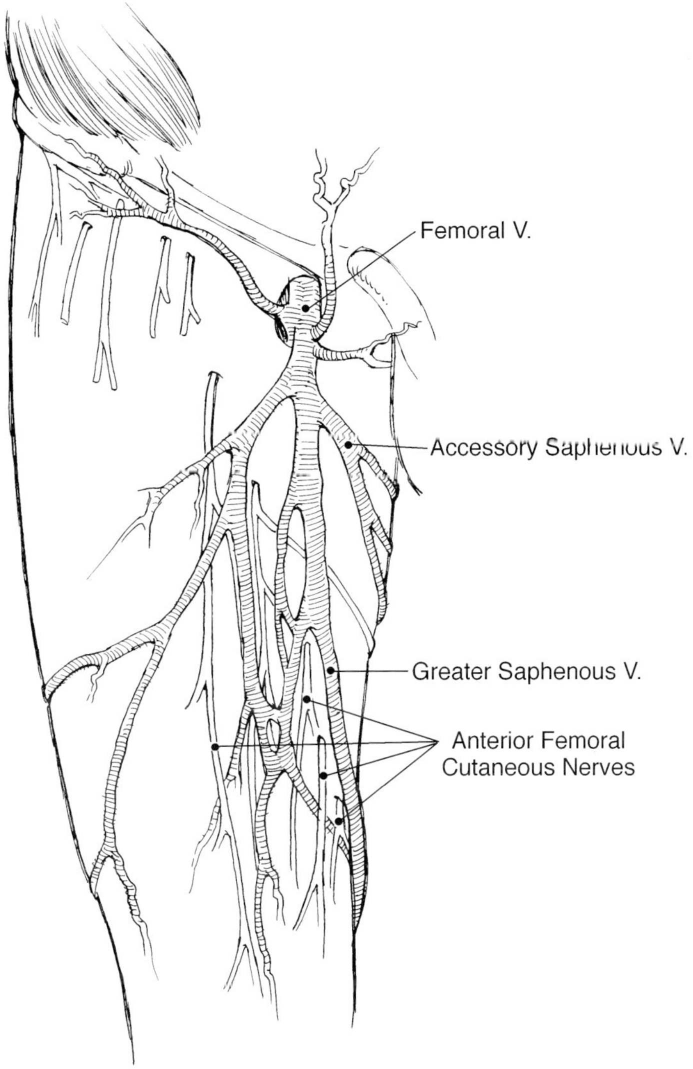
Femoral V.
Accessory Saphenous V.
Greater Saphenous V.
Anterior Femoral
Cutaneous Nerves

**FIGURE XI-3**

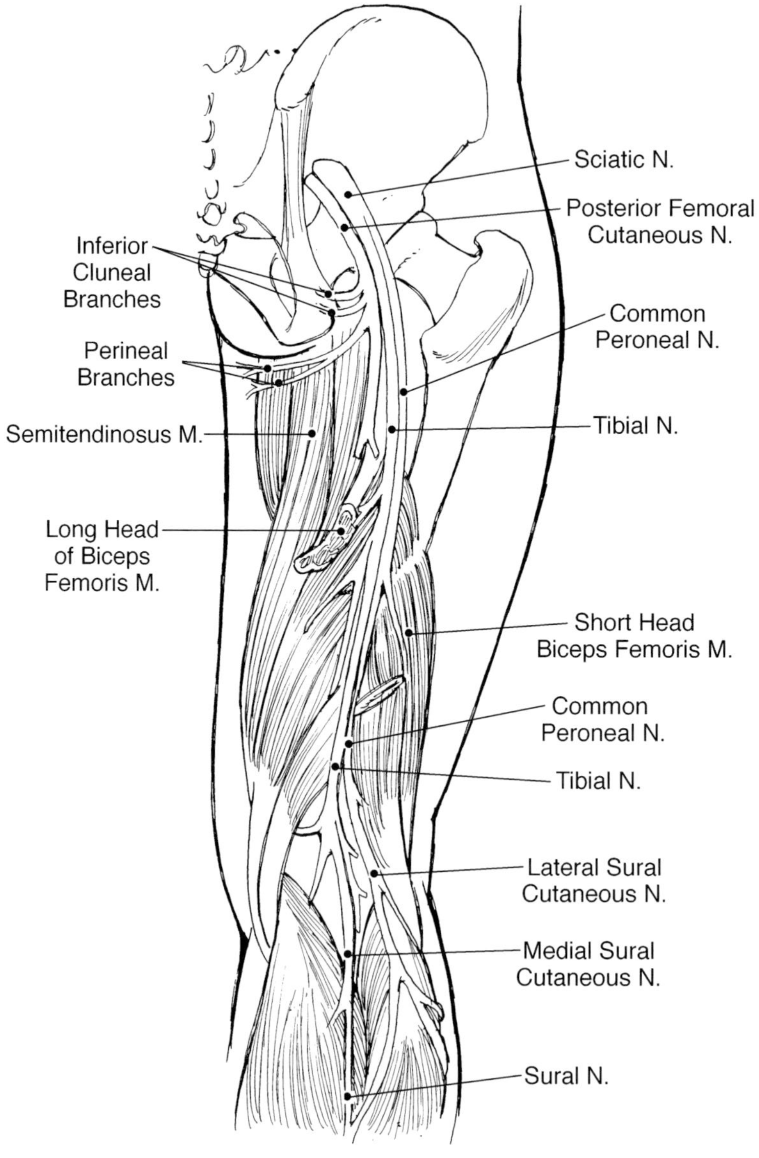
Sciatic N.
Posterior Femoral Cutaneous N.
Inferior Cluneal Branches
Common Peroneal N.
Perineal Branches
Semitendinosus M.
Tibial N.
Long Head of Biceps Femoris M.
Short Head Biceps Femoris M.
Common Peroneal N.
Tibial N.
Lateral Sural Cutaneous N.
Medial Sural Cutaneous N.
Sural N.

**FIGURE XI-4**

the greater trochanter to the lateral femoral condyle as needed (XI-5). The fascia lata is incised in line with the skin incision to expose the belly of the vastus lateralis. The muscle belly of the vastus lateralis is retracted anteriorly to expose its origin from the posterolateral femur and the broad external aponeurosis. The muscle is then split longitudinally along a line 1 cm anterior to the posterior edge of the aponeurosis (XI-6). As the muscle fibers are split, the perforating branches of the profunda femoris vessels are encountered and should be clamped, ligated, and transected. The vastus lateralis can be elevated from the anterior and lateral surface of the femur as necessary (XI-7).

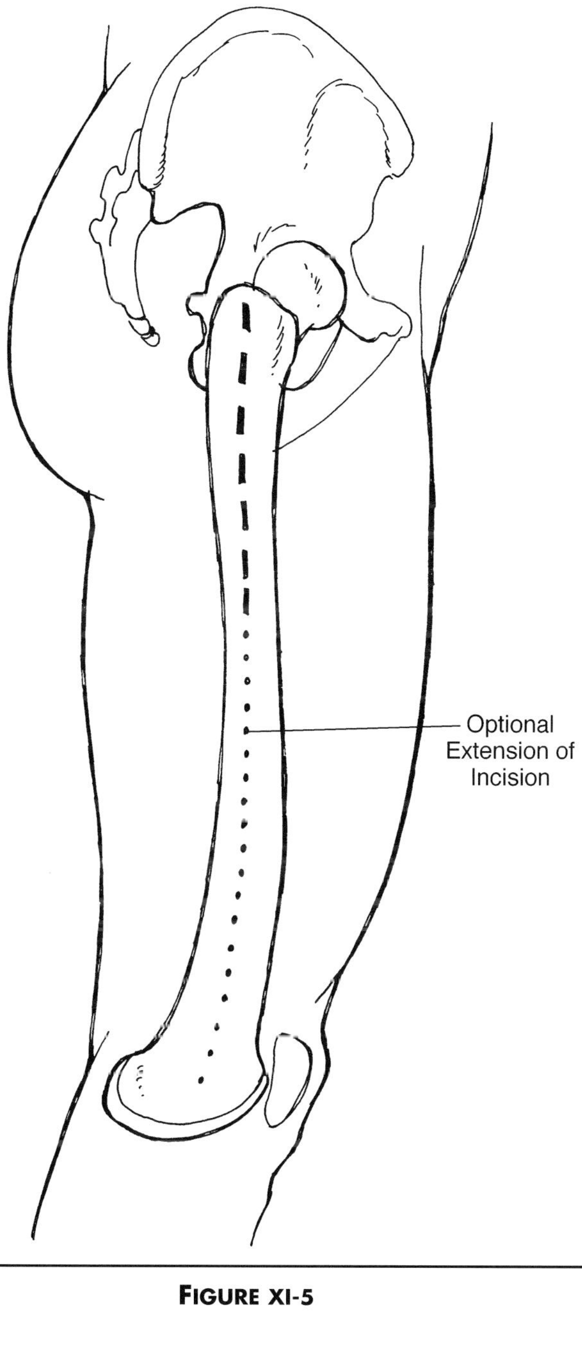


**FIGURE XI-5**

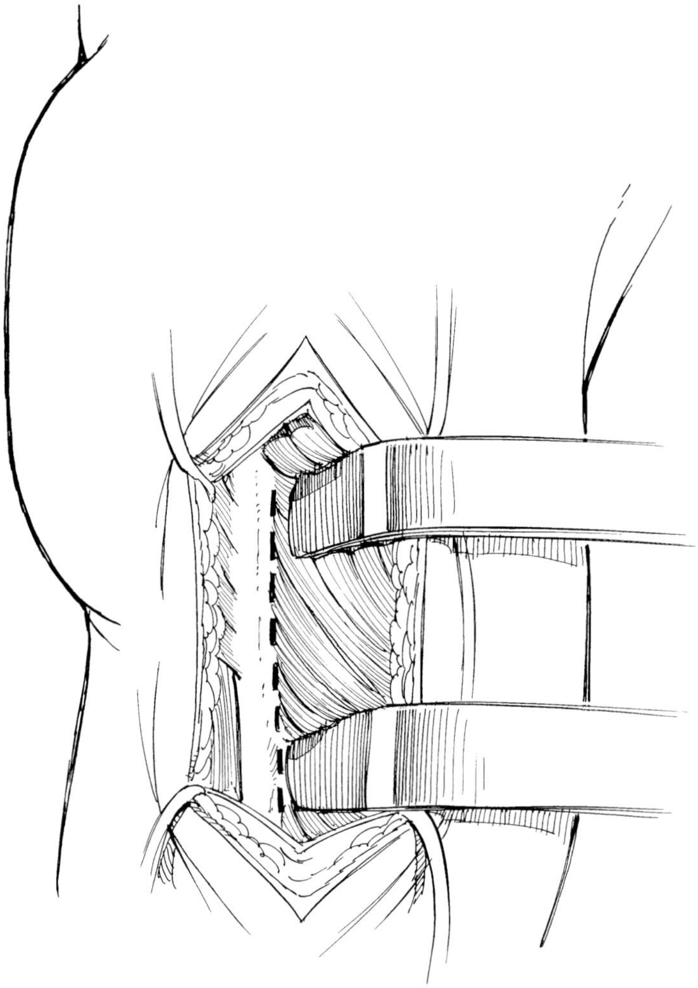

**FIGURE XI-6**

*Dangers*

The dissection is through a safe plane. However, brisk bleeding can be encountered from transected perforating vessels that may retract into the posterior compartment. Periosteal stripping should be minimized to preserve blood supply to the femur.

*Limitations*

This exposure can be extended over the hip and across the knee if necessary. The entire femur can be removed by circumferential elevation of the muscles.

## Anteromedial Approach to the Femur

*Applications*

The anteromedial approach is especially useful for access to the femoral shaft and knee in cases where access to the femoral artery is also necessary. This circumstance may occur in fractures associated with arterial injury or in nonunions or defects in the femur that require a vascularized bone transfer. This approach is also useful for open reduction and internal fixation of complex distal femur fractures such as intraarticular fractures of the condyles or for excision of tumors of the medial femoral condyle.

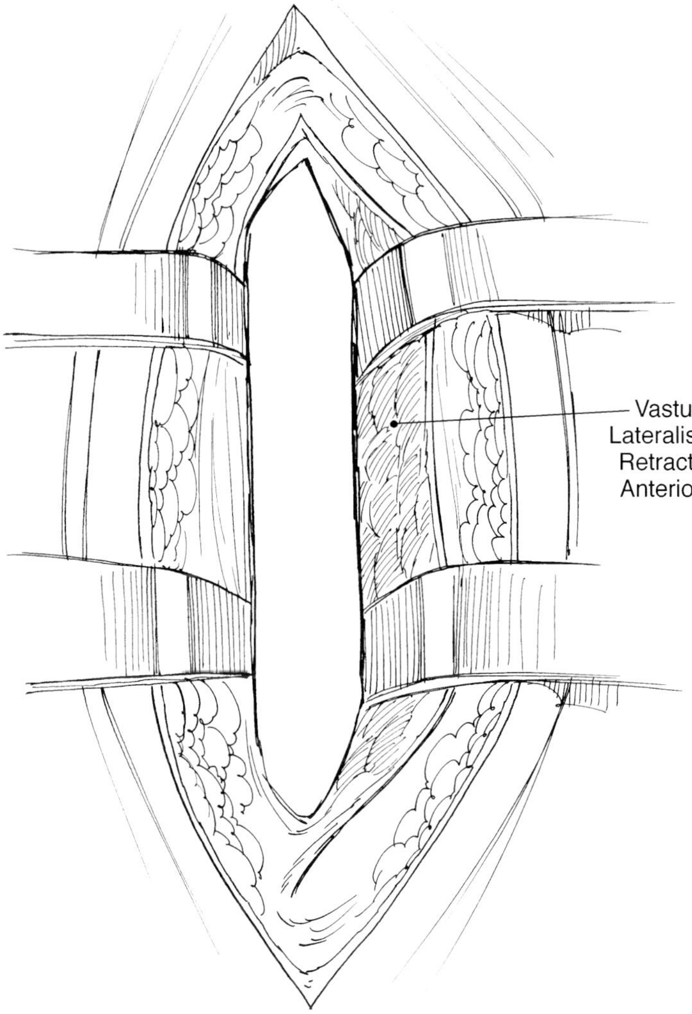


**FIGURE XI-7**

*Technique*

The patient is positioned supine with the limb externally rotated. A longitudinal incision is made from the anteromedial femoral condyle proximally, along the interval between the rectus femoris and vastus medialis. The fascia is incised in line with the skin (XI-8). The rectus femoris is retracted laterally to expose the vastus medialis. The vastus medialis may be elevated from distal to proximal, detaching its fibers of origin from the medial intermuscular septum (XI-9). If wider exposure is needed, the quadriceps tendon may be split longitudinally along its medial edge to open the interval between the vastus medialis and the intermedius. Access to the femoral artery may be obtained by extending the dissection proximally to expose the artery in the adductor canal or by opening the medial intermuscular septum to expose the vessel from the popliteal fossa proximally (XI-10). The superior medial genicular artery may be found by this technique and used as an arterial trunk for a microvascular anastomosis if needed. The bone is exposed by elevation of the vastus medialis and intermedius (XI-11).

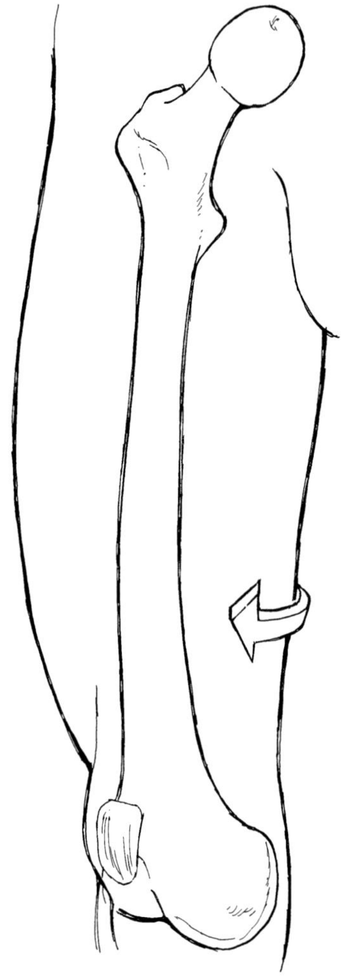

**FIGURE XI-8**

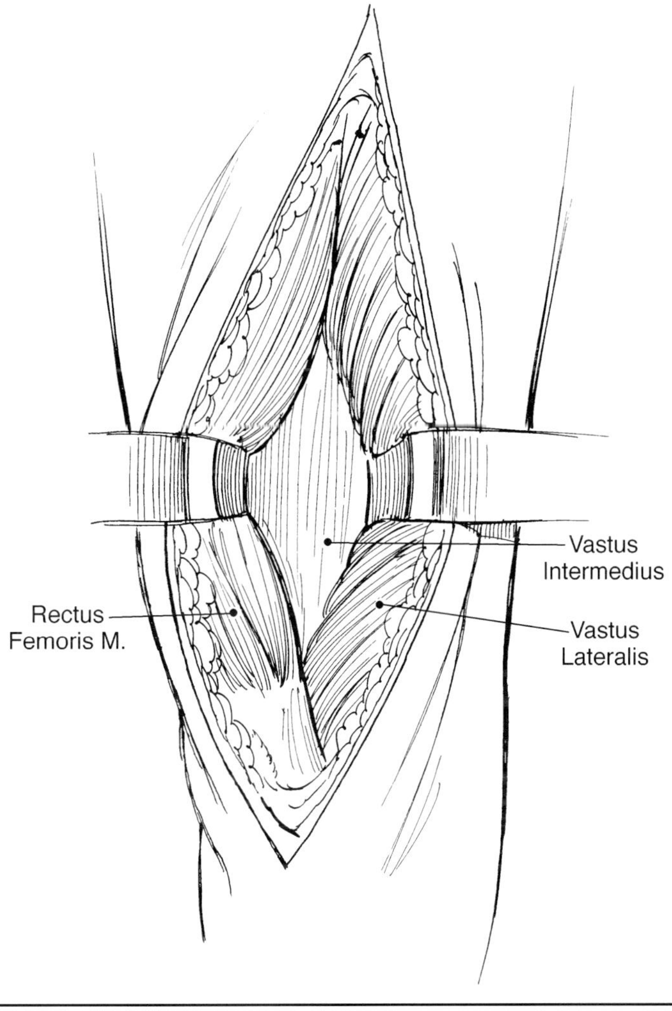


**FIGURE XI-9**

***Dangers***

The proximal end of this dissection encounters the femoral artery and vein. If the quadriceps tendon is incised, it should be carefully repaired to allow early motion to prevent adhesions of the muscle and loss of knee motion. The motor branch to the vastus medialis runs longitudinally within the muscle and can be damaged. Loss of strength in the vastus medialis can produce a sensation of weakness and giving way of the knee and may create lateral tracking of the patella that may produce anterior knee pain.

***Limitations***

This approach may be extended proximally toward the anterior superior iliac spine (ASIS) and distally across the knee as necessary. Proximal exposure of the femur requires extensive dissection of the femoral neurovascular bundle that may be avoided by use of a lateral approach.

## Posterior Approach to the Femur

***Applications***

This approach is rarely necessary for exposure of the femur. It is, however, useful for resection of tumors of the posterior compartment of the thigh or exploration of the sciatic nerve.

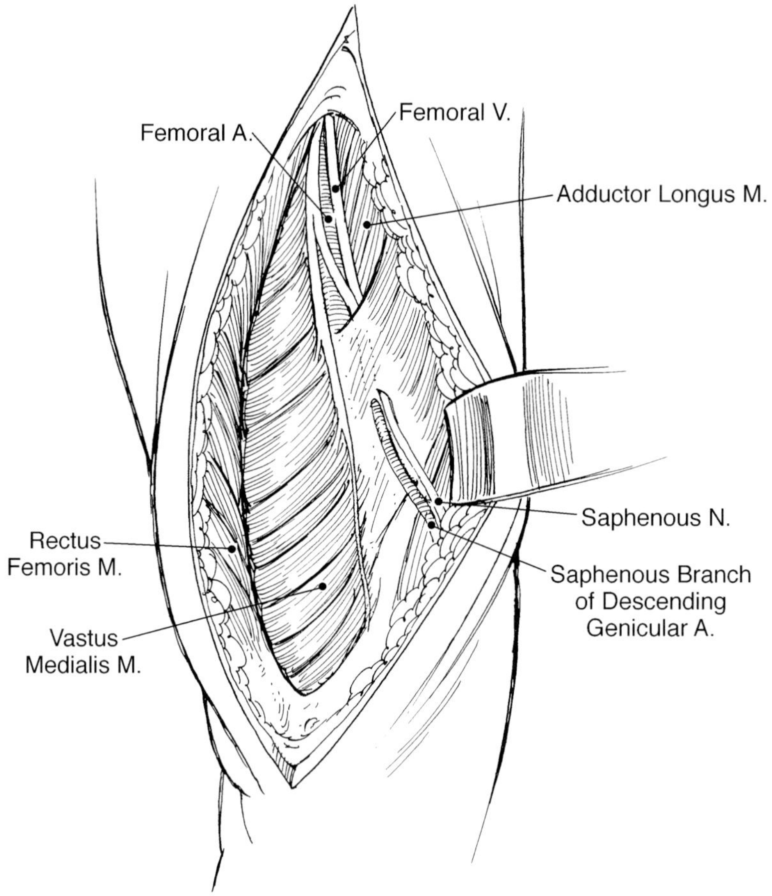


**FIGURE XI-10**

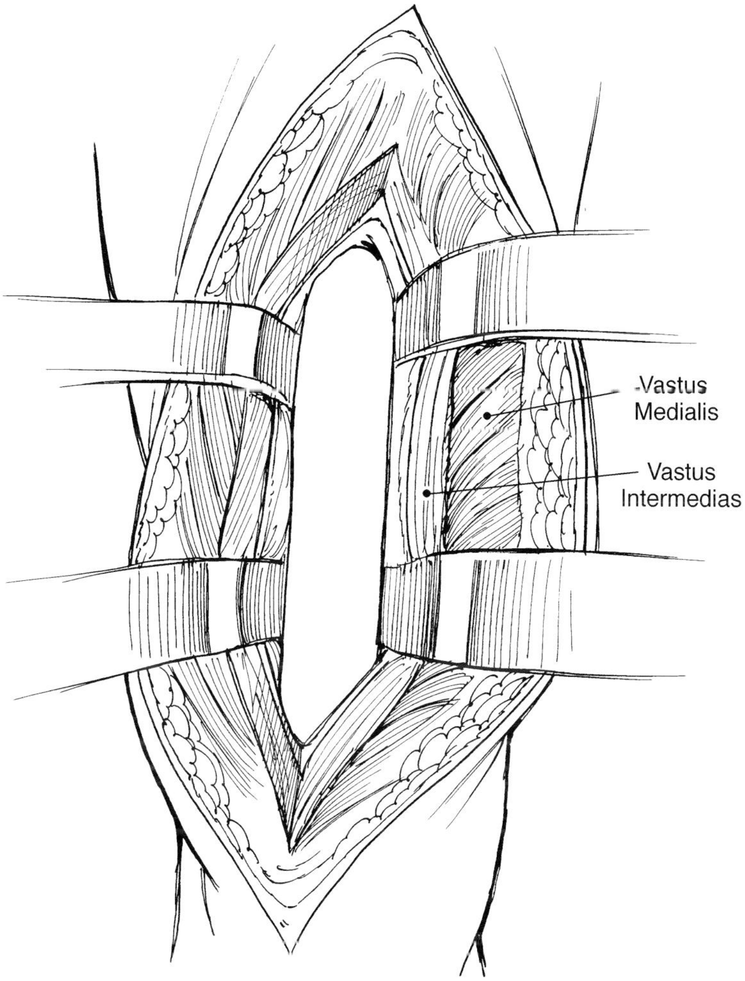


**FIGURE XI-11**

### *Technique*

The patient is placed prone with the knee flexed approximately 20°. A long S-shaped incision extends from the ischial tuberosity to the lateral edge of the flexor crease of the knee, medial to the biceps femoris tendon. The fascia is incised in line with the skin incision (XI-12). Flaps are elevated medially and laterally to expose as much of the posterior compartment as necessary. The sciatic nerve lies in a fat pad between the medial and lateral hamstrings and may be traced into the popliteal fossa. To expose the femur, the long head of the biceps is retracted medially in the proximal half of the wound and laterally in the distal half to expose the short head of the biceps (XI-13). The short head is detached from its origin and reflected medially subperiosteally to expose the femur (XI-14).

### *Dangers*

The sciatic nerve is exposed and mobilized. Retraction on the nerve should be minimal. The branch of the sciatic nerve to the biceps femoris arises in the proximal thigh and should be preserved. The posterior femoral cutaneous nerve runs on the

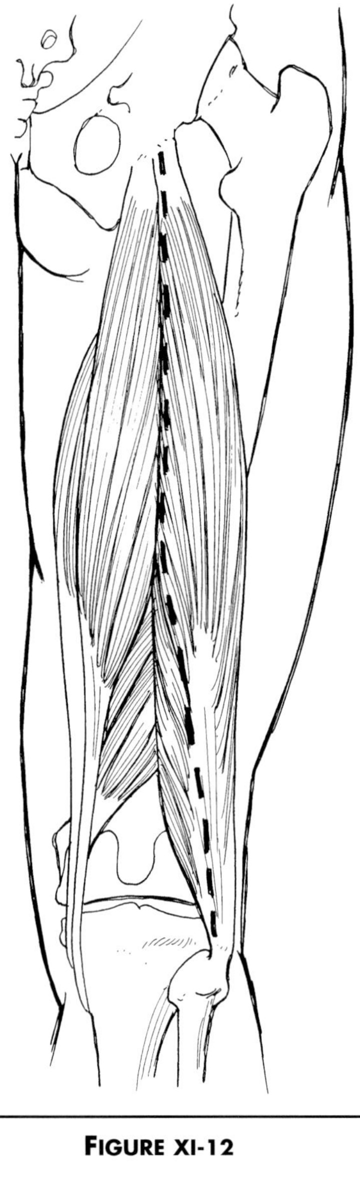

**FIGURE XI-12**

fascia on the posterior thigh and should be protected to avoid creating a painful neuroma.

*Limitations*

This exposure can be extended into the buttock by retracting and splitting the fibers of the gluteus maximus to expose as far proximally as the sciatic notch. The incision can be extended as an S-shaped extension across the popliteal fossa onto the calf if necessary.

# Compartment Resections of the Thigh

Each compartment of the thigh may be resected for malignant tumors. The adductor and extensor compartments are most commonly involved with soft tissue sarcomas. The skin incision is a gentle S extending over the middle of the compartment from the pelvis to the knee. The fascia and skin are reflected as a single layer

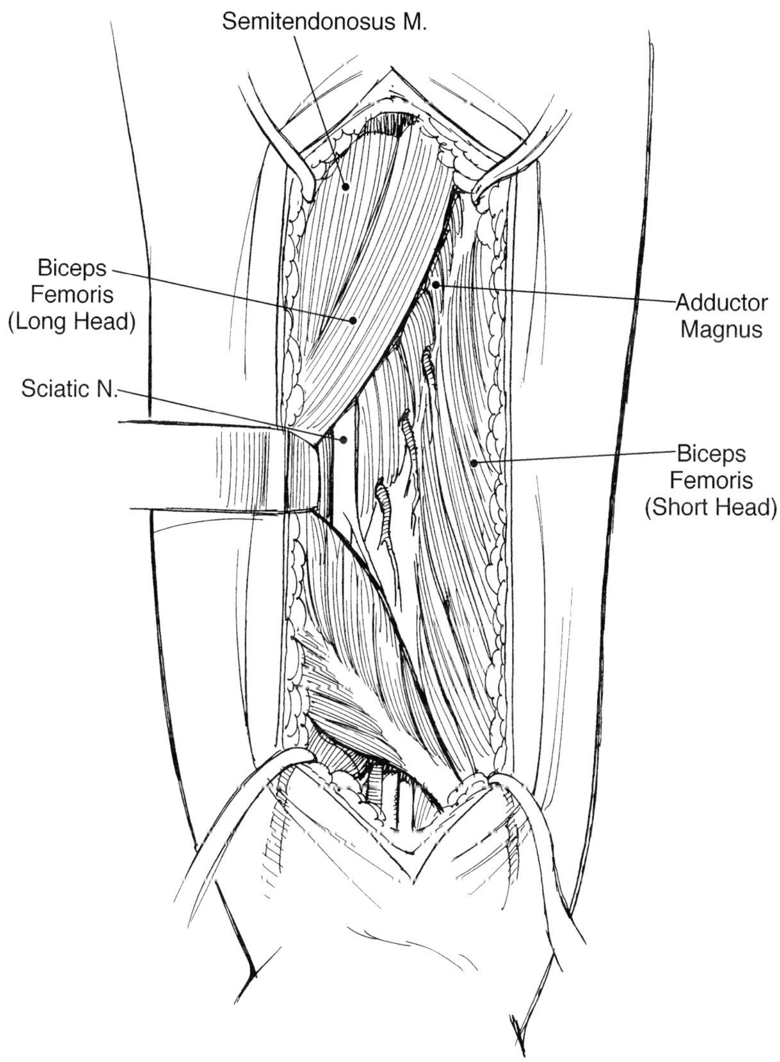


**FIGURE XI-13**

after ellipsing the biopsy tract and leaving the tract with the muscle to be resected (XI-15). The muscles are detached from the pelvis and reflected distally. The femoral artery must be preserved or reconstructed. The profunda femoris may be ligated if necessary, but doing so significantly diminishes collateral flow to the skin of the thigh. The femoral nerve and its extensions can be resected without reconstruction. The patient can walk with a reasonably smooth gait with a completely absent extensor mechanism. Conversely, preservation of the rectus femoris can significantly improve the function of the limb to allow active extension of the knee for ascending inclines and climbing ladders or stairs. The adductor compartment may be completely excised with little noticeable change in the function of the limb. Excision of the posterior compartment muscles produces minimal morbidity; however, excision of the sciatic nerve produces a major deficit with complete paralysis of the muscles below the knee and an insensate foot that may be a hazard to the

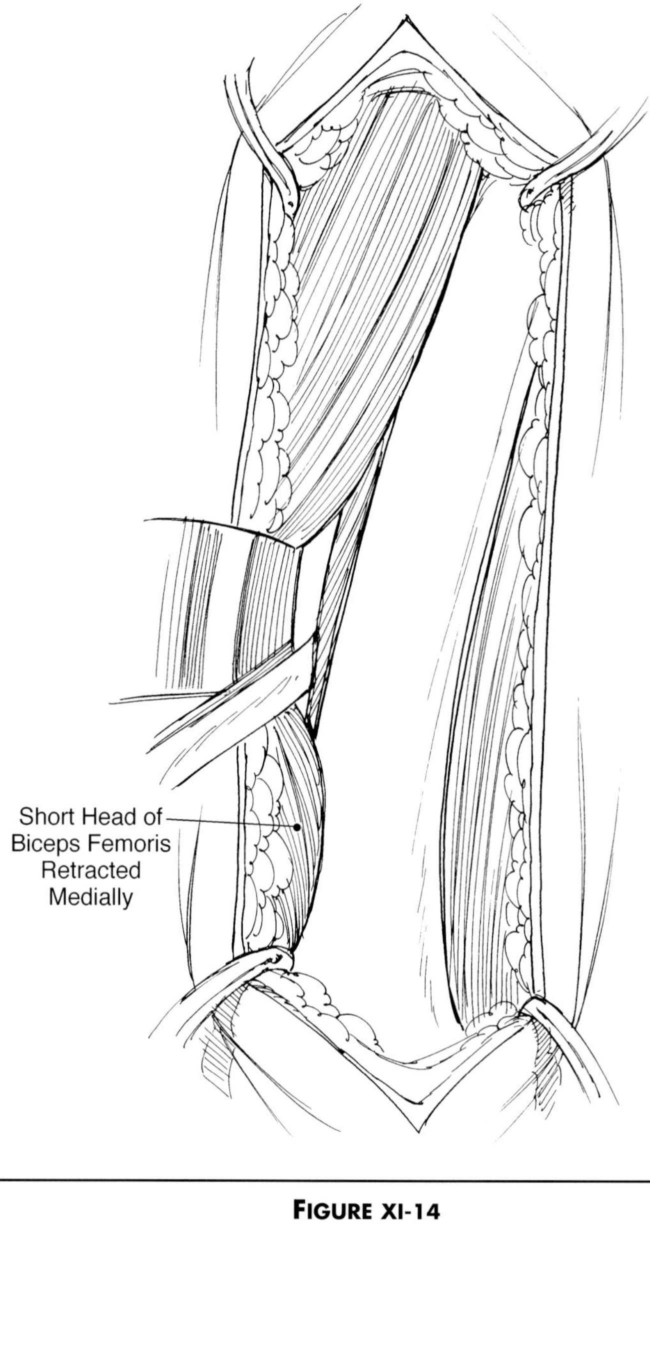


**FIGURE XI-14**

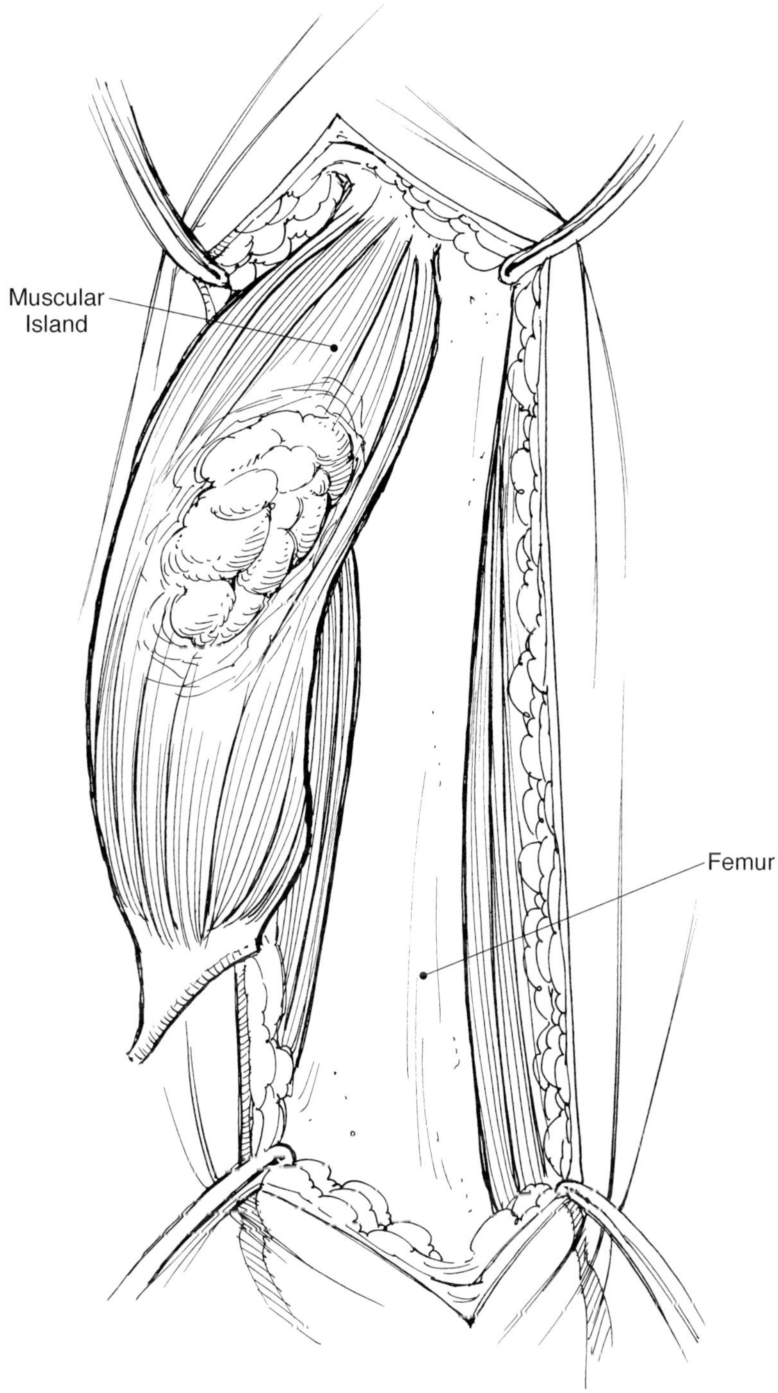


**FIGURE XI-15**

patient. Intercalary segments of the femur may be resected with the compartments and reconstructed with an allograft, an autologous fibular transfer, a prosthesis, or a composite of these. Reasonable soft tissue coverage of the distal thigh may be obtained with a gastrocnemius rotation flap. Large soft tissue defects in the proximal or middle thigh may require free flaps for coverage. Preservation of the blood supply to the skin and fascia and provision of adequate muscle coverage over implants in the thigh are critical to the long-term success of the limb salvage.

# References

1. Peltier LF. Fat embolism. Clin Orthop 66:241–253, 1969.
2. Bradford DS, Foster RR, Nossel HL. Coagulation alternatives, hypoxemia and fat embolism in fracture patients. J Trauma 10(4):307–321, 1970.
3. Gossling HR, Ellison LH, Degraff AC. Fat embolism. The role of respiratory failure and its treatment. J Bone Joint Surg 56(7):1327–1337, 1974.

# XII

# SURGICAL APPROACHES TO THE KNEE

*Robert C. Schenck, Jr.*

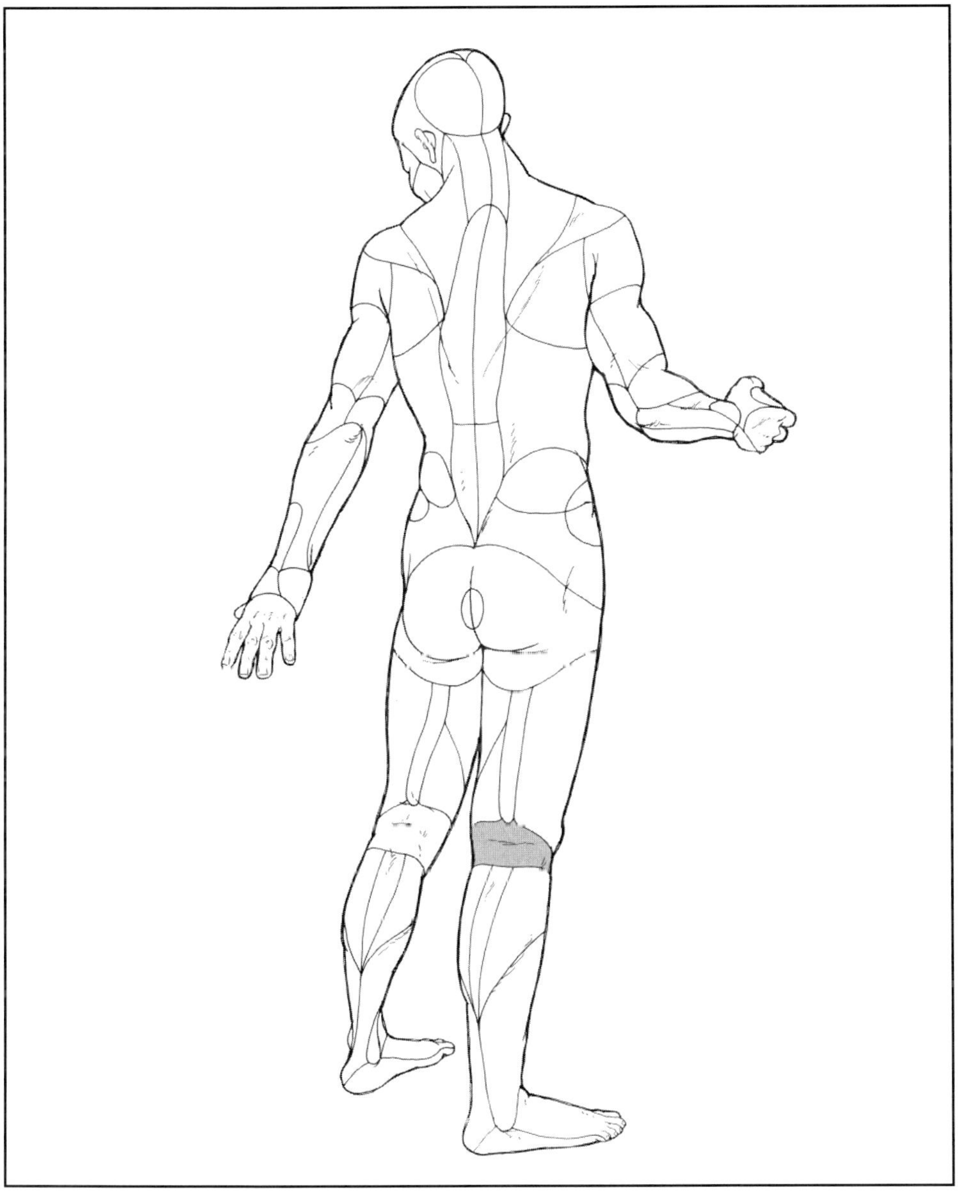

# General Principles and Complications

The development of arthroscopic knee surgery has dramatically decreased the need for knee arthrotomy. Most meniscal and cruciate ligament injuries can be evaluated and repaired by arthroscopic or arthroscopy-assisted techniques. If arthrotomy is necessary, most structures in the knee joint can be adequately exposed by an anterior approach. The skin over the anterior knee is mobile with its blood supply in the subcutaneous fat. Therefore, anterior approaches should be oriented longitudinally and carried deep to the investing fascia to preserve the collateral blood supply to the skin minimize the risk of devitalizing skin and making repeat operations safer (1). Longitudinal incisions have minimal tension on the wound with knee motion and are therefore compatible with early rehabilitation of the knee. The soft tissues of the knee can be well evaluated by noninvasive imaging such as magnetic resonance imaging (MRI). This allows the surgeon to decide preoperatively precisely where to place his incision.

Severe injuries to the knee, such as traumatic dislocations or tibial plateau fractures, are usually associated with significant crush injury to the skin overlying the knee. Therefore, surgery may need to be delayed or more limited procedures, such as percutaneous fixation or external fixation, may be used to allow adequate fixation without extensive soft tissue dissection.

# Surgical Anatomy

Most of the ligamentous restraining structures in the knee are in the posterior one-third of the joint. The medial and lateral collateral ligaments, as well as the cruciate ligaments, are positioned posteriorly and have the appearance of functioning as a hinge (XII-1). The knee joint is made up of three compartments: the patellofemoral, medial tibiofemoral, and lateral tibiofemoral joints.

The femoral condyles are asymmetric in size and shape (XII-2). The medial femoral condyle is 1.7 cm longer than the lateral in its outer curvature, the asymmetry causing rotation of the tibia on the femur during normal flexion and extension. In the sagittal axis of the condyles, the lateral femoral condyle is longer or taller when viewed end on (XII-3). The distal aspect of the femoral condyles forms a 6° to 7° valgus angle with respect to the long axis of the femoral shaft (XII-4).

The medial tibial condyle is larger than the lateral and provides for greater translation during the flexion/extension arc (XII-5). The articular surface of the lateral tibial condyle is nearly flat. The medial tibial articular surface may be slightly concave, flat, or slightly convex. The menisci function as extensions of the tibial surface, providing symmetric contact between the femur and tibia. The menisci are attached to the tibia by the coronary ligaments on the peripheral edges and attached anteriorly and posteriorly through their specific horns to the tibial eminence (XII-6). The medial meniscus is nonmobile and rigidly fixed to the proximal tibia. The lateral meniscus is more mobile due to its lack of circumferential coronary attachments. Posteriorly, the lateral meniscus has attachments from its posterior horn to the medial femoral condyle by two meniscal-femoral ligaments (2). The ligament of Humphrey courses anterior to the posterior cruciate ligament while the ligament of Wrisberg passes posterior to the posterior cruciate ligament (XII-7).

The joint capsule is divided into medial and lateral portions, each of which is further divided into thirds from anterior to posterior (XII-8). The anterior third of the capsule, both medial and lateral to the patellar ligament, functions as a restraint, providing control of the patella in the femoral trochlea. The medial mid-third of the joint capsule consists of the deep medial collateral ligament and the coronary ligaments, attaching the meniscus to the femur and tibia (XII-9). The posterior one-third of the medial joint capsule is referred to as the posterior oblique ligament. The middle one-third of the lateral capsular ligament is the coronary ligament which may be considered the deep lateral collateral ligament. The posterior one-third of the lateral knee joint capsule is a thickening designated the arcuate ligament (XII-10). The superficial medial collateral ligament originates from the medial femoral epicondyle and inserts 4 cm below the tibiofemoral joint line, deep and posterior to the pes anserinus tendon insertion (XII-11A and XII-11B). The lateral or fibular collateral ligament originates from the lateral femoral epicondyle and inserts onto the fibular head. It is intimately associated with the popliteus tendon that originates from the posterior aspect of the tibia and wraps around and deep to the fibular collateral ligament to insert on the distal lateral edge of the femur. The popliteus tendon sends insertions to the fibular head as well as to the femur (XII-12).

The iliotibial tract inserts on the lateral tibial flare known as Gerdy's tubercle, approximately halfway between the patellar tendon and lateral collateral ligament (XII-13).

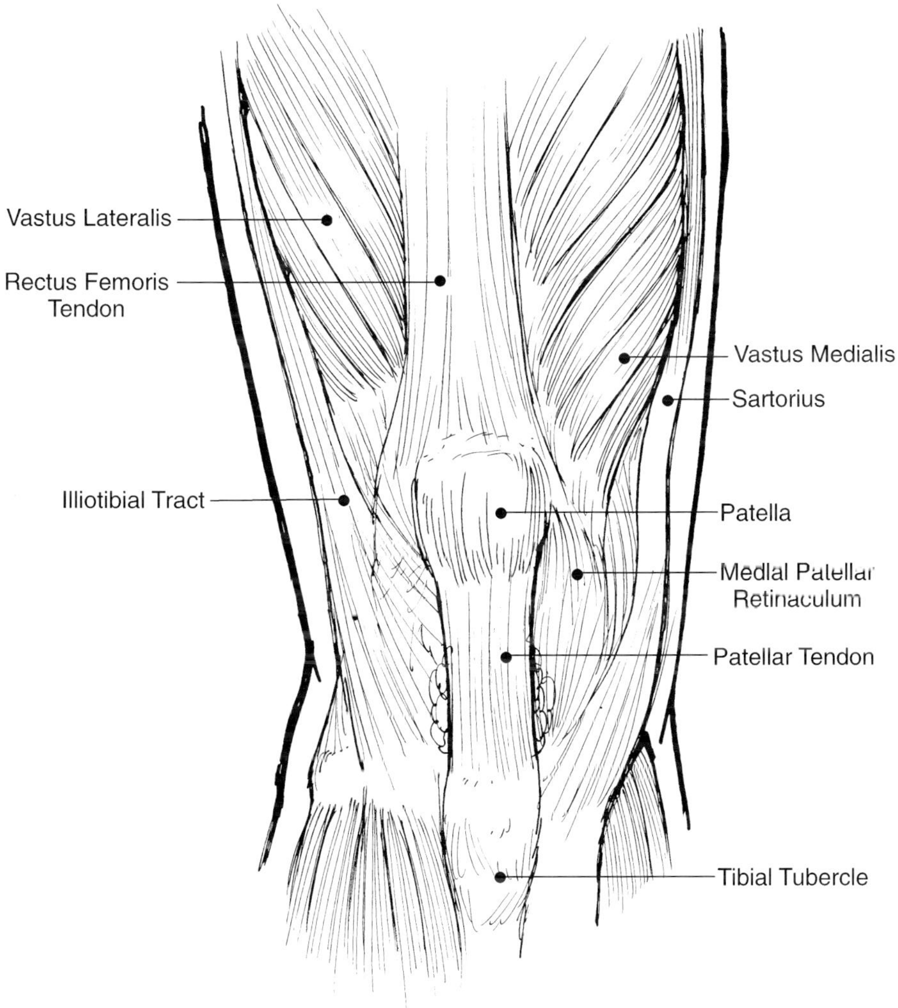


**FIGURE XII-1**

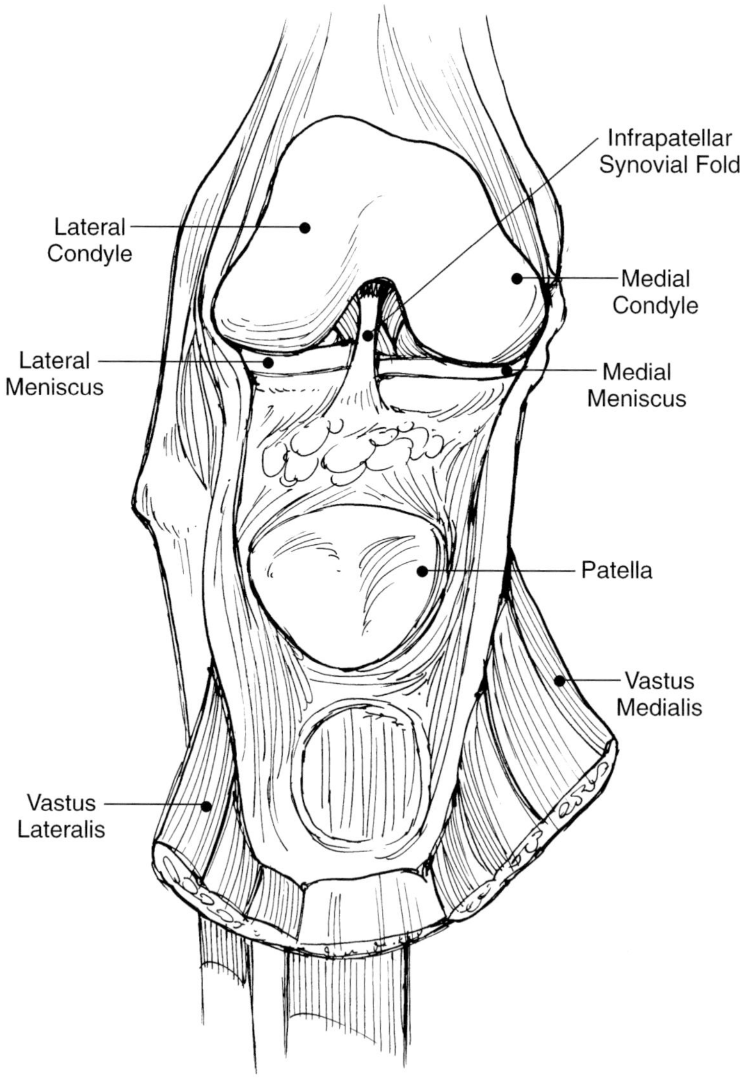
Infrapatellar
Synovial Fold
Lateral
Condyle
Medial
Condyle
Lateral
Meniscus
Medial
Meniscus
Patella
Vastus
Medialis
Vastus
Lateralis

**FIGURE XII-2**

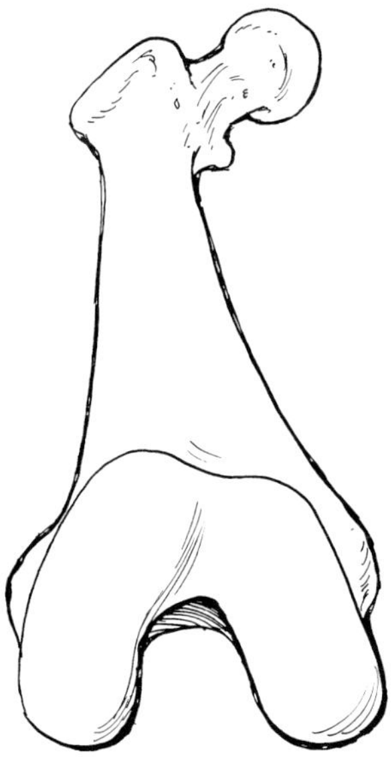

**FIGURE XII-3**

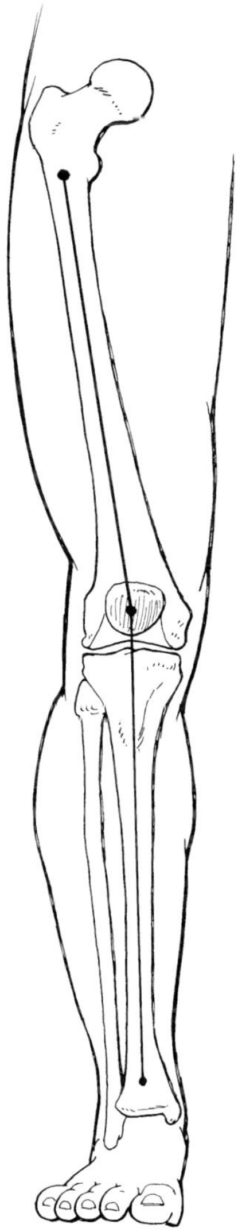

**FIGURE XII-4**

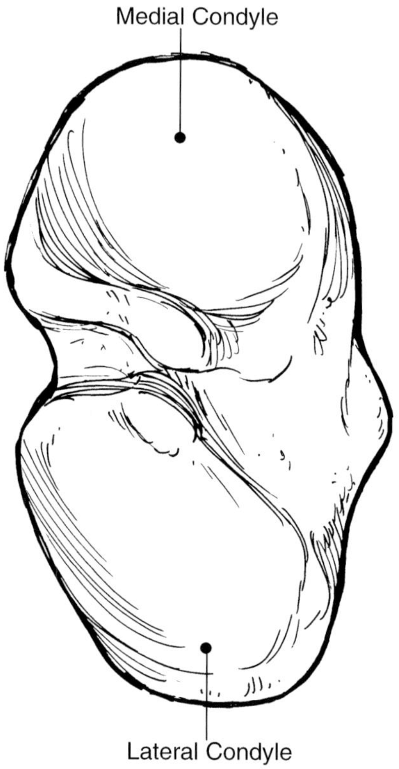


**FIGURE XII-5**

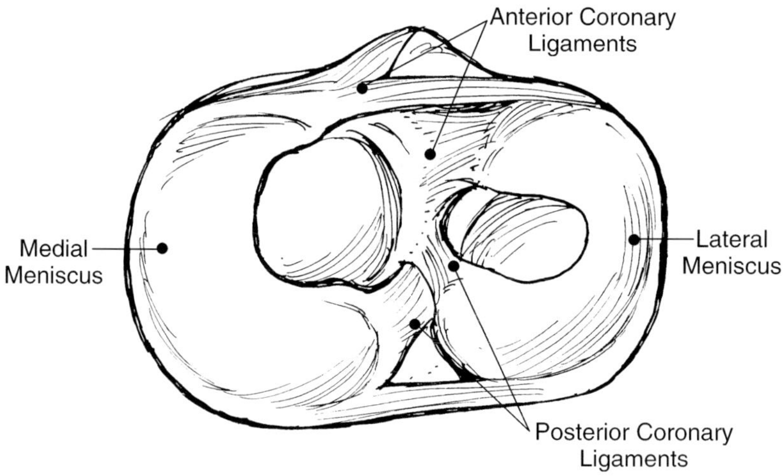


**FIGURE XII-6**

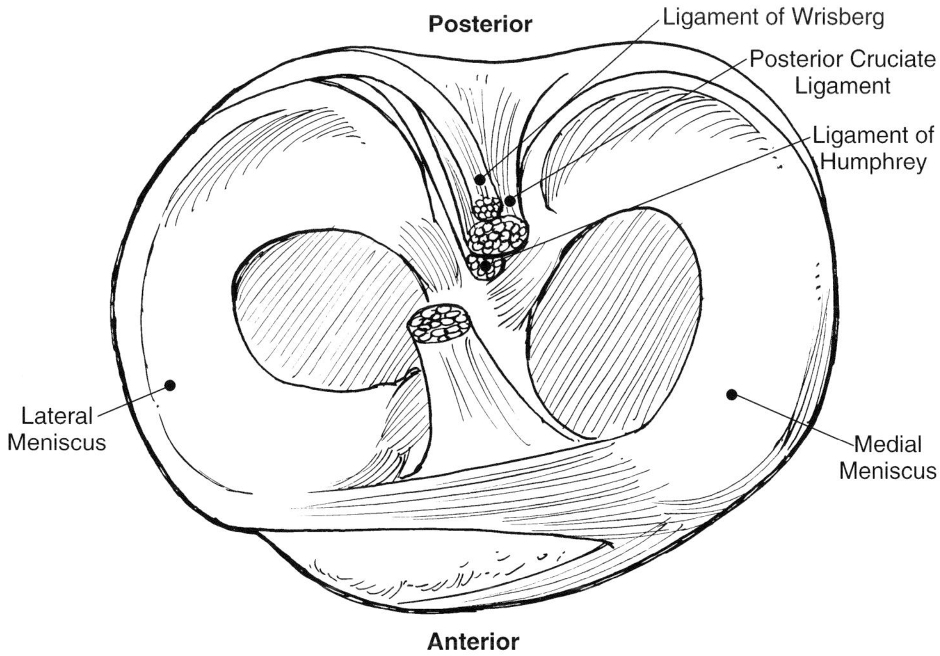


**FIGURE XII-7**

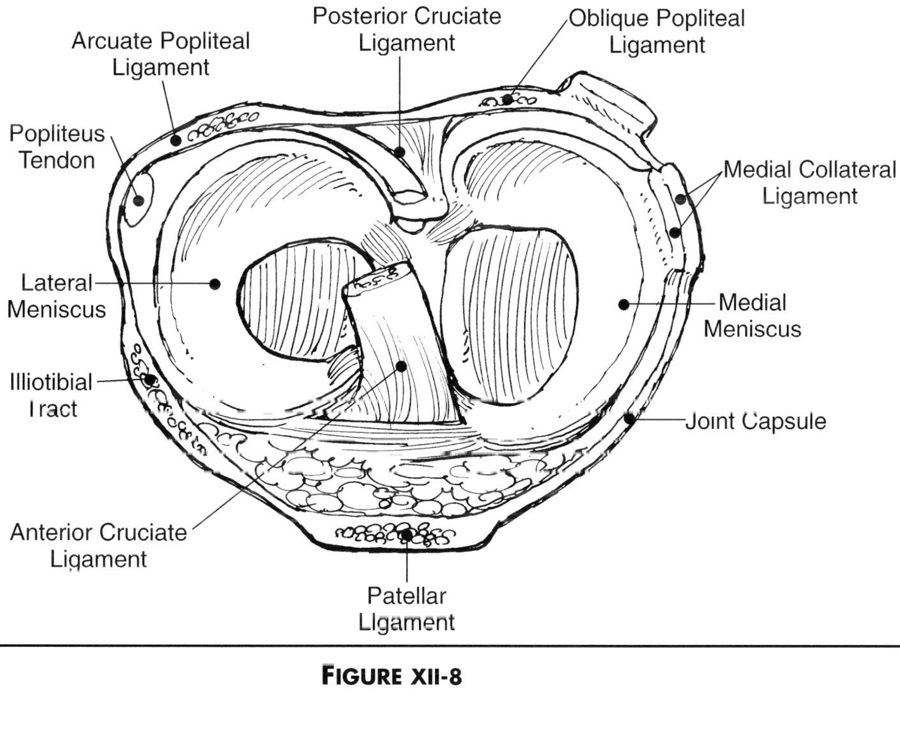


**FIGURE XII-8**

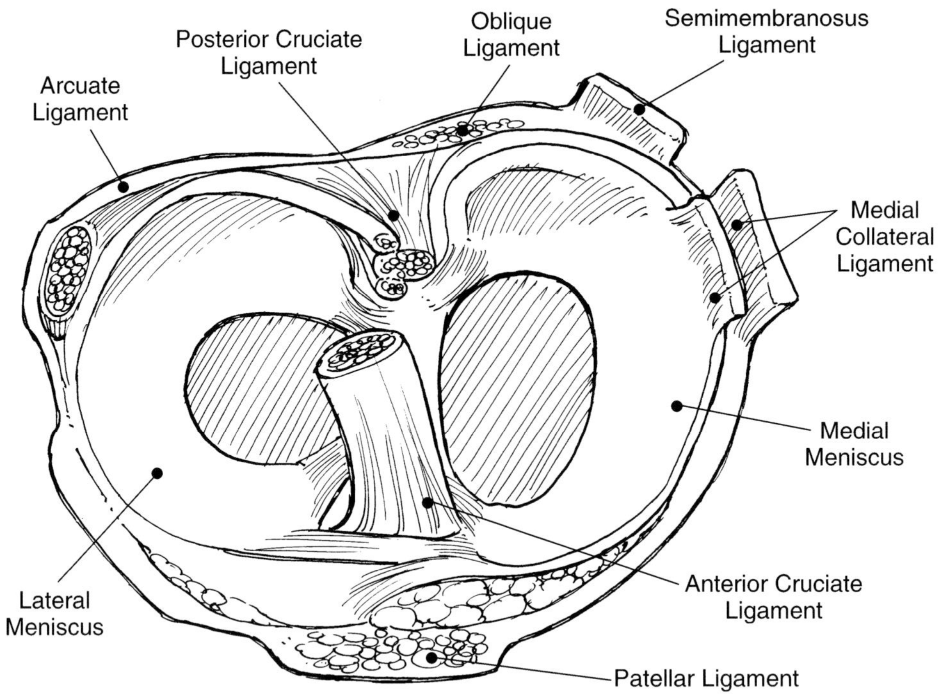


**FIGURE XII-9**

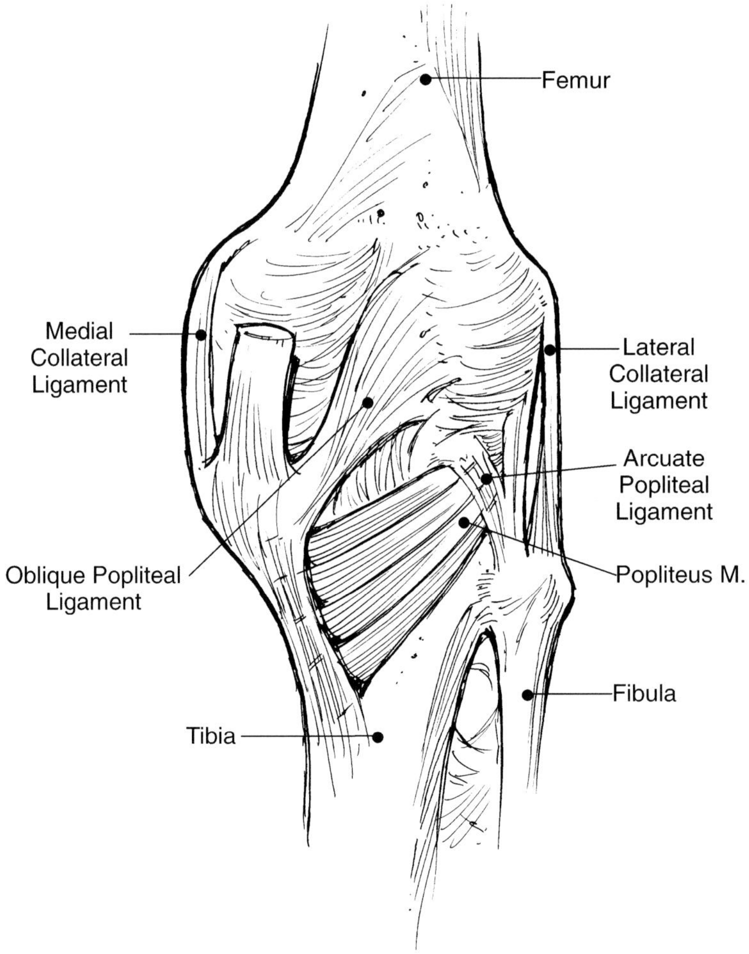


**FIGURE XII-10**

The anterior cruciate ligament originates from the medial aspect of the lateral femoral condyle posteriorly, coursing anteriorly through the notch and inserting into the anterior tibial spine (XII-11A and XII-11B).

The posterior cruciate ligament originates from the lateral surface of the medial femoral condyle approximately 11 mm posterior to the edge of the articular cartilage of the anterior notch. It courses to the posterior aspect of the tibia and inserts into the posterior surface of the tibia (XII-12).

The femoral artery becomes the popliteal artery at the adductor hiatus. The popliteal artery trifurcates at the level of the soleus leash (XII-13). Through its course in the popliteal fossa, the artery gives off numerous muscular branches and five articular branches. The middle genicular artery arises from the anterior aspect of the popliteal artery and pierces the knee joint, providing blood supply to the capsular structures and cruciate ligaments. The superior medial and lateral genicular arteries course anteriorly around the femoral condyles, supplying the patella and skin of the anterior knee. The inferior medial and lateral genicular arteries course anteriorly at the level of the joint line (XII-14). The popliteal vein courses through the popliteal fossa, changing from a lateral to a medial position in relationship to the artery. The common peroneal nerve arises from the sciatic nerve and courses around the lateral head of the gastrocnemius, posterior and medial to the biceps tendon to cross the neck of the fibula (XII-15). Because of its superficial course and exposure against the fibular neck, the peroneal nerve is prone to injury.

## Anterior Approach to the Knee

***Applications***

The anterior approach to the knee allows for exploration of the knee joint, synovectomy, fracture fixation, and. total knee arthroplasty.

***Technique***

The patient is placed in a supine position and a small linen roll is placed under the ipsilateral buttock. A tourniquet is applied on the proximal thigh. A straight. incision, beginning proximal to the superior pole of the patella is carried distally, directly over the patellar tendon and medial to the tibial tubercle (XII-16). The quadriceps tendon is incised, medial to the patella and then medial to the tibial tubercle (XII-17). A cuff of capsule at least 5 mm in width should be preserved on the medial edge of the patella for closure.

***Dangers***

Extensive subcutaneous dissection about the anterior knee can devitalize the skin. Inadequate longitudinal release of the quadriceps tendon can result in avulsion of the tendon from the tibial tuberosity.

***Limitations***

This incision allows exposure of the anterior knee, distal femur, and proximal tibia. The tibial tubercle and patellar tendon limit exposure of the lateral knee joint.

## Lateral Approach to the Knee

***Applications***

The lateral approach is useful for open reduction, internal fixation of distal femoral condyle fractures, and open anterior cruciate ligament reconstruction.

***Technique***

The patient is positioned supine with a small bolster under the ipsilateral hip. The incision is placed over the lateral side of the lateral femoral condyle, anterior to the iliotibial band and is carried distally over Gerdy's tubercle (XII-18). The fascia lata is opened parallel to the skin incision, anterior to the iliotibial band (XII-19). The vastus lateralis is elevated off of the lateral intermuscular septum, and perforating

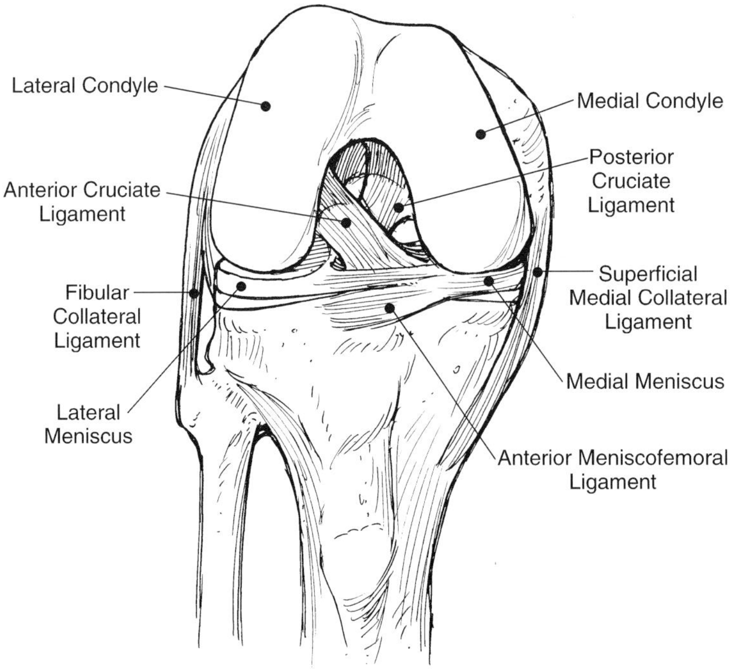


**FIGURE XII-11A**

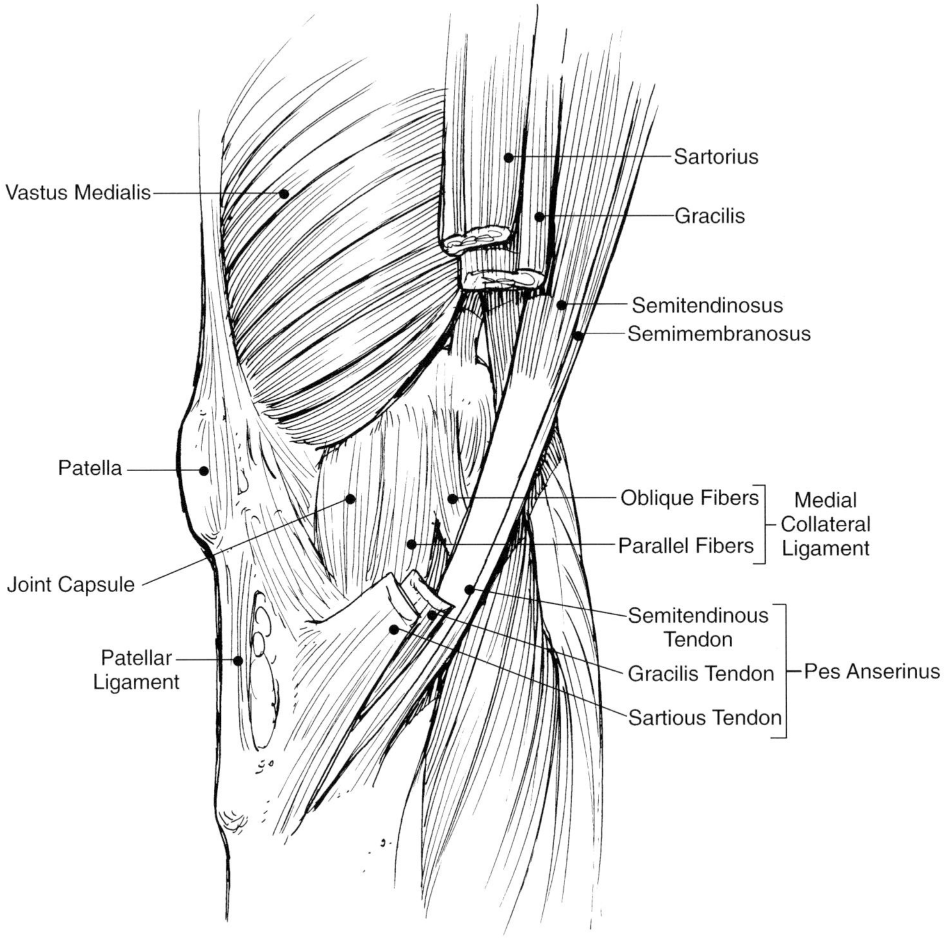


**FIGURE XII-11B**

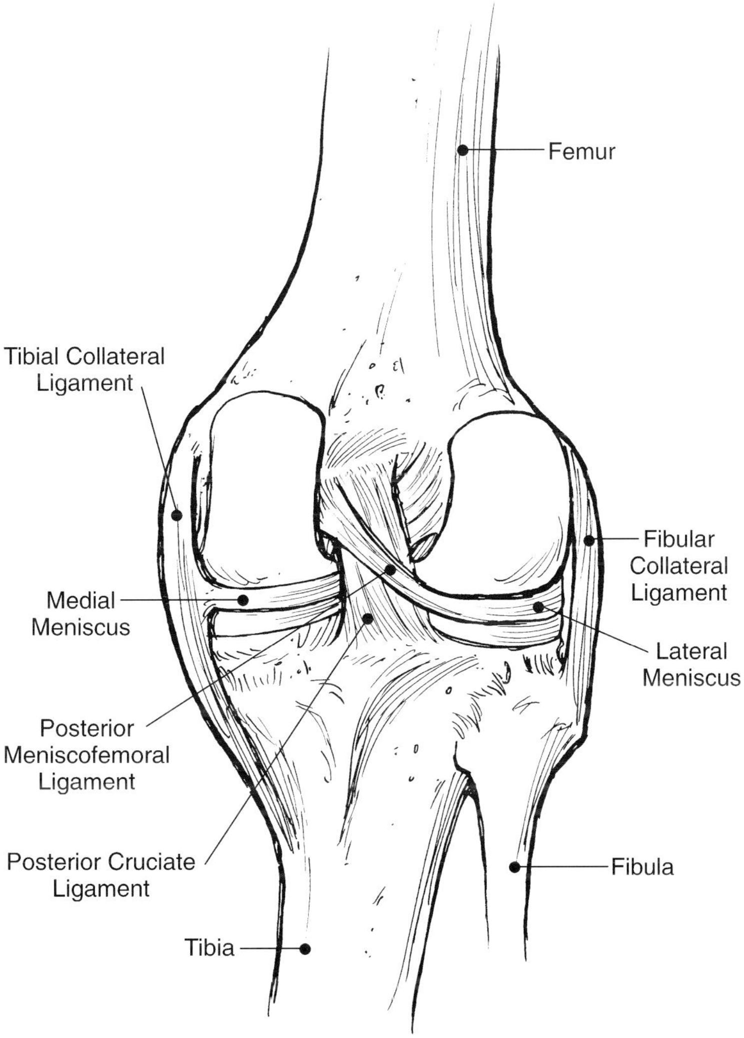


**FIGURE XII-12**

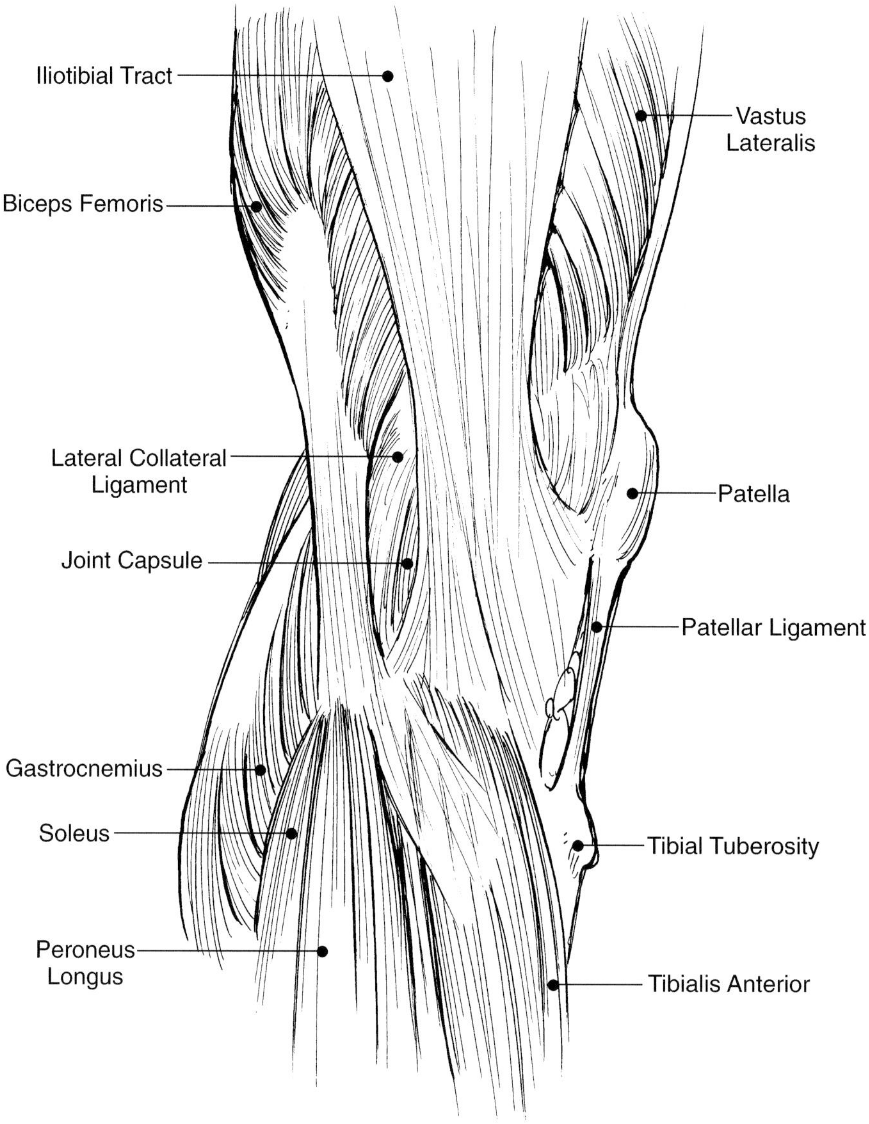


**FIGURE XII-13**

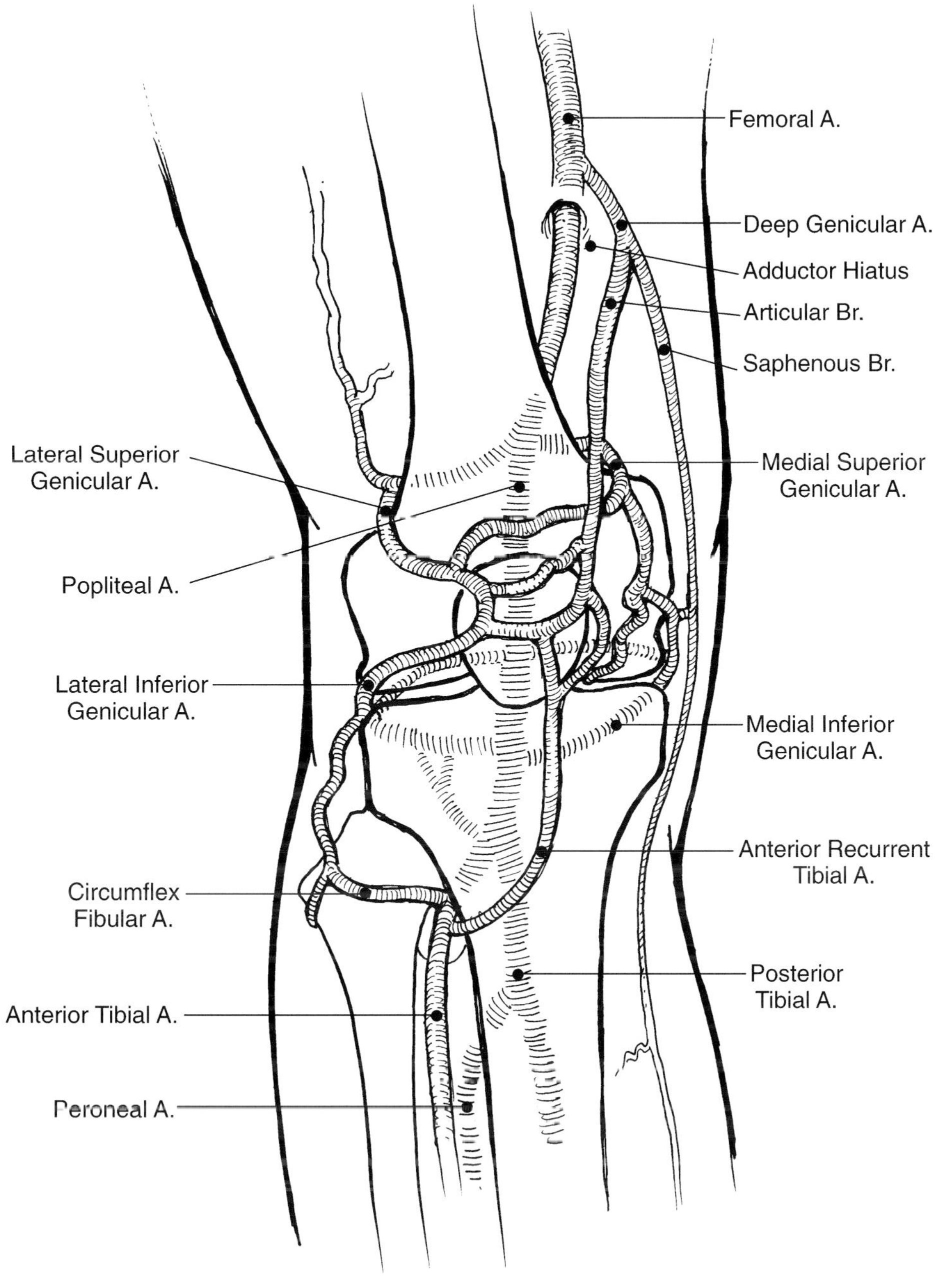


**FIGURE XII-14**

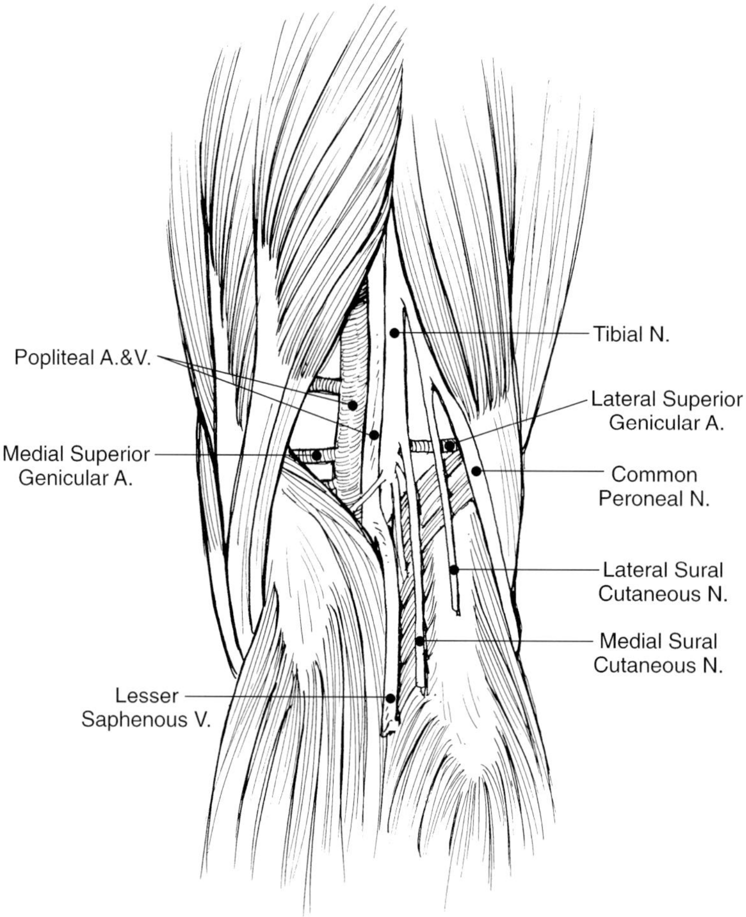


**FIGURE XII-15**

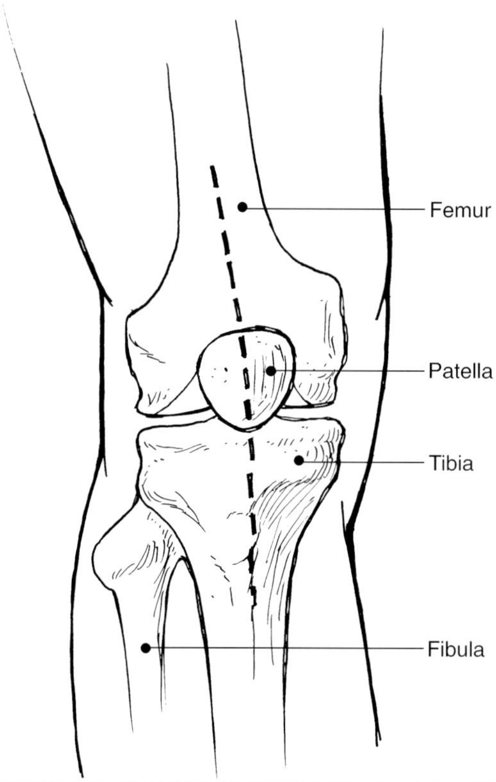


**FIGURE XII-16**

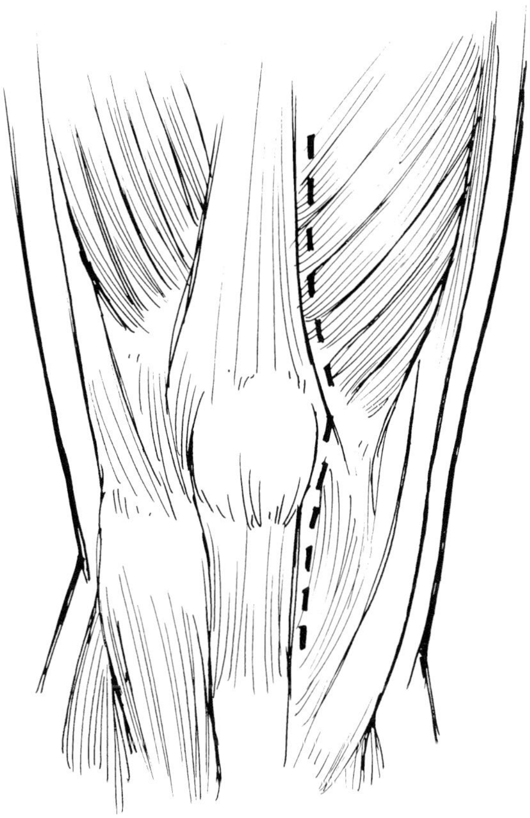

**FIGURE XII-17**

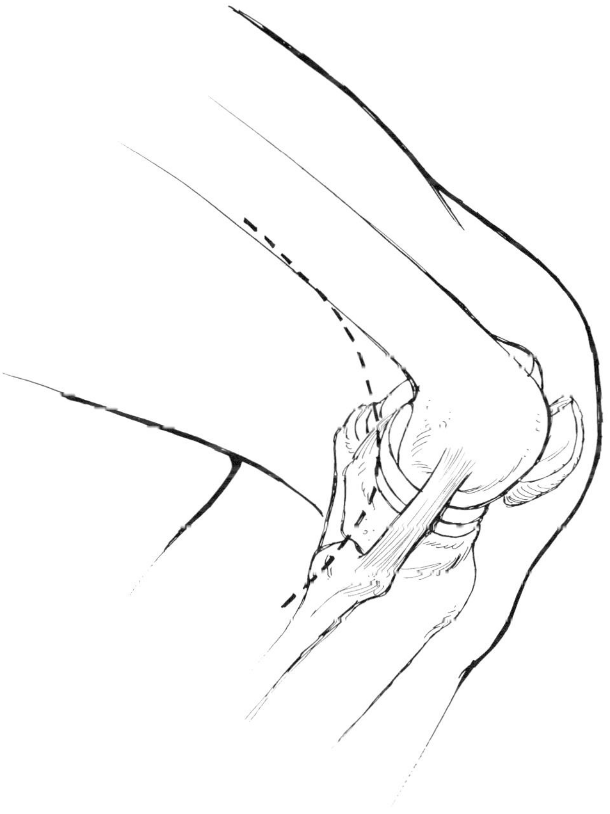

**FIGURE XII-18**

vessels are ligated. Retractors are placed subperiosteally over the anterior aspect of the femur, exposing the entire distal aspect of the lateral femur (XII-20). The patellofemoral joint can be exposed by incising the lateral transverse patellar ligament.

***Dangers***

Excessive bleeding can be caused by splitting the vastus lateralis muscle through its belly and losing control of the perforating vessels.

***Limitations***

Posterior exposure in the knee is limited by the fibular collateral ligament and common peroneal nerve.

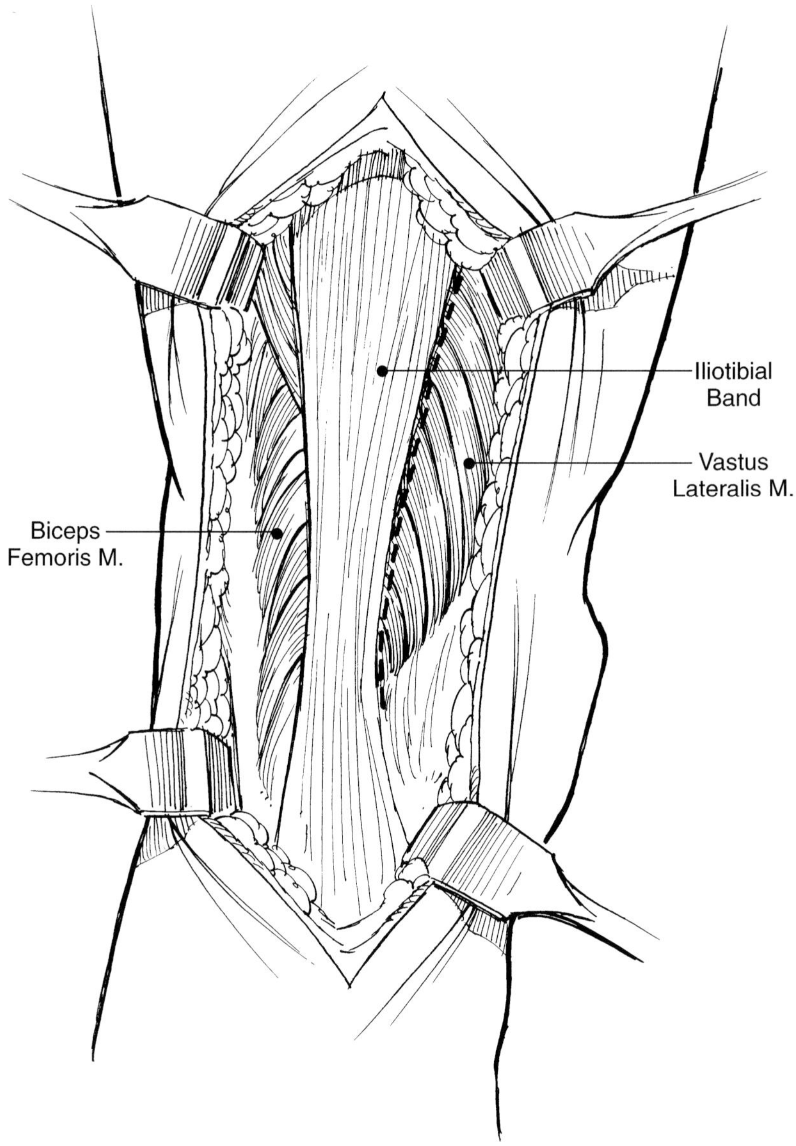


**FIGURE XII-19**

# Posteromedial Approach to the Knee

### *Applications*

The posteromedial approach is very useful for access to the vascular structures of the popliteal fossa and is the utilitarian approach to the vessels in the popliteal fossa. Therefore, it is especially useful for repair of vascular injuries associated with joint injuries such as traumatic dislocation. This exposure also allows exploration and repair of the knee joint structures including the menisci and the cruciate and medial collateral ligaments.

### *Technique*

The incision is placed along the posterior aspect of the medial femur, over the adductor (Hunter's) canal, and courses distally along the posterior edge of the proximal tibia, into the leg (XII-21). The saphenous vein is identified and should be protected if possible. The saphenous nerve should be retracted with the skin flap and saphenous vein to avoid neuroma formation. The tendons of the pes

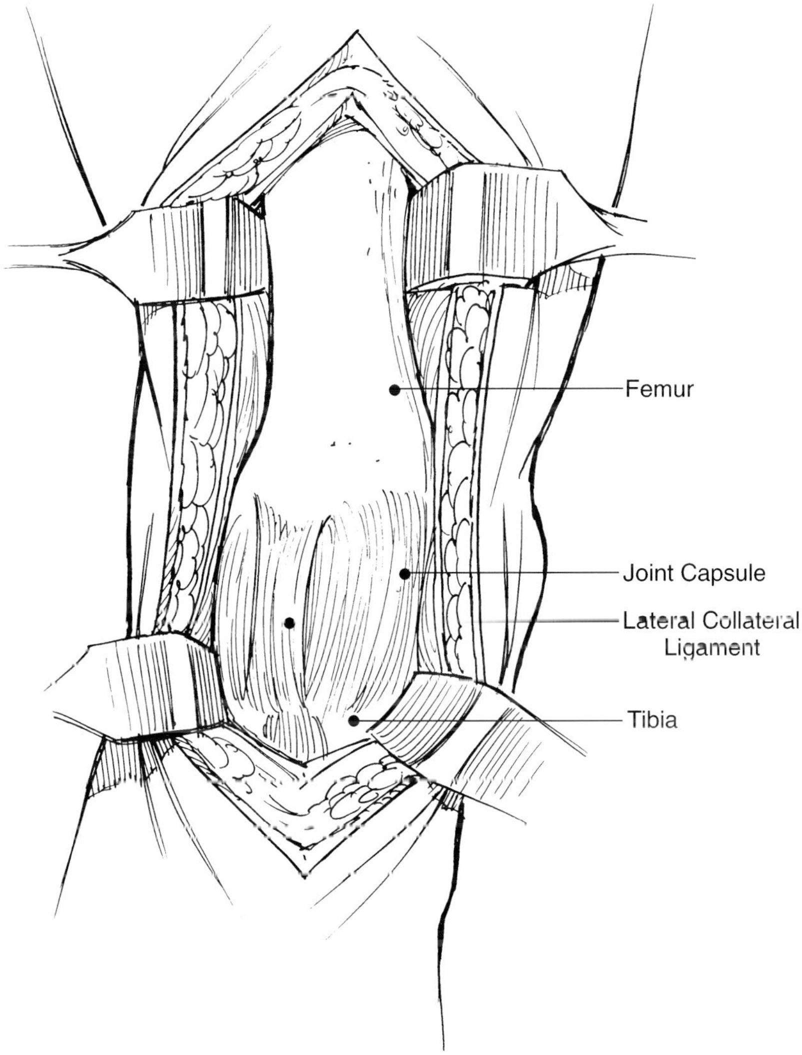


**FIGURE XII-20**

anserinus are transected 2 cm proximal to their tibial insertion. The proximal portion of the pes is reflected with the posterior flap, and the distal portion of the pes is reflected anteriorly. This allows exposure to the medial gastrocnemius (XII-22). The medial gastrocnemius head may be detached from the medial femur to allow exposure of the popliteal artery from Hunter's canal to the trifurcation (XII-23).

***Dangers***

It is easy to inadvertently dissect posterior to the medial gastrocnemius belly. Keeping the knee flexed to relax the muscle will make it easier to identify the plane anterior to the gastrocnemius. Damage to the saphenous nerve can produce persistent medial knee pain from a traumatic neuroma. The incision should be placed posteriorly, over the muscle bellies in the leg since incisions directly over the tibia can result in skin necrosis. .

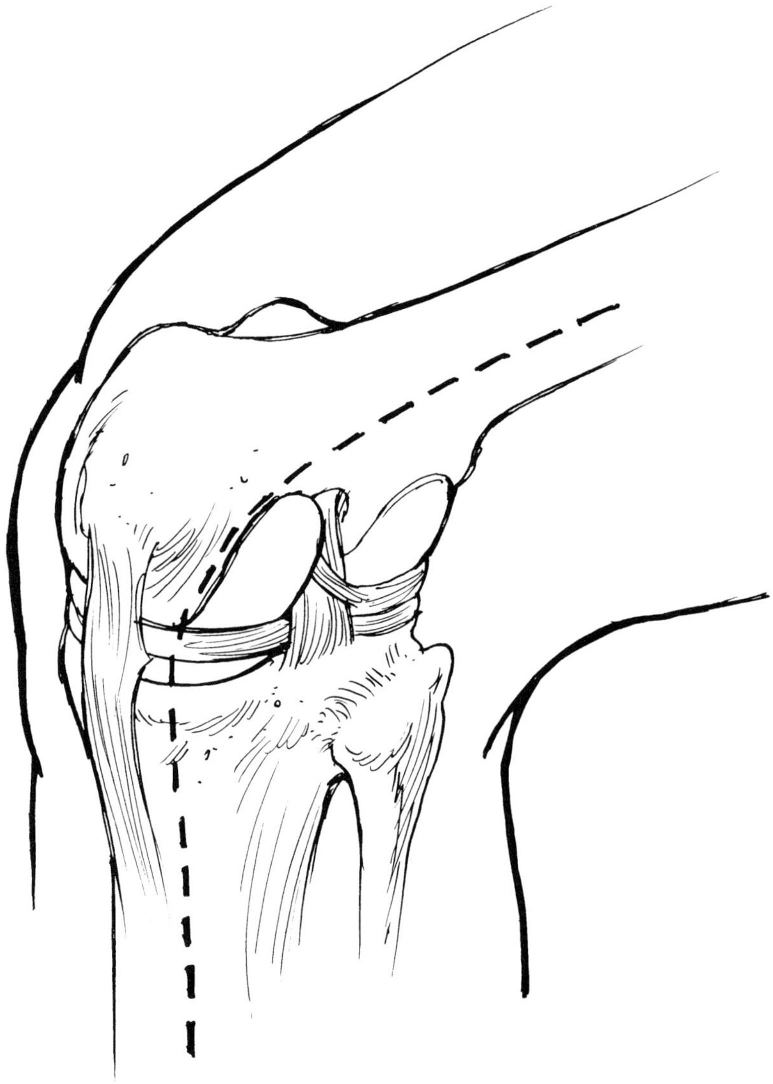

**FIGURE XII-21**

*Limitations*

Access to the lateral side of the knee is limited; however, in the presence of a knee dislocation and evidence of medial collateral ligament insufficiency, capsular structures are usually completely disrupted, allowing clear exposure of the knee joint.

# Posterolateral Approach to the Knee

*Applications*

This approach is useful for reconstruction of the posterolateral joint capsule, mobilization of the lateral gastrocnemius muscle for use as a muscle pedicle flap and exploration and repair of the common peroneal nerve. It is frequently useful in knee dislocations for reattachment or repair of the cruciate ligaments and the lateral collateral structures. The peroneal nerve is always isolated prior to deep joint exposure, and because of the injuries to the lateral knee in dislocations, the ligaments are frequently disrupted from the patellar tendon, posterior to the medial aspect of the knee joint. This allows exposure of the tibiofemoral joint by placing the tibia in varus.

*Technique*

The patient is placed in the lateral position with a tourniquet on the thigh. The skin incision is placed posterior to the fibular head and carried in a straight line posterior to the biceps femoris tendon onto the lateral thigh (XII-24). The incision is carried down to the deep fascia, which is then opened with scissors at the level of the fibular neck to mobilize the common peroneal nerve (XII-25). The nerve is mobilized proximally and distally. This allows exposure of the fibular collateral ligament and the lateral gastrocnemius muscle belly. The knee joint is best exposed

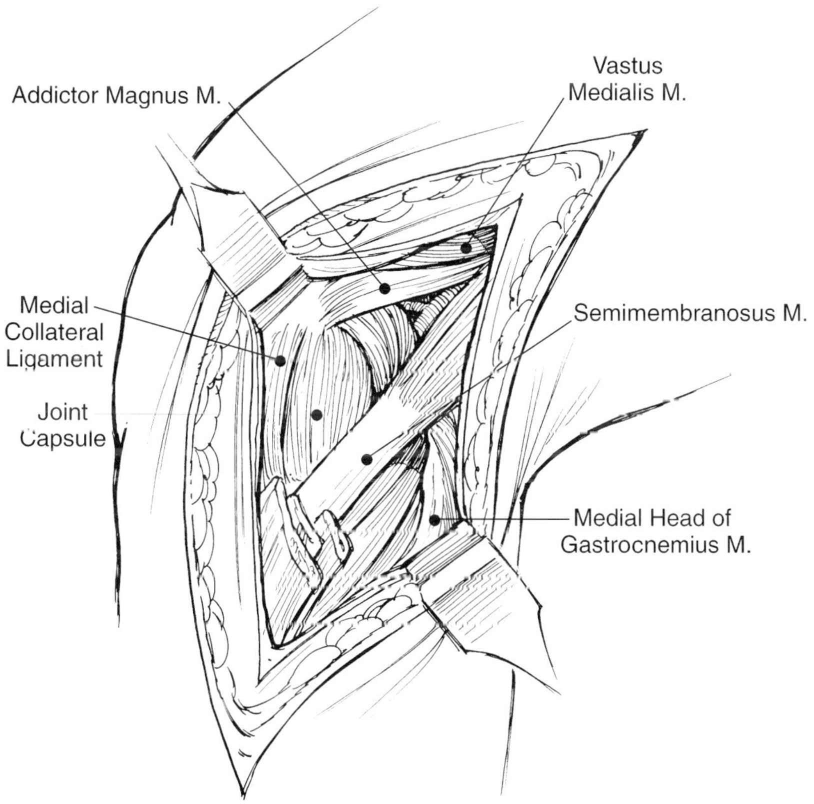


**FIGURE XII-22**

with the knee flexed to 90°. This allows relaxation of the peroneal nerve and makes visualization easier (XII-25).

Blunt dissection is used to define the plane anterior to the lateral gastrocnemius head.

***Dangers***

This approach should always include exposure of the peroneal nerve prior to deep dissection. The peroneal nerve is best isolated proximally and dissected distally as it winds along the fibular neck. Straying posterior to the gastrocnemius places the popliteal neurovascular structures at risk.

***Limitations***

This approach provides minimal access to the medial side of the knee. If the lateral collateral ligaments are intact, the posterior cruciate ligament cannot be identified from this approach.

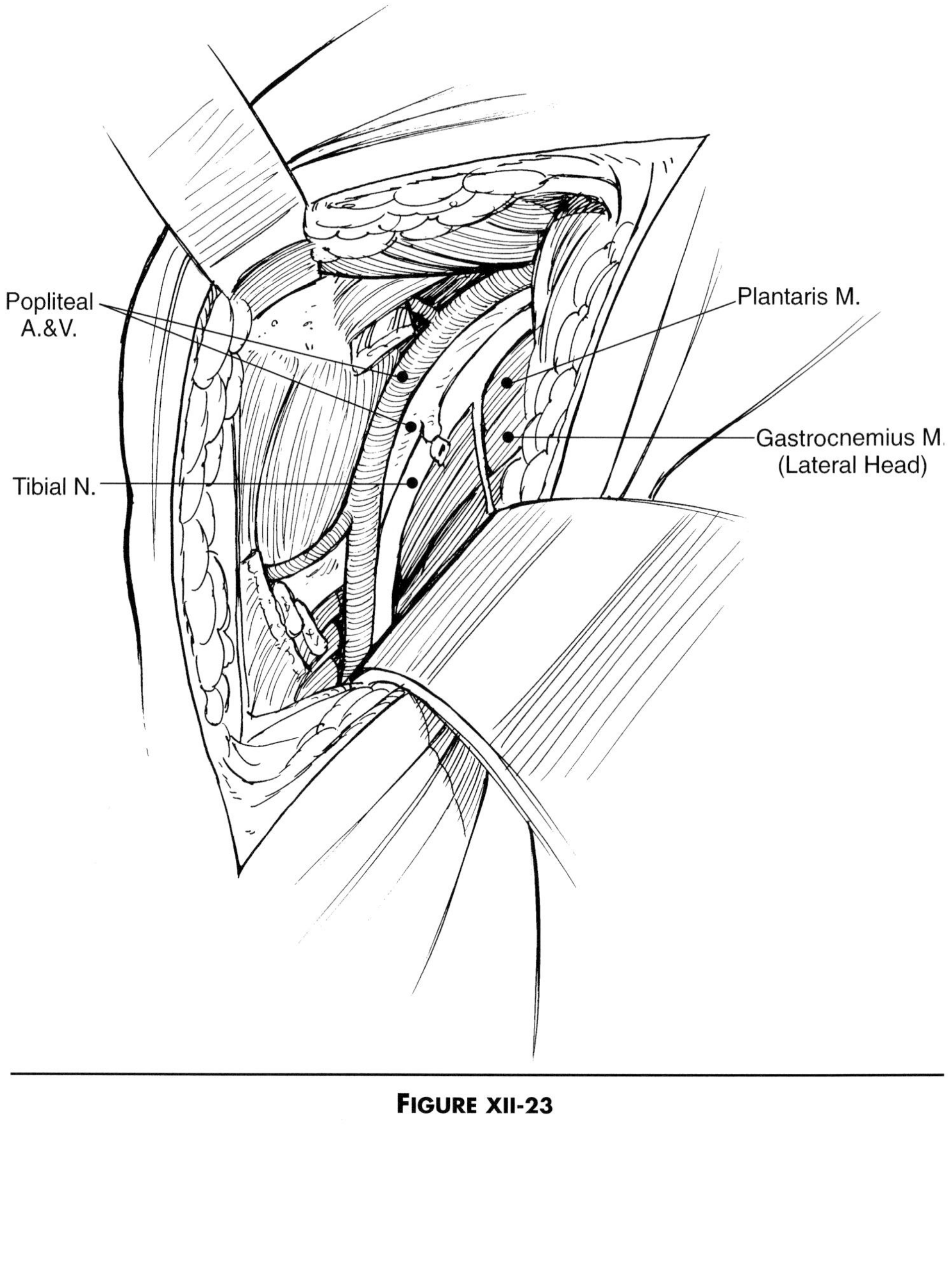


**FIGURE XII-23**

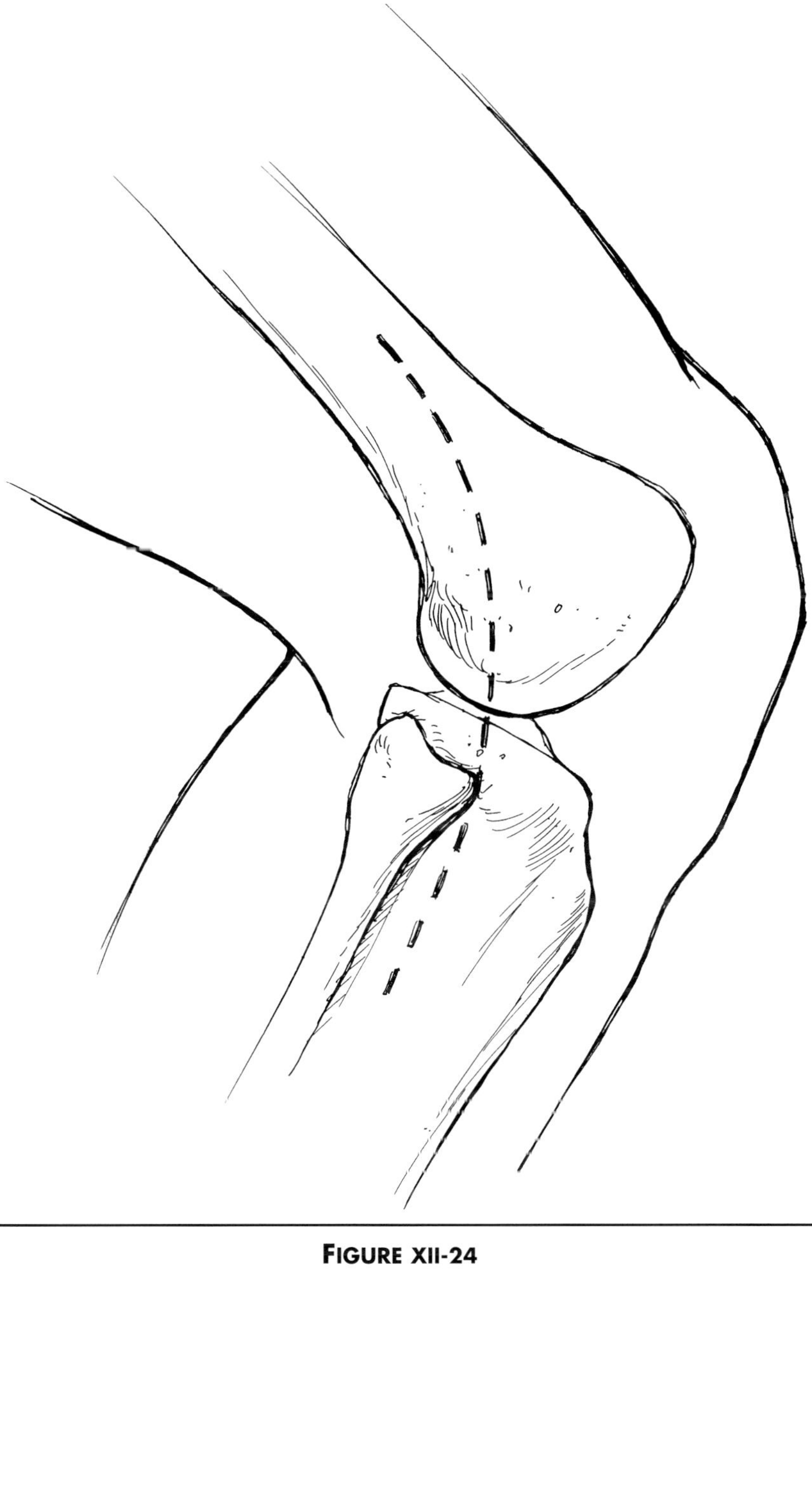

**FIGURE XII-24**

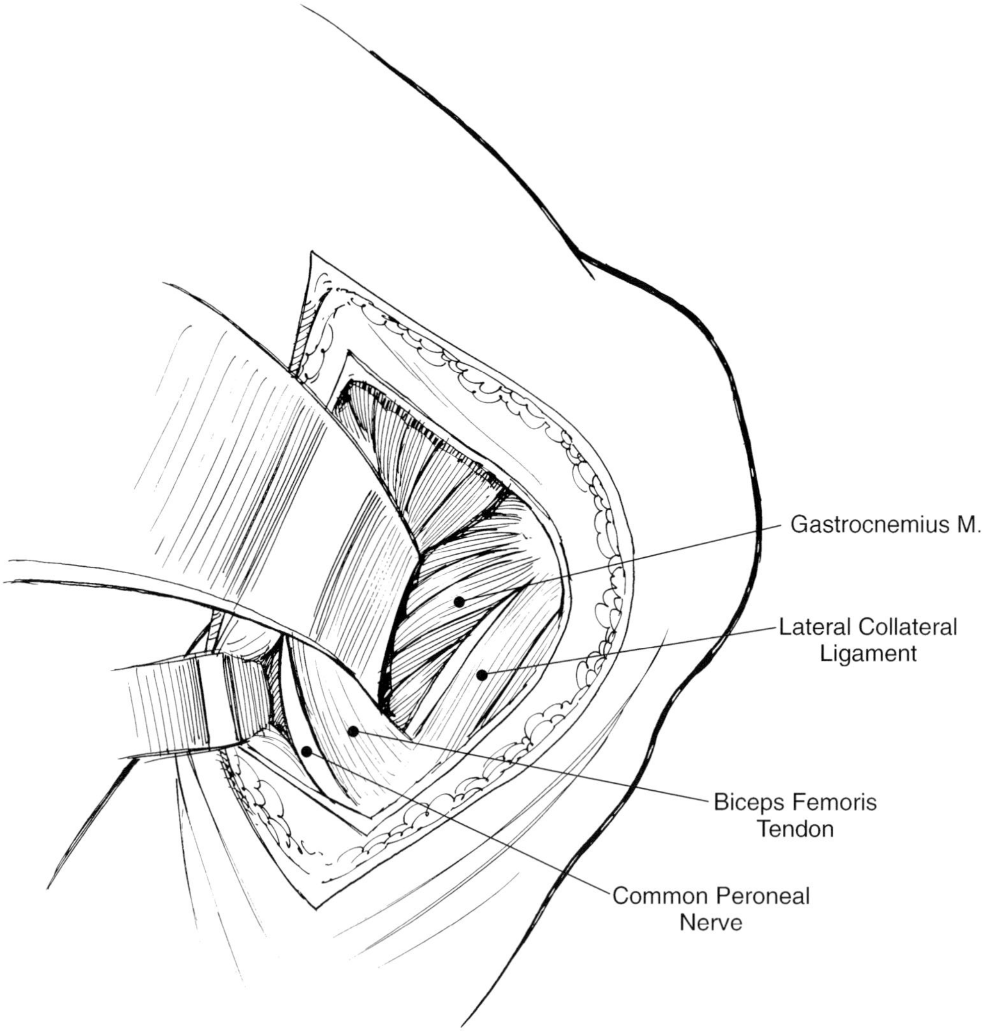


**FIGURE XII-25**

# Posterior Approach to the Knee

*Applications*

This approach provides access to the popliteal fossa, posterior surface of the femoral condyles, posterior knee capsule, and posterior aspect of the distal tibia. It is useful for resection of tumors from the popliteal fossa or posterior knee, nerve or blood vessel exploration, and reattachment of posterior cruciate ligament avulsions.

*Technique*

The patient is placed in a prone position. A tourniquet is placed on the thigh. The skin incision begins posteromedially over the semitendinous and semimembranosus tendons, curves transversely across the knee flexion crease, and then proceeds laterally over the fibular head and fibula (XII-26). The sural nerve and short saphenous vein are identified and followed proximally to the trunk of the popliteal vein (XII-27). The short saphenous vein and sural nerve pierce the fascia of the posterior knee in the area of the distal flexion crease. The medial and lateral gas-

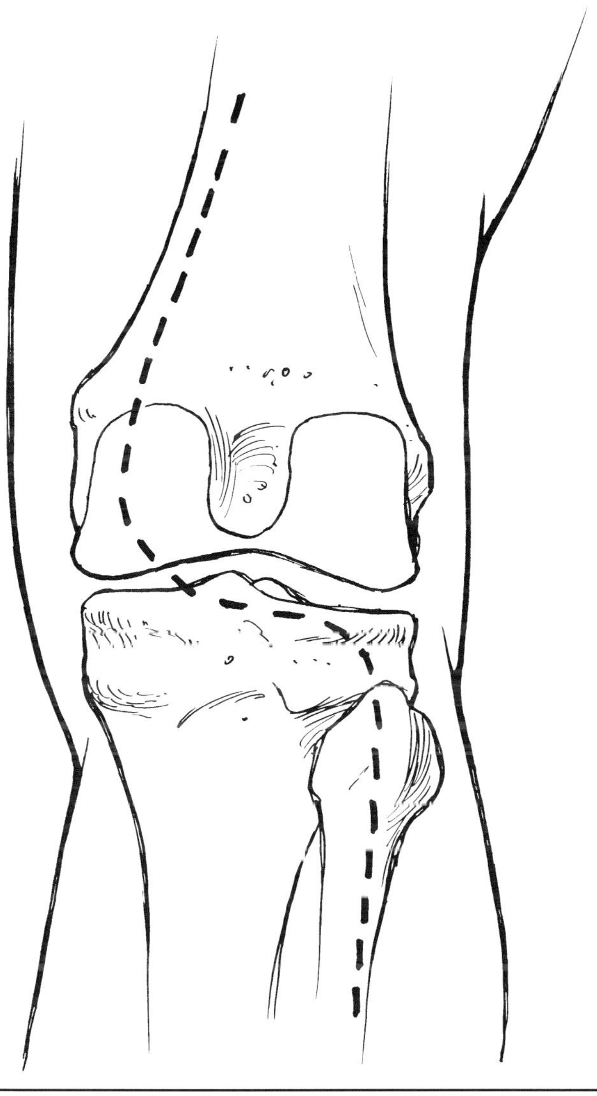

**FIGURE XII-26**

trocnemius muscle heads are identified. The popliteal nerve, vein, and artery are exposed with ligation of the genicular branches as required (XII-28). It is best to approach the vessels from the medial, proximal end, working distally. The vessels and nerve may be retracted together, or alternatively, the vessels may be retracted medially and the nerve laterally. Exposure of the femoral and tibial surface is performed through the neurovascular interval with care to protect these structures. Distally, the popliteus muscle is found on the posterior aspect of the tibia and can be retracted to allow exposure of the proximal tibia (XII-29). Blunt dissection is safest for access to the proximal tibia. This is best performed with a finger to avoid injury to the neurovascular bundle. Release of the medial gastrocnemius head can be performed to allow better exposure of the proximal tibia.

***Dangers***

The greatest danger is potential injury to the neurovascular structures of the popliteal fossa that are directly exposed in this approach.

***Limitations***

Because the patient is in a prone position, access to the anterior knee is difficult, making reconstruction of the posterior cruciate ligament impossible. This approach should not be used for biopsy of potentially malignant neoplasms because of the contamination of the neurovascular structures.

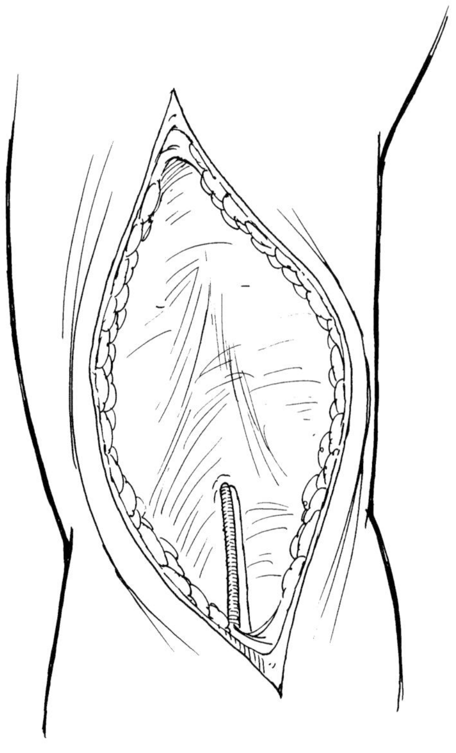

**FIGURE XII-27**

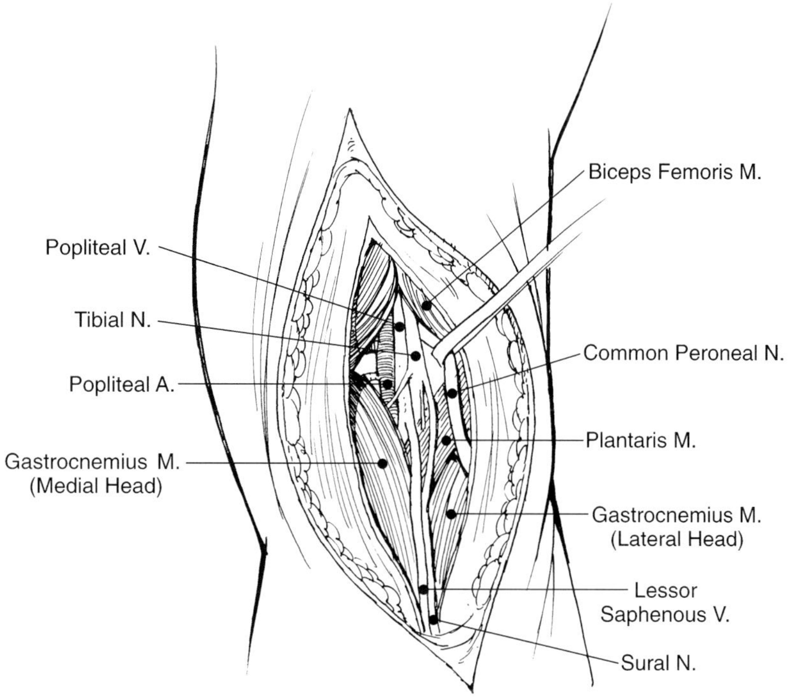


**FIGURE XII-28**

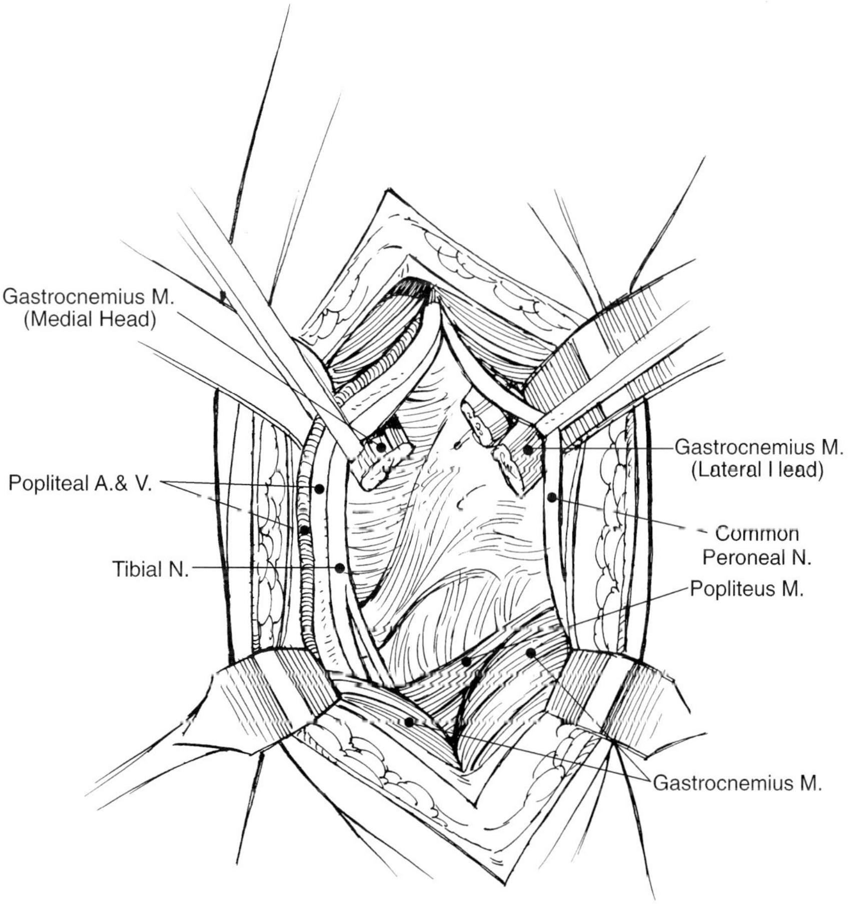


**FIGURE XII-29**

# References

1. Insall JN. Surgical approaches to the knee. In: Insall JN, ed. Surgery of the Knee. New York: Churchill Livingstone, 1984:41–54.
2. Insall JN. Anatomy of the knee. In: Insall JN, ed. Surgery of the Knee. New York: Churchill Livingstone, 1984:1–40.

# XIII

# SURGICAL APPROACHES TO THE LEG

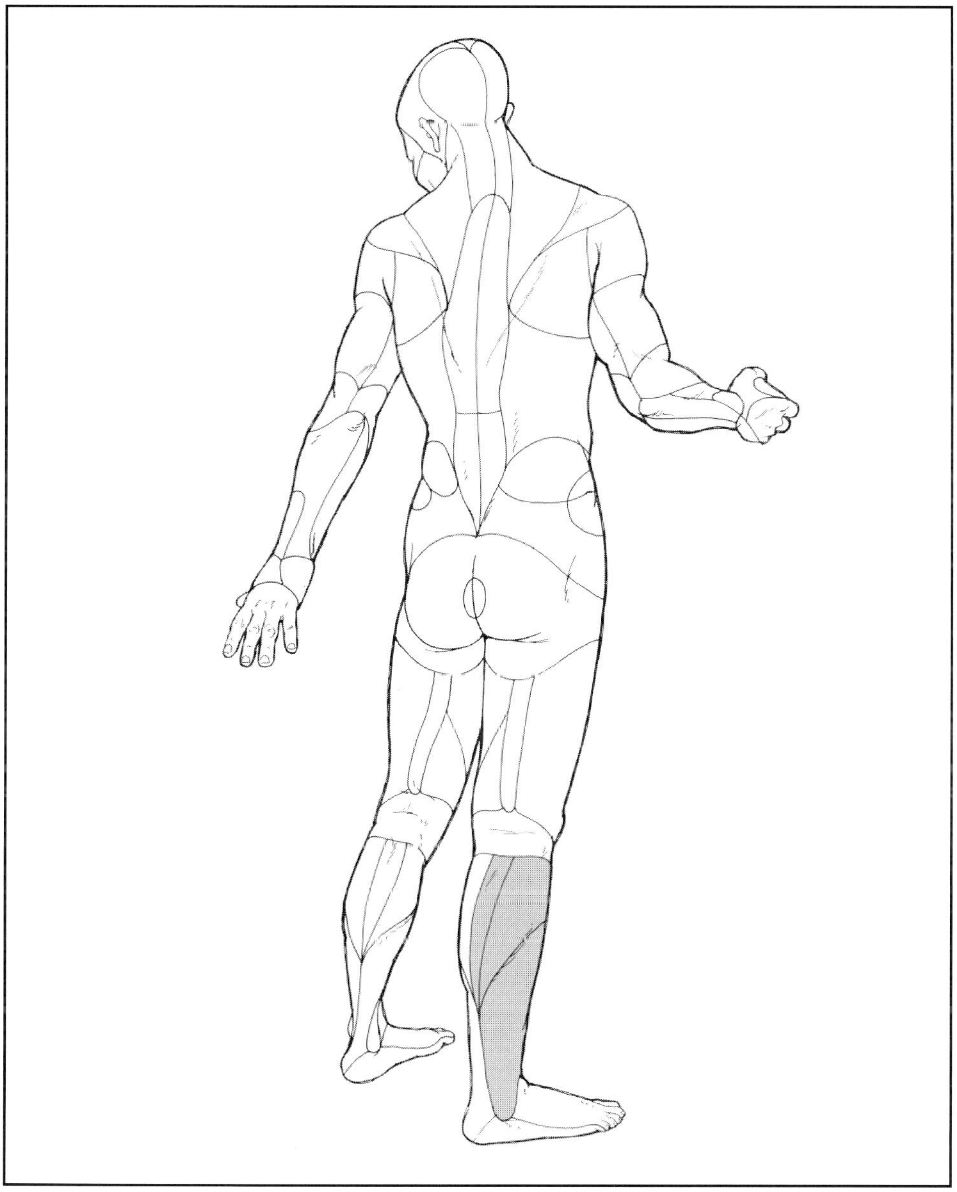

## General Principles and Complications

Most operations on the leg are done for acute management and reconstruction of tibial fractures. The tibia is the major weight-bearing bone of the leg. In contrast to the femur, it has much less muscle coverage and includes mostly cortical bone and, therefore, has a relatively poor blood supply. Thus, delayed healing, nonunion, and osteomyelitis are routine problems in dealing with tibial fractures. The proximal fibula (up to 20 cm in an adult) may be excised for use as a bone graft as long as the distal interosseous membrane and syndesmotic ligaments are left intact to preserve the ankle mortise. In general, the principles of management of tibial fractures involve: 1. prevention or eradication of infection, 2. provision of adequate blood supply and soft tissue coverage to the bone, and 3. reconstruction of bony defects. Preservation of the foot by multiple, staged reconstructions of the leg must be weighed against the functional results obtained with a below knee amputation. Even though it may be technically possible to reconstruct any or all of the components of the leg (bone, nerves, arteries, and muscle defects), the cost to the patient in terms of years off of work, limited mobility, and a painful, poorly functional foot may not be acceptable.

## Surgical Anatomy

The leg is divided into three compartments. The anterior (extensor) compartment contains the tibialis anterior, extensor hallucis longus, extensor digitorum communis, and peroneus tertius (XIII-1). It is bordered by the tibia, the fibula, and the anterior intermuscular septum. The muscles are supplied by the deep peroneal nerve and anterior tibial artery. The lateral (peroneal) compartment contains the peroneus longus and peroneus brevis (XIII-2). They are supplied by the superficial peroneal nerve and the perforating branches of the peroneal artery. The lateral compartment is bounded by the anterior and posterior intermuscular septa (XIII-3). The posterior (flexor) compartment is bounded by the posterior intermuscular septum, tibia, fibula, and interosseous membrane. The muscles of the posterior compartment are divided into a superficial group (XIII-4) (gastrocnemius, soleus, and plantaris) and a deep group (XIII-5) (tibialis posterior, flexor digitorum longus, and flexor hallucis longus). The muscles are supplied by the tibial nerve and posterior tibial artery, which run between the two groups (XIII-6). The long saphenous vein originates anterior to the medial malleolus and ascends subcutaneously along the medial leg.

The common peroneal nerve passes posterior to the tendon of the biceps femoris to enter the leg and then curves anteriorly deep to the fascia to wrap around the fibular neck. It enters the substance of the peroneus longus and splits into deep and superficial branches. The deep peroneal nerve continues anteriorly into the extensor digitorum longus to descend along the anterior surface of the interosseous membrane. The superficial peroneal nerve continues distally in the peroneus longus to supply the lateral compartment (XIII-7).

The anterior tibial artery is a terminal branch of the popliteal artery. It enters the anterior compartment by passing proximal to the interosseous membrane to run along the anterior surface of the membrane with the deep peroneal nerve. It continues into the foot as the dorsalis pedis artery. The posterior tibial artery, the longitudinal continuation of the popliteal artery, passes anterior to the soleus to descend in the posterior compartment. The peroneal artery arises from the posterior tibial artery close to its origin and passes anteriorly through the deep posterior compartment to descend on the posterior interosseous membrane just medial to the fibula. It sends perforating branches into the lateral compartment.

# Anterior Approach to the Tibia

***Applications***

The anterior approach provides safe, direct access to the tibia. It is useful for open reduction and internal fixation of fractures (1), biopsy of tumors, and sequestrectomy for osteomyelitis.

***Technique***

The patient is supine. The incision is placed approximately 1 cm lateral to the anterior crest of the tibia (XIII-8). It may be extended longitudinally as far as necessary. The fascia is incised in line with the skin incision. The lateral surface of the tibia is exposed by retracting and reflecting the tibialis anterior muscle subperiosteally

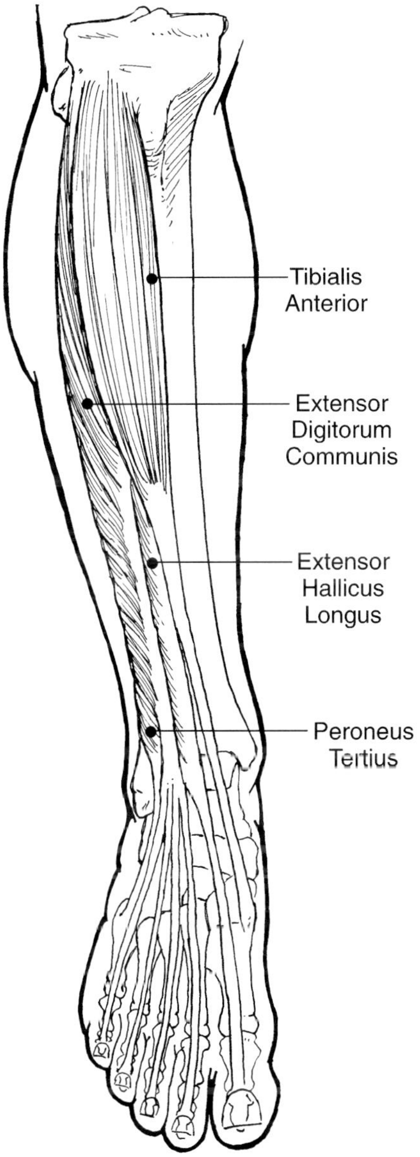


**Anterior (Extensor) Compartment**

**FIGURE XIII-1**

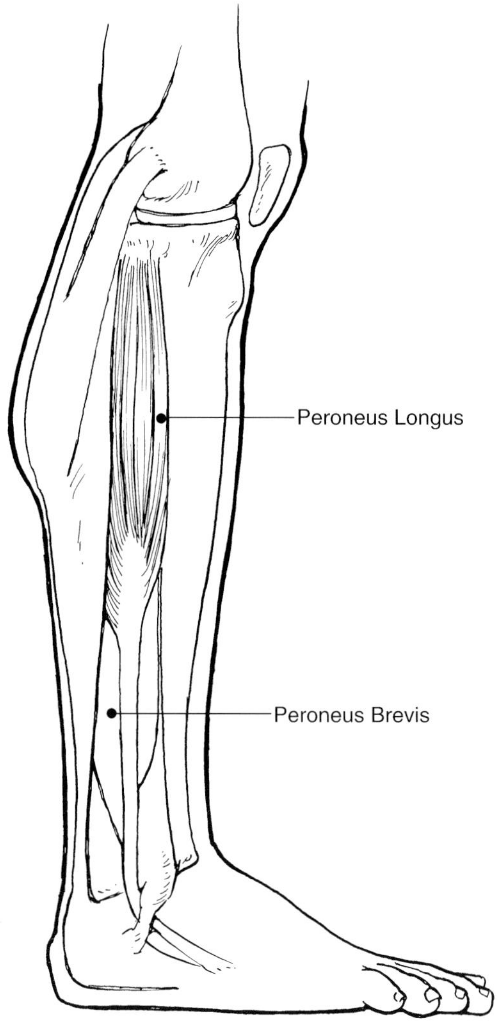


Lateral ( Peroneal) Compartment

**FIGURE XIII-2**

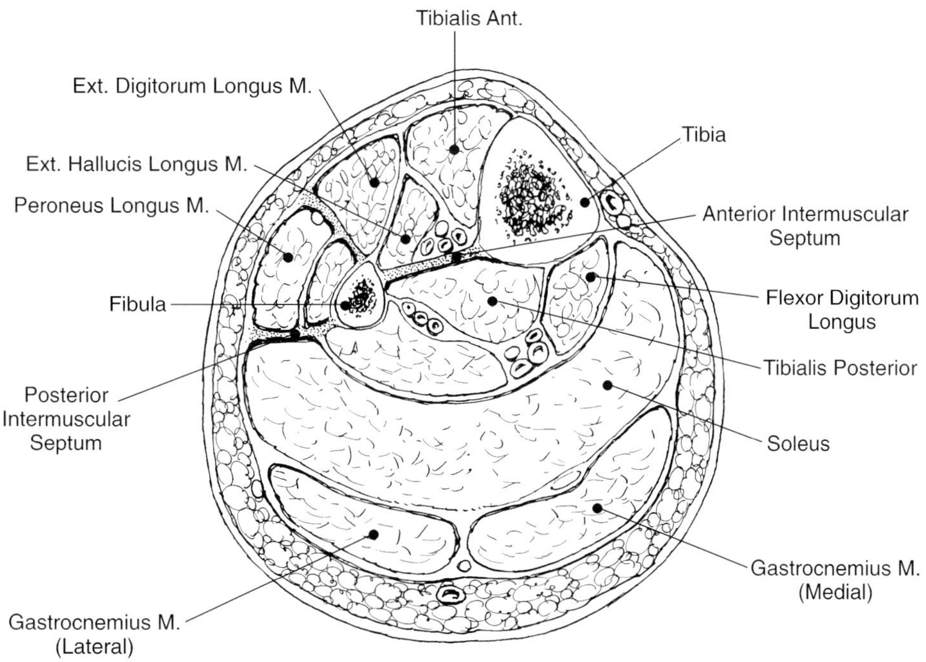


**FIGURE XIII-3**

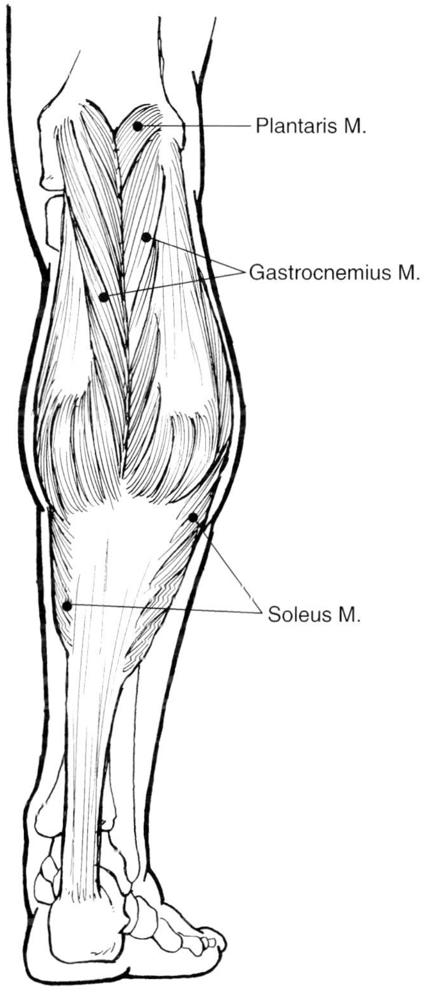


**Superficial Posterior Compartment**

**FIGURE XIII-4**

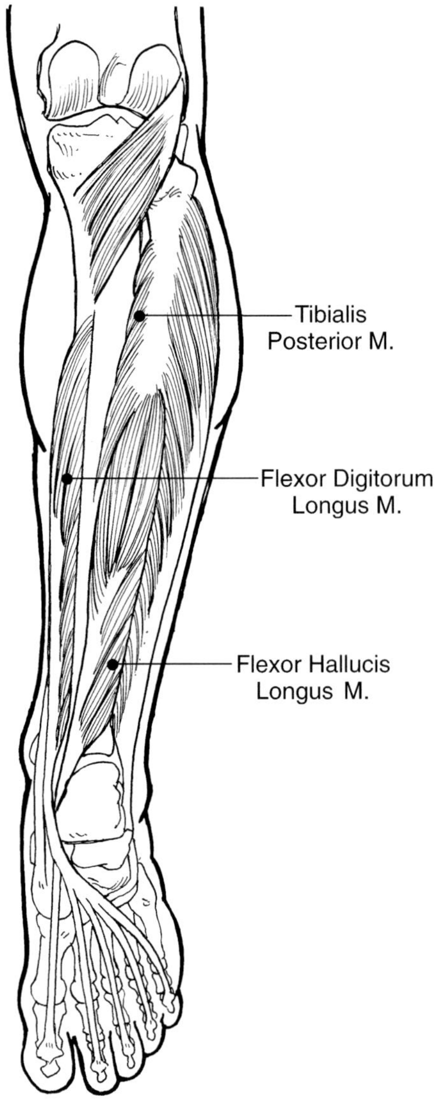


**Deep Posterior Compartment**

**FIGURE XIII-5**

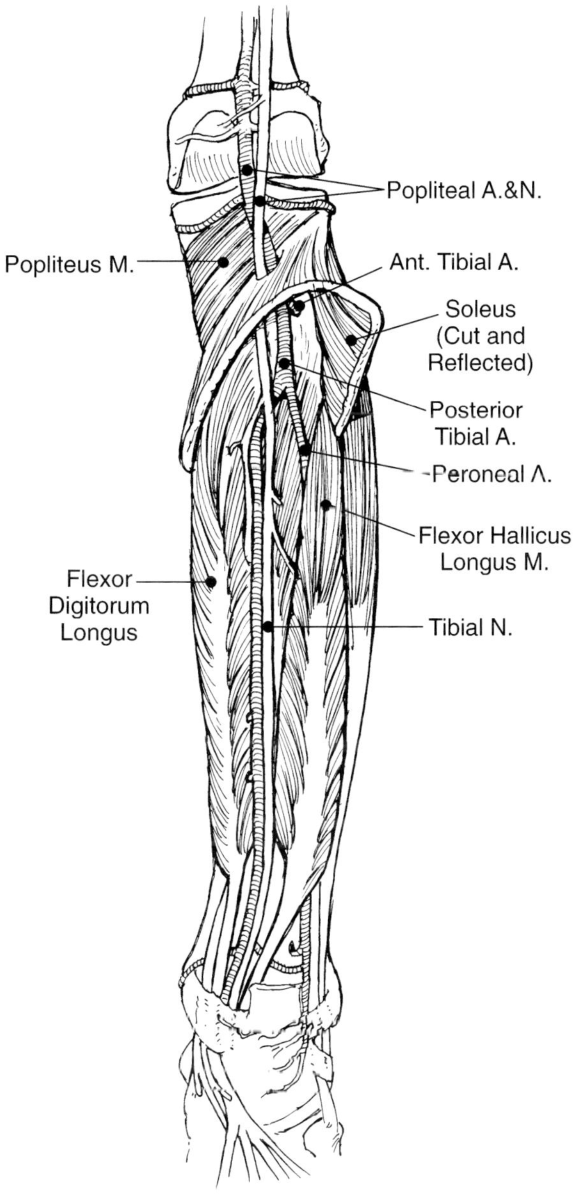


FIGURE XIII-6

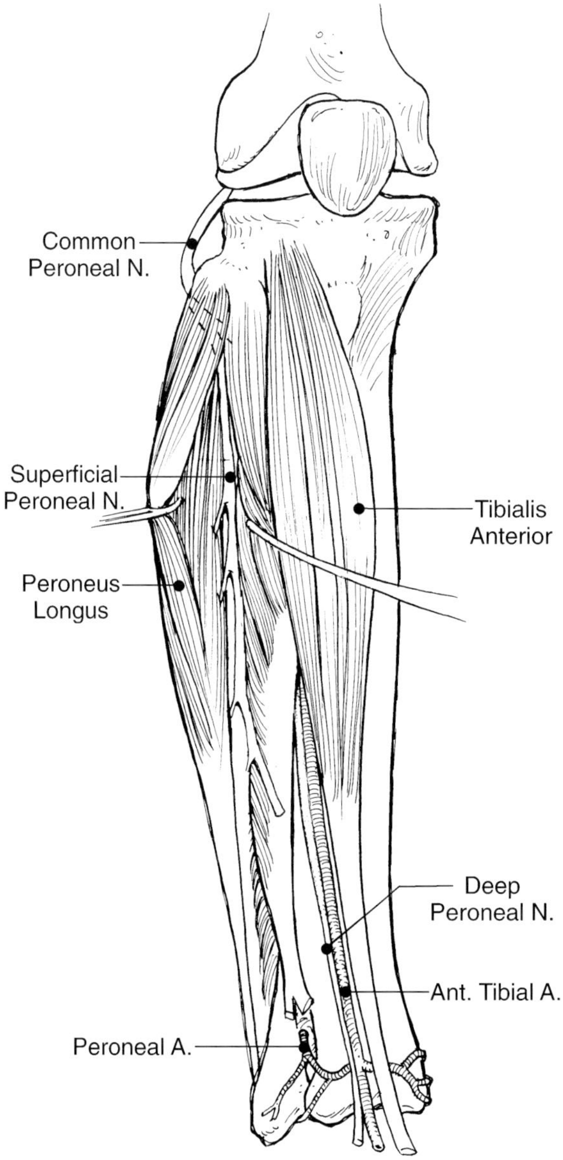


**FIGURE XIII-7**

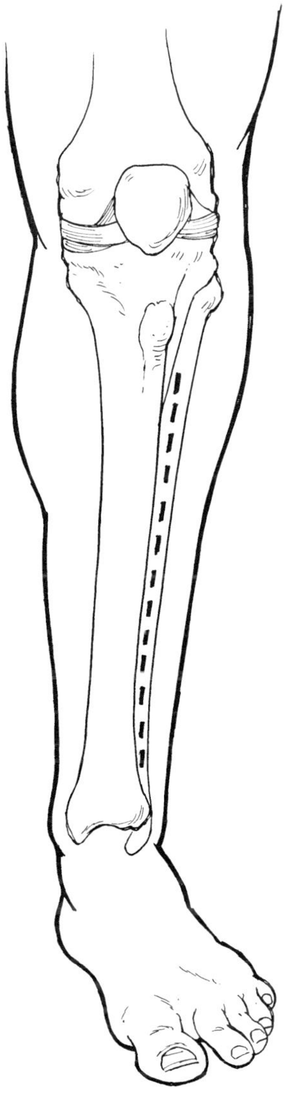

**FIGURE XIII-8**

(XIII-9). It may be extended as far posteriorly as the posterolateral edge of the tibia. Exposing the medial edge of the tibial shaft is not recommended because doing so may disrupt the limited periosteal blood supply.

***Dangers***

The skin incision is placed away from the subcutaneous surface of the tibia to preserve the blood supply to the skin. By making the incision over the muscle, the anterior compartment is entered and subcutaneous dissection can be avoided. Wound healing problems over the tibia can lead to infection and osteomyelitis that can lead to disastrous infected nonunions of fractures and amputations.

***Limitation***

This approach allows an exposure of the entire anterior compartment of the leg and the lateral surface of the tibia.

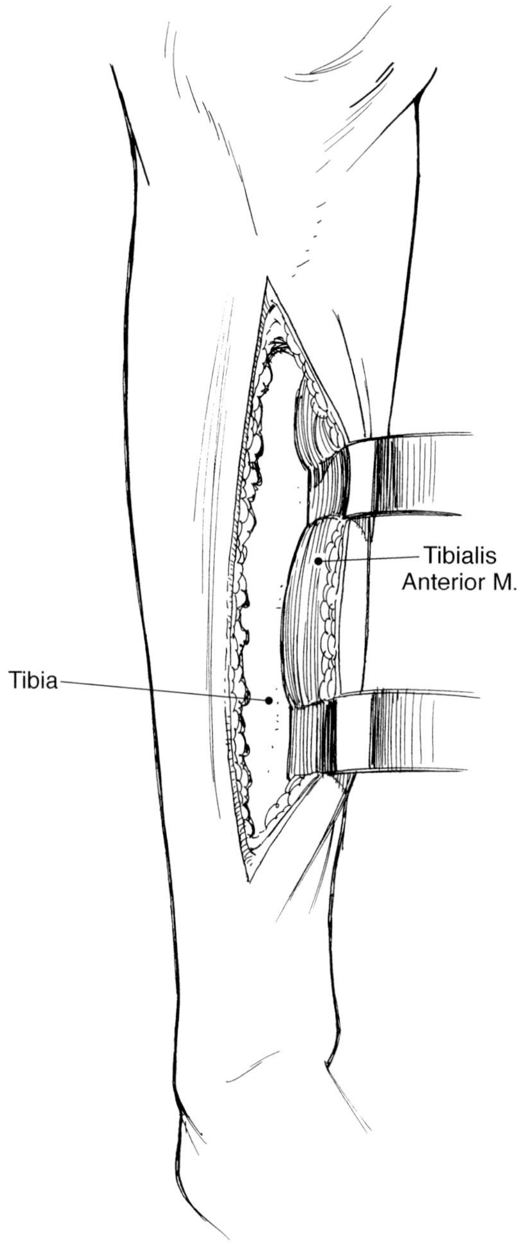


**FIGURE XIII-9**

# Posterolateral Approach to the Tibia

***Application***

This approach is specifically designed to provide access to the posterior surfaces of the tibia and fibula for bone grafting of tibial nonunions (2). The use of this technique with autologous iliac crest bone graft provides reliable healing of delayed union or nonunion of fractures of the tibia. It is one of the most precarious approaches because of scarring and distortion of the anatomy from the previous injury.

***Technique***

The patient is placed prone or in the lateral decubitus position. A thigh tourniquet should be used to allow clear visualization. The incision is made longitudinally, approximately 1 cm posterior to the fibula, and is extended at least 15 cm over the area to be exposed (XIII-10). The fascia is incised in line with the skin incision. The gastrocnemius and soleus are retracted posteriorly, opening the interval between

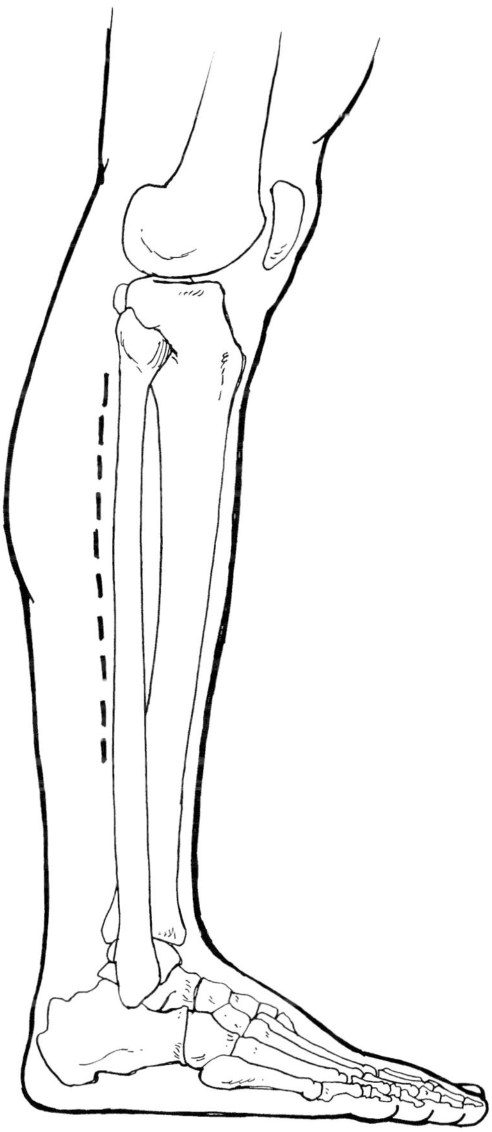

**FIGURE XIII-10**

the soleus and the peroneus longus and brevis. The origin of the soleus is elevated from the posterior surface of the fibula, leading anteriorly around the fibula to expose the interosseous membrane (XIII-11). Perforating branches of the peroneal artery may be ligated and transected as necessary. The flexor hallucis longus is elevated from the posterior fibula, and the tibialis posterior is elevated from the interosseous membrane and posterior tibia (XIII-12). The periosteum of the posterior tibia is incised longitudinally and elevated.

***Dangers***

The most common mistake is dissecting into the interspace between the superficial and deep compartments by going posterior to the tibialis posterior muscle. Doing so leads directly to the tibial nerve and posterior tibial artery which, if injured, will compromise the viability of the foot. Therefore, it is critical to find the interosseous membrane and stay on its surface. There is an extensive plexus of veins running with the peroneal artery along the posteromedial fibula. They can only be avoided by dissecting subperiosteally on the fibula.

***Limitation***

This approach should not be extended into the proximal tibial metaphysis because of risk to the common peroneal nerve, posterior tibial artery, and tibial nerve. The posterior aspect of the proximal tibia can be exposed by extending the posteromedial approach to the knee. This posterolateral approach can be extended as far distally as the ankle joint.

## Approach to the Fibula

***Applications***

This approach may be used to harvest the fibula for bone grafting, partial fibula ostectomy for tibial nonunions, and resection of tumors of the fibula. The entire bone can be exposed, but the distal 10 cm of the fibula should not be removed since it is necessary for preservation of the ankle mortise.

***Technique***

The patient is placed in the lateral decubitus position. The skin incision is made just posterior to the fibula, over the extent needed. The fascia is incised in line with the skin (XIII-13). At the proximal end, the common peroneal nerve can be seen and palpated as it passes around the fibular neck deep to the fascia. The nerve can be safely exposed by incising the fascia with dissecting scissors from proximal to distal directly over the surface of the nerve and splitting the fibers of the peroneus longus to allow free mobility of the nerve (XIII-14A and XIII-14B). Once the plane between the soleus and the peroneus longus and brevis is opened, the lateral edge of the fibula can be visualized. The periosteum can then be incised longitudinally and the muscles can be elevated subperiosteally (XIII-15).

***Dangers***

The common peroneal nerve is subject to injury, usually by traction during the procedure. Dissecting outside of the subperiosteal space is likely to damage the peroneal artery and the plexus of veins around it.

***Limitation***

The entire fibula can be exposed. The incision can be extended distally as an anterolateral approach to the foot.

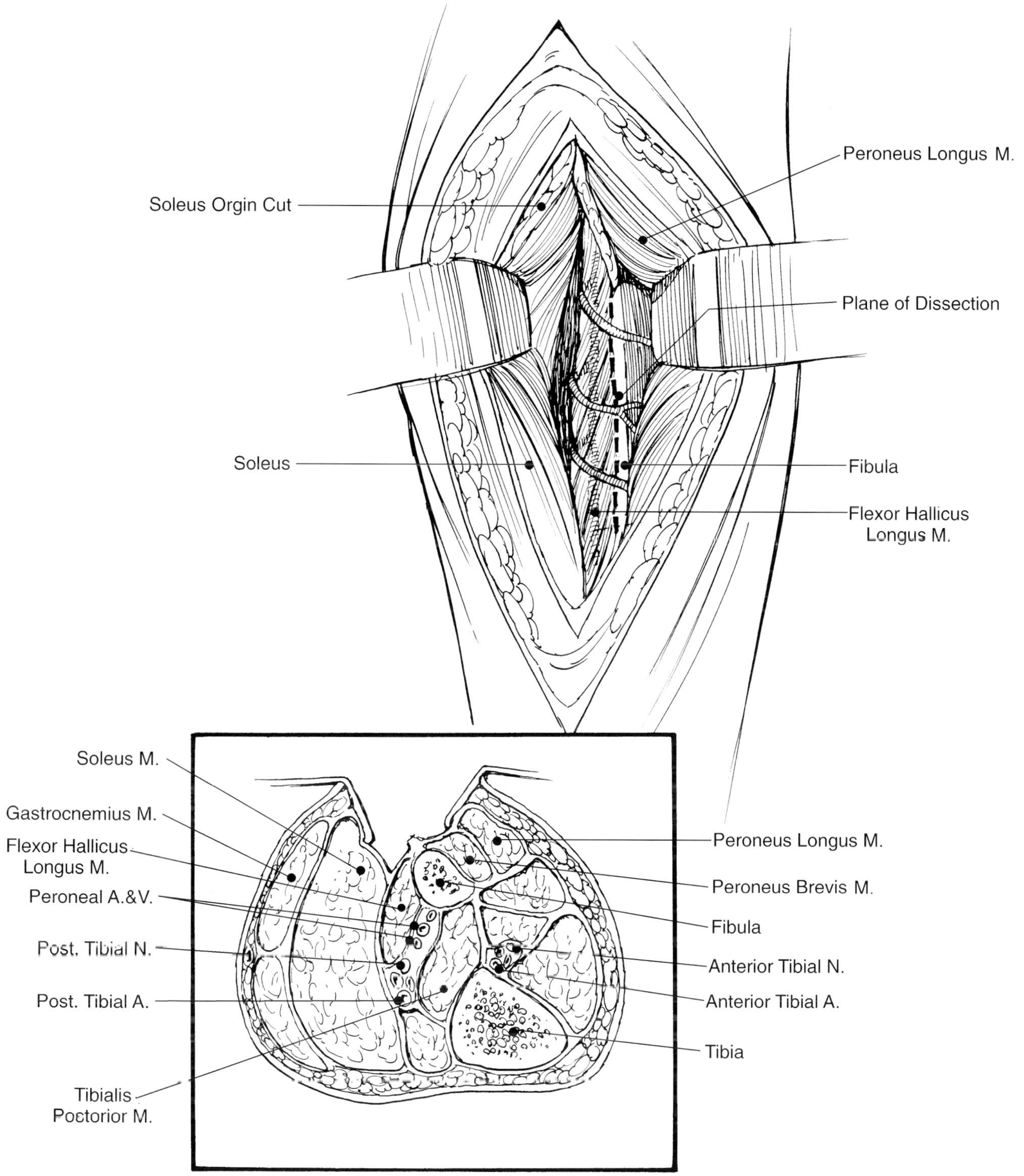


**FIGURE XIII-11**

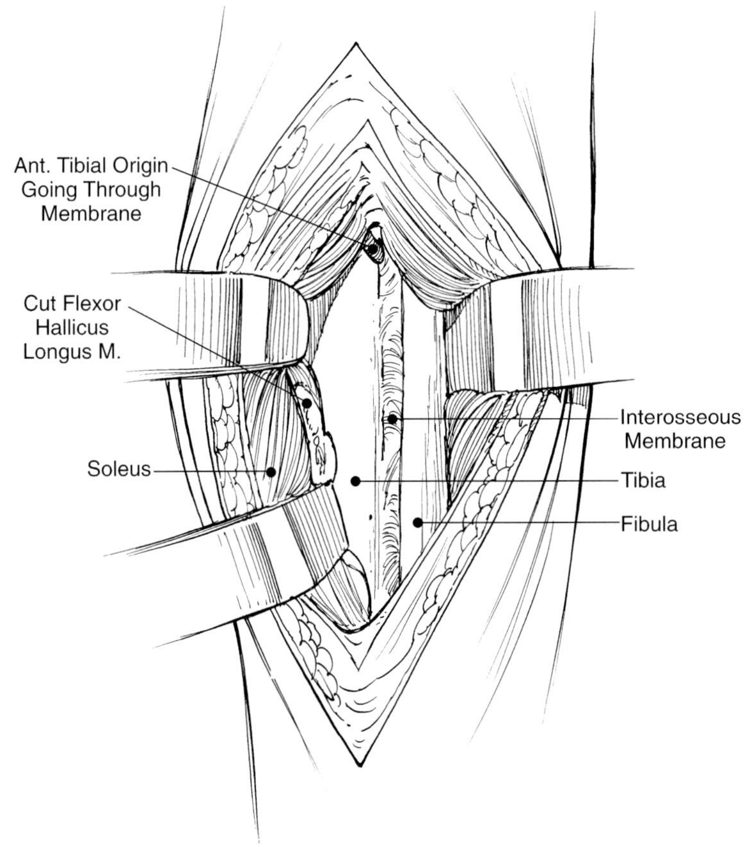


**FIGURE XIII-12**

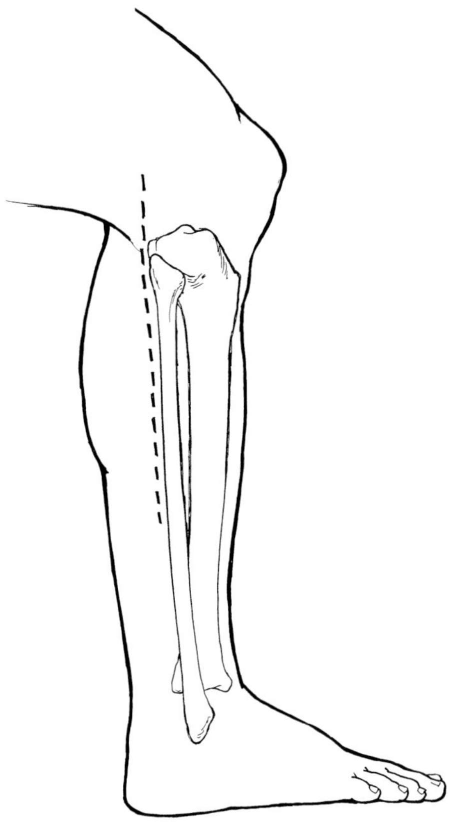

**FIGURE XIII-13**

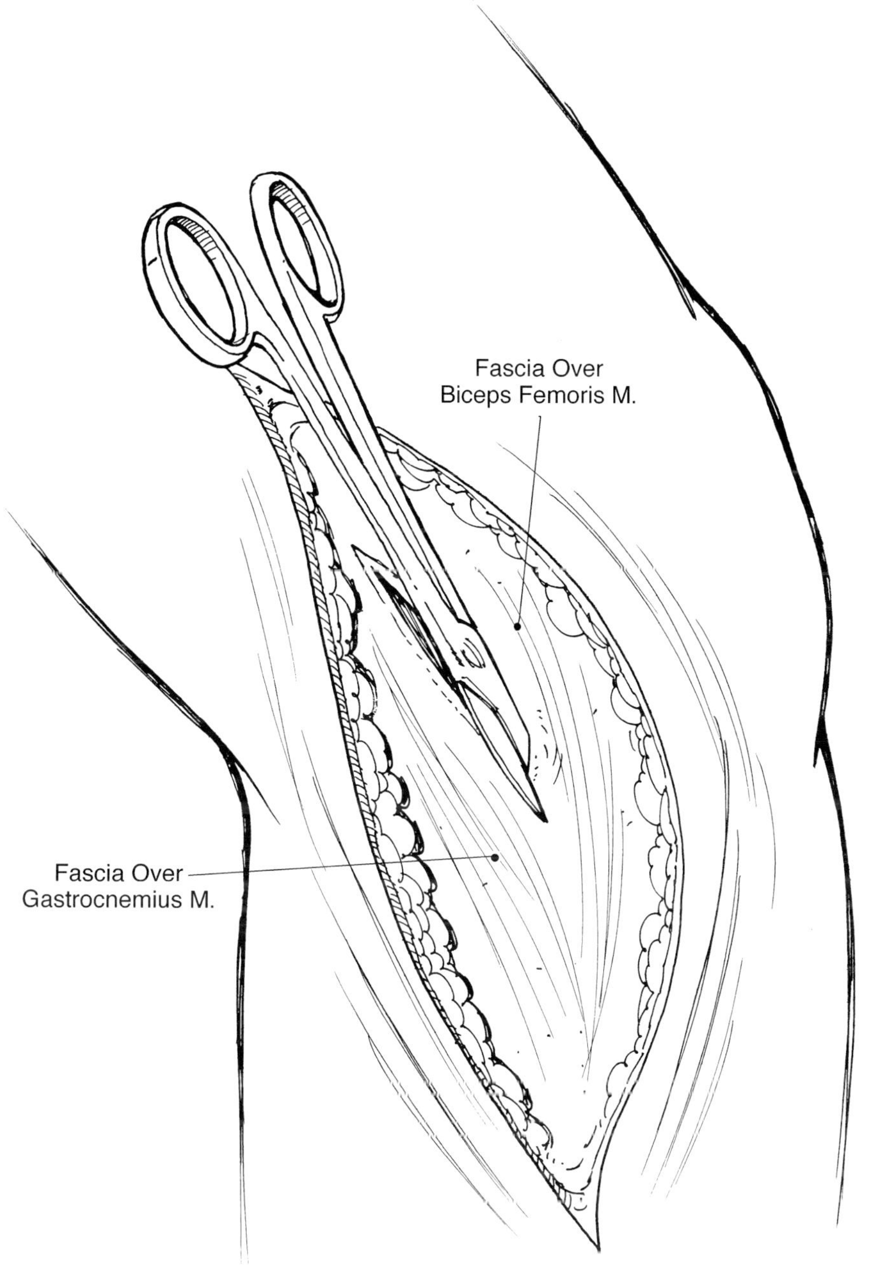


**FIGURE XIII-14A**

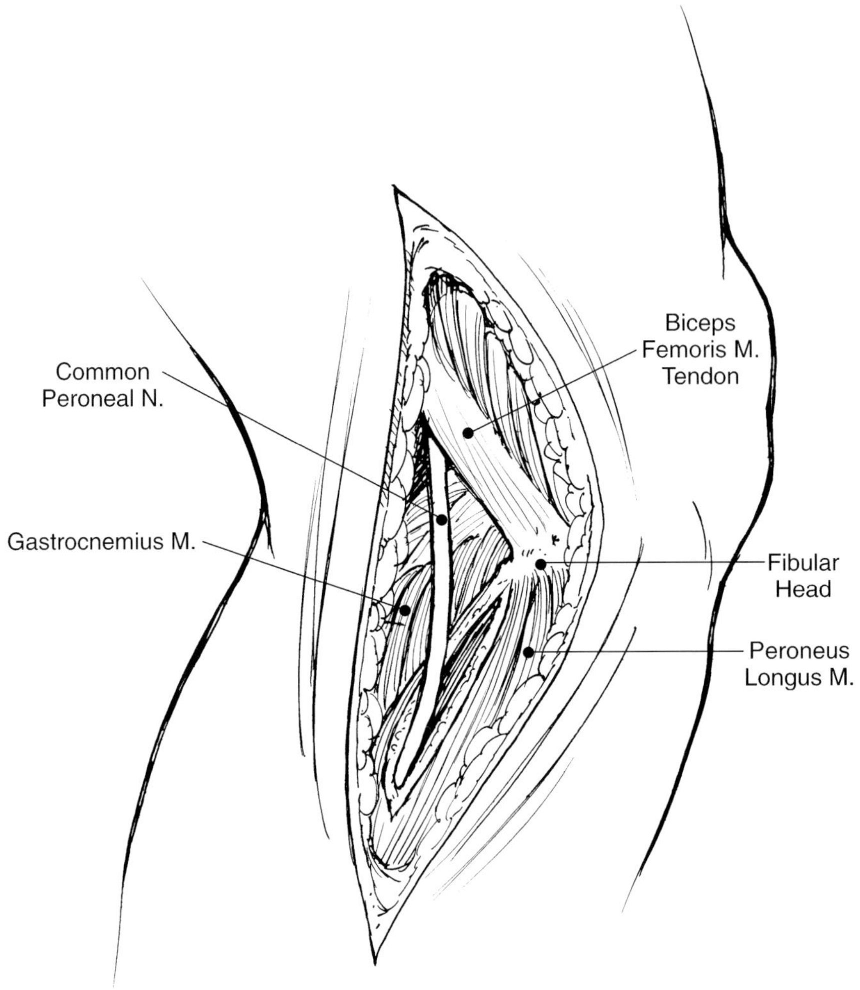


**FIGURE XIII-14B**

# Compartment Resections in the Leg

The anterior and lateral compartments of the leg can be resected individually or together, with or without resection of the fibula. Each compartment is exposed by a longitudinal S-shaped incision over its middle. The fascia is incised and the muscles are elevated from their origin, ligating the anterior tibial artery and its branches as they are encountered. The tendons are transected above the ankle. The peroneal tendons can be anchored to the periosteum of the fibula to stabilize the ankle. The extensor tendons can be anchored to the tibia with the toes and ankle in a neutral position. Alternatively, a split tibialis posterior tendon or flexor hallucis longus tendon may be transferred through the interosseous membrane to balance the foot and provide some dorsiflexion. Ankle dorsiflexion can also be provided by a dorsiflexion-assist ankle foot orthosis that can be worn inside of a shoe. Resection of the posterior compartment of the leg is impractical because loss of the posterior neurovascular bundle will produce an unbalanced muscle pull and an insensate foot with a poor blood supply. Large anterior soft tissue defects over the proximal third of the leg can be covered reliably with a gastrocnemius muscle rota-

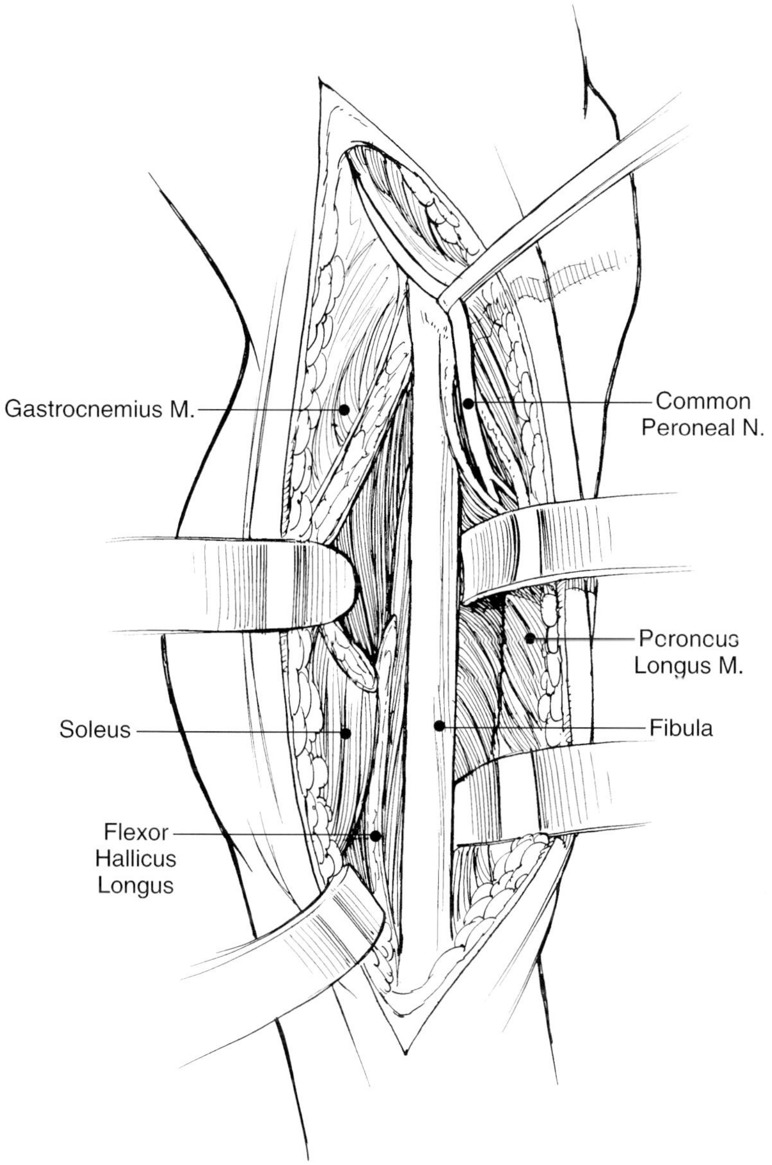


**FIGURE XIII-15**

tion flap. Defects over the middle third can be covered by a soleus muscle rotation flap. Coverage of the anterior distal third of the tibia will usually require a vascularized free flap.

## References

1. Müller ME, Allgover M, Willeneggen H. Manual of Internal Fixation. New York: Springer-Verlag, 1970.
2. Harmon PH. A simplified surgical approach to the posterior tibia for bone grafting and fibular transference. J Bone Joint Surg. 27:496, 1945.

# XIV

# SURGICAL APPROACHES TO THE FOOT AND ANKLE

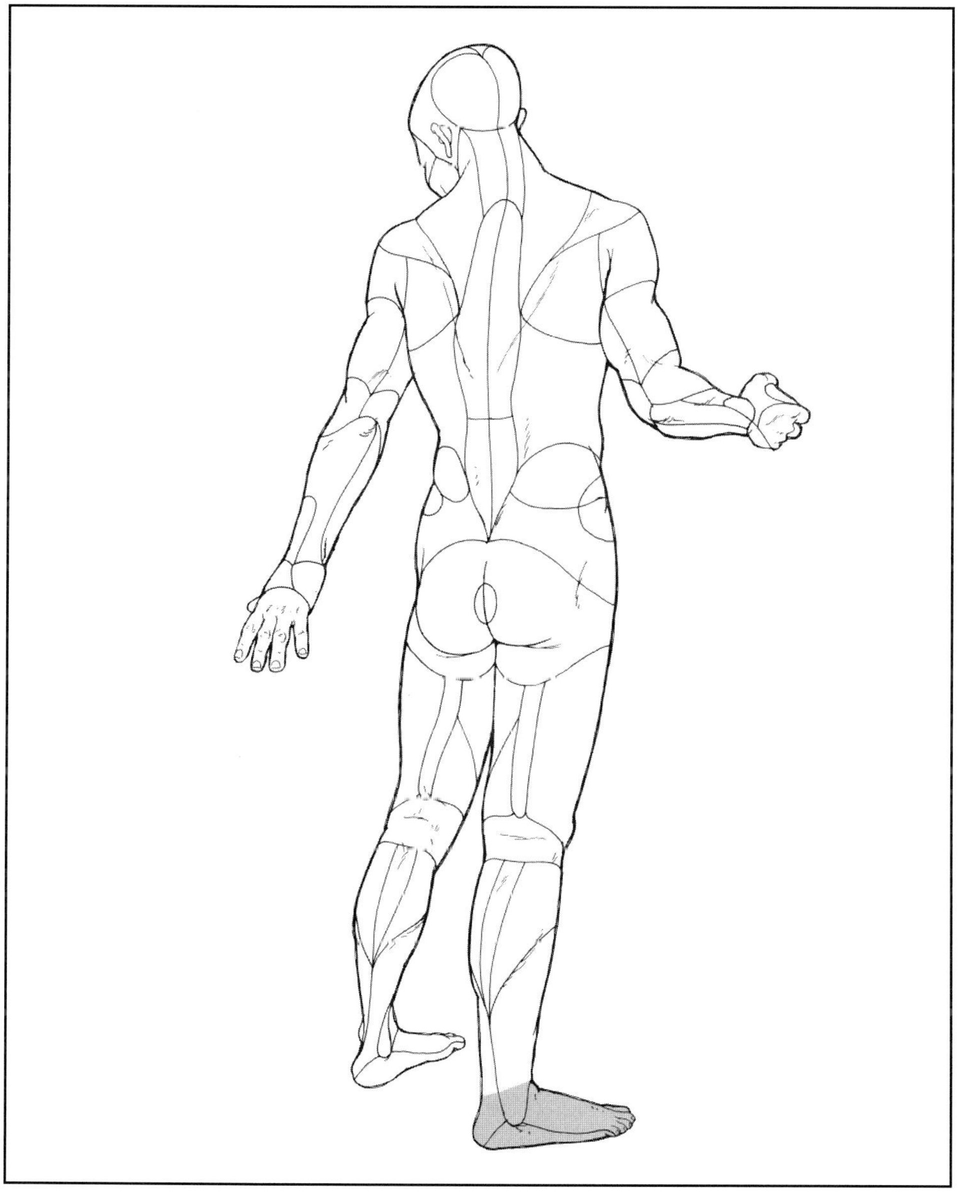

## General Principles and Complications

At the distal aspect of the limb, collateral vessels are fewer and terminal branches are more frequent. Extensile incisions should be placed longitudinally to minimize the risk of transecting these terminal vessels. Of particular concern in the ankle and foot is the preservation of adequate venous and lymphatic drainage. Surgical incisions should be placed parallel to the supplying arteries and, when possible, the incisions should lie at the perimeter of an angiosome. Incisions should go directly through the skin, subcutaneous tissue, and underlying fascia without dissection in the subcutaneous layer.

In the ankle and foot, there is less subcutaneous tissue, which limits the mobility of the skin and access to the underlying structures. Therefore, careful planning is needed and a clear understanding of the topographic anatomy is essential. When possible, the incision should be carried directly from the skin through the soft tissue to bone and a full thickness flap of skin, subcutaneous tissue, fascia, and periosteum should be created. Extensive subcutaneous dissection can result in skin and soft tissue ischemia with resultant severe tissue loss or chronic edema.

Numerous sensory nerves course along the ankle joint and extend into the foot. Because of the limited amount of subcutaneous tissue in this region, these nerves are relatively immobile and subject to direct injury. They are quite susceptible to stretch injury both acutely during surgical retraction and chronically as the scar contracts during the healing of the surgical wound. Some of the most dissatisfied patients are those with persistent neuritic symptoms following operations on the ankle and foot. While all of the superficial sensory nerves are vulnerable to injury or late scar entrapment, the sural nerve and the many branches of the superficial peroneal nerve (XIV-1) are most likely to be involved.

## Surgical Anatomy

Because the amount of muscle and subcutaneous tissue is limited in the ankle and foot, bony landmarks are relatively easy to see and palpate. The careful surgeon will take advantage of this fact to guide the surgical approach. The major landmarks are the medial malleolus, head of the talus, navicular tuberosity, head of the first metatarsal, lateral malleolus, anterior process of the calcaneus, and the tuberosity and head of the fifth metatarsal (XIV-2 and XIV-3).

The three major arteries supplying the ankle and foot are the anterior tibial, peroneal, and posterior tibial arteries. At the ankle, the posterior tibial artery divides into the medial and lateral plantar arteries to nourish the plantar aspect of the foot.

The anterior tibial artery supplies the skin over the anterior and lateral aspects of the ankle and the dorsum of the foot from the medial side of the little toe to the lateral side of the great toe. The peroneal artery supplies the skin over the lateral aspects of the ankle and heel. The posterior tibial artery supplies the posteromedial ankle, the rest of the heel, and the dorsomedial aspect of the foot distally to the medial aspect of the great toe. Its two major terminal branches, the medial and lateral plantar arteries, supply the medial and lateral aspects, respectively, of the sole of the foot (XIV-4 and XIV-5).

The critical relationships along the medial aspect of the ankle and the foot are:

1. The posterior tibial tendon lies in a groove on the posterior aspect of the medial malleolus. Sometimes it lies so deep in the groove that it is overlooked and the adjacent flexor digitorum longus tendon is mistaken for it.

2. The order in which the major structures lie behind the medial malleolus can be remembered by the mnemonic "Tom, Dick, And Not Harry" that identifies, in order, the tibialis posterior tendon, the flexor digitorum longus tendon, the posterior tibial artery, the tibial nerve, and the flexor hallucis longus tendon (XIV-6).
3. The flexor hallucis longus remains muscle until it reaches the level of the ankle joint. Just distal to this point, the tendon passes between the medial and lateral tubercles of the posterior process of the talus.
4. In the foot, at the level of the navicular tuberosity, the tendons of the flexor hallucis longus and the flexor digitorum longus cross in an area called the master knot of Henry, a thick, fibrous tunnel that, when cut, allows the flexors to be lifted away plantarward, giving access to the deeper structures of the foot (XIV-7).

The critical relationships along the lateral side of the ankle and foot are:

1. The peroneal tendons lie behind the lateral malleolus with the peroneus brevis lying deep and anterior to the longus (XIV-8).
2. The anterior process of the calcaneus is the origin of the extensor digitorum brevis muscle (XIV-9).

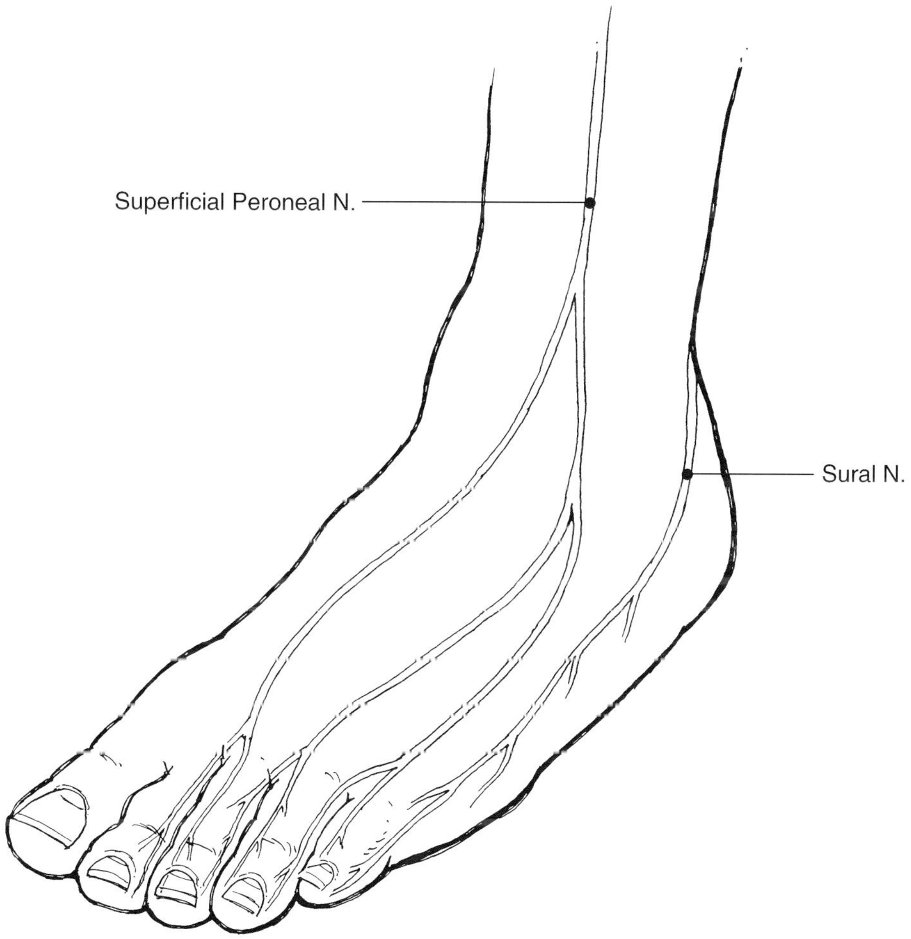


**FIGURE XIV-1**

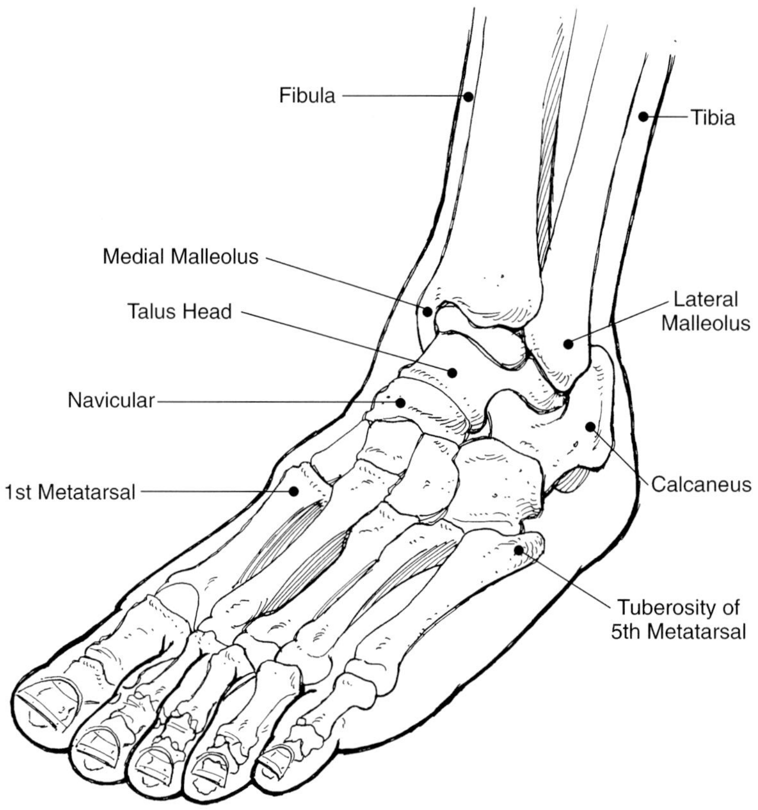


**FIGURE XIV-2**

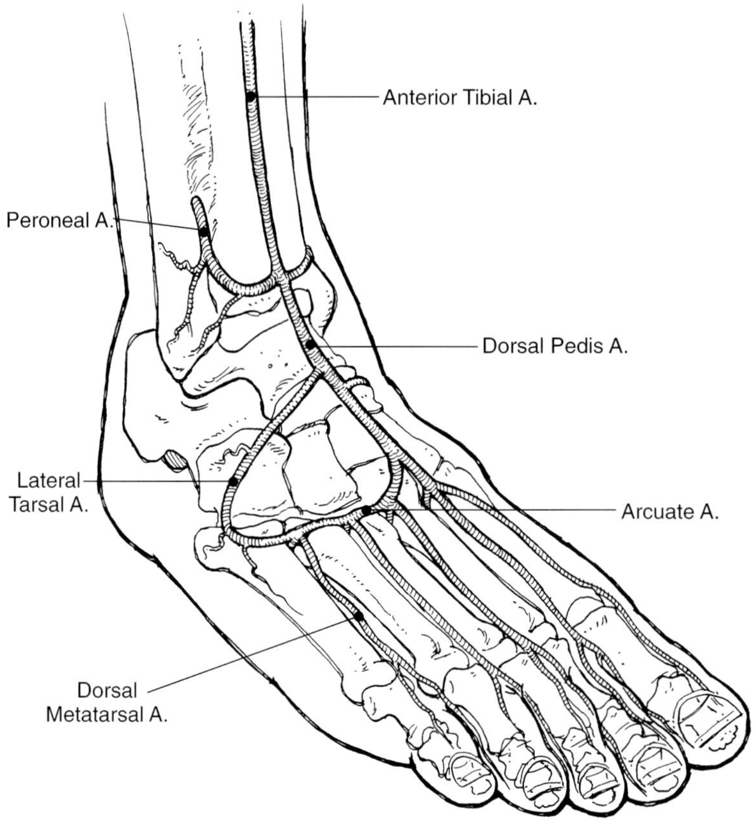


**FIGURE XIV-3**

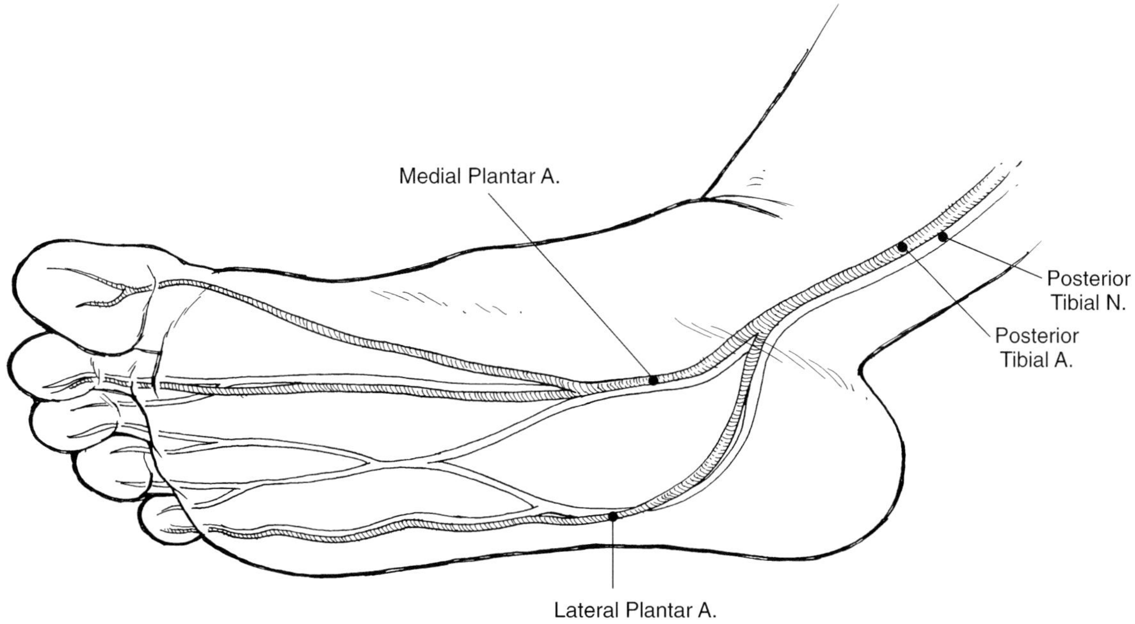


**FIGURE XIV-4**

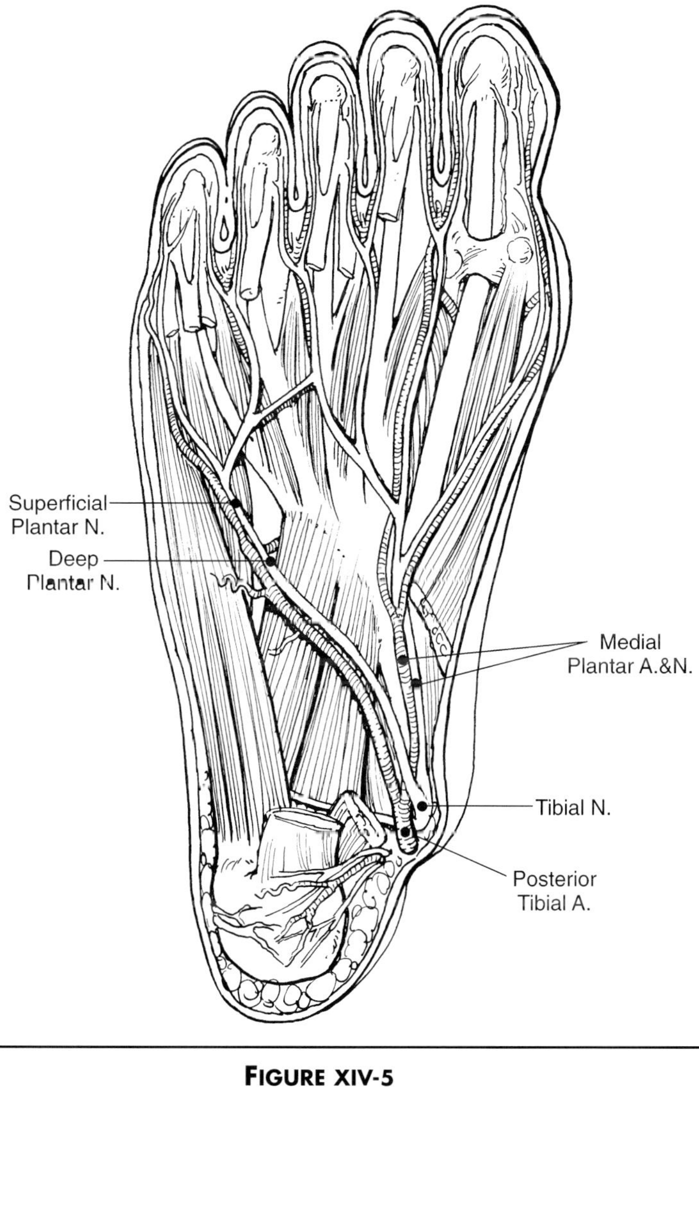


**FIGURE XIV-5**

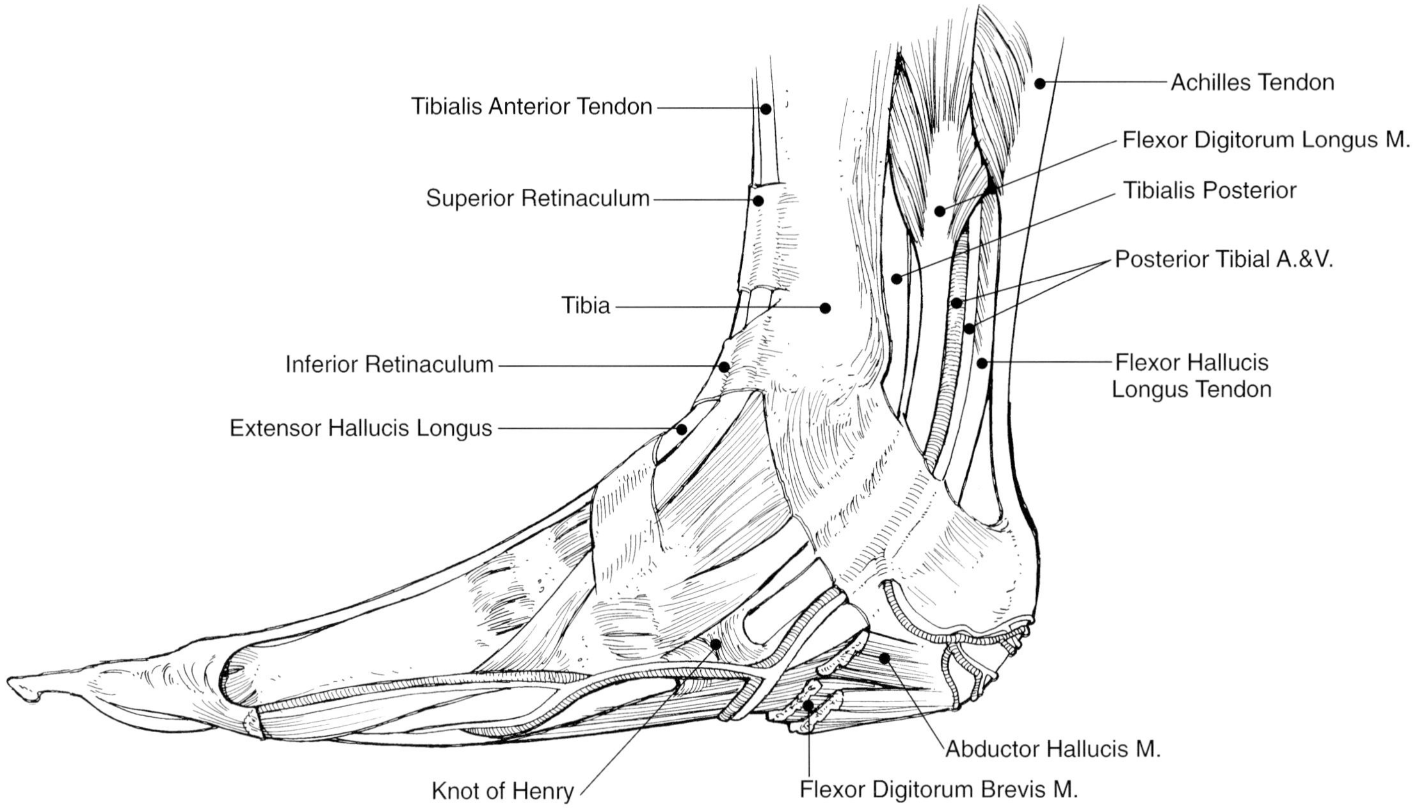


**FIGURE XIV-6**

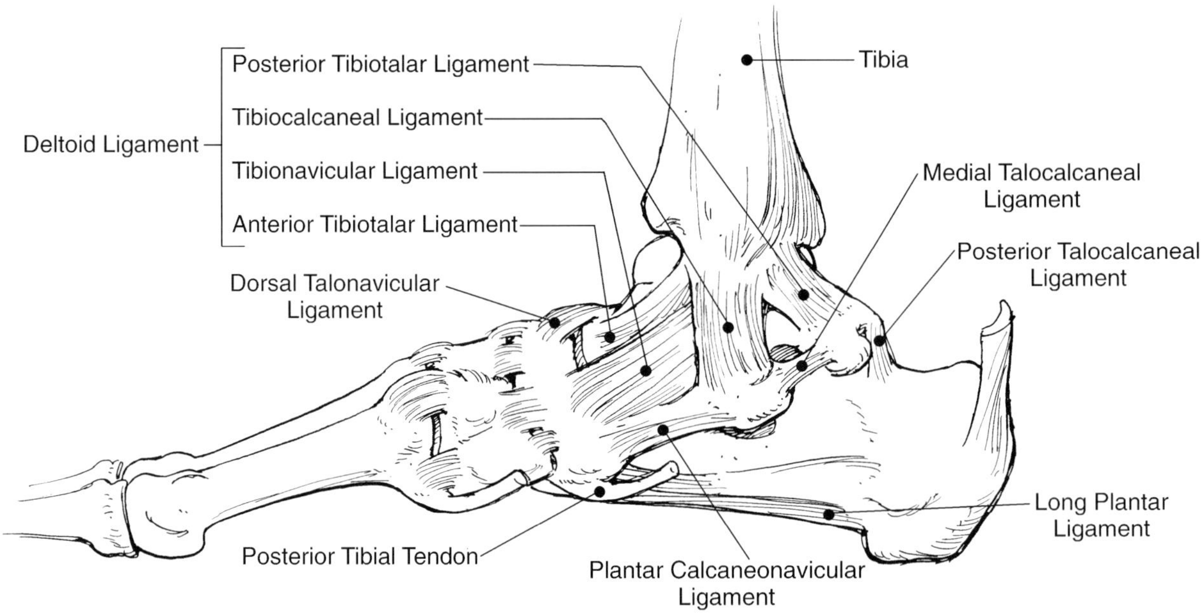


**FIGURE XIV-7**

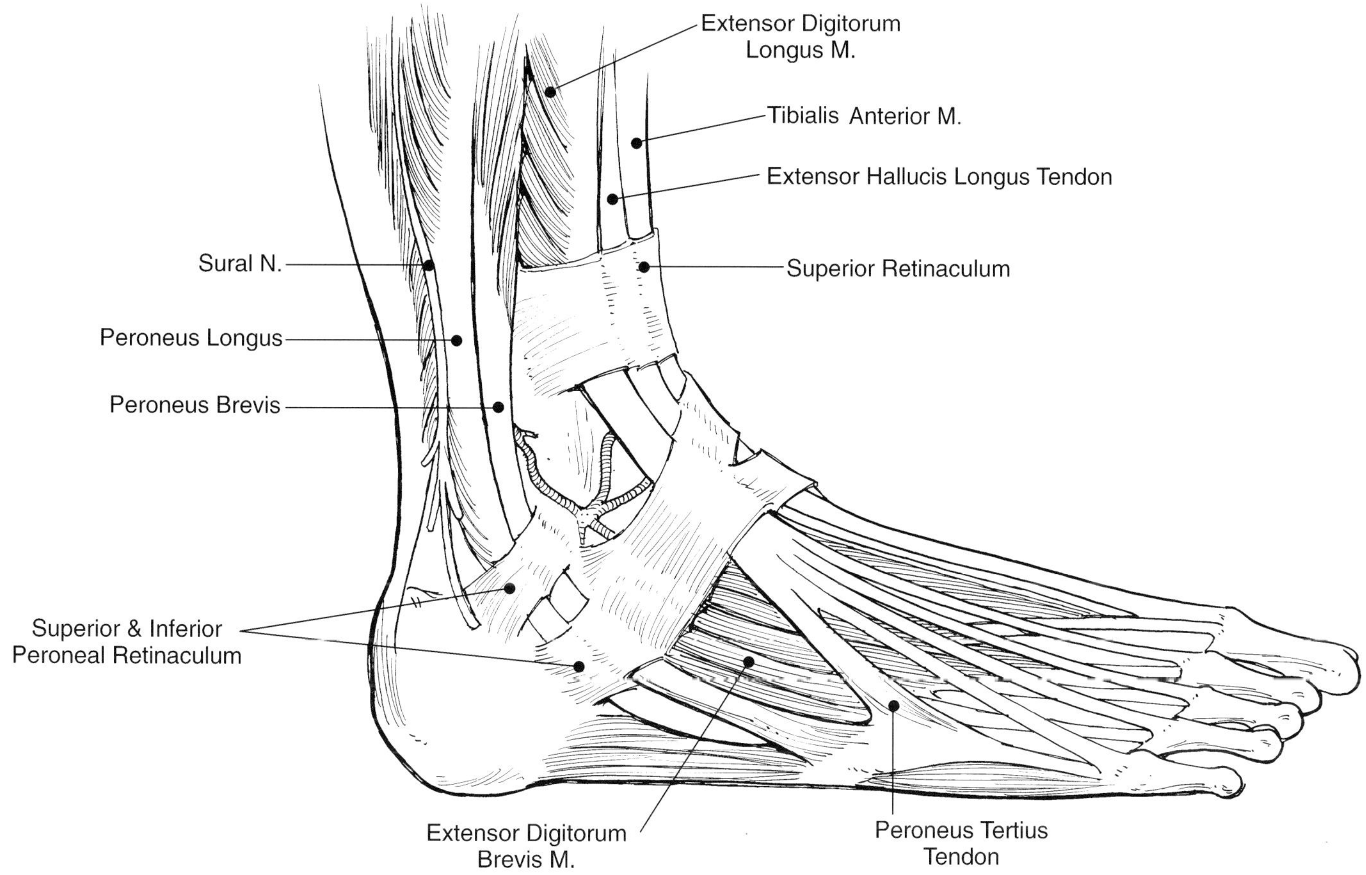


**FIGURE XIV-8**

The muscles of the foot are described as being divided into four layers. A dense plantar aponeurosis covers the middle of the plantar surface of the foot, analogous to the palmar aponeurosis (XIV-10A). The most superficial (first) layer of muscles includes the flexor digitorum brevis, abductor hallucis, and abductor digiti minimi (XIV-10B). The medial and lateral plantar nerves and arteries lie between the first and second layers. The second layer includes the flexor hallucis longus, flexor digitorum longus, flexor accessorius tendons, and the lumbricals (XIV-10C). The third layer consists of the flexor hallucis brevis, adductor hallucis, and flexor digiti minimi (XIV-10D). The fourth layer consists of the interossei and the tendons of the peroneus longus and tibialis posterior (XIV-10E).

# Posteromedial Approach to the Ankle

*Applications*

This approach allows access to the posterior tibial tendon, the flexor digitorum longus tendon, the flexor hallucis longus tendon, and the entire extent of the main neurovascular bundle to the foot. Deep to these structures and easily accessible once they have been mobilized, are the deltoid ligament, the medial malleolus, and the medial face of both the talus and the calcaneus. Through this approach, the tarsal tunnel can be exposed and decompressed. Tendons arising from the muscles of the deep posterior compartment can be transferred or released (as in a clubfoot), the deltoid ligament can be repaired, ununited fracture fragments from

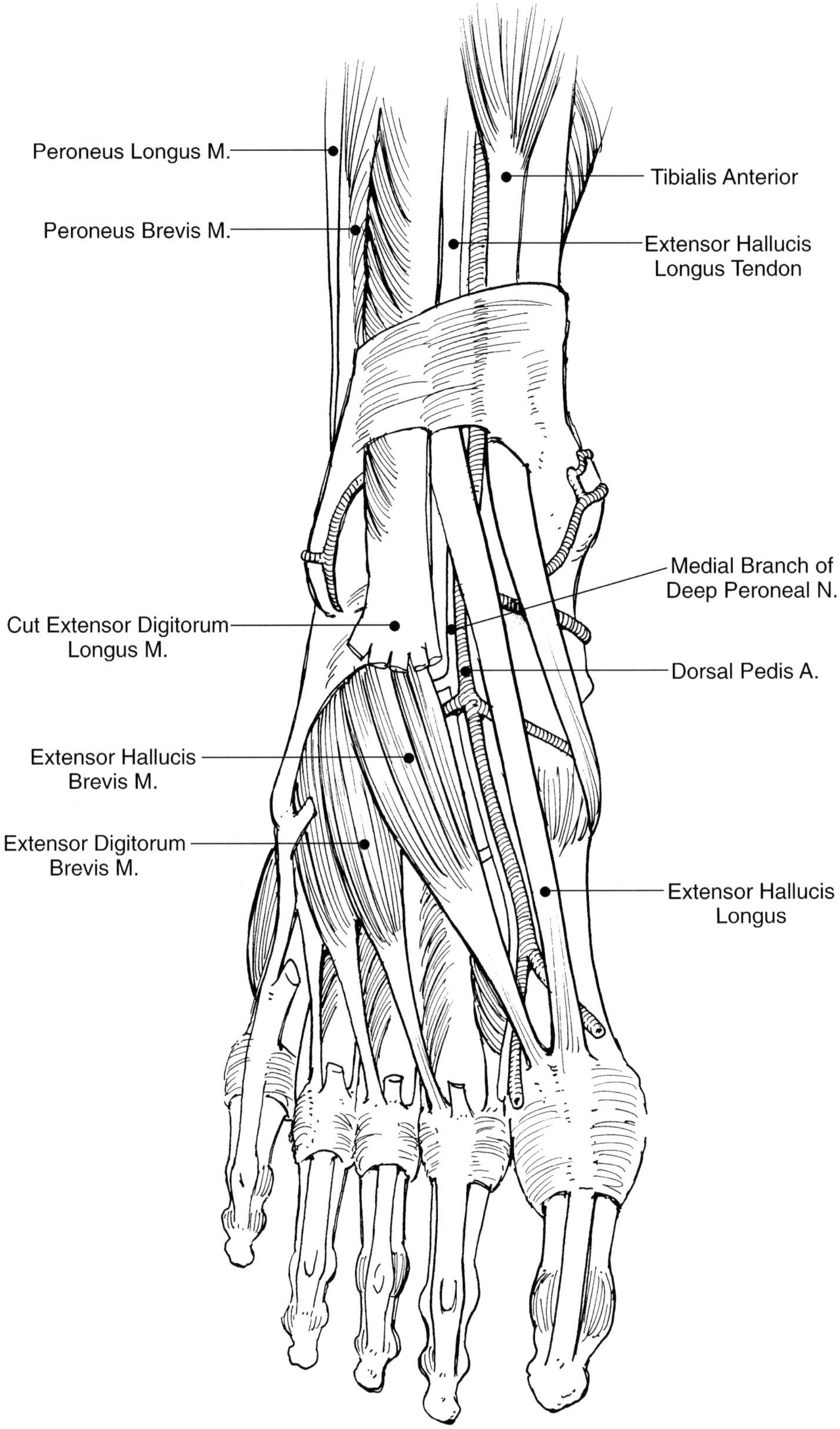
Peroneus Longus M.
Peroneus Brevis M.
Tibialis Anterior
Extensor Hallucis Longus Tendon
Medial Branch of Deep Peroneal N.
Cut Extensor Digitorum Longus M.
Dorsal Pedis A.
Extensor Hallucis Brevis M.
Extensor Digitorum Brevis M.
Extensor Hallucis Longus

**FIGURE XIV-9**

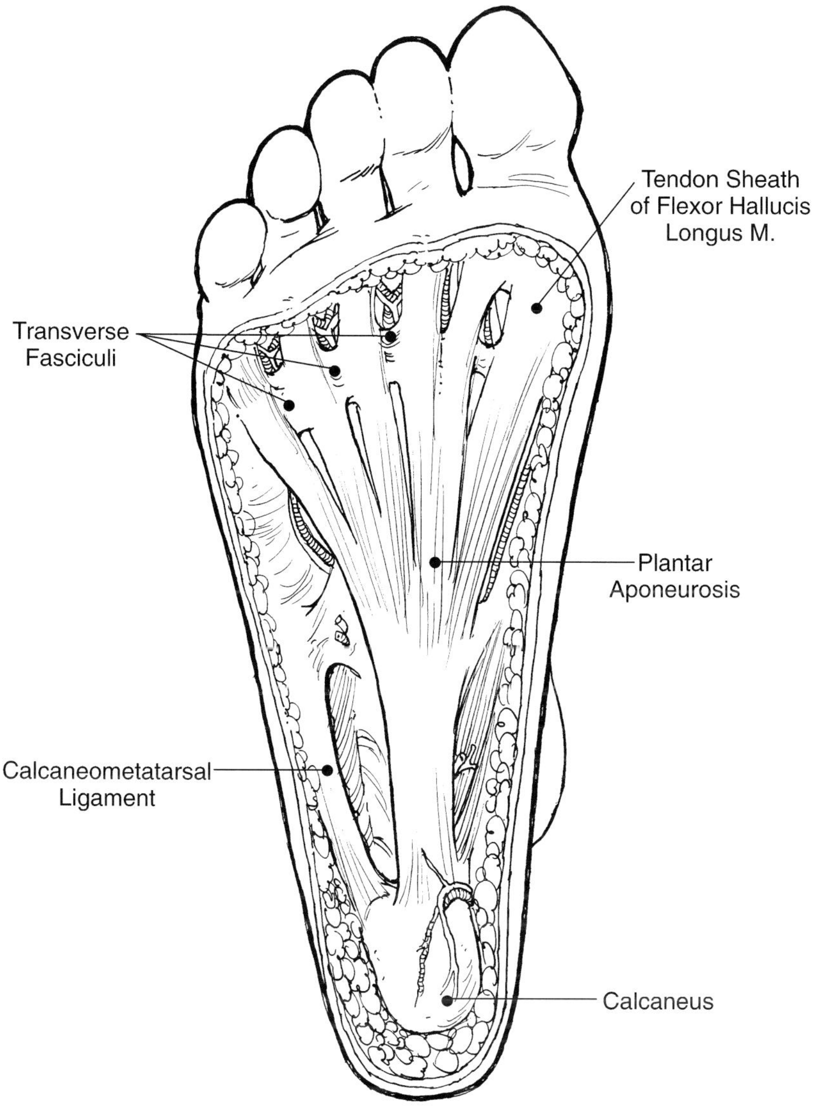


**FIGURE XIV-10A**

the medial aspect of the talus or calcaneus can be removed, or a tarsal coalition between the talus and the calcaneus can be resected.

## *Technique*

The patient should be positioned supine. The incision is longitudinal and begins 5 to 8 cm proximal to the tip of the medial malleolus, but it may be extended as far proximally as the midcalf if necessary. The incision is one finger's breadth posterior to the medial border of the tibia, equidistant from the medial edge of the tibia and the medial border of the Achilles tendon. It is extended distally to the level of the tip of the medial malleolus and then curved anteriorly toward the arch of the foot (XIV-11). Sharp dissection should be carried down to the level of the deep fascia without creating extensive skin flaps. The posterior tibial tendon lies anteriorly, against the edge of the distal tibia, sometimes lying in a deep bony groove behind the medial malleolus. The posterior tibial tendon should be approached proximally and distally, leaving intact a 1-cm long pulley at the tip of the medial malleolus (XIV-12). This allows access to the entire length of the posterior tibial tendon.

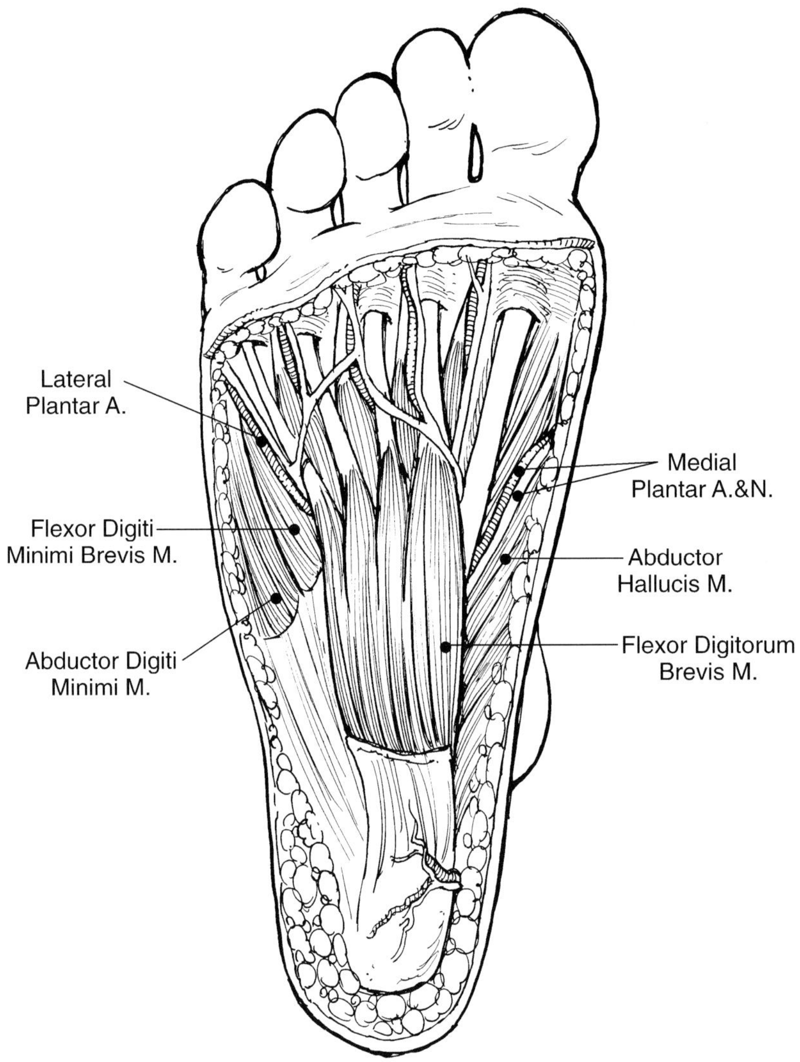


**FIGURE XIV-10B**

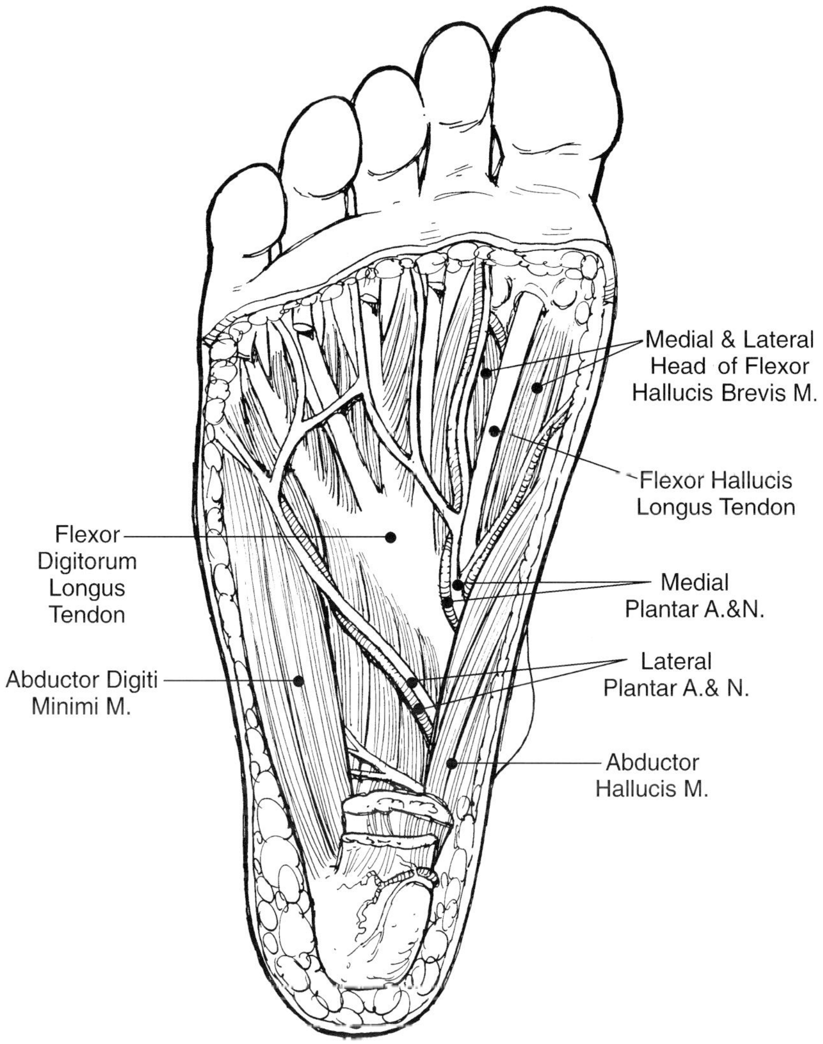


**FIGURE XIV-10C**

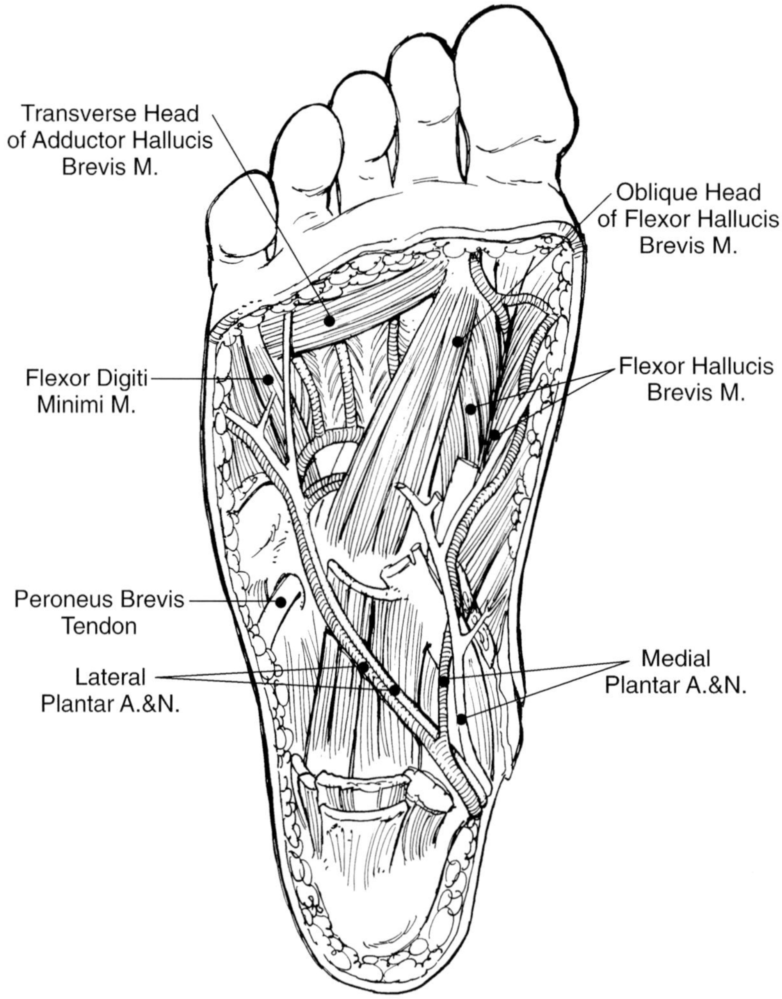


**FIGURE XIV-10D**

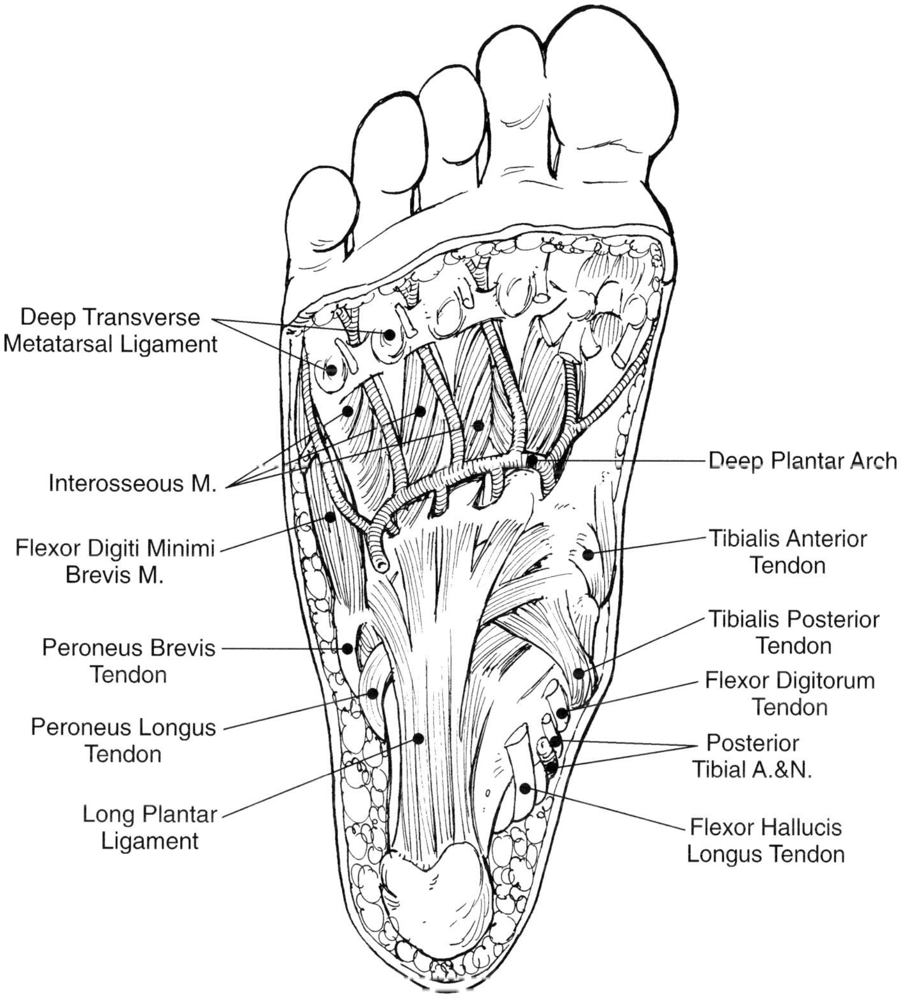


**FIGURE XIV-10E**

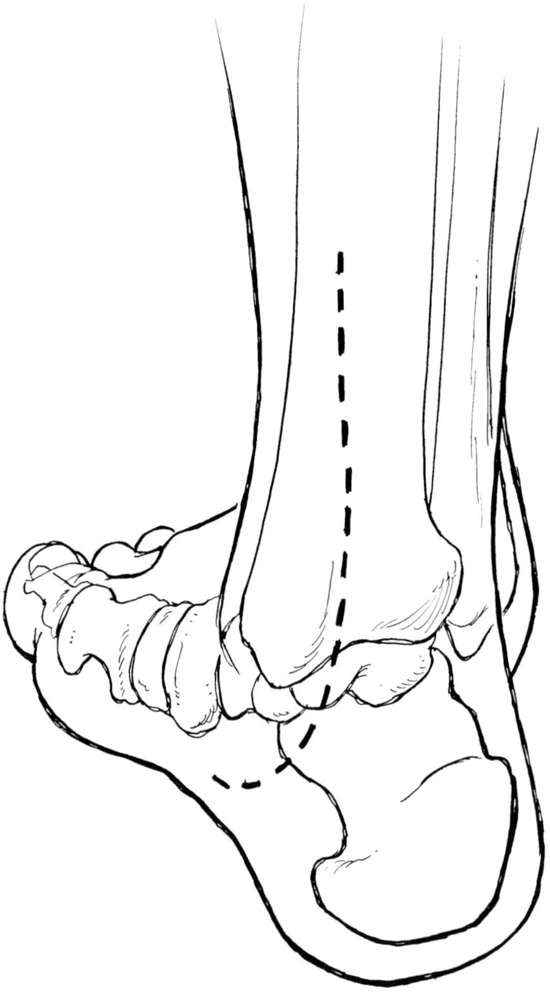

**FIGURE XIV-11**

Complete opening of the sheath allows the tendon to be displaced over the top of the medial malleolus and gives access to the deltoid ligament that is deep to the sheath (XIV-13). If the pulley is completely disrupted, it should be repaired during closure to prevent chronic subluxation of the tendon.

Immediately behind the posterior tibial tendon lies the flexor digitorum longus tendon in a separate sheath, and behind it is the tarsal tunnel containing the neurovascular bundle. The tibial nerve and its branches can be fully exposed. There are three major branches of the tibial nerve. The calcaneal branch usually leaves the main trunk before it enters the tarsal canal to innervate the medial aspect of the heel. The medial and lateral plantar nerves separate within the tunnel and then extend to innervate the sole of the foot. Posterior and lateral to the neurovascular bundle, also in its own sheath, lies the flexor hallucis longus, which is muscular until it reaches the level of the ankle joint (XIV-13).

The neurovascular bundle and the flexor hallucis longus tendon can be mobilized and retracted anteriorly. The deep portion of the vascular sheath can be incised longitudinally to expose the medial aspect of the middle and posterior facets of the subtalar joint and the medial face of both the talus and the calcaneus (XIV-14).

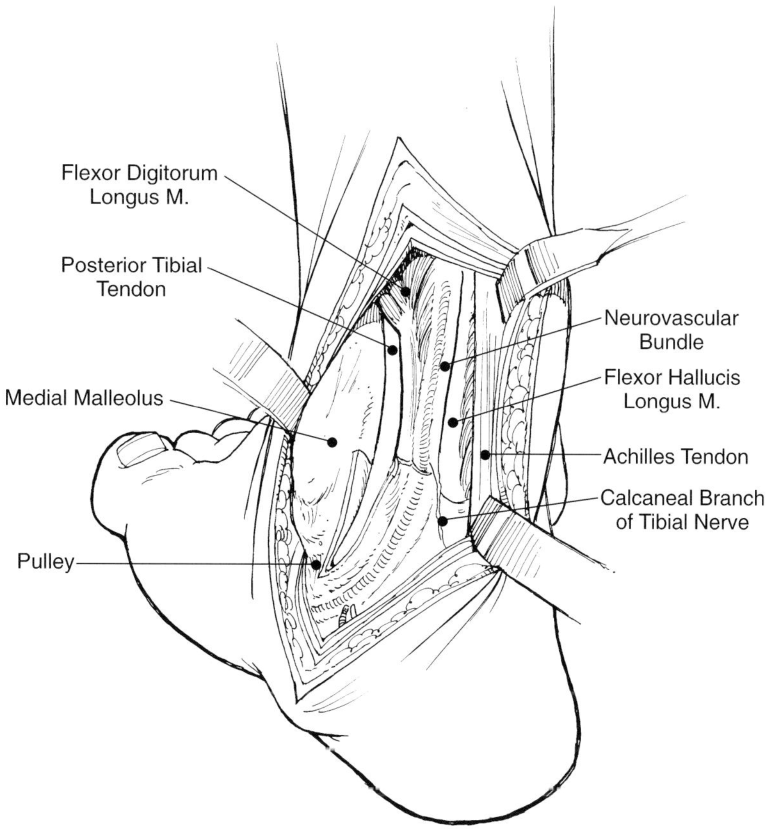


**FIGURE XIV-12**

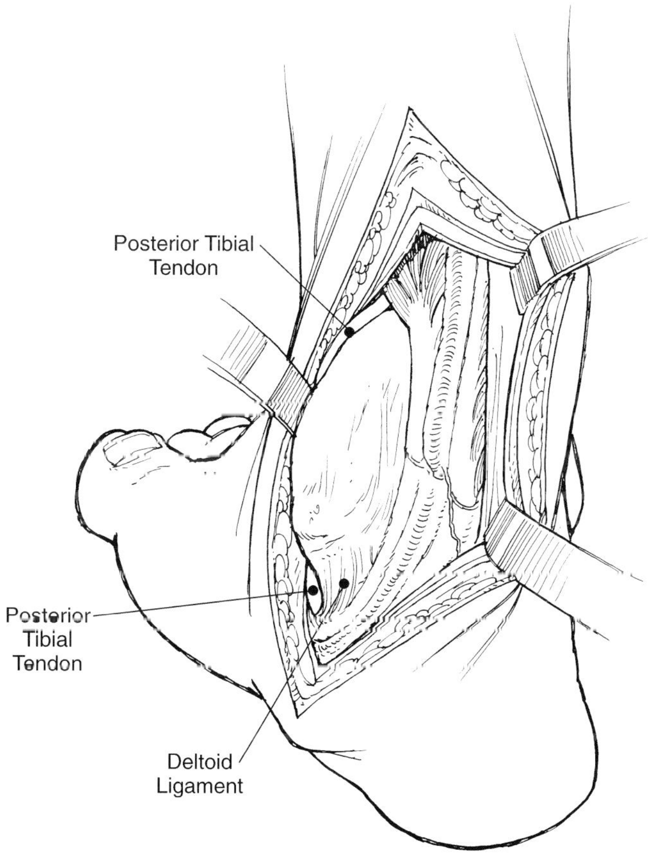


**FIGURE XIV-13**

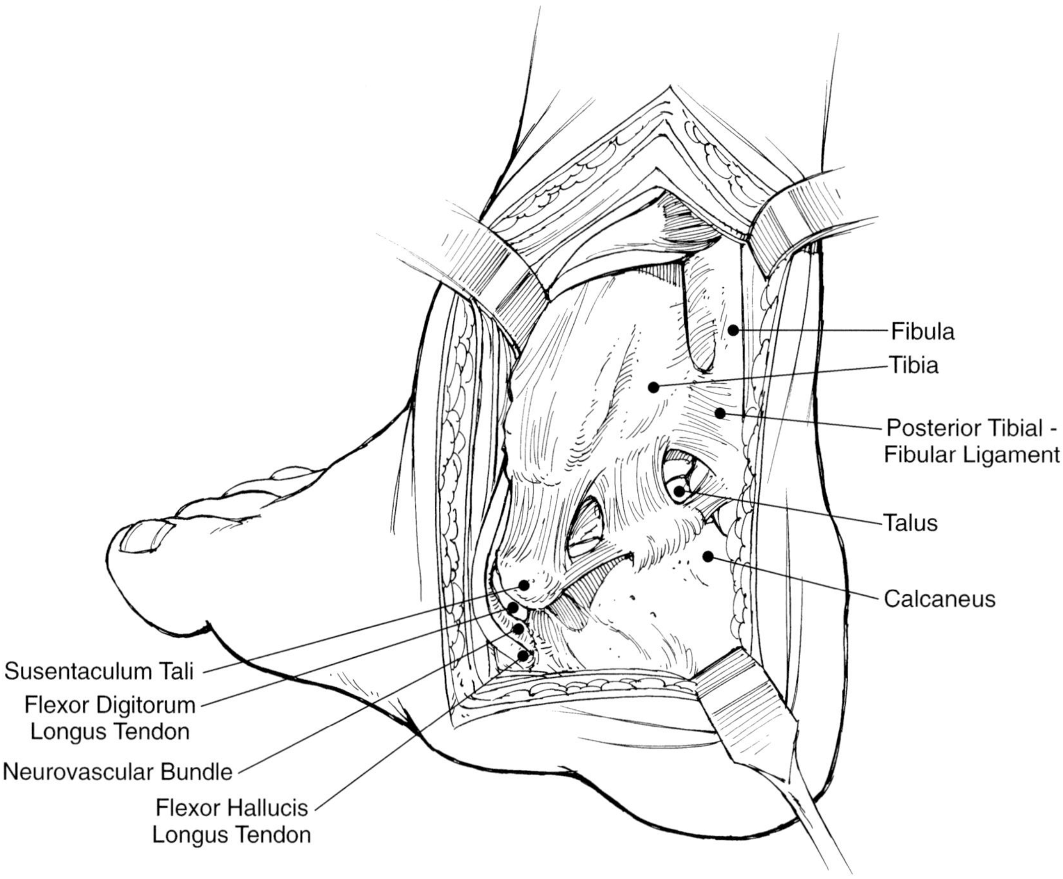


**FIGURE XIV-14**

Extending this incision proximally exposes the Achilles tendon for lengthening or repair. The posteromedial approach is preferable to a direct posterior approach to the Achilles tendon because the skin overlying the tendon has a poor blood supply and heals poorly. Vertical incisions made directly over the tendon also scar onto the tendon, creating heel cord contractures.

***Dangers***

Injury to the neurovascular bundle is the most serious complication of this approach. Dissection should always be performed from proximal to distal to minimize the risk of cutting a branch of an artery or nerve. Identifying the trunks proximal to the tarsal tunnel and then dissecting distally to identify the branches will minimize the risk of injury.

The flexor digitorum longus tendon can be easily mistaken for the posterior tibial tendon. The posterior tibial tendon lies in a firm, fibro-osseous tunnel posterior to the medial malleolus. Tension applied to a mobilized tendon can be used to help identify it. The toes will flex when tension is applied to the flexor digitorum longus tendons but they will move very little if tension is applied to the posterior tibial tendon.

Aggressive resection of a talocalcaneal coalition can jeopardize the flexor hallucis longus tendon as it courses beneath the sustentaculum tali. Before the talocalcaneal bar is resected, the course of the tendon through the pulley created by the posterior process of the talus and distally beneath the sustentaculum tali, should be defined.

Tight closure of an incision over the neurovascular bundle should always be avoided because there is a strong tendency for scarring and contracture of this wound. The contracture may lead to the development of a tarsal tunnel syndrome 6 to 12 months following closure.

*Limitations*

To extend this incision distally into the deeper layers of the foot, the origin of the abductor hallucis will have to be detached from the first metatarsal, giving access to the master knot of Henry.

Some authors have advocated the use of the distal portion of the posteromedial approach for open reduction and internal fixation of calcaneal fractures. This approach, however, does not allow the surgeon to visualize the subtalar joint well enough to assess the adequacy of reduction of posterior facet fractures.

# Posterolateral Approach to the Ankle

*Applications*

An extensile posterolateral approach to the ankle allows access to the peroneal tendons, the lateral malleolus, the Achilles tendon, and the posterior aspects of the ankle and subtalar joints. It is well suited for peroneal tendon repair, reconstruction, or transfer; for lateral clubfoot release; and for calcaneus fracture fixation.

*Technique*

The patient should be positioned prone or in a lateral decubitus position. The skin incision is made parallel to the posterior edge of the fibula, halfway between it and the Achilles tendon (XIV-15). There is no proximal limit to this incision. It can be extended distally into the foot through a gentle anterior curve to the level of the fifth metatarsal. Once through the skin, careful blunt dissection should be used to identify and protect the lesser saphenous vein and the adjacent sural nerve. Both of these structures should be identified throughout the length of the incision and gently retracted toward the fibula (XIV-16).

Behind the ankle, the muscle belly of the flexor hallucis longus lies deep to the Achilles tendon. The peroneal tendons are in the anterior edge of the wound. Deep dissection of the posterior aspect of the ankle and subtalar joints is pursued through the interval between the flexor hallucis longus and peroneal tendons (XIV-17A and XIV-17B. Remaining lateral to the flexor hallucis longus avoids injury to the neurovascular bundle (posterior tibial artery and tibial nerve) that lies just medial to the tendon. Mobilization of the peroneal tendons allows clear visualization of the lateral malleolus and the origin of the posterior tibiofibular ligament. In addition, the variably sized terminal branch of the peroneal artery lies in this interval (XIV-17C). The posterior margin of both the ankle and the subtalar joints can be palpated. The joints can be exposed by incising their posterior capsules.

*Dangers*

Two structures are particularly vulnerable to injury in this approach: the sural nerve and the terminal branches of the peroneal artery. Laceration of the sural nerve will leave an area of permanent numbness along the lateral border of the foot. Even worse, a partial laceration or a stretching injury (to which this nerve seems to be particularly vulnerable) will often create permanent and disabling dysesthesias in its sensory distribution. Careful identification of the nerve, thorough mobilization, and continuous protection during the operation will minimize these risks.

The last perforating branch of the peroneal artery is given off to anastomose with the anterolateral malleolar artery, approximately 5 cm above the tip of the lateral malleolus. The terminal branches of the peroneal artery lie on the periosteal

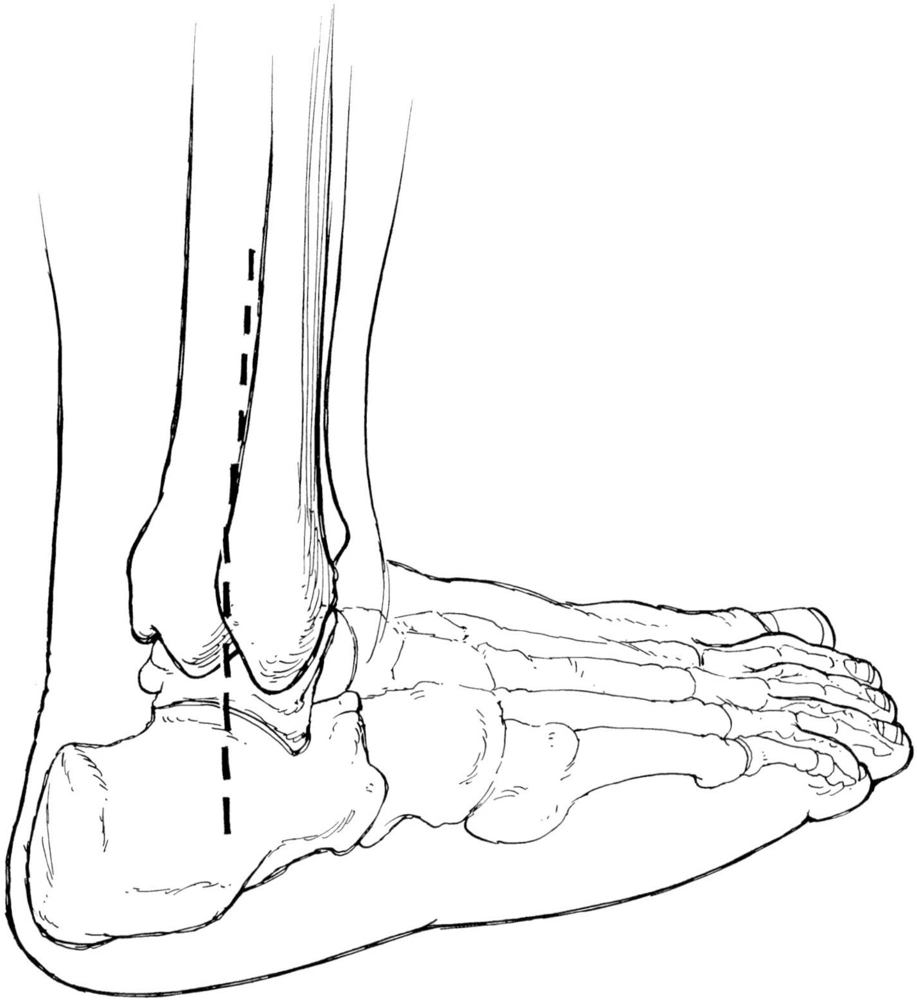

**FIGURE XIV-15**

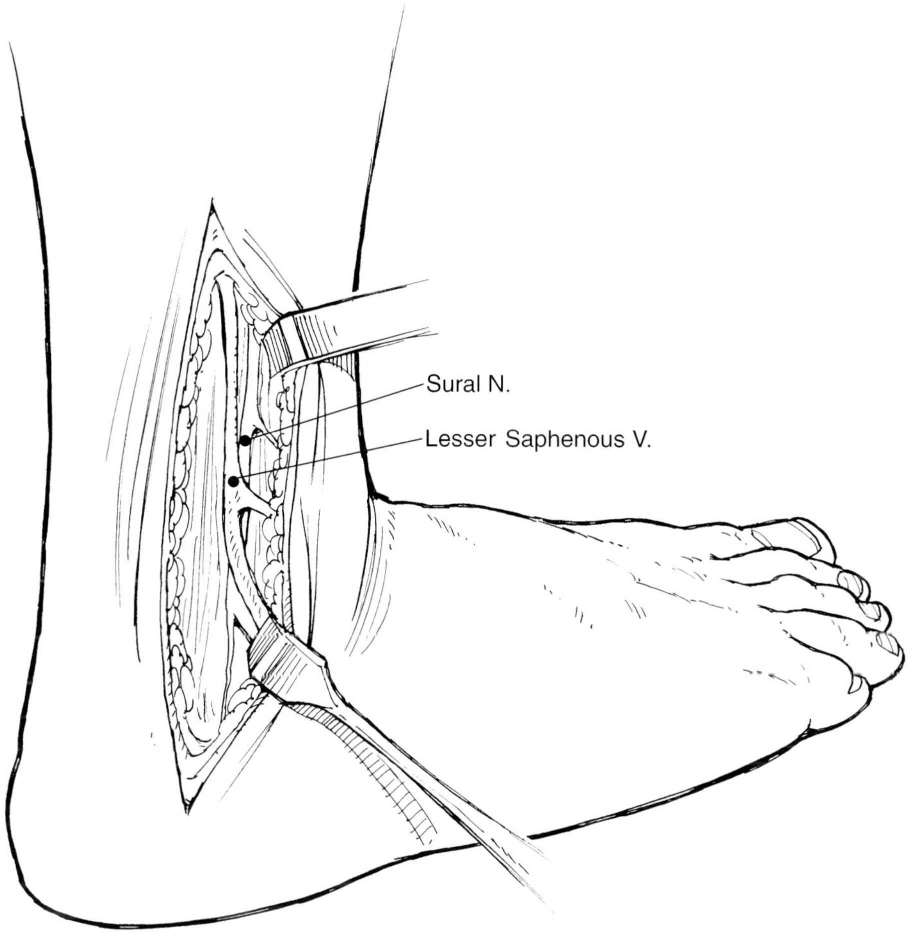


**FIGURE XIV-16**

surfaces of the tibia and fibula. The peroneal artery then terminates in the lateral calcaneal artery (XIV-18). On occasion, this vessel is of substantial size, and inadvertent injury to it may lead to significant bleeding.

The posteromedial neurovascular bundle lies just medial to the muscle belly of the flexor hallucis longus and dissection into or behind this muscle should always be avoided.

*Limitations*

While this extensile exposure is not restricted either proximally or distally, it is difficult to visualize any significant portion of the articular surfaces of either the ankle or the subtalar joint through this approach. The posterior process of the talus fills the space between the overhanging posterior lip of the tibia and the calcaneal tuberosity. Even forced dorsiflexion of the foot only exposes a small amount of the articular surfaces of the ankle and subtalar joints.

# Anterolateral Approach to the Ankle

*Applications*

The anterolateral approach to the ankle joint lies at the junction of the anterior tibial and peroneal angiosomes, just in front of the fibula. There is no proximal limit to this incision. It can extend across the ankle joint, over the anterior process of the calcaneus, and onto the dorsum of the foot. It allows access to the anterior

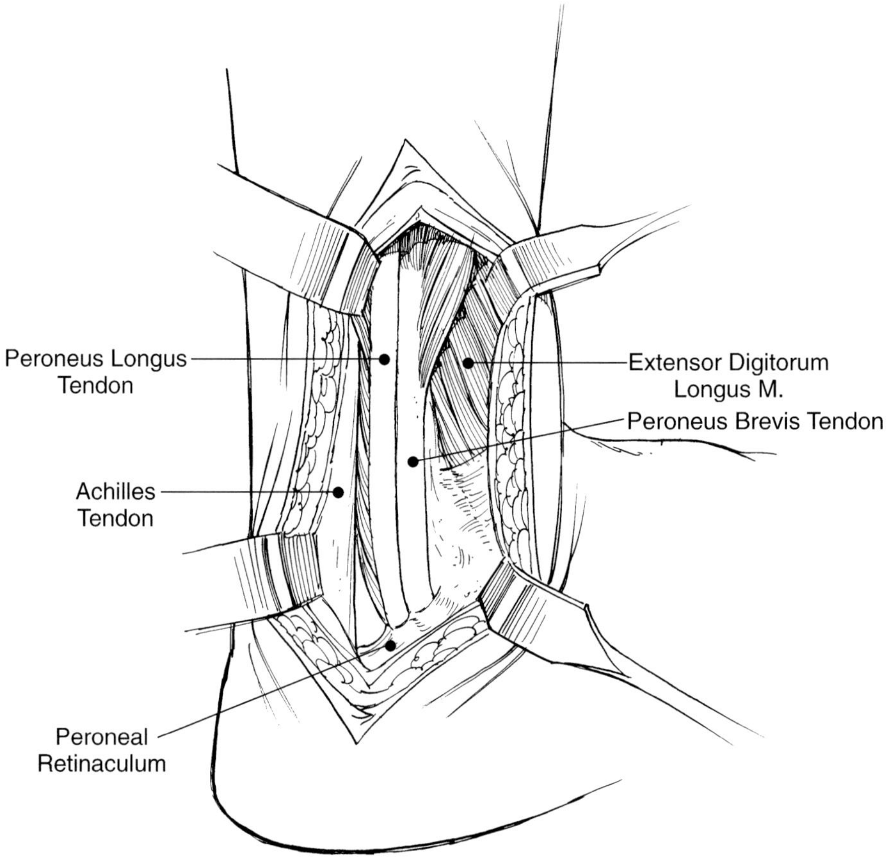


**FIGURE XIV-17A**

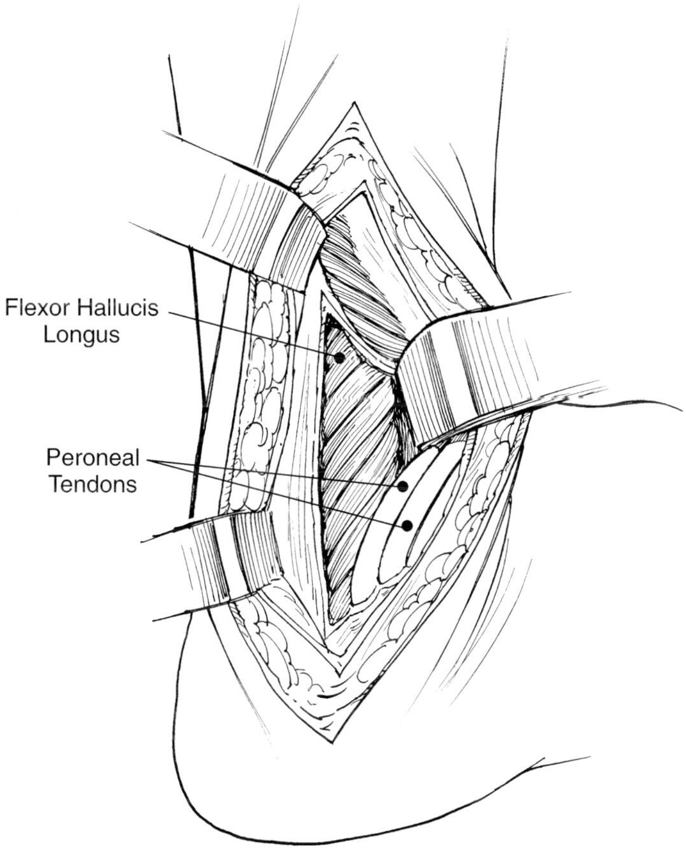


**FIGURE XIV-17B**

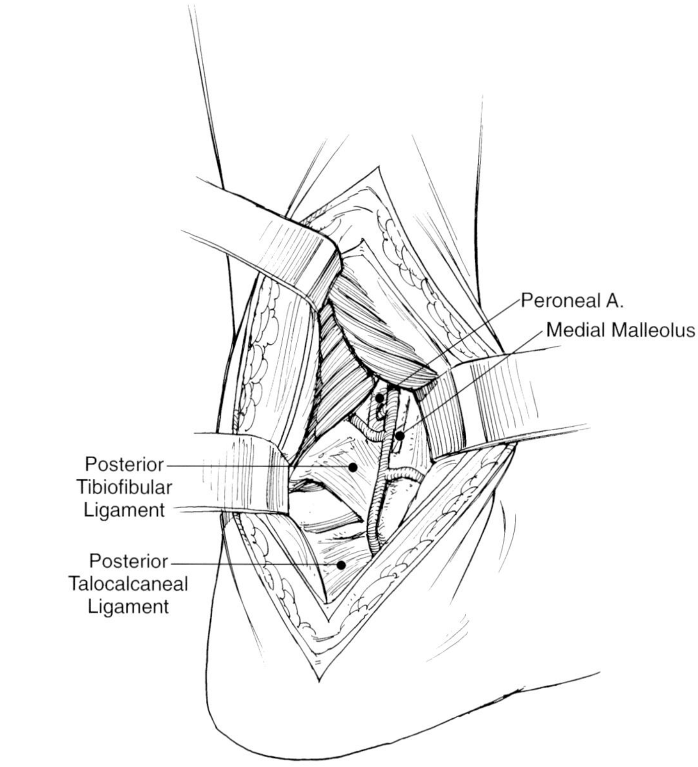


**FIGURE XIV-17C**

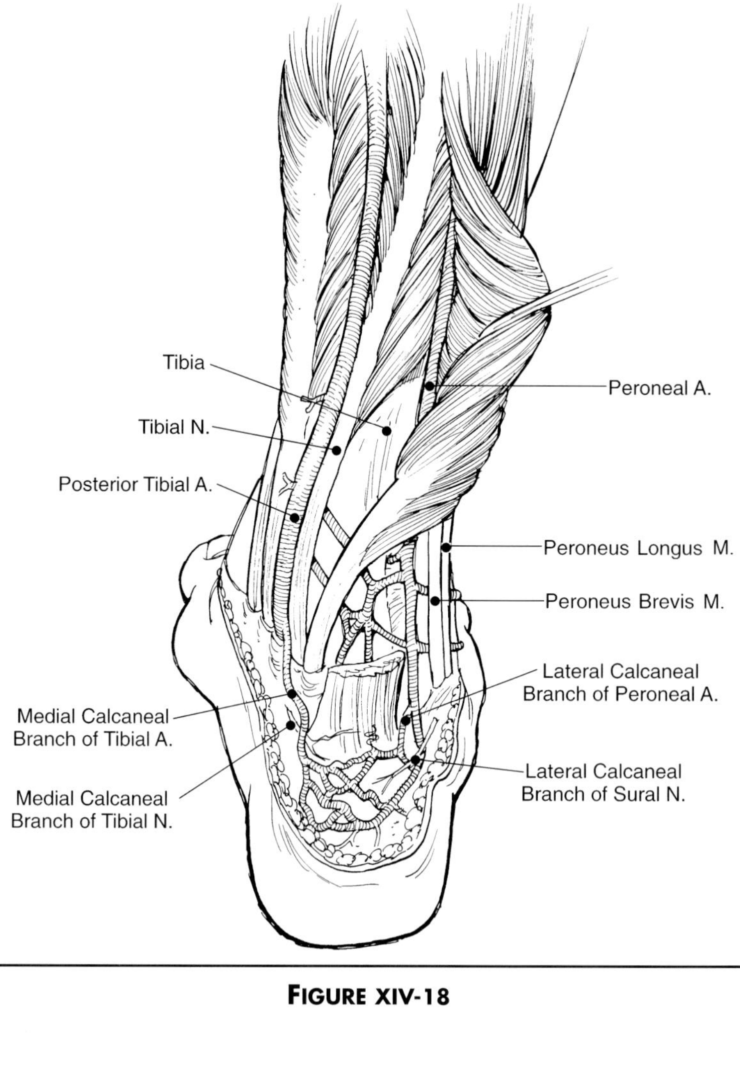


**FIGURE XIV-18**

aspect of the distal tibia and fibula, the anterior aspect of the ankle joint, and the dorsum of the talus. It is very useful for the treatment of acute and chronic lateral ankle ligament injuries. It can be used for open reduction and internal fixation of fractures of the distal fibula, lateral process of the talus, and anterior process of the calcaneus. In its course, at the level of the ankle joint, is the anterolateral portal for ankle arthroscopy.

*Technique*

The patient should lie supine with a small bolster under the ipsilateral hip. The skin incision is made in line with the anterior edge of the fibula and is extended distally toward the anterior process of the calcaneus. Prior to incising the skin, the ankle and toes should be passively plantar flexed to put tension on and show the branches of the superficial peroneal nerve (XIV-19A). When this maneuver shows the nerve, the skin incision should parallel it to avoid injury. Otherwise, careful extensile dissection of the subcutaneous tissue is required to avoid injury to a branch of this nerve (XIV-19B). Once through the subcutaneous layer, blunt dissection will expose the superficial extensor retinaculum which can be incised longitudinally to expose the lateral edge of the tendons of the extensor digitorum communis. Mobilizing the extensor digitorum communis tendons medially leads directly to the fibular periosteum and, at the level of the ankle joint, the oblique expanse of the anterior tibiofibular ligament (XIV-20). Blunt elevation of the soft tissues deep to the retinaculum, at the distal margin of the fibula, will demonstrate the anterior talofibular ligament (XIV-21). The ankle joint capsule lies immediately deep to it. The perforating branch of the peroneal artery lies in the interval between the tibia and fibula at this level and should be protected, cauterized, or ligated, depending upon its size. In the distal aspect of the wound, the origin of the extensor digitorum brevis muscle can be seen arising from the prominent anterior process of the calcaneus. Extending the skin incision proximally and distally allows more extensive mobilization of the soft tissues anteriorly to the extent that the entire anterior face of the tibia and the anterior aspect of the ankle joint can be exposed.

*Dangers*

Damage to a branch of the superficial peroneal nerve can occur in this approach. Careful identification and continuous protection of it is essential throughout the procedure. Uncontrolled bleeding from a perforating branch of the peroneal artery can lead to a postoperative hematoma. The subcutaneous tissue in this region is especially sparse and the creation of thin skin flaps should always be avoided.

*Limitations*

There are no significant limitations to this approach. It can be extended proximally to expose the anterolateral tibia and distally to expose the dorsum of the foot.

## Posteromedial Approach to the Foot

*Applications*

The posteromedial approach to the ankle can be readily extended into the foot. The incision between the angiosomes created by the medial and lateral plantar arteries can be extended from the arch of the foot to the web space between the third and fourth toes. This approach can be used to help control traumatic bleeding from the vessels, decompress tensely swollen plantar fascial compartments, or repair a lacerated nerve or tendon on the sole of the foot.

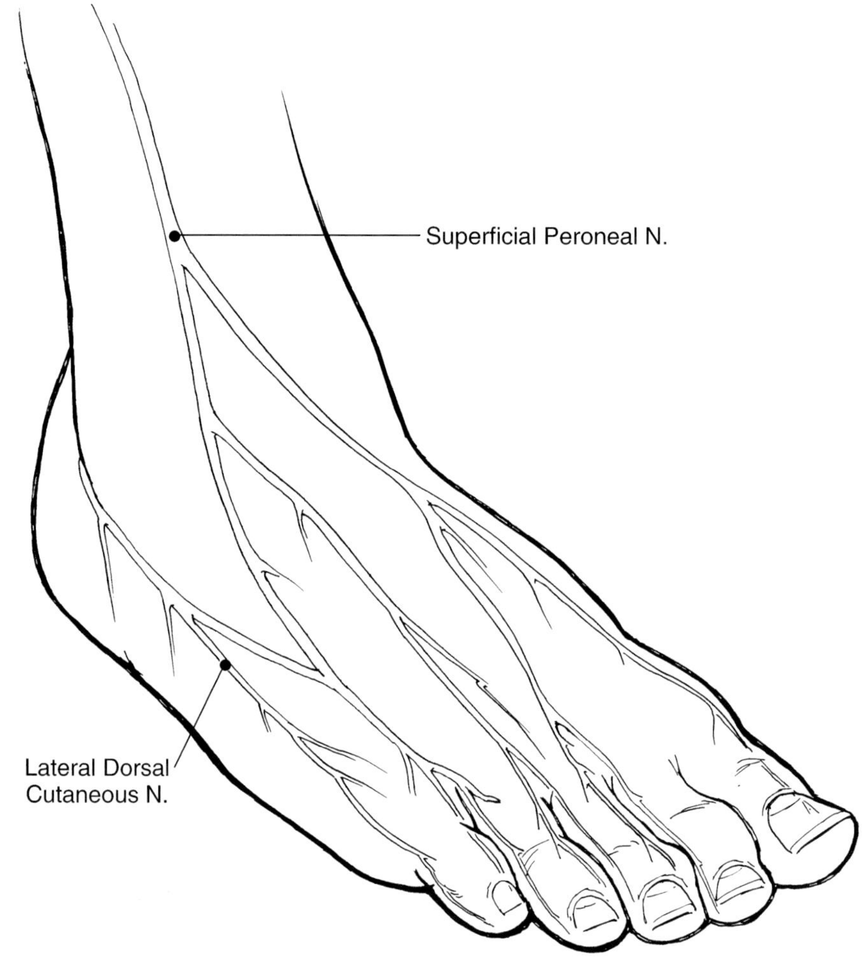


**FIGURE XIV-19A**

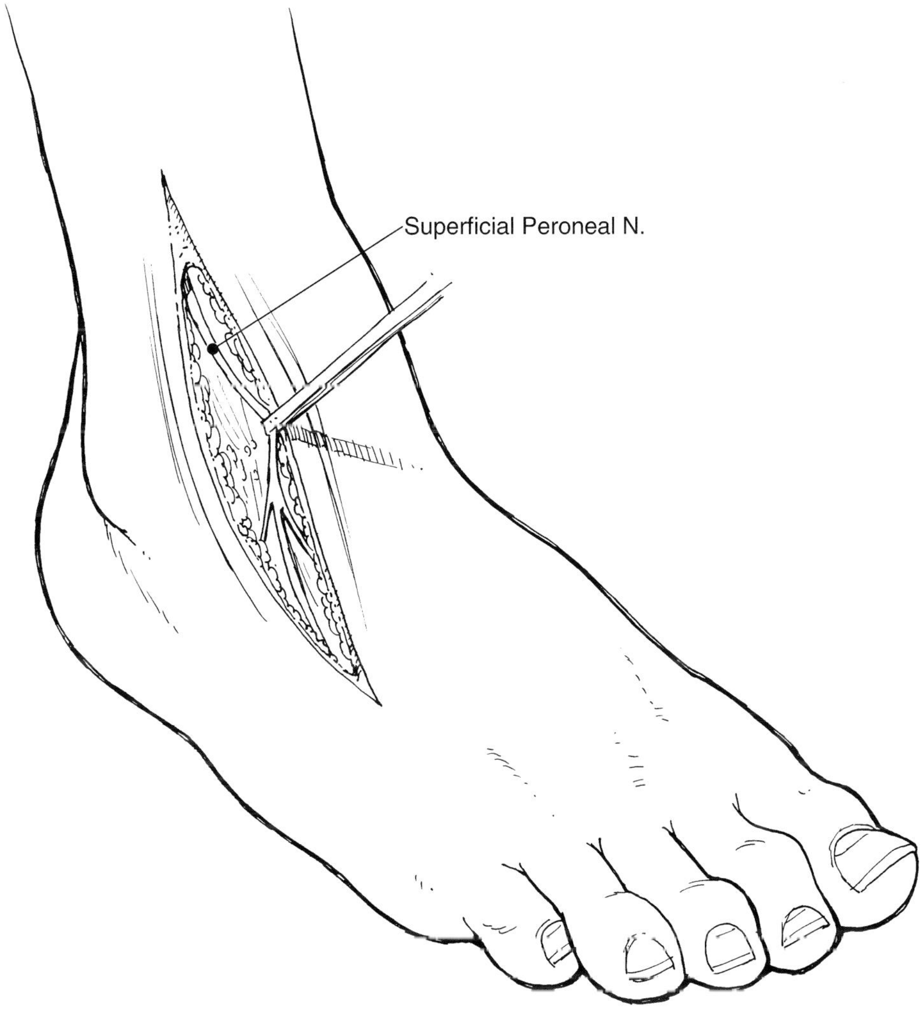


**FIGURE XIV-19B**

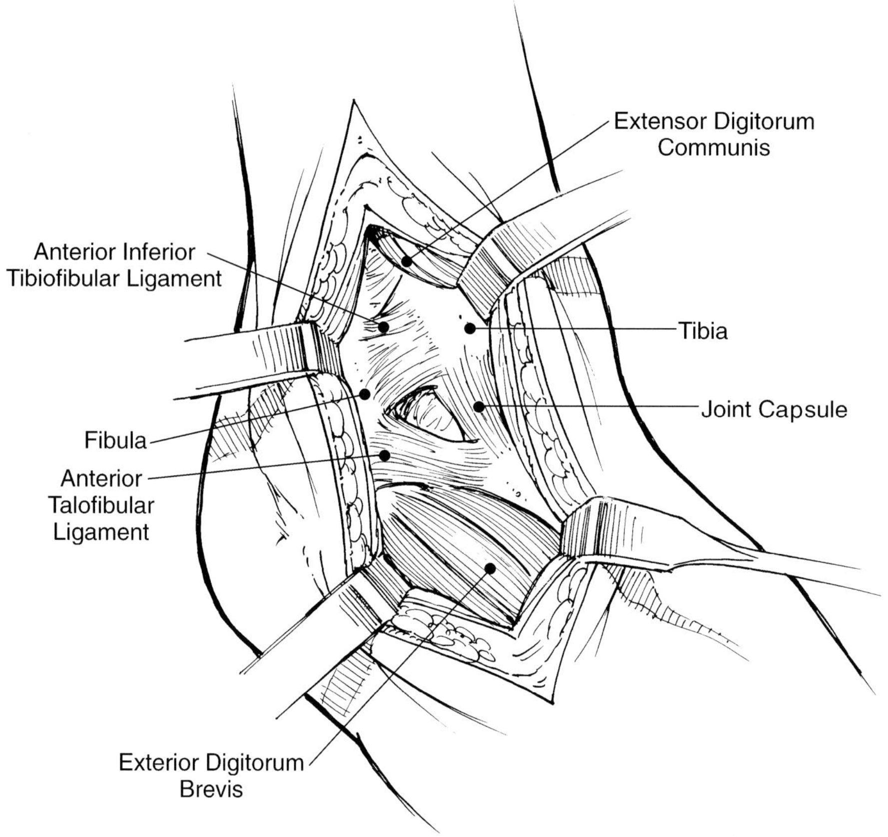


**FIGURE XIV-20**

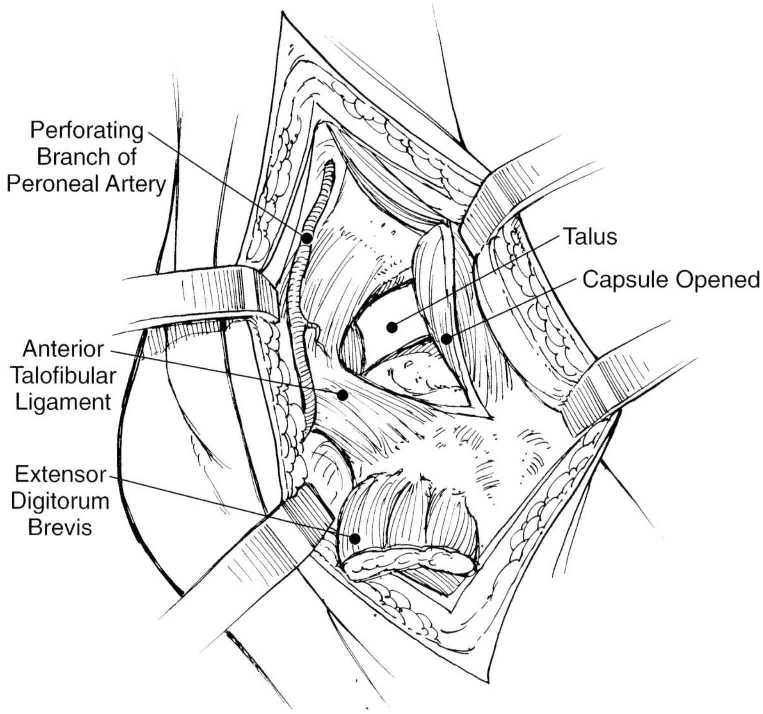


**FIGURE XIV-21**

### *Technique*

The posteromedial ankle approach is extended from the arch of the foot in a gentle curve along the plantar aspect of the length of the third ray, ending in the web space between the third and fourth toes (XIV-22). The dissection should be carried through the subcutaneous tissue to the level of the plantar fascia without creating skin flaps. This approach allows complete access to the plantar fascia (XIV-23). Deep to the plantar fascia lies the superficial layer of muscles of the sole of the foot: the abductor hallucis, the flexor digitorum brevis, and the abductor digiti minimi (XIV-10B). Careful reflection of the muscles provides access to the medial and lateral neurovascular bundles as well as the compartments immediately deep to them. Deep dissection in the distal aspect of this approach will lead to the common digital nerve to the third web space, an approach performed by many for excision of a recurrent interdigital neuroma.

### *Dangers*

Deep blind dissection using this approach can lead to serious problems. The critical neurovascular bundles lie deep to the three muscles of the first layer of the foot, and injudicious dissection may injure them.

### *Limitations*

This extensile exposure is limited by the attachments of the plantar fascia and the first layer of muscles to the calcaneus and by the many branches of the neurovascular bundles, particularly those of the lateral plantar artery as it forms the plantar arch.

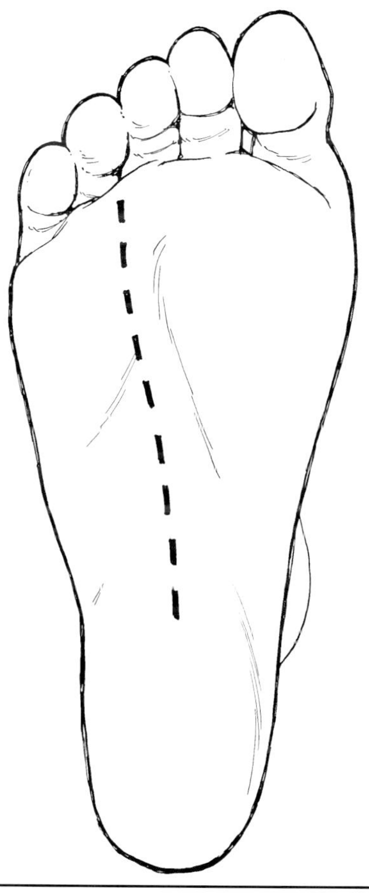

**FIGURE XIV-22**

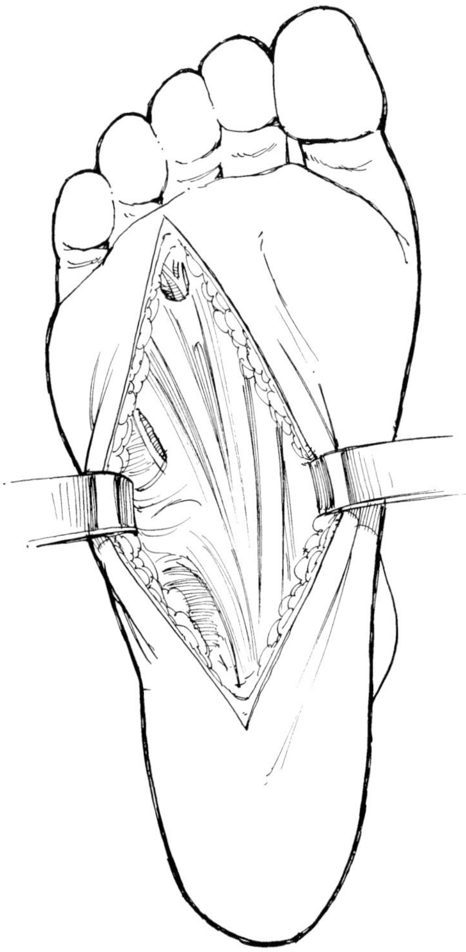

FIGURE XIV-23

## Medial Approach to the Plantar Aspect of the Foot

***Applications***

All of the plantar structures of the foot may be accessed through this medial extensile approach originally described by Henry (1).

***Technique***

A slightly dorsally curved incision parallel to the first ray is made beginning at the level of the first metatarsal head and extending proximally to the navicular tuberosity and then plantarly toward the medial aspect of the calcaneus (XIV-24). Beneath the subcutaneous tissue, the abductor hallucis muscle is identified and its superior border incised. The abductor is then rotated plantarward to expose the medial plantar neurovascular bundle (XIV-25). Deep to it, at the level of the navicular tuberosity, is the master knot of Henry, where the flexor hallucis longus and the flexor digitorum communis cross. Incision of the master knot will allow the flexor tendons and the neurovascular bundle to be mobilized plantarly along with the abductor, giving access to the deeper layers of the foot (XIV-26).

***Dangers***

All of the critical neurovascular structures to the sole of the foot lie in the plane of dissection of this approach. Special care must be taken to identify each one. Blunt dissection should be avoided because many of these structures are firmly tethered

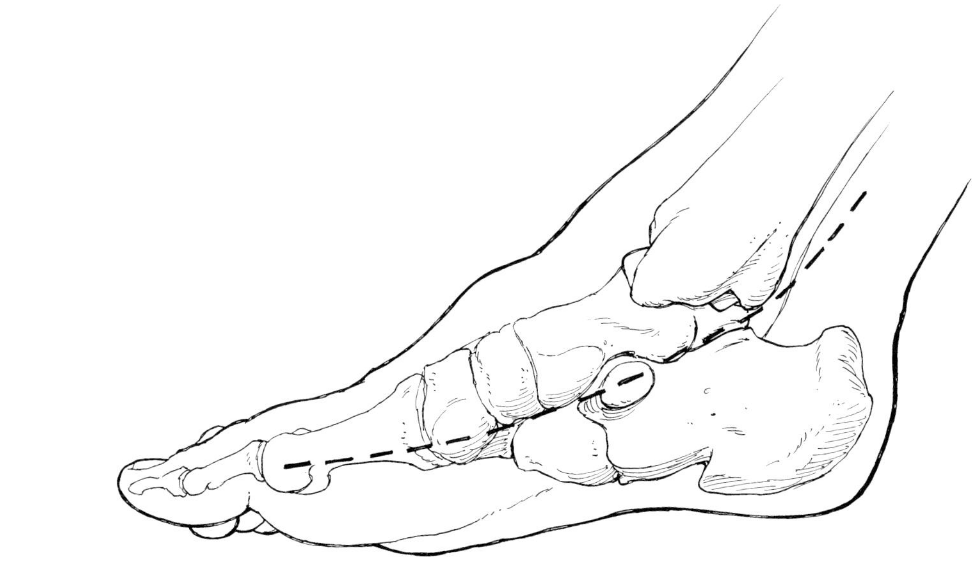

**FIGURE XIV-24**

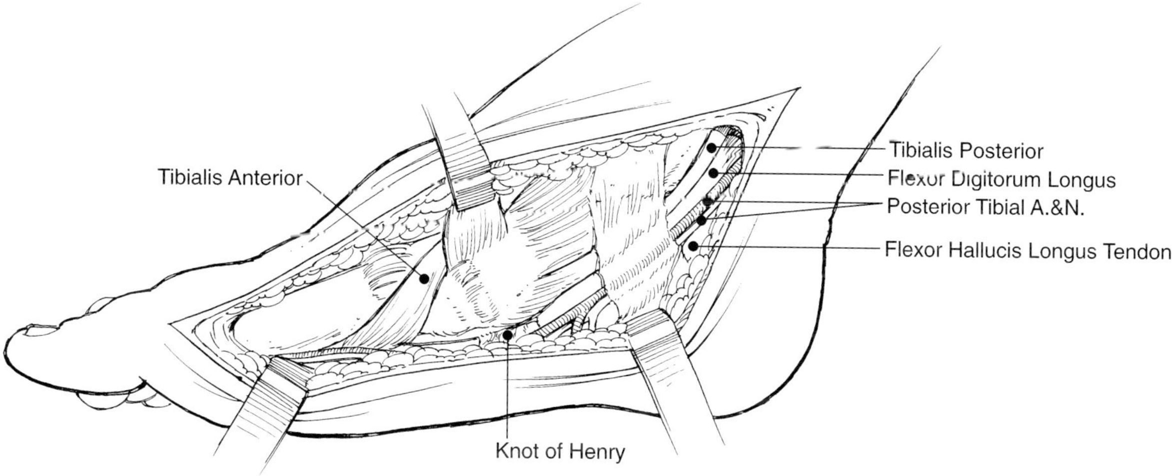


**FIGURE XIV-25**

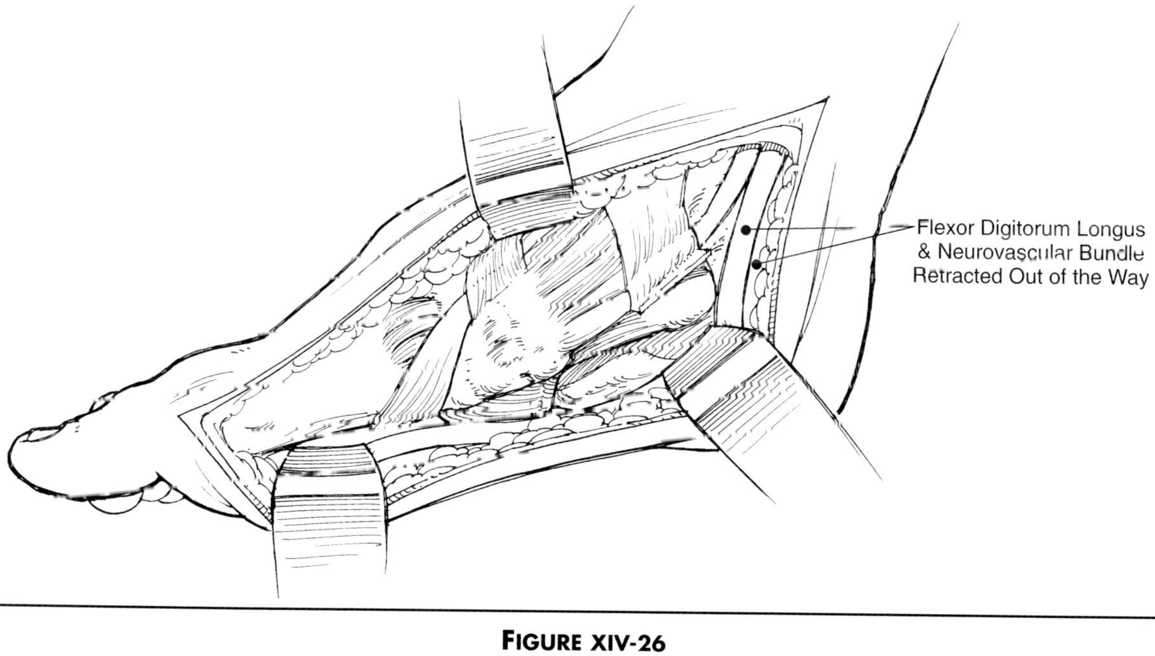


**FIGURE XIV-26**

in place and can be torn easily. Careful hemostasis should be achieved at the end of any procedure using this approach to avoid the formation of a hematoma and the creation of a compartment syndrome.

*Limitations*

There are no specific limitations to this approach. When fully extended, it allows access to all of the important structures on the plantar aspect of the foot.

## Lateral Approach to the Foot

*Applications*

The lateral approach to the foot is an extension of the posterolateral approach to the ankle. It allows access to the peroneal tendons, the entire lateral wall of the calcaneus, the calcaneocuboid joint, the sinus tarsi, the cuboid, and the fifth metatarsal. Any segment of this exposure may be used to access the structures of the lateral aspect of the foot. It is particularly appropriate for open reduction and internal fixation of fractures of the calcaneus, the cuboid, and the fifth metatarsal and provides adequate access to the subtalar joint.

*Technique*

With the patient prone or in the lateral decubitus position, the posterolateral ankle incision is curved gently anteriorly, paralleling the course of the peroneal tendons and directed toward the tuberosity of the fifth metatarsal (XIV-27). The sural nerve, running with the lesser saphenous vein, should be identified in the subcutaneous plane proximally (XIV-28). It should be mobilized, retracted, and assiduously protected. The inferior edge of the peroneal retinaculum can then be identified as it blends with the periosteum of the lateral calcaneus. Incision of the periosteum of the lateral wall of the calcaneus will allow the peroneal retinaculum

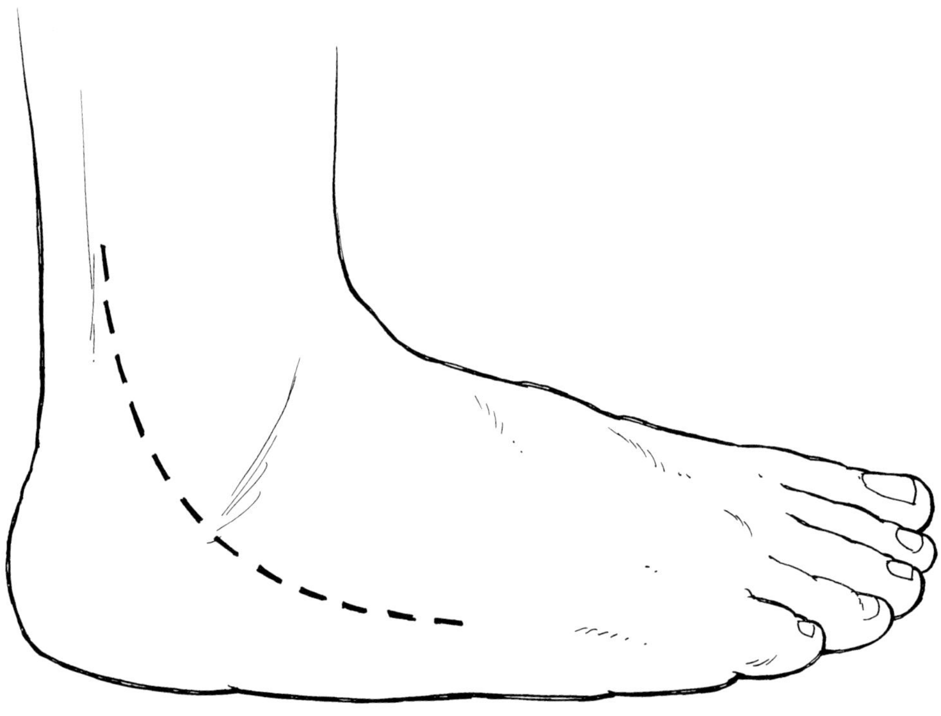

**FIGURE XIV-27**

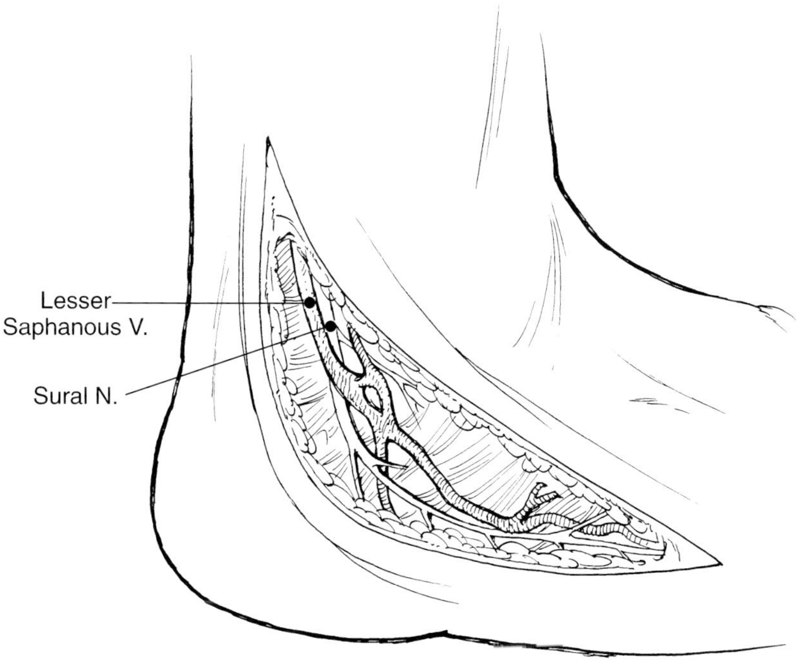


**FIGURE XIV-28**

to be elevated toward the subtalar joint, mobilizing along with it, as a unit, the peroneal sheath (XIV-29). As the periosteum is elevated, the insertion of the calcaneofibular ligament will be encountered. Its fibers can be dissected sharply from the calcaneus, allowing all of the lateral soft tissues to be elevated in a dorsal direction to expose the lateral wall of the calcaneus and the posterior facet of the subtalar joint completely (XIV-30).

Carrying the dissection distally over the anterior process of the calcaneus, the insertion of the extensor digitorum brevis can be released to expose the calcaneocuboid joint and the sinus tarsi. Further distal extension allows exposure of the cuboid, its articulation with the base of the fourth and fifth metatarsals, the dorsum of the fifth metatarsal base, and, eventually, the entire shaft of the fifth metatarsal.

***Dangers***

The sural nerve is always at risk of transection or traction injury. It should be identified early in the dissection and protected throughout. Aggressive periosteal elevation from the calcaneus can result in damage to its thin lateral wall. During exposure of a calcaneal fracture, some authors have recommended an L- or J-shaped (right angle) skin incision extending from the posterolateral ankle incision into the foot. On occasion, this approach has been complicated by slough of the corner of the anterior flap. Extending the posterolateral incision with a gentle curve (less than a right angle) minimizes circulatory embarrassment of this skin.

***Limitations***

The fibula overhangs the lateral process of the talus and it is sometimes difficult to mobilize the peroneal tendons sufficiently to achieve a good view of the posterior facet of the subtalar joint. In order to visualize the joint, the peroneal tendons must be dislocated anterior to the fibula. Plantarly, the fibrous septa of the fat pad insert onto the calcaneus. These septa should not be disturbed as they create compartments that contain fat lobules which provide the important shock absorbing func-

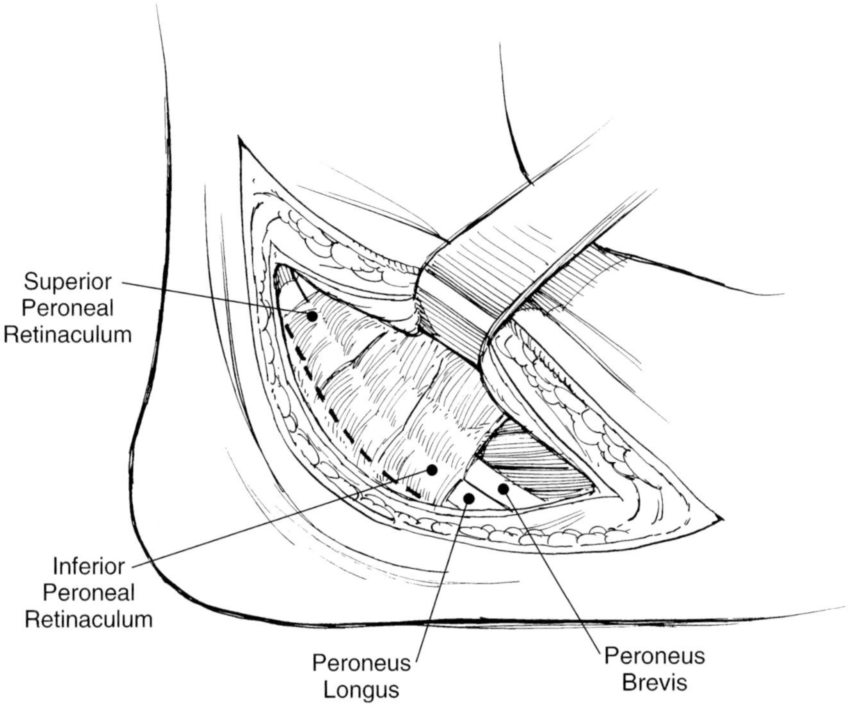


**FIGURE XIV-29**

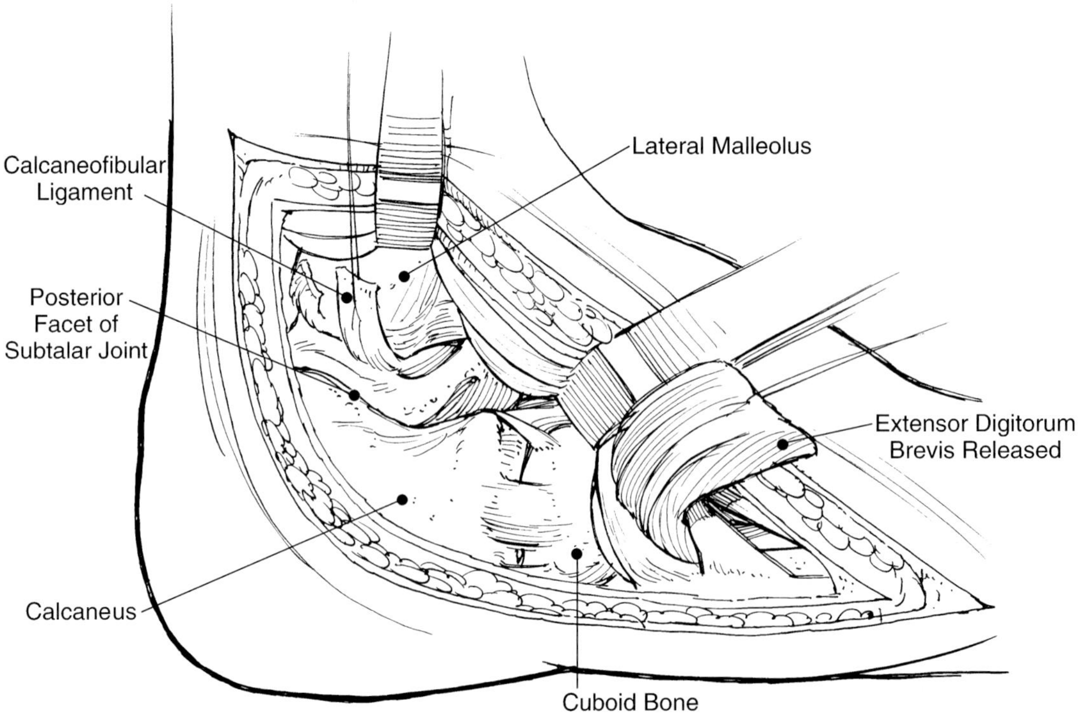


**FIGURE XIV-30**

tion of the heel pad. Distally and dorsally, the dissection is limited somewhat by the extensor tendons.

# Dorsal Approach to the Foot

*Applications*

There are three dorsal foot approaches: the dorsomedial, the central, and the dorsolateral (an extension of the anterolateral approach to the ankle joint).

Through part or all of one of these three approaches, one may access all elements of the dorsum of the foot. The dorsomedial approach lies in the interval between the anterior tibial and the extensor hallucis longus tendons. It allows access to both of these tendons as well as to the medial column of the foot (the talar head and neck, the navicular, the medial cuneiform, and the first metatarsal). Its extension to the great toe allows access to the first metatarsophalangeal joint.

The central approach is designed to access simultaneously the second and third metatarsals and their metatarsophalangeal joints. Lying between the second and third rays, it extends from the metatarsal bases into the second web space.

The dorsolateral approach to the foot extends the anterolateral ankle approach to the fourth web space.

*Techniques*

As the dorsomedial approach between the tibialis anterior and extensor hallucis longus tendons is extended distally, it courses along the shaft of the first metatarsal, curves slightly dorsally over the medial aspect of the head of the metatarsal, and then runs distally in the midlateral line of the great toe (XIV-31A). After incising the skin, care should be taken to identify and retract laterally the most medial branch of the superficial peroneal nerve that supplies sensation to the dorsomedial aspect of the great toe. Once through the subcutaneous tissue, this approach leads directly to periosteum and the joint capsules. Proximally, periosteal incision and elevation will expose the head and neck of the talus and the navicular. Distally, the entire first metatarsal, or any part of it, can be exposed to correct a hallux valgus deformity or reduce and fix a fracture (XIV-31B). Extension into the toe allows excellent exposure of the first metatarsophalangeal joint.

The central approach lies between the second and third rays. A straight skin incision extending to the web space will allow access to the distal two-thirds of the second and third metatarsals as well as to the metatarsophalangeal joints (XIV-32A). When blunt dissection is carried plantarly between the metatarsal heads, the transverse metatarsal ligament can be identified (XIV-32B). Transection of this ligament allows access to the common digital nerve supplying the web space. Thus it is the preferred approach for excision of a Morton's neuroma. A similar, parallel approach to the third web space can be used to remove a Morton's neuroma in that space.

The dorsolateral approach is a direct extension of the anterolateral ankle approach carried distally to the fourth web space. It overlies the superior margin of the sinus tarsi, the medial border of the cuboid, and the interosseous space between the fourth and fifth rays. After incising the skin, care must be taken to identify and protect the lateral branches of the superficial peroneal nerve (XIV-33A). Next, the long extensor tendon of the fifth toe will pass from medial to lateral across the incision (XIV-33B). This tendon should be identified and mobilized medially to access the fifth ray and laterally to access the fourth web space and the fourth ray. In the proximal portion of this approach, the contents of the sinus tarsi can be excised to expose the subtalar joint, and elevation of the origin of the extensor digitorum brevis from the anterior process of the calcaneus allows exposure of the calcaneocuboid joint (XIV-34).

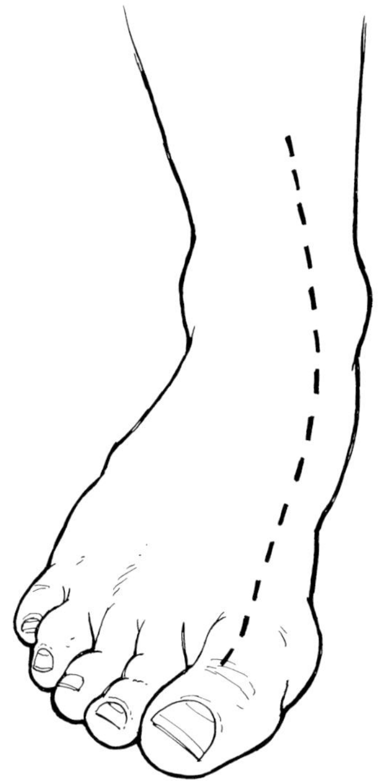

**FIGURE XIV-31A**

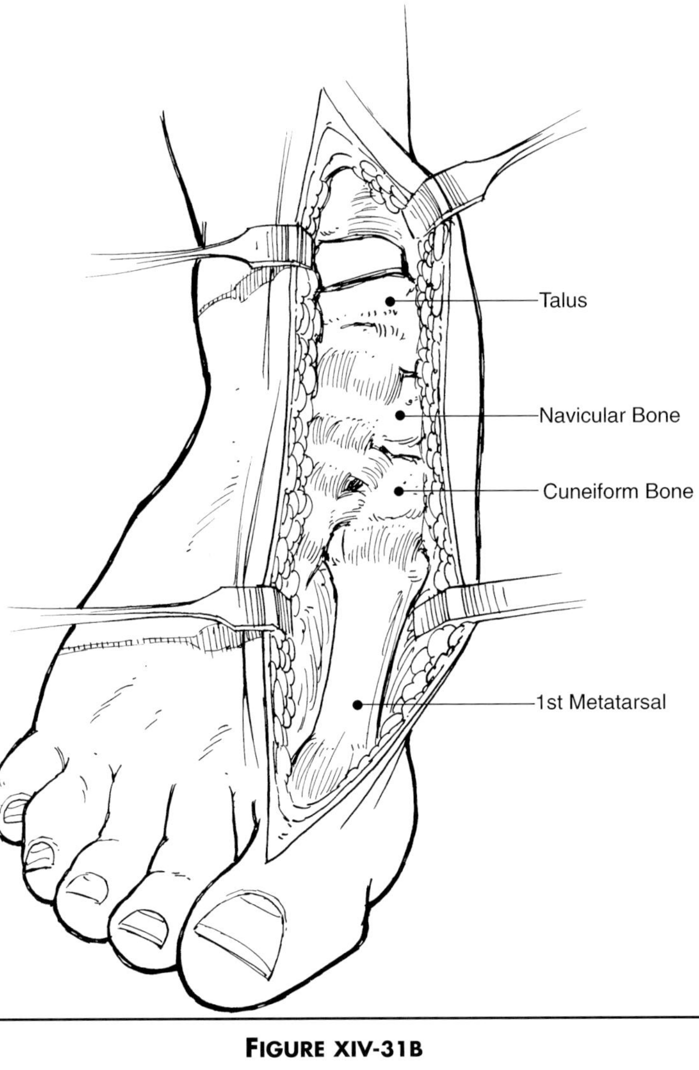


**FIGURE XIV-31B**

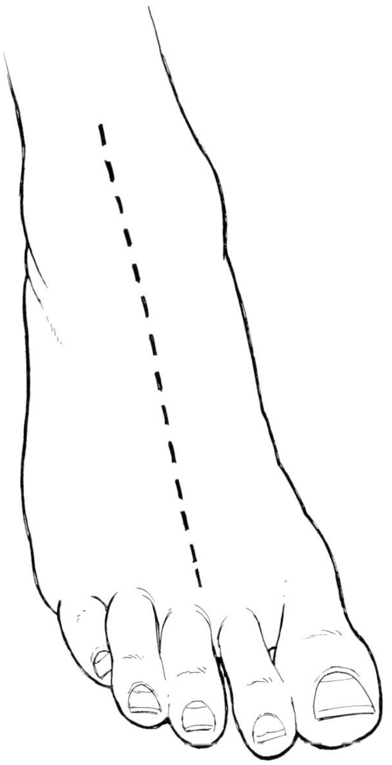

**FIGURE XIV-32A**

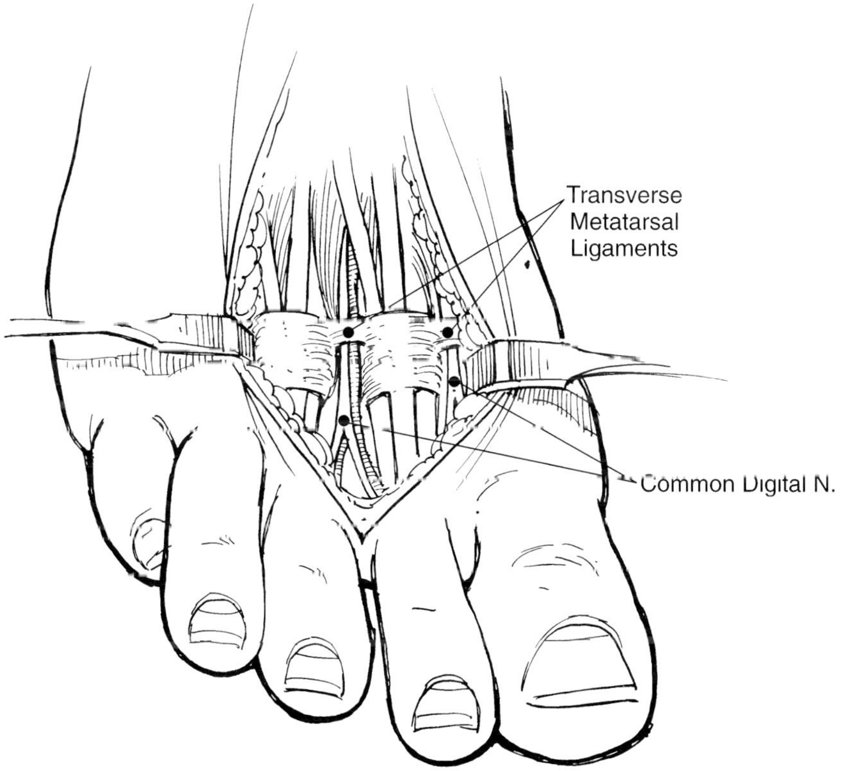


**FIGURE XIV-32B**

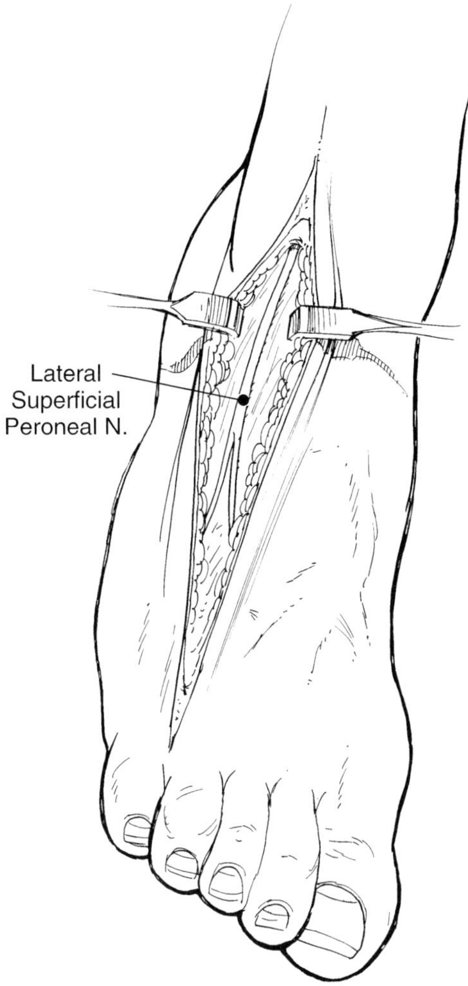


**FIGURE XIV-33A**

***Dangers***

With all three dorsal incisions, the branches of the superficial peroneal nerve are vulnerable to injury (2). Because of the limited amount of subcutaneous tissue dorsally, a neuroma resulting from stretch or transection of one of these branches becomes very susceptible to irritation from shoes. Great care must be taken to avoid injury to this nerve. The dorsalis pedis artery crosses the ankle between the tendons of the extensor hallucis longus and the extensor digitorum longus. Dissection on the medial side of the extensor hallucis longus tendon or the lateral side of the extensor digitorum longus will usually avoid injury to this vessel. Particular care must be taken to protect the artery where it dives between the bases of the first and second metatarsals to form the deep plantar arch.

***Limitations***

The skin on the dorsum of the foot has limited mobility and only a small amount of underlying subcutaneous tissue. Thus, it is difficult to undermine skin flaps to extend exposure laterally or medially in this area. Lengthening the incision in an extensile manner provides the best means of achieving additional exposure.

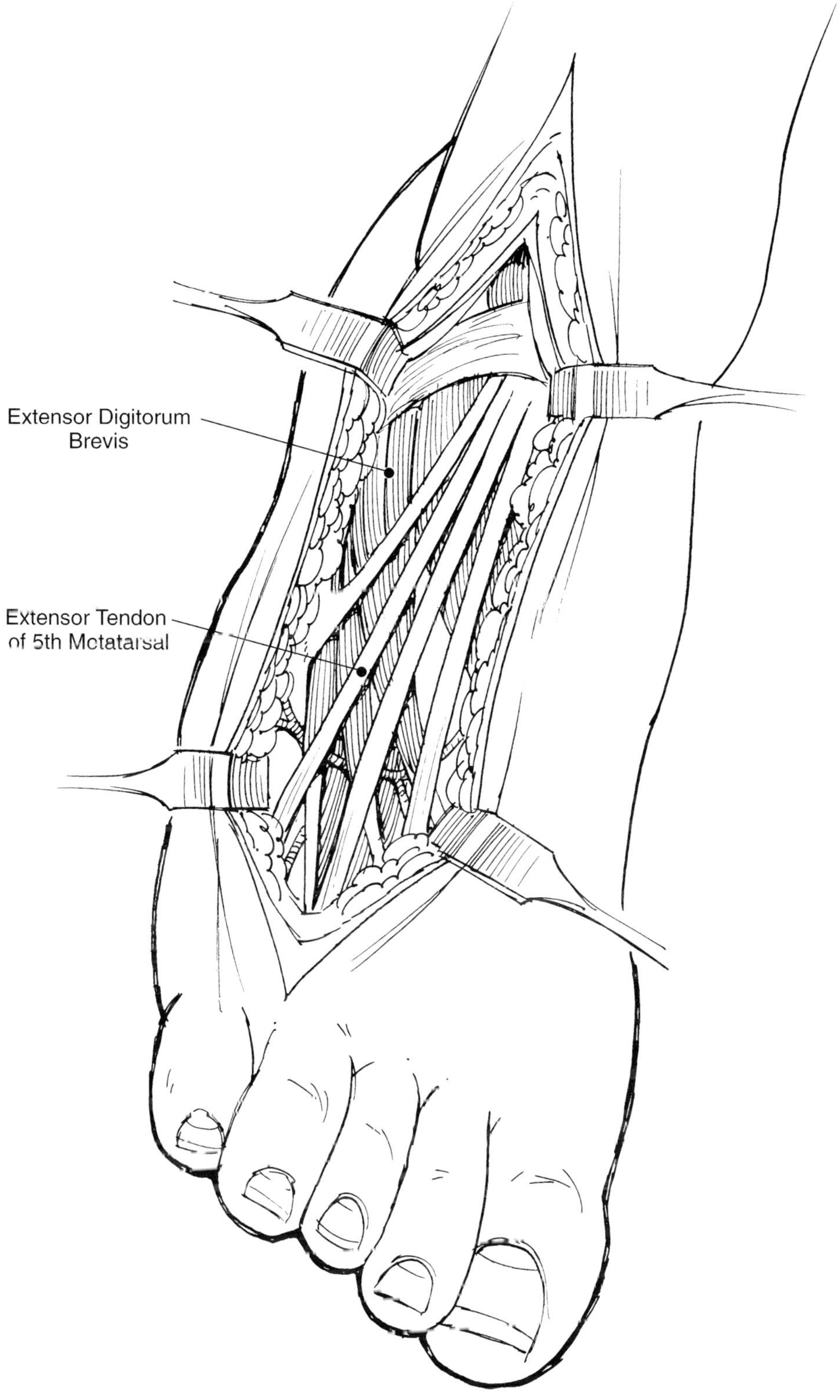


**FIGURE XIV-33B**

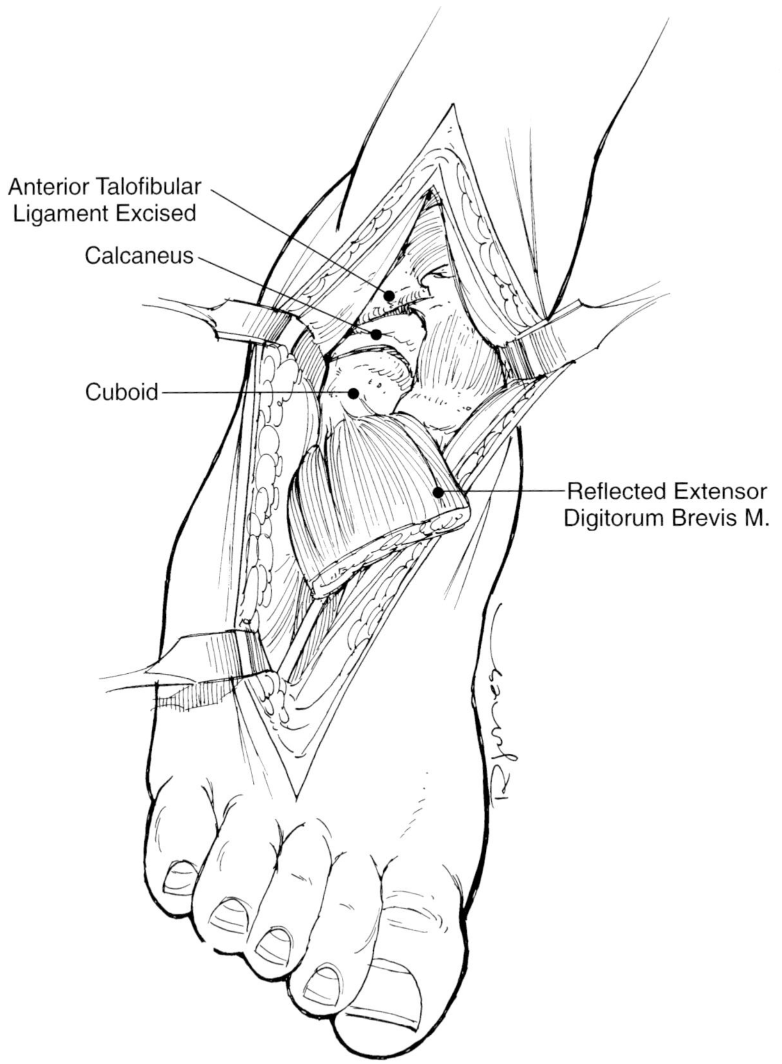


**FIGURE XIV-34**

# References

1. Henry AK, ed. Extensile Exposure Applied to Limb Surgery. Baltimore: Williams & Wilkins, 1950:165–171.
2. Blair JM, Botte MJ. Surgical anatomy of the superficial peroneal nerve in the ankle and foot. Clin Orthop 305:229–238, 1994.

# INDEX

Page numbers in *italics* refer to illustrations

## A

## D

## E

## G

## H

## I



## J



## K

## Q

## R



## S

## T

## U

## V



## W